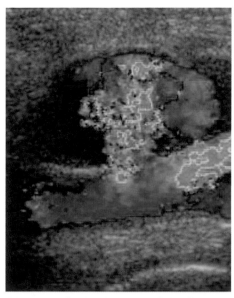

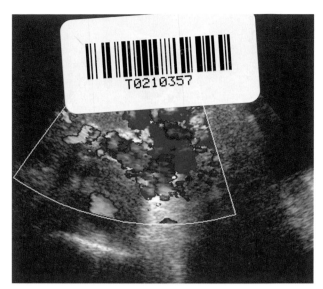

Color Plate 1 Sagittal image of the femoral artery

Color Plate 4 Doppler image of the left upper quadrant

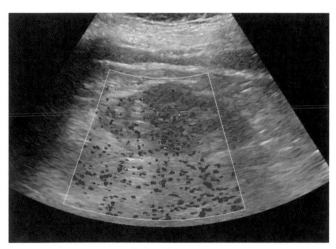

Color Plate 2

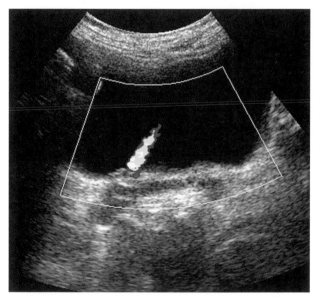

Color Plate 5 Transverse Doppler sonogram

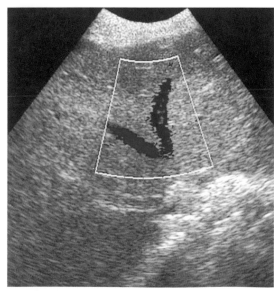

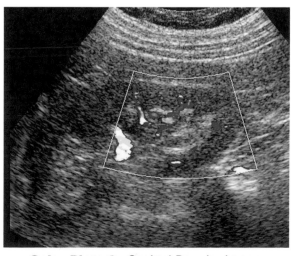

Color Plate 3 Sagittal image of the liver

Color Plate 6 Sagittal Doppler image

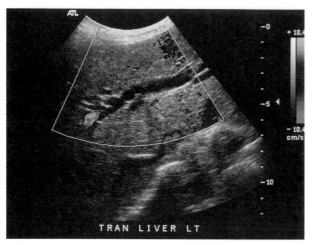

Color Plate 7   Transverse sonogram of the liver

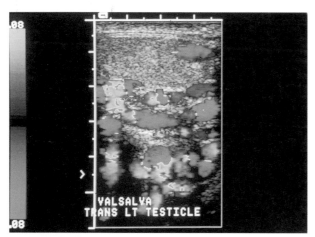

Color Plate 8   Duplex sonogram of the inferior portion of the left scrotum

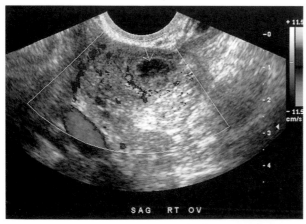

Color Plate 9   Endovaginal sonogram

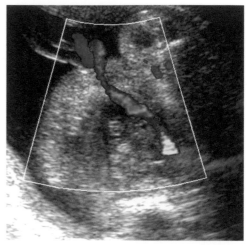

Color Plate 10

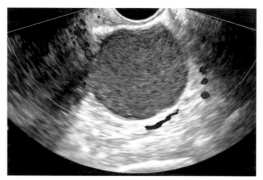

Color Plate 11   Sonogram of the adnexa

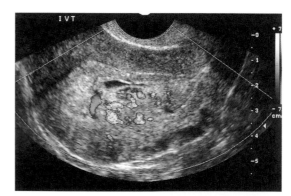

Color Plate 12

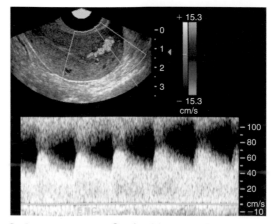

Color Plate 13   Sagittal image of the uterus

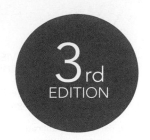

3rd EDITION

SONOGRAPHY EXAM REVIEW

PHYSICS, ABDOMEN, OBSTETRICS AND GYNECOLOGY

SUSANNA OVEL, RDMS, RVT, RT(R)
Clinical Instructor and Senior Sonographer
Sonography Consultant
Sacramento, California

ELSEVIER

SONOGRAPHY EXAM REVIEW: PHYSICS, ABDOMEN, OBSTETRICS AND GYNECOLOGY, THIRD EDITION

ISBN: 978-0-323-58228-5

Notice

Practitioners and researchers must always rely on their own experience and knowledge in evaluating and using any information, methods, compounds or experiments described herein. Because of rapid advances in the medical sciences, in particular, independent verification of diagnoses and drug dosages should be made. To the fullest extent of the law, no responsibility is assumed by Elsevier, authors, editors or contributors for any injury and/or damage to persons or property as a matter of products liability, negligence or otherwise, or from any use or operation of any methods, products, instructions, or ideas contained in the material herein.

Library of Congress Control Number: 2019935137

Senior Content Development Manager: Luke Held
Executive Content Strategist: Sonya Seigafuse
Publishing Services Manager: Deepthi Unni
Project Manager: Bharat Narang
Cover Design: Patrick Ferguson

Printed in India

Last digit in the printer: 9 8 7 6 5 4

ELSEVIER

3251 Riverport Lane
St. Louis, Missouri 63043

Working together
to grow libraries in
developing countries

www.elsevier.com • www.bookaid.org

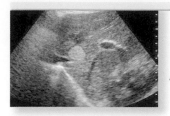

About the Author

Susanna Ovel, RDMS, RVT, RT(R), began her career in 1979 as a radiological technologist at Radiological Associates of Sacramento, California. She became a Registered Diagnostic Medical Sonographer (RDMS) in abdomen and obstetrics/gynecology in 1985 and pediatric sonography in 2016, a Registered Vascular Technologist (RVT) in 1993, and a Pioneer Breast Sonographer in 2002.

Susanna has lectured in both introductory and advanced courses in obstetrics/gynecology and abdominal sonography as well as sonography physics and instrumentation at Sacramento City Community College. She was the clinical coordinator for a new diagnostic medical sonography program for Kaiser Permanente Richmond Medical Center in Richmond, California.

She is a site visitor for the Joint Review Committee–Diagnostic Medical Sonography (JRC-DMS) and has been a member on the Continuing Medical Education Committee for SDMS. Susanna has written instructor materials and test bank ancillaries for Elsevier textbooks and continues to lecture on various sonographic subjects while working as a pediatric sonographer and clinical instructor in Sacramento.

In loving memory of Ashlee Hempt,
who would be first to say "You got this."

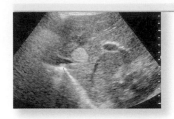

Reviewers

Jackie Bennett, BSRS, RDMS, RVS, RT (R)(CT)
Sonography Program Director
Tarrant County College
Fort Worth, Texas

Sandra E. Gepfert, AAS, BA, RDMS (AB, OB/GYN, BR), RT(R)
Program Director, Diagnostic Medical Sonography
Hudson Valley Community College
Troy, New York

Ziffie Thomas, DHSc, MHSA, RDMS, RT(R)(M)
Director, Diagnostic Medical Sonography Program
Southside Regional Medical Center Professional Schools (SRMCPS)
Colonial Heights, Virginia

Cheryl Zelinsky, MM, RT(R), RDMS
Diagnostic Medical Sonography
Program Director/Professor/Allied Health Faculty Lead
Merced College
Merced, California

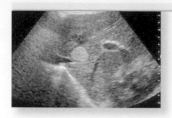

Preface

CONTENT AND ORGANIZATION

Sonography Exam Review: Physics, Abdomen, Obstetrics and Gynecology is designed for students preparing for the American Registry of Diagnostic Medical Sonography (ARDMS) examinations.

The text is divided into three major sections covering these general topics: *Physics, Abdomen,* and *Obstetrics and Gynecology.* Each section follows and thoroughly covers the ARDMS examination outline.

- **Part I:** *Physics* includes the most recent material covered on the ARDMS examination beginning in spring of 2009. Patient Care and Communications is included along with information on Doppler ultrasound and hemodynamics.
- **Part II:** *Abdomen* divides the material into specific organs, vascular structures, and associated areas within the abdominal cavity. Superficial structures and extracranial arteries are also included. Each chapter includes associated laboratory values, congenital anomalies, and normal and pathological sonographic appearance of specific structures. Differential considerations are also included. Additional information on Patient Care is included in Chapter 18.
- **Part III:** *Obstetrics and Gynecology* divides the material into smaller sections, enabling the sonography student to review specific areas. Each chapter includes laboratory values, sonographic appearance, and differential considerations. Additional information on Patient Care is included in Chapter 29

Individual chapters follow a consistent format using tables whenever possible. Differential considerations and laboratory values are included in the *Abdomen* and *Obstetrics and Gynecology* sections, allowing use of the text as a reference and study guide.

FEATURES

Registry-Level Questions

Fifty multiple-choice Registry-level questions follow each chapter. Rationales accompany all answers, pointing out key words within the question and/or reasons why the correct answer is right and the distracters are wrong for the specific question. Rationales increase comprehension and retention of specific material and allow for focus on areas needing more review.

A mock Registry examination follows each of the three sections to help students assess accumulated knowledge in each part. Each examination includes images, rationales, and the exact number of questions in the actual Registry exam.

Images and Illustrations

More than 350 anatomical illustrations and scans demonstrating normal anatomy and pathologic conditions are utilized in the Abdomen and Obstetrics and Gynecology sections within the text and in the mock examinations. Three-dimensional images are included in the Obstetrics and Gynecology section. These help with recognition of sonographic findings in both normal and abnormal cases. Because color images are now included on the Registry exams, color Doppler images are also included to help identify blood flow and can be found in a special color insert at the front of the book.

Evolve

Evolve is an interactive learning environment designed to work in coordination with Sonography Exam Review. One of the most valuable features of this review resource is the accompanying mock exam on the student Evolve website. This program is designed to simulate the computer-based exam administered by the ARDMS. It contains 645 questions—all different from the 1815 questions in the text and all relevant to preparation for the ARDMS examinations. In practice mode, particular topics that need review can be chosen. For example, if the student is preparing for the Abdomen Registry exam and is a bit uncertain of his or her knowledge of anatomy and sonography of the liver and gastrointestinal tract, he or she can choose Practice Mode and answer only questions on these two topics. Rationales provide immediate feedback, and questions can be bookmarked for later reference. In test mode, a virtually unlimited number of randomly generated multiple-choice questions are available in a timed format that replicates the actual time constraints of the Registry exams. More than one-third of these mock exam questions include images, some in color.

On Evolve, students can also find two entertaining review games, Sonography Millionaire and Tournament of Sonography, which make studying for the Registry exam more fun and less stressful. The games can be played in timed or untimed versions. Timed games and examinations help students practice time-management skills.

The Evolve resources, along with the text, make this the premier general sonography review book, reference, and study guide, all in one product.

How to Use

The text provides information on the common three general sonography ARDMS examinations and is an effective study guide to use throughout the general sonography program. The content outline may be referenced as a supplement to most courses in the general sonography curriculum.

As a review book, this text provides a logical, well-thought-out approach to preparing for the Registry examinations. The content outline, so effective throughout the educational program, is particularly appreciated at review time. All content that may be tested is presented in a format that is easy to use and understand. Because I have taught these subjects, my approach to the reader is the same as if class were being held each time the book is opened.

Care has been taken to create multiple-choice questions that cover the primary information taught in general diagnostic sonography programs and are therefore relevant to the ARDMS examinations. This philosophy, along with the outline and table formats, help students make optimal use of study time. All questions in this text and on Evolve are written in the multiple-choice style used on the Registry examinations. Explanations of answers describe key words and/or reasons why distracters are incorrect. This approach increases comprehension of the subject material.

Information provided in each individual chapter should be reviewed before attempting the subject's examination. Tests and files can be dated for later review. Reviewing the answers from previous examinations can demonstrate repetitive problem areas, guiding the student on which subjects or areas are in need of additional review.

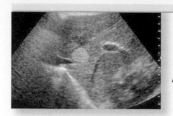

Acknowledgments

I would like to recognize and thank several people for their contributions. My sincere thanks to Jeanette Burlbaw (3D fetal face) and Ravi D. Kadasne, MD (renal hydrone-phrosis) for contributing excellent sonographic images for my cover. You two rock!

A warm thank you to Sonya Seigafuse and Luke Held for your encouragement and support during the development of my third edition. I would also like to thank the Elsevier staff for their professional contributions to this text.

I extend special thanks to L. Todd Dudley, MD, and the late Thomas K. Bellue, MD, for their encouragement and for helping me to progress in my career and life.

Susanna Ovel

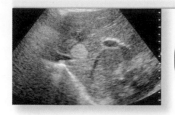

Contents

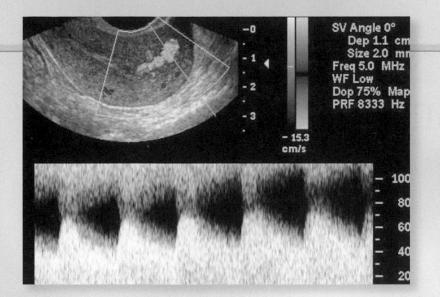

Physics

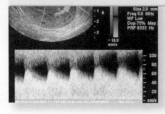

CHAPTER 1

Clinical Safety

KEY TERMS

acoustic exposure amount of acoustic energy the patient receives.

ALARA principle as low as reasonably achievable; used to reduce the potential for biological effects in humans and the fetus.

biological effect effect of ultrasound waves on living organisms, including their composition, function, growth, origin, development, and distribution.

cavitation interaction of the sound wave with microscopic gas bubbles found in tissues.

epidemiology studies of various factors determining the frequency and distribution of diseases in the human community.

ergonomic study of the human body at work.

ex vivo refers to experimentation done in or on living tissue in an artificial environment outside the organism.

in vitro refers to the technique of performing a given experiment in a test tube or, generally, in a controlled environment outside a living organism.

in vivo refers to experimentation done in or on the living tissue of a whole, living organism as opposed to a partial or dead one. Animal testing and clinical trials are forms of in vivo research.

mechanical index (MI) describes the likelihood of cavitation occurring.

Occupational Safety and Health Act (OSHA) an act passed by Congress to assure safe and healthful working conditions.

pulse average (PA) average intensity throughout the pulse duration.

pulse repetition duration portion of time from the beginning to the end of the pulse.

pulse repetition period time between the beginning of one cycle and the beginning of the next cycle.

radiation force force exerted by the sound beam on an absorber or reflector.

spatial average (SA) average intensity across the entire sound beam.

spatial peak (SP) peak intensity found across the sound beam.

temporal average (TA) average intensity during the pulse repetition period.

temporal peak (TP) greatest intensity during the pulse.

thermal index (TI) relates to the heating of tissue.

thermal index for bone (TIB) relates to the heating of bone.

thermal index for cranium (TIC) relates to the heating of the cranium.

thermal index for soft tissue (TIS) relates to the heating in soft tissue.

Work-Related Musculoskeletal Disorders (WRMSD) injuries that result in restricted work, time away from work, or that involves symptoms that last for 7 days or more. Include muscles, tendons, and joints.

OCCUPATIONAL SAFETY AND HEALTH ACT (OSHA)

- Act passed by Congress in 1970 to assure safe and healthful working conditions.
- An agency of the U.S. Department of Labor.
- Covers employers and their employees either directly through federal OSHA or through an OSHA-approved state program.
- Assures safe and healthful working conditions for workers by setting and enforcing standards and providing training, outreach, education, and assistance.

ERGONOMICS

- Study of the human body at work.
- Primary goal is to increase productivity while decreasing worker injury.
- Accomplished by modifying products, tasks, and worker environment.
- Prevention of injury is the key, and the key to prevention is education.

WORK-RELATED MUSCULOSKELETAL DISORDERS (WRMSD)

- Defined as injuries that:
  1. Result in restricted work.
  2. Result in days away from work.
  3. Involve musculoskeletal disorder symptoms that remain for 7 days or more.
  4. Involve musculoskeletal disorder symptoms that require medical treatment beyond first aid.
- Include injuries of the muscles, tendons, and joints.
- Almost 90% of sonographers have some form of WRMSD, with the highest percentages of injuries in the upper extremity and neck.

Contributing Causes and Risk Factors of WRMSD in Sonography

- Workspace design.
- Infrequent breaks or rest periods.
- Static work posture.
- Awkward scanning posture (e.g., bending, twisting).
- Forceful and repetitive movements.
- Prolonged abduction of upper extremity.
- Inappropriate monitor height.
- Incorrect or continual grip of the transducer.
- Staff shortages.

Signs and Symptoms of WRMSD

- Pain.
- Cramping of the hand/wrist.
- Loss of grip.
- Stiffness.
- Tingling.
- Swelling.

Types of Injuries

Types of Musculoskeletal Injuries

TYPE	DESCRIPTION	CAUSE
Bursitis	Inflammation of a joint bursa, commonly the shoulder	Repetitive motion Repeated arm abduction restricts blood flow to the soft tissues
Carpal tunnel syndrome	Entrapment of the median nerve as it runs through the carpal bones of the wrist	Repeated flexion and extension of the wrist Mechanical pressure against the wrist
Cubital tunnel syndrome	Entrapment of the ulnar nerve as it runs through the elbow	Repeated twisting of the forearm Mechanical pressure against the elbow as it rests on the examination table
de Quervain's disease	Specific type of tendonitis of the thumb	Repeated gripping of the transducer
Epicondylitis	Inflammation of the periosteum area of the insertion of the biceps tendon into the distal humerus	Repeated twisting of the forearm

Continued

Types of Musculoskeletal Injuries—(cont'd)

TYPE	DESCRIPTION	CAUSE
Rotator cuff injury	Fraying or tearing of the rotator cuff of the shoulder	Repeated arm abduction Repetitive motion
Spinal degeneration	Intervertebral disk degeneration	Awkward postures Static posture
Tendonitis	Inflammation of the tendon and the sheath around the tendon	Repetitive motion Repeated arm abduction
Thoracic outlet syndrome	Nerve entrapment that can occur at different levels	Repetitive motion Awkward postures
Trigger finger	Inflammation and swelling of the tendon sheath in a finger entraps the tendon and restricts the motion of the finger	Repeated gripping of the transducer

Prevention of Injury

- Position examination table at a proper height with the patient close enough to avoid bending and reaching.
- Place monitor directly in front of operator, positioning the monitor height so eyes are even with the top of the monitor.
- Ergonomic chair positioned for proper back alignment and foot support to avoid twisting and reaching.
- Keep elbow close to body with shoulder abduction at an angle ≤30 degrees.
- Maintain neutral hand position.
- Avoid resting wrist on the keyboard.
- Wear properly fitting glove to maintain a loose grip on the transducer (avoid pinch grip).
- Never place transducer cord around the neck.
- Neutral position of neck to avoid bending or twisting.
- Avoid static work posture; alternate between standing and sitting positions.
- Use of ergonomic support cushions.
- Position ultrasound system close to body.
- Regular stretching and strengthening exercises.
- Proper nutrition and sleep.

BIOEFFECTS AND ALARA PRINCIPLE

Safety

- Knowledge of bioeffects is important for the safe and prudent use of ultrasound.
- The Food and Drug Administration (FDA) regulates ultrasound instruments according to application, output intensities, and thermal and mechanical indexes.
- The American Institute of Ultrasound in Medicine (AIUM) recommends prudent use of ultrasound in the clinical environment by minimizing exposure time and output power.

ALARA Principle

- *As Low As Reasonably Achievable* (ALARA).
- Achieve information with the least amount of energy exposure to the patient.
- Use of high amplification (gain) and low output power.
- Power should be decreased in obstetric and pediatric examinations.
- Exposure time should be kept to a minimum.
- Benefit must outweigh risks.

Acoustic Output Quantities

QUANTITIES	DEFINITION	UNITS	RELATIONSHIP
Acoustic exposure	Amount of acoustic energy the patient receives High amplification (gain) and low output power is recommended	s	Directly related to the intensity of the sound beam and exposure time Operator-controlled using power or output control
Intensity	Power divided by area	W/cm^2 mW/cm^2	Proportional to acoustic output and amplitude squared Determined by a hydrophone or force balance system
Power	Rate at which work is performed	mW	Proportional to the amplitude squared Determined by a hydrophone
Pressure	Force divided by area	Pa MPa mm Hg	Areas of compression and rarefaction are measured Determined by a hydrophone

INTENSITY OF ULTRASOUND

- Intensity varies across the sound beam.
- Intensity is highest in the center of the sound beam and falls off near the periphery.
- Intensity varies with time and is zero between pulses.
- Intensity varies within a pulse, starting high and decreasing near the end of the pulse.
- Lowest- to highest-intensity values for various imaging modalities include:
  - 1–200 mW/cm^2 spatial peak–temporal average (SPTA) for gray-scale imaging.
  - 70–130 mW/cm^2 SPTA for M-mode imaging.
  - 20–290 mW/cm^2 SPTA for pulsed-wave Doppler.
  - 10–230 mW/cm^2 SPTA for color Doppler.
- Intensity of pulsed-wave Doppler is greater than continuous-wave Doppler.
- Spatial values describe intensity as it relates to distance or space.
- Temporal values are used to describe intensity over time.

Spatial Peak (SP)

- Greatest intensity found across the sound beam.
- Usually located at the center of the sound beam.

Spatial Average (SA)

- The average intensity across the entire sound beam.
- Equal to the total power across the beam divided by the beam area.

Temporal Peak (TP)

- Greatest intensity during the pulse.

Temporal Average (TA)

- The average intensity during both the transmitting and receiving times (pulse repetition period).
- Equal to the PA intensity multiplied by the duty factor (DF).

Pulse Average (PA)

- The average intensity over the entire duration of the pulse (pulse duration).
- For continuous wave, the pulse average is equal to the temporal peak.

INTENSITY VALUES (Lowest to Highest)

Spatial Average–Temporal Average (SATA)

- Averages the spatial and temporal intensities of the sound beam.
- Lowest intensity value for a given sound beam.
- Measured during the pulse repetition period.
- Heat is most dependent on SATA intensity.

Spatial Peak–Temporal Average (SPTA)

- The average intensity at the center of the beam.
- Used to describe pulse ultrasound intensities and determine biological effects.
- Measured during the pulse repetition period.
- Typically higher than SATA values by a factor of 2 to 3 for unfocused and 5 to 200 for focused transducers.

Spatial Average–Pulse Average (SAPA)

- Average intensity within the beam throughout the duration of the pulse.
- Measured during the pulse duration.

Spatial Peak–Pulse Average (SPPA)

- Average intensity that occurs during the pulse.
- Measured during the pulse duration.

Spatial Average–Temporal Peak (SATP)

- The average intensity within the beam at the highest intensity in time.
- Used to describe pulse ultrasound intensities.
- Measured during pulse duration.

Spatial Peak–Temporal Peak (SPTP)

- Peak intensity of the sound beam in both space and time.
- Highest intensity value for a given sound beam.
- Measured during pulse duration.

INSTRUMENT OUTPUT

- Imaging instruments have the lowest output intensity.
- Pulsed-wave Doppler has the highest output intensity.
- Determined by a hydrophone.

Biological Effects

- As a form of energy, ultrasound has a small potential to produce a biological effect.
- Ultrasound is absorbed by tissue, producing heat.
- Adult tissues are more tolerant of temperature increases than fetal or neonatal tissues.
- Lower in unfocused transducers because of a larger beam area.
- No confirmed significant biological effects in mammalian tissue for exposures below 100 mW/cm^2 with an unfocused transducer and 1 W/cm^2 with a focused transducer.
- Higher intensities are needed to produce bioeffects with a focused transducer.
- Exposure duration up to 50 hours has not demonstrated significant bioeffects.

Cavitation

- Result of pressure changes in soft tissue causing formation of gas bubbles.
- Can produce severe tissue damage.
- Highest rate in tissues with collagen.
- Relevant parameters include pressure, amplitude, and intensity.
- The introduction of bubbles into the tissues and circulation from contrast agents may increase the risk for cavitation.

Stable Cavitation

- Involves microbubbles already present in tissue.
- Bubbles that oscillate in diameter with the passing pressure variations of the sound wave.
- Bubbles can intercept and absorb a large amount of acoustic energy.
- Shear stressing and microstreaming may be produced in surrounding fluid.

Transient Cavitation

- Dependent on the pressure of the ultrasound pulse.
- May occur with short pulses.
- Bubbles expand and collapse violently.
- Pulses with peak intensity greater than 3300 W/cm^2 (10 MPa) can induce cavitation in mammals.

Studies on the Bioeffects of Ultrasound

STUDY	PURPOSE	FINDINGS
Animals	Determination of the conditions under which thermal and nonthermal bioeffects occur	Postpartum mortality Fetal abnormalities and weight reduction Tissue lesions Hind-limb paralysis Blood flow stasis Slow wound healing Tumor regression
Cells	Useful for identifying cellular effects	Ultrasonically induced changes of the cytoskeleton seem to be nonspecific and temporary
Epidemiology	Long-term studies on the fetus or humans with a history of previous sonograms Evaluation of birth weight, anomalies, intelligence, and overall health	No significant biological differences have been detected between exposed and unexposed patients
In vitro	Performing experiment in a test tube Limits testing on live tissue	Suggest endpoints found serve as guideline to design in vivo experiments Can disclose fundamental intercellular or intracellular interactions
In vivo	Observation of living tissue Ability to explore and evaluate specific tissues or areas	Focal lesions can occur at spatial peak–temporal average intensities greater than 10 W/cm^2
Plants	To understand cavitational effects in living tissue	When tissues contain micrometer-sized, stabilized gas bodies, pulse ultrasound can produce damage

ACOUSTIC OUTPUT LABELING STANDARDS

- Voluntary output display standard.
- Includes two types of indexes: mechanical and thermal.

Acoustic Output Indexes

- Energy is not lost but converted.
- Harmonics, cross beam, number of focal zones, and increase in depth can increase power to an area increasing the indices.

INDEX	DESCRIPTION	RELATIONSHIP
Mechanical index (MI)	Indicator of cavitation Equal to the peak rarefactional pressure divided by the square root of the operating frequency Dependent on thresholds	Value <1 indicates a low risk of adverse effects or cavitation Proportional to the output Inversely proportional to the operating frequency Relates to temporal peak intensity
Thermal index (TI)	Ratio of acoustic power produced by the transducer and the power required to raise tissue temperature 1° C Relates to attenuation (heat) and the spatial peak–temporal average intensity Continuous wave has the highest heat potential	Value <2 indicates a low risk of adverse effects A rise in temperature exceeding 2° C is significant Above 39° C biological effects are determined by the temperature and exposure time In situ, above 41° C is dangerous to the fetus Proportional to exposure time Calculated by analyzing acoustic power, beam area, operating frequency, attenuation, and thermal properties of soft tissue
Thermal index for bone	Relates to the heating of bone	Increases with focal diameter Absorption is higher in bone than soft tissue, especially in the fetus
Thermal index for cranium	Relates to the heating of the cranium	Exposure must not exceed 33 continuous minutes to avoid thermal damage to the brain surface Transcranial Doppler (TCD) demonstrates a rapid rise in temperature
Thermal index for soft tissue	Relates to the heating in soft tissue	Increases with an increase in frequency

PATIENT CARE

- Intravenous (IV) equipment
  - Keep area of needle placement straight.
  - Use caution when moving patient to avoid tangling of the tubing.
  - Plug into an electrical outlet to minimize risk of the battery running out.
  - Report when encountering one or more of the following:
    - IV alerts (e.g., air in line)
    - blood appears in tubing
    - needle has accidently been removed
    - patient complains of pain near needle placement
    - raised skin near needle placement
    - tubing becomes disconnected.
- Nasogastric tube
  - Use caution when moving patient and during scanning to avoid pulling on tubing.
- Oxygen therapy
  - Check flowmeter to ensure oxygen is being delivered.
  - Do not allow patient to lie on tubing.
  - Check for any kinks in tubing that could inhibit delivery of oxygen.
  - Use caution when moving patient to avoid tangling of tubing.

- Urinary catheters
  - Caution not to pull or tangle tubing when moving patient.
  - Keep drainage bag below the level of the urinary bladder.
  - Tubing can be clamped when necessary for an ultrasound examination.
  - Report when encountering one or more of the following:
    - drainage bag is full
    - catheter has accidently been removed.

INFECTION CONTROL

- Prevent the spread of communicable diseases and microorganisms among patients, personnel, and visitors.
- Includes:
  - Hand washing—best protection to stop the spread of pathogens.
  - Gloves—should only be used once, then discarded.
  - Gowns—most protective clothing.
  - Masks—used for airborne particle and droplet protection.
  - Eye and face shields—protect the mucous membranes of the face from pathogens.

STERILE TECHNIQUE

- Wash hands thoroughly.
- Place sterile wrapped package on a clean and stable work surface.
- Open sterile wrapped package starting with the outmost flap of the drape, placing it on the work surface. Repeat with adjacent flap of the drape, placing it on the work surface.
- Additional sterile items should be "dropped" directly onto the sterile portion of the package.
- Sterile gloves must be used when touching any item in the sterile field.
- A sterile transducer sheath may be necessary to cover the transducer and cord.
- Sterile ultrasound gel should be used on patient's skin.

SYSTEM MAINTENANCE

- Transducers and keyboard are cleaned with an approved disinfectant after each patient examination.
- Transducer cables and connections, display monitor, and fan filters are cleaned and evaluated on a weekly or biweekly basis.
- Preventive maintenance service is generally completed two to three times per year.
- Avoid products with acetone, mineral oil, iodine, oil-based perfume, and chlorine bleach.
- Never autoclave or use heat sterilization.
- Except for endocavity transducers, ultrasound transducer should not be immersed in liquid.

COMMUNICATION SKILLS

- Listen to the patient. (Look him/her in the eyes whenever possible.)
- Observe the patient's nonverbal communication.
- Respond appropriately:
  - Think and prepare your thoughts before you speak.
  - Analyze the intent of each message.
  - Adapt to your physical settings.
  - Consider your tone of voice, rate of speech, and body language.
- Clarify:
  - Check your understanding and/or the patient's understanding of verbal and nonverbal communication before, during, and after the ultrasound examination.

- Gather information:
  - Obtain pertinent information from the patient regarding symptoms and concerns.
- Touching:
  - A pat on the shoulder or touch of the hand is a nonverbal gesture of support.
- Communicating with physicians:
  - Speak with courtesy and respect.
  - Within professional guidelines answer questions directly.
  - Relay only technical information not your impression to the referring physician. Your impression of the examination is for the reading physician only.
  - It is up to the reading physician to diagnose the examination and relay this information to the referring physician.

CLINICAL SAFETY REVIEW

1. Which of the following are types of cavitation?
   a. stable and thermal
   b. in vivo and in vitro
   c. transient and stable
   d. spatial and transient

2. Which of the following displays the lowest intensity value in pulsed-wave ultrasound?
   a. SPTP
   b. SAPA
   c. SPTA
   d. SATA

3. With a focused transducer, for which of the exposures that follow are there no confirmed significant biological effects in mammalian tissue?
   a. 1 W/cm^2
   b. 1 mW/cm^2
   c. 100 W/cm^2
   d. 100 mW/cm^2

4. The acronym SPPA denotes:
   a. spatial pulse–peak average
   b. spatial peak–pulse average
   c. spatial pulse–pressure average
   d. spatial pulse–pulse amplitude

5. Which of the following imaging modalities demonstrates the highest intensity?
   a. color Doppler
   b. real-time imaging
   c. pulsed-wave Doppler
   d. continuous-wave Doppler

6. Cleaning of transducers should be performed:
   a. daily
   b. hourly
   c. weekly
   d. after each patient

7. Plant studies are useful for understanding:
   a. the effects on wound healing
   b. when focal lesions will occur
   c. the thermal effects on living tissues
   d. the cavitational effects on living tissues

8. The highest percentage of sonography-related injuries involve the:
   a. foot
   b. thumb
   c. lower back
   d. upper extremity

9. The study of various factors determining the frequency and distribution of diseases in the human community describes:
   a. cavitation
   b. epidemiology
   c. mechanical index
   d. biological effects

10. Mechanical index indicates the:
    a. likelihood cavitation will occur
    b. peak intensity of the sound beam
    c. amount of heat absorbed by human tissues
    d. likelihood tissue temperature will rise 2° C

11. When researching the biological effects of diagnostic ultrasound, which intensity is most commonly used?
    a. SATA
    b. SPTA
    c. SATP
    d. SPTP

12. Clinical trials are examples of which of the following?
    a. in situ studies
    b. in vivo studies
    c. ex vivo studies
    d. in vitro studies

13. Which intensity is the greatest during the pulse?
    a. spatial peak
    b. pulse average
    c. temporal peak
    d. spatial average

14. Pulse average is defined as the average intensity:
    a. of the pulse
    b. over the pulse area
    c. throughout the duration of a pulse
    d. across the entire sound beam

15. Cavitation is the interaction of the sound wave with:
    a. living organisms
    b. an acoustic reflector
    c. gas bubbles in the aqueous gel
    d. microscopic gas bubbles found in tissues

16. The best protection to stop the spread of pathogens is:
    a. wearing gloves
    b. wearing a mask
    c. proper handwashing
    d. wiping down the equipment with disinfectant

17. The AIUM recommends:
    a. ultrasound as a safe obstetric procedure
    b. decreasing amplification and increasing acoustic power
    c. prudent use of ultrasound in the clinical environment
    d. obstetric examinations for sex determination of a fetus

18. Cavitation is the result of:
    a. a rise in tissue temperature exceeding 1° C
    b. the attenuation of the sound wave as it travels through soft tissue
    c. pressure changes in soft tissue causing the formation of gas bubbles
    d. introduction of bubbles into the tissues and circulation from contrast agents

19. Absorption of the sound beam is highest in:
    a. air
    b. bone
    c. fluids
    d. muscle

20. Heating of soft tissue is proportional to the:
    a. tissue thickness
    b. mechanical index
    c. operating frequency
    d. spatial peak intensity

Using Figure 1.1, answer question 21.

21. The sonographer in this image is demonstrating which of the following?
    a. twisting of the neck and reaching of the arm
    b. abduction of the shoulder and twisting of the trunk
    c. twisting of the trunk and reaching of the arm
    d. reaching of the arm and abduction of the shoulder

22. Work-related musculoskeletal disorders (WRMSD) are defined as injuries that involve musculoskeletal symptoms that remain for:
    a. 7 days or longer
    b. 2 weeks or longer
    c. 7 weeks or longer
    d. 1 month or longer

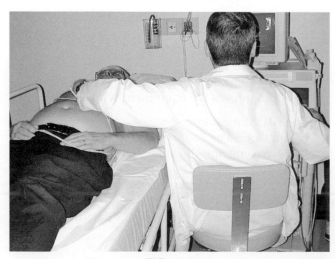

FIG. 1.1

23. Repeated gripping of the transducer is more commonly associated with:
    a. carpal tunnel syndrome
    b. de Quervain's disease
    c. cubital tunnel syndrome
    d. thoracic outlet syndrome

24. Which of the following denotes the likelihood cavitation will occur?
    a. thermal index
    b. radiation force
    c. SATA intensity
    d. mechanical index

25. Which of the following intensities is greatest across the sound beam?
    a. spatial peak
    b. temporal peak
    c. spatial average
    d. temporal average

26. Research has shown transcranial Doppler (TCD) imaging results in:
    a. a minimal amount of cavitation
    b. tissue lesions in small mammals
    c. a rapid increase in the temperature of the cranium
    d. a minimal increase in the temperature of the cranium

27. Ultrasound has a small potential to produce a biological effect because:
    a. it is a form of energy
    b. of the frequency range employed
    c. contrast agents introduce bubbles into the tissues
    d. fetal tissue is less tolerant to temperature increases

28. Biological studies of the cytoskeleton have shown:
    a. ultrasound increases the risk of cavitation
    b. ultrasound-induced changes are temporary
    c. ultrasound produces long-term tissue damage
    d. ultrasound increases the risk of tissue hyperplasia

29. The use of contrast agents in diagnostic sonography:
    a. has induced cell changes
    b. may increase the risk of cavitation
    c. demonstrates a rapid increase in tissue temperature
    d. determines the conditions under which thermal effects occur

30. Limiting the exposure time to a fetus is an example of:
    a. Snell's law
    b. mechanical index
    c. ALARA principle
    d. Huygens principle

31. Experimentation on living tissue in an artificial environment describes which of the following?
    a. in situ
    b. in vivo
    c. ex situ
    d. ex vivo

32. Heat is most dependent on which of the following intensities?
    a. SPTP
    b. SATP
    c. SATA
    d. SPTA

Using Figure 1.2, answer question 33.

33. Which of the following is demonstrated in this image?
    a. The examination table is too low.
    b. The monitor is too high.
    c. The sonographer is reaching with her elbow.
    d. The sonographer is demonstrating proper ergonomics.

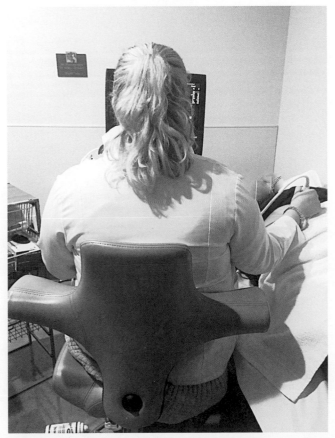

FIG. 1.2

34. Higher intensities are necessary to produce bioeffects with a(n):
    a. focused transducer
    b. unfocused transducer
    c. multifrequency transducer
    d. three-dimensional transducer

35. To avoid a WRMSD, the shoulder should not be abducted more than:
    a. 15 degrees
    b. 20 degrees
    c. 30 degrees
    d. 40 degrees

36. With an unfocused transducer, for which of the exposures listed here are there no confirmed significant biological effects in mammalian tissue?
    a. 1 W/cm^2
    b. 1 mW/cm^2
    c. 100 W/cm^2
    d. 100 mW/cm^2

37. The average intensity during the pulse repetition period defines:
    a. spatial average
    b. temporal average
    c. spatial average–pulse average
    d. spatial average–temporal average

38. Which of the following reduces occupational injuries?
    a. chin is slightly raised
    b. eyes are even with the middle of the monitor
    c. chin is slightly tucked
    d. eyes are even with the top of the monitor

39. Which of the following may result in spinal degeneration?
    a. static posture
    b. repetitive motion
    c. de Quervain's disease
    d. thoracic outlet syndrome

40. Repeated twisting of the forearm may result in which of the following work-related injuries?
    a. carpal tunnel syndrome
    b. rotator cuff tear
    c. cubital tunnel syndrome
    d. de Quervain's disease

41. The common intensity during the extent of a pulse defines:
    a. duty factor
    b. pulse average
    c. spatial average
    d. temporal average

42. Exposure of a fetus to ultrasound is dangerous above:
    a. 10° C
    b. 35° C
    c. 39° C
    d. 41° C

43. Epidemiology studies on the biological effects of diagnostic ultrasound have determined:
    a. pulse ultrasound damages soft tissue
    b. no significant biological effects
    c. temperatures above 35° C are dangerous to the fetus
    d. focal lesion can occur at SPTA intensities greater than 10 W/cm²

44. Pressure changes in soft tissue are most likely to result in:
    a. cavitation
    b. tissue lesions
    c. blood flow stasis
    d. fetal abnormalities

45. Microbubbles will expand and collapse when:
    a. pressure is applied
    b. the thermal index reaches 2.0
    c. the temperature of bone increases by 1° C
    d. the temperature of soft tissue increases by 2° C

46. Which of the following is consistent with the ALARA principle?
    a. limited exposure time and high acoustic output
    b. low acoustic output and limited exposure time
    c. low acoustic output and high operating frequency
    d. high operating frequency and limited exposure time

47. Use of ultrasound for entertainment is:
    a. approved by the FDA
    b. a medically approved examination
    c. discouraged by the medical community
    d. an excellent bonding tool for mother and fetus

48. Power is defined as:
    a. energy between two points
    b. rate at which work is performed
    c. rate of motion with respect to time
    d. amount of force applied to a specific area

49. Animal testing is a form of what type of research?
    a. in situ
    b. in vivo
    c. ex vivo
    d. in vitro

50. The intensity of M-mode imaging is greater than the intensity of:
    a. color Doppler
    b. gray-scale imaging
    c. pulsed-wave Doppler
    d. continuous-wave Doppler

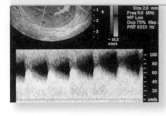

CHAPTER 2

Physics Principles

KEY TERMS

absorption   process whereby sound energy is dissipated in a medium, primarily in the form of heat.

acoustic   having to do with sound.

acoustic impedance   resistance of sound as it propagates through a medium.

acoustic variables   effects on the sound beam caused by the medium; includes pressure, density, and particle motion (distance and temperature).

amplitude   relating to the strength of the compression wave; maximum variation of an acoustic variable.

area   amount of space within a specific boundary.

attenuation   weakening of sound as it propagates through a medium.

attenuation coefficient   attenuation occurring with each centimeter that sound travels.

backscatter   sound scattered back in the direction from which it came.

bandwidth   range of frequencies found in pulse ultrasound.

circumference   distance around the perimeter of an object.

compression   region of high pressure or density in a compression wave.

continuous wave   a nonpulsed wave in which cycles repeat indefinitely.

cycle   one complete variation in pressure or other acoustic variable.

decibel   a unit used to compare the ratio of intensities or amplitudes of two sound waves or two points along the wave.

density   concentration of mass, weight, or matter per unit volume.

dispersion   dependence of velocity or other physical parameters on frequency.

distance   amount of space from one object to another.

duty factor   fraction of time that pulse ultrasound is on.

electromagnetic wave   transverse waves of electric and magnetic fields that involve no particle motion and can travel through a vacuum at the speed of light.

energy   capability of doing work.

fractional bandwidth   describes how large a bandwidth is compared with operating frequency; unitless.

fundamental frequency   original operating frequency.

half value layer (HVL)   thickness of tissue required to reduce the intensity of the sound beam by one-half; also known as depth of penetration, half boundary layer, or penetration depth.

harmonic frequency   echoes of twice the frequency transmitted into the body that reflect back to the transducer, which improves image quality.

hertz (Hz)   one cycle per second; unit of frequency.

impedance   determines how much of an incident sound wave is reflected back from the first medium and how much is transmitted into the second medium.

incident angle   direction of incident beam with respect to the media boundary.

incident beam   initial or starting beam.

intensity   rate at which energy transmits over a specific area.

kilohertz (kHz)   one thousand cycles per second.

longitudinal wave   wave motion occurs when the particles vibrate in a motion that is parallel to the direction of wave propagation.

mechanical wave   wave that passes through a medium causing the molecules of the medium to vibrate.

oblique incidence   incident ultrasound traveling at an oblique angle to the media boundary.

perpendicular incidence   incident ultrasound traveling at an angle perpendicular to the media boundary.

pressure   concentration of force.

propagation speed   speed at which a wave moves through a medium.

pulse   a collection of a number of cycles that travel together.

pulse duration   portion of time from the beginning to the end of a pulse; sonography generally uses 2 to 3 cycles whereas Doppler uses 5 to 30 cycles per pulse.

pulse repetition frequency   number of pulses per second.

pulse repetition period   time between the beginning of one cycle and the beginning of the next cycle.

pulse ultrasound   a few pulses of ultrasound followed by a longer pause of no ultrasound. During this "silence," returning echoes are received and processed.

quality factor (Q factor)   for short pulses, the Q factor is equal to the number of cycles in a pulse; the lower the Q factor, the better the image quality. Reciprocal of fractional bandwidth.

rarefaction   regions of low pressure or density in a compression wave.

Rayleigh's scatter   occurs when the reflector is much smaller than the wavelength of the sound beam.

reflected beam   the beam redirected back to the transducer after striking a media boundary.

KEY TERMS—cont'd

reflection redirection (return) of a portion of the sound beam back to the transducer.

reflection angle angle between the reflected sound and a line perpendicular to the media boundary.

refraction change in direction of the sound wave after passing from one medium to another.

scattering redirection of sound in several directions on encountering a rough surface; also known as nonspecular reflections.

sound a traveling variation of acoustic variables.

spatial relating to space.

speckle multiple echoes received at the same time generating interference in the sound wave, resulting in a

grainy appearance of the sonogram. Also known as acoustic noise.

specular reflections these comprise the boundaries of organs and reflect sound in only one direction; specular reflections are angle dependent.

stiffness resistance of a material to compression.

temporal relating to time.

transmitted beam the sound beam continuing on to the next media boundary.

transverse wave motion occurs when particle motion is perpendicular to the direction of the wave propagation.

volume amount of occupied space of an object in three dimensions.

SOUND CATEGORIES

Infrasound

- Below 20 Hz.
- Below human hearing.

Audible Sound

- Above 20 Hz and below 20,000 Hz.
- Within human hearing.

Ultrasound

- Above 20,000 Hz (20 kHz).
- Above human hearing.

SOUND WAVES

- A traveling variation of acoustic variables (pressure, density, and particle motion).
- Longitudinal, mechanical, pressure waves produced by a vibrating source.
- Matter must be present for sound to travel; it cannot travel through a vacuum.
- Sound waves carry energy—not matter—from one place to another.
- Vibrations from one molecule carry to the next molecule along the same axis. These oscillations continue until friction causes the vibrations to cease.
- Contain regions of compression (high pressure or density) and rarefaction (low pressure or density).

Metric Prefixes

METRIC PREFIX	VALUE	SYMBOL
Tetra	10^{12} (trillion)	T
Pico	10^{-12} (trillionth)	p
Giga	10^{9} (billion)	G
Nano	10^{-9} (billionth)	n
Mega	10^{6} (million)	M
Micro	10^{-6} (millionth)	μ
Kilo	10^{3} (thousand)	k

Metric Prefixes—(cont'd)

METRIC PREFIX	VALUE	SYMBOL
Milli	10^{-3} (thousandth)	m
Hecto	10^{2} (hundred)	h
Centi	10^{-2} (hundredth)	c
Deca	10^{1} (ten)	Da
Deci	10^{-1} (tenth)	d

Wave Variables
Wavelength (λ) = Propagation Speed (c)/Frequency (f)

WAVE VARIABLE	DEFINITION	UNITS	DETERMINED BY	RELATIONSHIP
Frequency (f)	Number of cycles in 1 s	Hz kHz MHz	Transducer	Proportional to image quality and attenuation Inversely proportional to the wavelength, period, and penetration depth Determines resolution and penetration depth
Period (T)	Time to complete one cycle Peak to peak	s ms μs	Transducer	Proportional to the wavelength Inversely proportional to frequency
Propagation speed (c)	Speed with which a wave travels through a medium	s ms μs	Stiffness and density of the medium Primarily by the stiffness of the medium	Proportional to the stiffness of the medium Inversely proportional to the density of the medium Dense structures or pathologies decrease propagation speed Stiff structures increase the propagation speed (bone) Soft tissue—propagation speed is equal to 1.54 mm/μs Range from 1.44 to 1.64 mm/μs 13 μs for sound to travel 1 cm in soft tissue round-trip
Wavelength (λ)	Distance it takes to complete one cycle	m mm	Transducer Medium	Proportional to the period and penetration depth Inversely proportional to frequency

Properties of Ultrasound

PROPERTY	DEFINITION	UNITS	DETERMINED BY	RELATIONSHIP
Amplitude	Relates to sound strength Maximum variation that occurs in an acoustic variable Magnitude from the neutral value to the maximum extent in an oscillation	Depends on the acoustic variable	Ultrasound system Operator-adjustable using output or power control	Proportional to power Decreases as the wave propagates through tissue
Intensity	Relates to the strength of the sound beam Rate at which energy passes through unit area Equal to the total power of the beam divided by the area over which the power is spread	W/cm^{2} mW/cm^{2}	Ultrasound system Operator-adjustable using output or power control	Proportional to power and amplitude of the wave squared Inversely proportional to the beam area
Power	Rate at which energy is transmitted into the body Rate at which work is done	W mW	Ultrasound system Operator-controlled using output or power control	Proportional to intensity Energy transferred divided by the time required to transfer
Pressure	Amount of force over a specific area Acoustic variable	Pascal (Pa) MPa	Operator-adjustable using output or power control	Proportional to amount of force and volume of the sound wave Inversely proportional to the area covered

PULSE ULTRASOUND

- Electrical energy applied to the transducer produces short bursts of acoustic energy.
- A pulse must have a beginning and an end.
- There are two components to a pulse: transmitting (on) and receiving (off).
- Ultrasound systems use soft tissue propagation speed to display returning echoes on the display.

Properties of Pulse Ultrasound

PROPERTY	DEFINITION	UNITS	DETERMINED BY	RELATIONSHIP
Bandwidth	Range of frequencies contained in a pulse	MHz	Transducer Ultrasound system Cannot be adjusted by the operator	Inversely proportional to the length of the pulse (SPL) and Q factor Portion of the bandwidth used is adjusted with the multi-Hertz or harmonic control
Duty factor (DF)	Percentage of time that pulsed ultrasound is transmitting (on-time)	None	Transducer Operator-adjustable with depth control	Proportional to PRF and PD Inversely proportional to PRP
Pulse duration (PD)	Time it takes for one pulse to occur On-time of phase	s	Ultrasound system Transducer Cannot be adjusted by the operator	Proportional to the duty factor and number of cycles in a pulse Inversely proportional to PRF
Pulse repetition frequency (PRF)	Number of pulses occurring in 1 s	kHz	Ultrasound system Operator-adjustable with depth control	Proportional to the duty factor Inversely proportional to imaging depth and PRP Determines the number of scan lines and images produced per second (frame rate)
Pulse repetition period (PRP)	Time from the start of one pulse to the start of the next pulse	s	Ultrasound system Operator-adjustable with depth control	Proportional to imaging depth Inversely proportional to the PRF
Spatial pulse length (SPL)	Length of a pulse from start to finish Length of space occupied by a pulse SPL and PD measure the same thing only in different units	mm	Ultrasound system Medium Cannot be adjusted by the operator	Proportional to the wavelength and number of cycles in a pulse Inversely proportional to the frequency Shorter pulse lengths improve image quality

PROPAGATION OF ULTRASOUND

- Sound travels through tissues at different speeds depending on the density and stiffness of the medium.
- Impedance determines how much of the wave will transmit to the next medium.

Impedance (rayls) = medium density (kg/m^3) × medium propagation speed (m/s).

- The greater the impedance difference the stronger the echo.
- The similar the impedance the weaker the echo.
- Sound travels faster in media that are denser than air because of their reduced compressibility.

Propagation Speeds

MEDIUM	PROPAGATION SPEED
Air	330 m/s
Fat	1459 m/s
Soft tissue	1540 m/s or 1.54 mm/μs
Blood	1570 m/s
Muscle	1580 m/s
Bone	4080 m/s

Propagation of Sound

PROPERTY	DEFINITION	UNITS	RELATIONSHIP

Attenuation	Progressive weakening in the intensity of the sound wave as it propagates in the human body
	Compensated by overall gain and time gain compensation (TGC).
	Result of:
	    Absorption*: conversion of sound to heat
	    Reflection: redirection of the sound beam back toward the transducer
	    Scattering: redirection of sound in multiple directions
		dB	Proportional to the frequency and penetration depth

Attenuation coefficient	Amount of attenuation per cm traveled In soft tissue, equal to half of the transducer frequency (MHz)	dB/cm	Proportional to the frequency and penetration depth
Density	Concentration of mass per unit volume Weight of 1 cm³ of material	kg/m³	Proportional to impedance and propagation speed
Half value layer	Thickness of tissue required to reduce the intensity of the sound beam by one-half Equal to an intensity reduction of -3 dB	cm	Inversely proportional to the frequency
Impedance (Z)	Equal to the density of the medium multiplied by its propagation speed Determines how much of the incident beam is reflected and how much continues to transmit	rayls	Proportional to the density and propagation speed of the medium

*Most common cause.

DECIBEL (dB)

- Compares the relationship between two values of intensity or amplitude along the sound wave.
- Does not represent an absolute value.
- Based on a logarithmic scale with a wide range of values.
- Positive decibels arise when the final intensity exceeds the initial intensity (e.g., increasing the gain control).
- Negative decibels arise when the final intensity is less than the initial intensity (e.g., attenuation).

Decibel Values

DECIBEL	VALUE
3 dB	Increased by 2×
6 dB	Increased by 4×
9 dB	Increased by 8×
10 dB	Increased by 10×
20 dB	Increased by 100×
30 dB	Increased by 1000×
40 dB	Increased by 10,000×
−3 dB	Decreased by ½ (half value layer)
−6 dB	Decreased by ¼
−9 dB	Decreased by ⅛
−10 dB	Decreased by 1/10
−20 dB	Decreased by 1/100
−30 dB	Decreased by 1/1000
−40 dB	Decreased by 1/10,000

ATTENUATION

- Progressive weakening of the amplitude or intensity of the sound wave as it propagates through a medium.
- Owing to absorption, reflection, and scattering of the incidental sound beam.

$$\text{Total attenuation (dB)} = \text{Attenuation coefficient (dB/cm/MHz)} \times \text{Path length (cm)}$$

Attenuation Values

TISSUE	ATTENUATION
Fat	0.6 dB/cm/MHz
Liver	0.9 dB/cm/MHz
Kidney	1.0 dB/cm/MHz
Muscle	1.2 dB/cm/MHz
Air	12.0 dB/cm/MHz
Bone	20.0 dB/cm/MHz

ATTENUATION COEFFICIENT

- Amount of attenuation in the sound beam for every centimeter traveled.

$$\text{Attenuation coefficient (dB/cm)} = \frac{1}{2}\text{ Frequency (MHz)}$$

HALF VALUE LAYER

- Thickness of tissue required to reduce the intensity of the sound beam by one-half.
- Also known as depth of penetration, half boundary layer, penetration depth.

$$\text{Half value layer (cm)} = \frac{3}{\text{Attenuation coefficient (dB/cm)}}$$

OR

$$\text{Half value layer (cm)} = \frac{6}{\text{Frequency (MHz)}}$$

RANGE EQUATION

- Distance to the reflector.
- Time (μs) is equal to distance (cm).
- Must know the direction of the echo and the distance traveled.
- Proportional to the round-trip time.

$$\text{Distance (mm)} = \frac{1}{2}\text{ propagation speed (mm/μs)} \times \text{round-trip time (μs)}.$$

OR

$$\text{Distance (cm)} = \frac{\text{Round-trip time (μs)}}{13\,(\text{μs/cm})}$$

PULSE ROUND TRIP TIME	DISTANCE TO REFLECTOR
0.5 cm	6.5 μs
1.0 cm	13 μs
5.0 cm	65 μs
10 cm	130 μs
15 cm	195 μs

INCIDENT BEAM = REFLECTED BEAM + TRANSMITTED BEAM

- *Incident beam* is the initial beam transmitting from the transducer.
- *Reflected beam* is the portion of beam returning to the transducer.
- *Transmitted beam* is the portion of the beam that continues to travel.

PERPENDICULAR INCIDENCE

- Perpendicular direction of the incident beam in relation to the boundary between two media.
- Allows reflection of the sound beam.
- Transmitted beam continues to travel along the path of the incident beam.
- Intensity of reflected and transmitted sound is dependent on the impedance difference between the two media.

REFLECTION OF ULTRASOUND

- Redirection of a portion of the sound beam back toward the transducer.
- A difference in acoustic impedance between two structures and striking the media boundary at a perpendicular angle MUST take place for reflection to occur.
- The *greater* the impedance difference between the media, the *greater* the reflection.
- The percentage of the incident beam reflected back toward the transducer after the sound beam passes from one tissue to the next is termed the *intensity reflection coefficient* (IRC).
- IRC is determined by the following formula:

$$IRC = \left[\frac{Z_2 - Z_1}{Z_2 + Z_1}\right]^2 = \frac{\text{Reflected intensity (W/cm}^2)}{\text{Incident intensity (W/cm}^2)}$$

- Z1 = impedance of medium 1.
- Z2 = impedance of medium 2.

Reflection of Sound

INTERFACE	REFLECTION
Fat–muscle	1%
Fat–bone	50%
Tissue–air	100%

Specular Reflections

- Occur when the wave strikes a large, smooth surface at a 90-degree angle (e.g., diaphragm).
- Highly angle dependent.

TRANSMISSION OF ULTRASOUND

- With perpendicular incidence, approximately 99% of the incident beam is transmitted.
- The percentage of the incident beam intensity that is transmitted after the beam passes from one tissue to the next is termed the *intensity transmission coefficient* (ITC).
- ITC is determined by the following formulas:

$$ITC = \frac{\text{Transmitted intensity (W/cm}^2)}{\text{Incident intensity (W/cm}^2)}$$

OR

$$ITC = 1 - IRC$$

OBLIQUE INCIDENCE

- Nonperpendicular direction of the incident beam in relation to the boundary between two media.
- The reflected sound does not travel back to the transducer but in some other direction.
- Direction of the incident beam with respect to the media boundary is termed the *incidence angle.*
- Incidence angle is equal to the reflection angle.
- Reflected and transmitted directions are given by the reflection angle and the transmission angle.
- Transmission angle depends on the propagation speeds in the media.

Scatter

- Redirection of sound in many directions by rough surfaces or heterogeneous media allowing the definition of organ parenchyma and tissue boundaries.
- A nonspecular reflector that is smaller, more irregular, or rougher than the incident beam will demonstrate scattering.
- Not angle dependent.
- Proportional to the frequency.

Rayleigh's Scatter

- Occurs when the reflector is much smaller than the wavelength of the sound beam (e.g., red blood cells).
- Is directed equally in all directions.

REFRACTION OF ULTRASOUND

- Redirection or bending of the transmitting beam after it passes through one medium to another.
- Oblique incidence and a change of velocity or propagation speed between two media MUST take place for refraction to occur.
- If the propagation speed in the second medium is *greater* than the speed in the first medium, the transmitted beam will bend *away* from the incident beam. The transmission angle is *greater* than the incident angle and vice versa.
- May cause lateral displacement of structures or shadowing.
- Refraction of a sound beam obeys Snell's law and is used to determine the amount of refraction at an interface.

Critical Angle

- An angle of incidence where there is no transmission and 100% internal reflection.
- Transmission angle is at 90 degrees.
- Causes edge shadowing.

HARMONIC FREQUENCIES

- Even and odd multiples of the fundamental frequency (2 MHz transducer has harmonics of 4, 6, and 8 MHz).
- Harmonic beams are weaker than the fundamental sound beams so they attenuate quickly.
- Lower frequency during transmission gives more imaging depth and higher frequency during reception, which improves resolution.
- Harmonic beams are narrower, improving lateral resolution.
- Degradation of axial resolution due to the increased spatial pulse length needed for transmission.
- Eliminates grating lobes.
- Harmonic energy is nonexistent in near field decreasing the amount of noise and reverberation artifact in this area.
- Do not use harmonics when measuring in the axial plane. Not as accurate as fundamental frequency.

Types of Harmonic Frequencies

Tissue Harmonics

- Sound waves become distorted while traveling through the medium due to uneven speeds, faster during compression and slower during rarefaction, which creates harmonic energy.
- Created during **transmission** as the beam travels further into the body.

- Due to an increase of pressure there is an increased amount of harmonic energy within the focal zone.
- Sound beam diverges in the far field decreasing the pressure, causing harmonic energy to decrease.

Contrast Harmonics

- As the sound wave encounters the microbubbles of the contrast agent, the bubble contracts and expands, which creates harmonic energy.
- Created during **receiving** when the sound beam reflects off the microbubbles causing it to expand and contract.
- Sound wave must have enough strength or pressure to change the shape of the bubble.
- The strength is measured by the Mechanical Index (MI); MI needs to be greater than 0.1 for harmonics to occur.
- Lower frequency transducers and increased beam strength create a higher MI, therefore more harmonics.

System Requirements for Harmonics

- Wide bandwidth: necessary to encompass both the bandwidth of the fundamental frequency and the bandwidth of the harmonic signal together.
- Must transmit at a lower frequency and receive at a higher frequency.
- Contain a bandpass filter within the receiver of the ultrasound system that acts to eliminate the fundamental frequency, allowing better resolution of the harmonic frequency.

CONTRAST AGENTS

- Injected into the body to enhance anatomic structures.
- Must be capable of:
  - Easy administration.
  - Nontoxic.
  - Stable for sufficient examination time.
  - Small enough to pass through the capillaries and large and echogenic enough to improve image resolution.
- Almost all contain microbubbles although free gas microbubbles and particle suspension have been used.
- Contrast agents improve lesion detection when lesion echogenicity is similar to surrounding tissue, lesions demonstrating arterial and portal phases in real time, and weak Doppler signals.
- Opacify anechoic regions from impedance mismatch.
- Contrast agents approved in the United States include Definity (octafluoropropane-containing liposomes), Imagent (dimyristoyl lecithin), and Optison (perfluoropropain-filled albumin).
- Contrast agents approved in Canada, Europe, and Japan include Sonazoid, Lenovist, and Sonovue.

PHYSICS PRINCIPLES REVIEW

1. In soft tissue, if the frequency of a wave increases, the propagation speed will:
   a. double
   b. increase
   c. decrease
   d. remain the same

2. The range of frequencies found within a pulse describes which of the following terms?
   a. duty factor
   b. bandwidth
   c. harmonics
   d. pulse repetition frequency

3. In gray-scale imaging, how many cycles per pulse are generally used?
   a. 2 to 3
   b. 4 to 5
   c. 5 to 10
   d. 10 to 30

4. Which of the following frequencies is within the audible range?
   a. 15 Hz
   b. 15 kHz
   c. 20 kHz
   d. 25,000 Hz

5. Propagation speed through a medium is determined by the:
   a. pulse repetition period
   b. intensity and amplitude of the wave
   c. density and stiffness of the medium
   d. impedance difference between the media

6. Which of the following is an acoustic variable?
   a. intensity
   b. wavelength
   c. particle motion
   d. propagation speed

7. Which of the following improves sonographic image quality?
   a. duty factor
   b. long pulse length
   c. shorter pulse length
   d. lower operating frequency

8. If the stiffness of a medium increases, the propagation speed will:
   a. double
   b. increase
   c. decrease
   d. remain the same

9. The length of a pulse from beginning to end is termed the:
   a. wavelength
   b. pulse duration
   c. spatial pulse length
   d. pulse repetition period

10. In which of the following media does sound propagate the fastest?
    a. air
    b. bone
    c. muscle
    d. soft tissue

11. Which of the following will occur when penetration depth is increased?
    a. propagation speed will increase
    b. pulse repetition period will decrease
    c. pulse repetition frequency will decrease
    d. spatial pulse length will decrease

12. If the amplitude of a wave doubles, the intensity will:
    a. double
    b. quadruple
    c. decrease by one-half
    d. decrease by one-quarter

13. The time for one pulse to occur defines:
    a. period
    b. pulse duration
    c. spatial pulse length
    d. pulse repetition period

14. Which of the following is associated with a broader bandwidth?
    a. a lower Q-factor
    b. an increase in amplitude
    c. a longer spatial pulse length
    d. a decrease in the number of frequencies within the pulse

15. Regions of low density in a compression wave are termed:
    a. cycles
    b. bandwidth
    c. rarefactions
    d. compressions

16. Which of the following formulas calculates the duty factor?
    a. power of the source divided by the area
    b. pulse duration divided by the pulse repetition period
    c. pulse repetition frequency divided by the pulse duration
    d. frequency of the source multiplied by the propagation speed

17. Resistance to the propagation of sound through a medium defines:
    a. reflection
    b. attenuation
    c. acoustic impedance
    d. Rayleigh's scatter

18. Which of the following units quantify pressure?
    a. rayls
    b. pascal
    c. decibels
    d. milliwatts

19. Overall compensation gain is set at 36 dB. If the gain is reduced by one-half, what will the new gain be?
    a. 18 dB
    b. 25 dB
    c. 30 dB
    d. 33 dB

20. Attenuation occurring as sound propagates through each centimeter of soft tissue is equal to:
    a. ½ operating frequency
    b. attenuation coefficient × path length
    c. medium density × propagation speed
    d. ½ (propagation speed × round-trip time)

21. *Spatial* is a term used to describe:
    a. time
    b. speed
    c. space
    d. distance

22. Which of the following units measures the attenuation of sound in soft tissue?
    a. μs
    b. dB
    c. rayls
    d. dB/cm

23. If the frequency is increased, pulse duration will:
    a. double
    b. increase
    c. decrease
    d. remain unchanged

24. Which of the following metric prefixes denotes 1 billion?
    a. deca
    b. mega
    c. tetra
    d. giga

25. Which of the following units of measurement represents the number of pulses occurring in 1 second?
    a. μs
    b. kHz
    c. mW
    d. W/cm²

26. Which of the following formulas determines the impedance of a medium?
    a. attenuation multiplied by the propagation speed of the medium
    b. propagation speed of the medium multiplied by the round-trip time
    c. density of the medium multiplied by the attenuation coefficient
    d. density of the medium multiplied by the propagation speed of the medium

27. Weakening of a sound wave as it travels through a medium defines:
    a. scattering
    b. harmonics
    c. attenuation
    d. acoustic impedance

28. Which of the following occurs when a sound wave strikes a large, smooth surface at a 90-degree angle?
    a. refraction
    b. specular reflection
    c. Rayleigh's scatter
    d. nonspecular reflection

29. With perpendicular incidence, what percentage of the incident beam continues to the next medium?
    a. 50%
    b. 85%
    c. 99%
    d. 100%

30. The unit of measurement used to describe the amplitude of a pressure wave is:
    a. rayl
    b. watt
    c. joule
    d. variable

31. Which of the following properties is proportional to the pulse repetition frequency?
    a. period
    b. duty factor
    c. penetration depth
    d. spatial pulse length

32. Which of the following will most likely decrease the propagation speed of a wave?
    a. increasing the penetration depth
    b. increasing the stiffness of the medium
    c. decreasing the transducer frequency
    d. increasing the density of the medium

33. For short pulses, the quality (Q) factor is equal to:
    a. the distance of one pulse
    b. one-half of the frequency
    c. the number of cycles in a pulse
    d. the intensity of the sound beam

34. The positive half of a pressure wave corresponds to:
    a. amplitude
    b. intensity
    c. rarefaction
    d. compression

35. Which of the following contrast agents is approved in the United States?
    a. Imagent
    b. Echovist
    c. Lenovist
    d. Sonovue

36. Bending of a transmitting sound beam after it passes through one medium into another describes:
    a. scattering
    b. refraction
    c. reflection
    d. reverberation

37. Attenuation is most commonly a result of:
    a. reflection
    b. scattering
    c. absorption
    d. transmission

38. Half value layer is equal to an intensity reduction of:
    a. 3 dB
    b. 6 dB
    c. 10 dB
    d. 50 dB

39. Propagation speed is directly related to:
    a. density
    b. stiffness
    c. frequency
    d. wavelength

40. Which of the following is proportional to the impedance of a medium?
    a. wavelength
    b. propagation speed
    c. stiffness of the medium
    d. attenuation coefficient

41. Which of the following units compares the ratio of amplitudes along two points of a sound wave?
    a. W
    b. dB
    c. rayl
    d. dB/cm

42. Attenuation of the sound beam is proportional to the:
    a. frequency of the sound wave
    b. direction of the incident beam
    c. reflected intensity of the sound wave
    d. transmitted intensity of the sound wave

43. Which of the following is responsible for determining the amount of reflection and transmission of the sound wave?
    a. density
    b. stiffness
    c. impedance
    d. propagation speed

44. Dissipation of heat in a medium primarily in the form of heat describes:
    a. reflection
    b. refraction
    c. absorption
    d. half value layers

45. Which of the following most accurately describes harmonic imaging?
    a. Harmonic imaging exists throughout the image.
    b. Harmonic imaging improves axial resolution.
    c. Harmonic beams are stronger than fundamental sound beams.
    d. Contrast harmonics are created during receiving.

46. Snell's law determines the amount of:
    a. reflection at an interface
    b. refraction at an interface
    c. transmission through a medium
    d. scattering distal to a dense medium

47. Direction of the incident beam with respect to the media boundary is termed the:
    a. specular angle
    b. reflection angle
    c. propagating angle
    d. transmission angle

48. Demonstration of boundaries between organs is a result of:
    a. refraction
    b. transmission
    c. specular reflection
    d. Rayleigh scattering

49. Angle of incidence, where there is no transmission and 100% reflection, describes:
    a. refraction
    b. critical angle
    c. specular angle
    d. reflection angle

50. With perpendicular incidence, the larger the impedance difference between the media, the greater the:
    a. scattering
    b. reflection
    c. absorption
    d. transmission

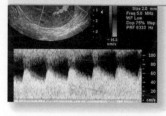

CHAPTER 3

Ultrasound Transducers

KEY TERMS

angle of divergence   the widening of the sound beam in the far field.

aperture   size of the transducer element(s).

array   collection of active elements connected to individual electronic currents in one transducer assembly.

axial resolution   ability to distinguish two structures along a path parallel to the sound beam.

channels   multiple transducer elements with individual wiring and system electronics.

constructive interference   occurs when two waves in phase with each other create a new wave with amplitude greater than the original two waves

convex array   curved linear transducer containing multiple piezoelectric elements.

crystal   piezoelectric element.

Curie point   temperature to which a material is raised, while in the presence of a strong electrical field, to yield piezoelectric properties. If the temperature exceeds the Curie point, the piezoelectric properties will be lost.

damping   material attached to the rear of the transducer element to reduce the pulse duration.

destructive interference   occurs when two waves out of phase with each other create a new wave with amplitude less than the two original waves.

detail resolution   includes both axial and lateral resolution.

diffraction   deviation in the direction of the sound wave that is not a result of reflection, scattering, or refraction.

dynamic aperture   aperture that increases as the focal length increases; minimizes change in the width of the sound beam.

dynamic damping   electronic means to suppress the element from ringing.

dynamic focusing   variable receiving focus that follows the changing position of the pulse as it propagates through tissue; the electrical output of the elements can be timed to "listen" in a particular direction and depth.

element   piezoelectric component of the transducer assembly.

elevation resolution   detail resolution located perpendicular to the scan plane; it is equal to the section thickness and is the source of the section thickness artifact.

far zone   region of the sound beam in which the diameter increases as the distance from the transducer increases.

focal length   distance from a focused transducer to the center of the focal zone; distance from a focused transducer to the spatial peak intensity.

focal point   concentration of the sound beam into a smaller area.

focal zone   area or region of the focus.

Fraunhofer zone   far zone.

Fresnel zone   near zone.

fundamental frequency   operating frequency.

grating lobes   additional weak beams emitted from a multi-element transducer that propagate in directions different from the primary beam.

Huygens principle   all points on a wave front or at a source are point sources for the production of spherical secondary wavelets.

interference phenomenon   interference occurring when two waves interact or overlap, resulting in the creation of a new wave.

lateral resolution   ability to distinguish two structures lying perpendicular to the sound path.

lead zirconate titanate (PZT)   a ceramic piezoelectric material.

matching layer   material attached to the front face of the transducer element to reduce reflections at the transducer surface.

near zone   region of the beam between the transducer and focal point, which decreases in size as it approaches the focus.

operating frequency   natural frequency of the transducer; it is determined by the propagation speed and thickness of the element in pulse ultrasound and by the electrical frequency in continuous wave.

piezoelectricity   conversion of pressure to electric voltage.

phased   applying voltage pulses to all elements in the assembly as a group, but with minor time differences. Phased pulses allow multiple focal zones, beam steering, and beam focusing.

sequenced array   operated by applying voltage pulses to a group of elements in succession.

side lobes   additional weak beams traveling from a single-element transducer in directions different from the primary beam.

transducer   device that converts energy from one form to another.

transducer assembly   transducer element, damping, matching layers, and housing; also known as probe, scan head, or transducer.

DIAGNOSTIC ULTRASOUND TRANSDUCERS

- Convert electrical energy into acoustic energy during transmission and acoustic energy into electrical energy for reception.
- Operate on the principle of piezoelectricity.
- Driven typically by one cycle of alternating voltage.
- Diagnostic frequencies range between 2.0 and 20 MHz.
- More frequencies (bandwidth) and wavelengths are present in shorter pulses.

PIEZOELECTRICITY (Piezoelectric Effect)

- Piezoelectric principle states that some materials produce a voltage when deformed by an applied pressure.
- Various forms of ceramics and quartz are naturally piezoelectric.
- Lead zirconate titanate (PZT) is the most common manufactured piezoelectric element.
- PZT placed in a strong electric field while at a high temperature acts as an element with piezoelectric properties (Curie point).
- If the material exceeds the Curie point, the element will lose its piezoelectric properties (e.g., autoclave sterilization).
- Dipole alignment process: this very high temperature permits the molecules within the material to move more freely. When the electrical field is introduced, the positive and negative poles align in opposite directions. When the heat and electrical field are removed the molecules remain in this new polarized position.

Transducer Assembly

COMPONENT	FUNCTION	DESCRIPTION	RELATIONSHIP
Piezoelectric element, also called: Crystal Active element Transducer element	Converts electrical voltage into ultrasound pulses and the returning echoes back to electric voltage Electrical energy is applied to the element, increasing or decreasing the thickness according to the polarity of the voltage	*Natural Materials:* Rochelle salt, quartz, and tourmaline *Manufactured Materials:* Lead zirconate titanate (PZT), barium titanate, lead metaniobate, and polyvinylidene difluoride *Piezoelectric composites* Mixture of polymer and piezoceramic material allows: Wider bandwidth Increased sensitivity Harmonic imaging Lower element impedance increases the efficiency of the backing layer Single elements are in the form of a disk Array transducers contain numerous elements with separate electrical wiring Contain a bandwidth of frequencies Impedance is much greater than soft tissue	Propagation speed of the element is directly related to the operating frequency Thickness of the element is inversely related to the operating frequency (thinner elements operate at higher frequencies) Thickness is equal to half of the wavelength of the element material Impedance is 20× greater than that of the skin
Damping, also called: Backing	Reduces the number of cycles in each pulse An electronic means to suppress the crystal from ringing Reduces pulse duration and spatial pulse length	Attached to the rear face of the element Made of metal powder and a plastic or epoxy High absorption coefficient Reduces amplitude, sensitivity and Q-Factor Impedance should be equal to that of the element for maximum energy transfer	Increases the bandwidth and axial resolution

Continued

Transducer Assembly—(cont'd)

COMPONENT	FUNCTION	DESCRIPTION	RELATIONSHIP
Matching layers	Reduce the impedance difference between the element and skin Improve sound transmission across the element–tissue boundary Reduces reflection at element surface	Located in front of the element Composed of aluminum powder in an epoxy resin Two layers are typically used Aqueous gel is a matching layer between the transducer face and the skin	Increase the transmission of sound into the body Thickness equal to one-fourth of the wavelength of the element Impedance of matching layer is less than that of the crystal and greater than the impedance of the skin
Transducer housing	Protects the components of the transducer Protects the operator and patient from electrical shock Prevents the transducer from outside interference Provides orientation using identifying markers (grooves, notches)	Covering for transducer components Made of metal or plastic	Damage to the housing can increase risk of electrical shock and decrease image quality

TYPES OF TRANSDUCERS

Continuous Wave

- Produces a continuous wave of sound.
- Is composed of separate transmit and receiver elements housed in a single transducer assembly.
- Frequency of the sound wave is determined by the electrical frequency of the ultrasound system.
- Demonstrates a narrow bandwidth.
- Transducer does not contain a damping layer.
- Width of the sound beam varies with distance.

Pulse Wave

- Transmits pulses of sound and receives returning echoes.
- Classified by the thickness and propagation speed of the element.
- Demonstrates a wide bandwidth and short pulse length.
- Linear, convex, and annular are types of transducer construction.
- Sequenced, phased, and vector are types of transducer operation.
- Produces a 2-cycle to 3-cycle pulse for gray-scale imaging and a 5-cycle to 30-cycle pulse for Doppler techniques.
- Multihertz transducers utilize the range of frequencies in a pulse (bandwidth).
- Minor or secondary beams traveling in directions different from the primary beam are termed *side* or *grating* lobes.
- Frequency of the sound pulse is equal to the operating frequency.

Operating frequency (MHz) = Propagation speed of the element (mm/μs) × Element thickness (mm)

Pulse Wave Transducers

TYPE	DESCRIPTION	FOCUSING	BEAM STEERING
Annular array	Multiple elements are arranged in concentric rings with a motor assembly that are rotating or vibrating back and forth Sector-type image	Electronic	Mechanical
Convex sequenced array	Multiple elements arranged in a curved line (arc) Operated by applying voltage pulses to groups of elements in succession Pulses travel in different directions, producing a curved or arc-shaped image Also called: curved array, convex array, curvilinear array	Electronic	Electronic
Intracavital	Mechanical, linear array, or phased array transducers mounted on probes designed to insert into the vagina, rectum, or esophagus Crystal is mechanically swept up and down to produce a 45- to 110-degree sector image High frequency with rapid frame rates optimizing axial and lateral resolution Also called: endocavital, transcavital	Electronic	Electronic
Intraluminal	Extremely small crystal arrays are mounted on the end of a catheter designed to insert into a fetal, vascular, or anatomical structure (e.g., umbilical cord, artery, fallopian tube) High frequency (up to 50 MHz) Also called: transluminal	Electronic	Electronic
Linear sequenced array	Straight line of rectangular elements about one wavelength wide Operated by applying voltage pulses to groups of elements in succession Pulses travel in straight parallel vertical scan lines producing a rectangular image Also called: linear array	Electronic	Electronic
Linear phased array	Contains a compact line of elements about one-quarter–wavelength wide Operated by applying voltage pulses to most or all of the elements using minor time differences (delays) Resulting pulses can be shaped and steered producing a rectangular image Received echoes follow the changing position of the pulse Permits multiple focal zones	Electronic	Electronic
Sector	Each pulse originates from the same starting point Pie-shaped image	Electronic	Electronic
Vector array	Emits pulses from different starting points and in different directions Combines linear sequential and linear phased array technologies Converts the format of a linear array into a trapezoidal image	Electronic	Electronic

UNFOCUSED SOUND BEAM (Figs 3.1 and 3.2)

- Some beam narrowing will occur.
- The near-zone length is equal to one-half of the beam diameter.
- Two near-zone lengths are equal to the transducer diameter.

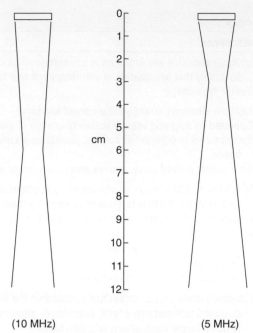

(10 MHz)   (5 MHz)

FIG. 3.1 Beams for disk transducers have a diameter of 6 mm at two frequencies. Higher frequencies produce smaller beam diameters (at a distance greater than 4 cm in this case) and longer near-zone lengths.

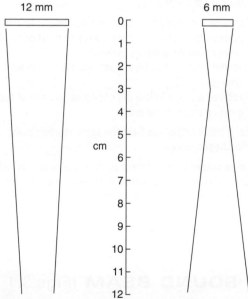

FIG. 3.2 Beams for 5-MHz disk transducers of two diameters. The larger transducer *(left)* produces the longer near-zone length. A smaller transducer *(right)* can produce a larger-diameter beam in the far zone. In this example, the beam diameters are equal at a distance of 8 cm.

Beam Focus Characteristics

- *Ultrasound beam consists of a near zone and far zone.*
- *The intensity of the sound beam is not uniform throughout the beam.*
- *Some intensity travels outside the main beam termed side lobes (single element) or grating lobes (multiple elements).*

CHARACTERISTIC	DESCRIPTION
Far zone	Region distal to the focal point where the sound beam diverges Intensity of the beam is more uniform Inversely related to the operating frequency and diameter of the element (increasing the frequency decreases the angle of divergence) Also called Fraunhofer zone, far field
Near zone length	Also called focal length Distance from the transducer to the narrowest portion of the beam Determined by the operating frequency and the diameter of the element $\text{NZL (mm)} = [\text{crystal diameter}\,(\text{mm}^2)] \times \text{frequency}\,(\text{MHz})$ $\text{NZL (mm)} = \dfrac{(\text{crystal diameter})^2}{4 \times \text{wavelength}}$ Directly related to the operating frequency and diameter of the element Inversely related to the divergence of the beam in the far zone
Focal point	Narrowest portion of the beam Width at the focal point is equal to half of the transducer width Area of maximum intensity in the beam Also called focus
Focal zone	Area where the beam is focused on each side of the focal point One-half of the focal zone is located in the near zone, and the other half is located in the far zone Also called focal area, focal region
Focal zone length	Distance between equal beam widths that are some multiples of the minimum value (at the focus) Also called field length, depth of field
Near zone	Region between the transducer and focus Beam width decreases with increasing distance from the transducer (conical in shape) Intensity variations are the greatest Length of the near zone is directly related to the frequency of the transducer and diameter of the element Additional focusing can be added in this region Also called Fresnel zone, near field

FOCUSING OF THE SOUND BEAM (Fig. 3.3)

- Improves lateral resolution by reducing beam width.
- Only accomplished within the near zone.
- Creates a narrower sound beam over a specified area.
- Beam diameter in the near zone decreases in size toward the focal point.
- Beam diameter in the far zone (angle of divergence) increases in size after the focal point.
- Increasing the frequency or diameter of the element will produce a narrower beam, longer focal length, and less divergence in the far zone.

Types of Focusing

Dynamic Receive Focusing

- Controlled by ultrasound system.
- Focusing occurring during reception.
- Introduces variable time delays to some electrical signals during reception.
- Delay times depend on depth of reflector.
- Delay patterns change continuously.
- Improves lateral resolution.

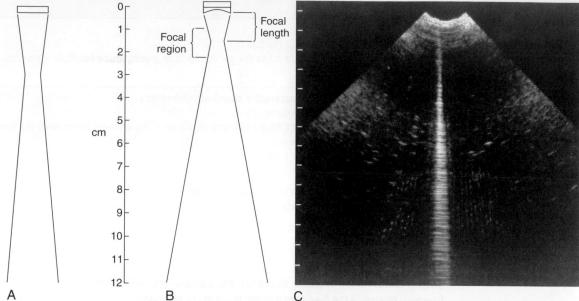

FIG. 3.3 Beam diameter for a 6-mm, 5-MHz transducer without **(A)** and with **(B)** focusing. Focusing reduces the minimum beam width compared with that produced without focusing. However, well beyond the focal region, the width of the focused beam is greater than that of the unfocused beam. **(C)** A focused beam. This is an ultrasound image of a beam profile test object containing a thin vertical scattering layer down the center. Scanning this object generates a picture of the beam (the pulse width at all depths). In this case the focus occurs at a depth of about 4 cm (this image has a total depth of 15 cm). Depth markers (in 1-cm increments) are indicated on the left edge of the figure.

Electronic

- Operator controlled.
- Allows multiple focal zones.
- Uses the interference phenomenon to focus the sound beam.
- Accomplished with a curved pattern of phased delays.
- An increase or decrease to the curvature of the delay pattern moves focus shallower or deeper, respectively.
- Applied to individual beams to improve slice thickness and lateral resolution.
- Improves spatial resolution within the focal point.

External

- Predetermined focal range.
- An acoustic lens is placed in front of the crystal to focus the sound beam.

Internal

- Predetermined focal range.
- Piezoelectric element(s) are shaped concavely to focus the sound beam.
- Beam diameter is reduced in the focal point.

Multizone Focusing

- Selecting to focus the sound beam in more than one location.
- A separate beam is fired for each focal zone.
- Decreases temporal resolution (decreases frame rate).

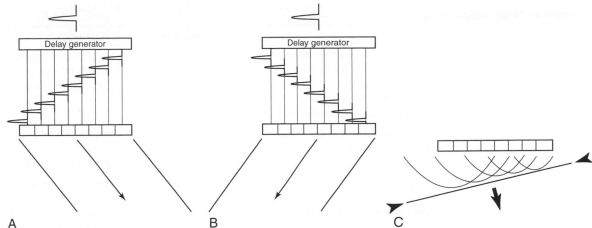

FIG. 3.4   A linear phased array (side view). **(A)** When voltage pulses are applied in rapid progression from left to right, one ultrasound pulse is produced that is directed to the right. **(B)** Similarly, when voltage pulses are applied in rapid progression from right to left, one ultrasound pulse is produced that is directed to the left. **(C)** The delays in **(A)** produce a pulse whose combined pressure wave front *(arrowheads)* is angled from the lower left to the upper right. A wave always travels perpendicular to its wave front, as indicated by the *arrow.*

STEERING OF THE SOUND BEAM (Fig. 3.4)

- Created by the beam former.
- Electronic steering is operator adjustable.
- Used to sweep the sound wave over a specific area.
- System alters the electronic excitation of the elements, steering the beam in various directions.
- The returning echoes are also delayed.

RESOLUTION

- The ability to distinguish two adjacent reflectors as two separate structures.

Types of Resolution

RESOLUTION	DESCRIPTION	DETERMINED BY	RELATIONSHIP

Axial, also called:
Longitudinal
Range
Depth
	Ability to distinguish two structures
	  in a path parallel to the sound beam
	Does not vary with distance
	Improves with transducer damping
	Always better than lateral resolution
		Transducer
		Medium
			Equal to $\frac{1}{2}$ SPL
			Directly related to the operating
			  frequency
			Increasing operating frequency will
			  reduce penetration depth
			Inversely related to the spatial pulse
			  length
			Smaller is better

Contrast	Ability to differentiate between echoes
	  of slightly different amplitude
	High contrast demonstrates fewer
	  shades of gray
	Low contrast demonstrates more
	  shades of gray
		Ultrasound system	Directly related to axial and lateral
			  resolution

Elevation, also called:
Z-axis
Slice or section thickness
	Thickness of the scanned tissue
	  perpendicular to the scan plane
	Z-axis has the poorest measure
	  of resolution for array transducers
	  (excluding annular array)
		Transducer	Related to the beam thickness
			Thinner slice thicknesses produce
			  better image quality

Continued

Types of Resolution—(cont'd)

RESOLUTION	DESCRIPTION	DETERMINED BY	RELATIONSHIP
Lateral, also called: Angular Transverse Azimuthal	Ability to distinguish two structures in a path perpendicular to the sound beam Varies with distance Improves with focusing Best resolution at the focal point	Transducer	Equal to beam diameter Directly related to beam diameter, frequency, focusing, and distance
Spatial	Ability to see detail on the image Includes axial, elevational, and lateral resolution	Transducer	Directly related to the number of scan lines Indirectly related to temporal resolution
Temporal	Ability to precisely position moving structures Ability to separate two points in time	Frame rate	Directly related to the frame rate Indirectly related to the number of focal zones, imaging depth, and spatial resolution

Optimizing Resolution

RESOLUTION	OPTIMIZING TECHNIQUE
Axial	Increase transducer frequency *Additional Options:* Increase number of focal zones Decrease imaging depth
Contrast	Increase compression (dynamic range) *Additional Options:* Increase transducer frequency Decrease beam width Postprocess mapping
Lateral	Proper focal placement *Additional Options:* Decrease beam width Decrease imaging depth
Temporal	Decrease number of focal zones Decrease imaging depth *Additional Options:* Decrease beam width Decrease persistence

TRANSDUCER CARE

- Do not heat-sterilize (auto-clave).
- Do not drop transducer or run over transducer cables.
- Use cleaning agents recommended by the transducer manufacturer.
- Avoid products with acetone, mineral oil, iodine, oil-based perfumes, and chlorine bleach.
- Routinely check for damage to the transducer assembly.

TRANSDUCER REVIEW

1. Widening of the sound beam is demonstrated in the:
   a. focal point
   b. focal zone
   c. Fresnel zone
   d. Fraunhofer zone

2. Weak beams emitted from a linear sequenced array transducer are termed:
   a. side lobes
   b. harmonics
   c. grating lobes
   d. mechanical waves

3. The fundamental frequency of a pulse wave is determined by the:
   a. diameter of the beam
   b. impedance of the matching layer
   c. electrical frequency of the ultrasound system
   d. thickness and propagation speed of the element

4. Heat sterilization is not recommended for diagnostic transducers because:
   a. apodization will occur
   b. the housing may be damaged
   c. the epoxy in the backing will melt
   d. the piezoelectric properties will be lost

5. Which of the following components is unnecessary in the construction of a continuous wave transducer?
   a. matching layer
   b. damping layer
   c. electrical wiring
   d. two active elements

6. Lateral resolution is determined by the:
   a. beam width
   b. near-zone length
   c. spatial pulse length
   d. thickness of the active element

7. An electronic means to suppress the elements from ringing describes:
   a. damping
   b. dynamic focusing
   c. dynamic damping
   d. dynamic aperture

8. More frequencies and wavelengths are present in:
   a. longer pulses
   b. shorter pulses
   c. thinner elements
   d. smaller diameter elements

9. On which of the following principles do diagnostic ultrasound transducers operate?
   a. Snell's law
   b. ALARA principle
   c. Huygens principle
   d. piezoelectric effect

10. If the width of the transducer is 5.0 cm, what is the width at the focal point?
    a. 1.0 cm
    b. 2.5 cm
    c. 5.0 cm
    d. 10.0 cm

11. Constructive interference will create a wave with amplitude:
    a. equal to the original waves
    b. less than the original waves
    c. shorter than the original waves
    d. greater than the original waves

12. Reducing the impedance difference between the crystal and the skin is the primary function of which of the following transducer components?
    a. aqueous gel
    b. damping layer
    c. matching layer
    d. backing layer

13. A sound beam demonstrates the most uniform intensity in the:
    a. far zone
    b. near zone
    c. focal zone
    d. focal length

14. Depth of field is also known as:
    a. focal zone
    b. far field
    c. near zone length
    d. focal zone length

15. Which of the following changes will improve temporal resolution?
    a. increase in beam width
    b. increase in focal zone depth
    c. decrease in imaging depth
    d. decrease in dynamic range

16. A disadvantage of multizone focusing is a reduction in:
    a. dynamic range
    b. lateral resolution
    c. detail resolution
    d. temporal resolution

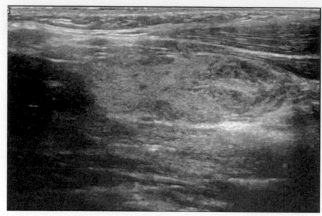

FIG. 3.5   Sagittal sonogram.

Using Figure 3.5, answer question 17.

17. Which of the following transducers is demonstrated in this sonogram?
    a. vector array
    b. annular array
    c. convex array
    d. linear array

18. The distance from the face of a focused transducer to the point of spatial peak intensity is termed the:
    a. focal region
    b. pulse duration
    c. near zone length
    d. spatial pulse length

19. The narrowest diameter of a sound beam is termed the focal:
    a. zone
    b. area
    c. point
    d. region

20. Which of the following best describes channels?
    a. interference occurring when two waves interact or overlap
    b. apertures that increase as the focal length increases
    c. multiple transducer elements with individual wiring and system electronics
    d. additional weak beams emitted from a multi-element transducer

21. Which of the following determines the diameter of the focus?
    a. spatial pulse length
    b. thickness of the element
    c. diameter of the transducer
    d. propagation speed of the element

22. The impedance of the damping layer is:
    a. less than the element's
    b. similar to the element's
    c. greater than the element's
    d. twice that of the element's

23. The purpose of backing material in the transducer assembly is to:
    a. decrease the bandwidth
    b. increase the pulse duration
    c. protect the components from moisture
    d. reduce the number of cycles in a pulse

24. Vector array is a type of transducer:
    a. assembly
    b. operation
    c. construction
    d. composition

25. Focusing of the sound beam is directly related to:
    a. axial resolution
    b. lateral resolution
    c. contrast resolution
    d. elevation resolution

26. Steering of the sound beam is accomplished by:
    a. constructive interference
    b. focusing of the sound beam
    c. increasing the fundamental frequency
    d. altering the excitation of the active elements

27. Exceeding the Curie point of a transducer element will result in:
    a. a broader bandwidth
    b. a higher propagation speed
    c. a higher operating frequency
    d. the loss of all piezoelectric properties

28. Axial resolution is equal to:
    a. the spatial pulse length
    b. the width of the sound beam
    c. one-half of the spatial pulse length
    d. one-half of the beam diameter

29. Which of the following would optimize contrast resolution?
    a. decreasing imaging depth
    b. increasing compression
    c. increasing the beam width
    d. decreasing the number of focal zones

30. Temporal resolution is determined by the:
    a. medium
    b. frame rate
    c. beam width
    d. element thickness

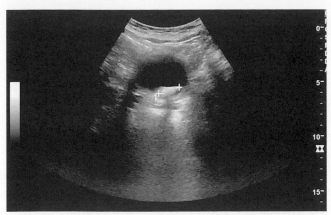

FIG. 3.6   Transverse sonogram of the gallbladder.

Using Figure 3.6, answer question 31.

31. Which of the following operator controls will most likely aid in demonstrating acoustic shadowing posterior to the gallstone?
    a. decrease operating frequency and imaging depth
    b. increase number of focal zones and beam width
    c. decrease the imaging depth and depth of the focus
    d. increase operating frequency and depth of focus

32. Which of the following transducers operates by applying voltage pulses to groups of linear elements in succession?
    a. vector array
    b. linear phased array
    c. convex phased array
    d. linear sequenced array

33. Focusing of the sound beam is only accomplished within the:
    a. focal area
    b. focal zone
    c. near zone
    d. focal region

34. What is the diameter of the sound beam at one near-zone length?
    a. equal to the transducer diameter
    b. one-half of the transducer diameter
    c. one-quarter of the transducer diameter
    d. variable depending on transducer frequency

35. The ability to distinguish two structures in a path perpendicular to the sound beam describes:
    a. spatial resolution
    b. contrast resolution
    c. temporal resolution
    d. azimuthal resolution

36. The most common piezoelectric material used in diagnostic ultrasound transducers is:
    a. quartz
    b. tourmaline
    c. barium titanate
    d. lead zirconate titanate

37. Beam steering is accomplished in an annular array:
    a. electronically
    b. mechanically
    c. using phase delays
    d. using sequential delays

38. Diagnostic frequencies range between:
    a. 1.0 and 10.0 MHz
    b. 2.0 and 12.0 MHz
    c. 2.0 and 20.0 MHz
    d. 3.5 and 15.0 MHz

39. Which of the following changes will improve axial resolution?
    a. increase in beam width
    b. increase in transducer frequency
    c. increase in imaging depth
    d. decrease in number of focal zones

40. During transmission, diagnostic ultrasound transducers convert:
    a. kinetic energy into thermal energy
    b. acoustic energy into electrical energy
    c. electrical energy into thermal energy
    d. electrical energy into acoustic energy

41. Which of the following states, "Some materials produce a voltage when distorted by an applied pressure"?
    a. Snell's law
    b. Huygens principle
    c. Ohm's acoustic law
    d. piezoelectric principle

42. Which of the following is a negative effect of using a damping material in the transducer assembly?
    a. low-quality factor
    b. reduced sensitivity
    c. narrowed bandwidth
    d. increased pulse duration

43. How many cycles per pulse are typically used in Doppler imaging?
    a. 2 to 20
    b. 3 to 15
    c. 5 to 30
    d. 6 to 40

44. The sonographer can determine the depth of the focal zone when using a transducer with a(n):
    a. internal focus
    b. external focus
    c. electronic focus
    d. mechanical focus

45. The impedance of the matching layer is:
    a. less than the impedance of the skin
    b. equal to the impedance of the skin
    c. less than the impedance of the crystal
    d. equal to the impedance of the crystal

46. Which of the following transducers displays a trapezoidal image?
    a. convex array
    b. vector array
    c. annular array
    d. curvilinear array

47. Which of the following differentiates similar or dissimilar tissues?
    a. axial resolution
    b. lateral resolution
    c. contrast resolution
    d. temporal resolution

48. Section thickness is related to the:
    a. frame rate
    b. beam thickness
    c. penetration depth
    d. operating frequency

49. Operating frequency of a transducer is directly related to the:
    a. thickness of the element
    b. diameter of the element
    c. impedance of the element
    d. propagation speed of the element

50. The matching layer is composed of a(n):
    a. metal or plastic
    b. metal powder and an epoxy
    c. aluminum powder in an epoxy resin
    d. mixture of polymer and piezoceramic material

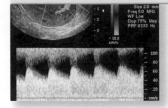

CHAPTER 4

Pulse-Echo Instrumentation

KEY TERMS

apodization nonuniform driving (excitation) of inner and outer elements in an array. Reduces grating lobes.

artifact anything not properly indicative of anatomy or motion imaged.

binary number group of bits typically expressed as 0 or 1.

bit binary digit; smallest amount of computer memory.

byte group of eight bits of computer memory.

channel an independent signal path consisting of a transducer element, delay, and other electronic components.

cine loop storage of the last several real-time frames.

code excitation a series of pulses and gaps allowing multiple focal zones and harmonic frequencies.

comet tail a series of closely spaced reverberation echoes behind a strong reflector.

dynamic range the ratio of the largest to the smallest amplitude that the ultrasound system can handle.

edge shadowing loss in intensity from bending of the sound beam at a curved surface.

enhancement the increase in reflection amplitude from structures that lie behind a weakly attenuating structure.

field of view displayed image of the returning echoes.

frame a complete scan of the ultrasound beam; individual image composed of multiple scan lines.

frame rate the number of complete scans (images) displayed per second.

freeze frame holding and displaying one frame of the real-time sequence.

gain ratio of amplifier output to input of electric power.

grating lobes secondary sound beams produced by a multielement transducer.

line density number of scan lines per frame; scan-line density.

matrix denotes the rows and columns of pixels in a digital image.

memory storage of echo information.

mirror image an artifactual gray-scale, color-flow, or Doppler signal appearing on the opposite side of a strong reflector.

multipath the path toward and away from a reflector are different.

noise disturbance that reduces the clarity of the signal.

Nyquist limit the minimum number of samples required to avoid aliasing; Doppler shift frequency above which aliasing occurs.

panoramic image an expanded image display beyond the normal limits of the transducer.

pixel picture element; smallest portion of a digital image.

pixel density number of picture elements per inch.

pixel interpolation assigning a brightness value to a missing pixel.

pulse inversion a harmonic imaging technique using two pulses per scan line where the second pulse is an inverse of the first pulse.

pulse repetition frequency (PRF) the number of voltage pulses sent to the transducer each second.

pulse repetition period (PRP) time from the beginning of one voltage pulse to the start of the next voltage pulse.

random-access memory (RAM) allows access of stored data in an unsystematic order.

range ambiguity produced when echoes are placed too superficially because a second pulse was emitted before all reflections have returned from the first pulse.

read-only memory (ROM) stored data that cannot be modified.

real-time imaging two-dimensional imaging of the motion of moving structures.

receiver receives, amplifies, and modifies echo information returning from the transducer. Parts of the receiver are incorporated into the reception side of the beam-former and the signal processor.

reflection portion of the sound reflected from the boundary of a medium.

refraction change of sound direction on passing from one medium to another.

reverberation multiple reflections between a structure and the transducer or within a structure.

scattering redirection of sound in several directions on encountering a rough surface.

shadowing reduction of reflective amplitude from reflectors that lie behind a strongly reflecting or attenuating structure.

signal-to-noise ratio comparison of meaningful information in an image (signal) to the amount of signal disturbance (noise).

spatial compounding averaging of frames that view anatomy from different angles.

specular large, flat, smooth surface.

subdicing dividing each element into small pieces and tying them together electronically so they function as one element. Reduces grating lobes.

voxel the smallest distinguishable part of a three-dimensional image; picture element with length, width, and thickness.

DISPLAY MODES

A-Mode

- Amplitude mode.
- One-dimensional (1-D) quantitative image using a single sound beam.
- Displays vertically the amplitude of the returning echo (y-axis), and distance is along the horizontal axis (x-axis).
- Best mode for precise measurements.

B-Mode

- Brightness mode.
- Creates a 2-D qualitative, cross-sectional image using multiple sound beams.
- Displays the strength of the returning echoes as pixels in various shades of gray.
- The vertical or the y-axis represents increasing depth and the horizontal or the x-axis represents the side-to-side or superior-to-inferior aspects of the body.
- The stronger the reflection, the brighter the pixel.

M-Mode

- Motion mode.
- 1-D quantitative series of B-mode pixels.
- The vertical or the y-axis represents reflector depth and demonstrates motion of the reflecting echoes, and the horizontal or the x-axis represents time.
- Used to document and evaluate the motion pattern of moving structures.

Volumetric Scanning

- 3-D mode demonstrates length, width, and thickness.
- 2-D display of a 3-D volume of echo information.
- Slower acquisition of information.
- Presentation of 3-D data includes surface rendering, 2-D slices through a 3-D volume, and transparent views.

REAL-TIME IMAGING

- Consists of frames or pictures displayed in rapid sequence creating the impression of constant motion of anatomy.
- Multiple frames per second make up multiple scan lines per frame.
- Imaging depth determines when the next pulse is transmitted.
- Echo brightness increases with echo amplitude.
- Echo position is determined by the round-trip time of the reflector.

Advantages

- Rapid location of anatomy.
- Movement can be observed.
- Structures or vessels can be followed.

Limitations

- Penetration depth is limited by the propagation speed of the medium.
- Exact imaging plane cannot be systematically reproduced.
- Measurement of structures larger than the field of view is estimated.

Real-Time Parameters

PARAMETER	DESCRIPTION	UNITS	RELATIONSHIP
Field of view	Size of the displayed image	N/A	Directly related to the pulse repetition frequency (PRF) Inversely related to frame rate and temporal resolution Operator-adjustable using depth and region-of-interest settings
Frame rate	Number of images per s Typically, 30-60 frames/s are used in real-time imaging Human eye detects fewer than 15-20 frames/s	Hz Frames/s	Determines temporal resolution Determined by the propagation speed of the medium and imaging depth Proportional to the PRF Inversely proportional to the number of focal zones used, imaging depth, and lines per frame (beam width) Operator adjustable using depth and PRF settings
Line density	Number of scan lines within the field of view	Lines/cm Lines/degrees	Directly related to PRF, image width, and spatial resolution Inversely related to the frame rate and temporal resolution
Maximum imaging depth	Maximum penetration depth for the overall parameters used	cm	Dependent on the frame rate, number of lines per frame, and the number of focal zones used Inversely related to the PRF
Pulse repetition frequency	Determines the number of scan lines per frame Equal to the voltage PRF	Hz kHz	Inversely related to the operating frequency and imaging depth Indirectly adjusted by the operator using imaging depth setting

Real-Time Imaging Techniques

TYPE	DESCRIPTION
Coded excitation	Mathematical technique designed for production of higher quality images Uses a series of pulses and gaps rather than a single driving pulse (occurs in the pulser) Ensembles of pulses drive the transducer to generate a single scan line Separates harmonic bandwidth from transmitted pulse bandwidth Allows for multiple focal zones Reduces speckle, frame rate, and temporal resolution Improves contrast, spatial, and axial resolution
Extended field of view (panoramic)	Expansion of the image display beyond the normal limits of the transducer diameter Manual sliding of the transducer parallel to the scan plane Retains previous echo information while adding new echo information parallel to the scanning plane
Four-dimensional imaging	Real-time presentation of a three-dimensional image Fourth dimension of time is combined with rapidly acquired volumetric data
Frequency compounding	Technique used to reduce noise and speckle Separates the received radiofrequencies into subbands Each subband creates an image that are combined into one assimilated image being created with different frequency transducers
Harmonic frequencies (MHz)	Even and odd multiples of the fundamental frequency Generated at a deeper imaging depth reducing reverberation artifact Generated in the highest intensity and narrowest portion of the beam Returning harmonic signals are processed separate from the operating signals Improves lateral resolution Reduces grating lobes and contrast resolution
Multifocal imaging	Ability to use multiple focal zones during real-time imaging Directly related to lateral resolution and pulse repetition frequency Inversely related to the frame rate and temporal resolution
Pixel interpolation	Assigns a brightness value to missed pixels Based on the average brightness of adjacent pixels Commonly used in sector scanning
Presets	Setup of grayscale, depth, and Doppler imaging controls to examination to be performed

Continued

Real-Time Imaging Techniques—(cont'd)

TYPE	DESCRIPTION
Pulse inversion	A technique in harmonic imaging using two pulses per scan, where the second pulse is the inversion of the first pulse Allows for a broader bandwidth and shorter pulses Improves axial resolution Reduces temporal resolution
Spatial compounding	Scan lines are directed in multiple directions Uses phasing to interrogate the structures more than once by the ultrasound beam Improves visualization of structures beneath a highly attenuating structure Smooths specular surfaces Reduces speckle and noise
Volume imaging	Acquired by assembling many parallel 2-D scans into a 3-D volume of echo information Acquired at rates of up to 30 volumes per s Obtained by: 1. Manual scanning with transducer position sensors 2. Automated mechanical scanned transducers 3. Electronic scanning with a 2-D element array transducer

PULSE-ECHO INSTRUMENTATION

Functions

1. Prepare and transmit electronic signals to the transducer to produce a sound wave.
2. Receive electronic signals from reflections.
3. Process the reflected information for display.
4. Produce audio signals from reflections.

POWER (Output)

- Controls the amplitude of transmitted sound beam and the amplitude of the received echoes.
- Directly related to the signal-to-noise ratio.
- Directly related to the intensity of acoustic exposure to the patient.
- Acoustic exposure is measured by mechanical index (MI) and thermal index (TI).
- May be shown as a percentage on the ultrasound display.

TRANSDUCER

- Produces ultrasound pulses for each electrical pulse applied.
- Receives returning echo reflections, producing an electrical voltage.
- Delivers electrical voltages to the memory.
- Generates a small voltage signal (radio frequency) proportional to the amplitude of the returning echo.
- Radio frequency signals are processed by the system.
- Preamplification can occur.

Channels

- An independent signal path consisting of a transducer element, delay, and possibly other electronic components.
- An increase in the number of channels equal to the number of transducer elements allows more precise control of the beam characteristics.

- Controlling the characteristics of the sound beam is directly related to the number of channels employed.
- In ultrasound, typically 64, 128, or 192 channels are used.
- Each independent pulse delay and element combination constitutes a transmission channel.
- Each independent element, amplifier, digitizer, and delay path constitutes a reception channel.

MASTER SYNCHRONIZER

- Brain or manager of the ultrasound system.
- Coordinates all components of the ultrasound system.
- Clock that instructs the pulser to send an electrical signal to the transducer.

BEAMFORMER

- Where the action originates,
- Consists of a pulser, pulse delays, transmit/receive (T/R) switch, amplifiers, digitizer, echo delays, and a summer.
- Functions:
  - Generate voltages that drive the transducer.
  - Determine PRF, coding, frequency, and intensity.
  - Scanning, focusing, and apodizing the transmitted beam.
  - Amplify the returning echo voltages.
  - Compensate for attenuation.
  - Digitize the echo voltage stream.
  - Directing, focusing, and apodizing the reception beam.
  - Determines the firing sequence, delay patterns, and delays during reception.
  - Controls electronic steering and focusing in array transducers.
- Advantages: software programming and extremely stable with a wide range of frequencies.

PULSER (Transmitter)

- Generates the electric pulses to the crystal producing pulsed ultrasound waves.
- In response, the transducer produces ultrasound pulses that travel into the patient (medium).
- Determines the pulse repetition frequency, pulse repetition period, and pulse amplitude.
- Drives the transducer through the pulse delays with one voltage pulse per scan line.
- Adjusts the PRF appropriately for imaging depth. Adjust the PRF appropriately for imaging depth (achieves the highest possible PRF while avoiding echo misplacement).
- Communicates with the signal processor the moment the crystal is excited to help determine the distance to the reflector.

Pulse Delays

- Allows electronic control of beam scanning, steering, transmission focusing, aperture, and apodization.
- Controls the size of the element and apodization in phased array operation.

Transmit and Receiver Switch (T/R Switch)

- Directs the driving voltages from the pulser and pulse delays to the transducer during transmission.
- Directs the returning echo voltages from the transducer to the amplifiers during reception.
- Protects the amplifier components from the large driving voltages of the pulse.

Amplifiers

- Units—dB.
- Increases small electric voltages received from the transducer to compensate for the loss of echo strength caused by the depth of the reflector.
- Attenuation and maximum amplifier gain determine maximum imaging depth.

Overall Gain

- Allows identical amplification no matter the depth.
- Operator adjustable using overall gain setting (adjusts entire image).
- Does NOT improve the signal-to-noise ratio.
- Typically, 60 to 100 dB of gain is available.

Time Gain Compensation (Fig. 4.1)

- Compensates for attenuation by boosting amplitudes of deep reflections and suppressing superficial reflections.
- Operator adjustable using time gain compensation or depth gain compensation centimeter division slide controls (adjusts variable depths of the image).
- Provides equal amplitude for all similar structures regardless of depth.
- Compensate for approximately 60 dB of attenuation.

Time Gain Compensation Curve (Fig. 4.1)

- Near field—area of minimum amplification.
- Delay—depth at which variable compensation begins.
- Slope—available region for depth compensation.
- Knee—deepest region attenuation compensation can occur.
- Far field—area of maximum amplification.

Lateral Gain Compensation

- Allows adjustment of gain laterally across the image.

Digitizer

- Analog-to-digital converter changes the analog voltages representing echoes to numbers for digital signal processing and storage.
- Further mathematical manipulation of the echoes is accomplished as digital signal processing.

Echo delays

- After amplification and digitizing the echo voltages pass through digital delay lines to accomplish reception dynamic focused steering functions.

FIG. 4.1
Time gain compensation curve.

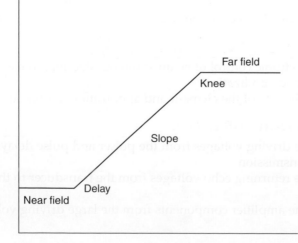

Summer (Adder)

- Adds the delayed channel signals together to produce the resulting scan lines that will be displayed after signal and image processing.
- Reception apodization and dynamic aperture functions are accomplished by the summing process.

SIGNAL PROCESSOR

- Receives the stream of echoes returning from each transmitted pulse.
- Operations include:
  - Digital filtering—bandpass.
  - Detection—amplitude.
  - Compression—dynamic range reduction.
- Filtering is usually done first followed by detection and compression in any order.

Filtering

- Amplifiers with a bandpass filter (tuned amplifiers) are used to reduce noise in the electronics.
- Bandpass filter rejects those frequencies above and below the accepted bandwidth while retaining those that are most useful in a given situation.

Detection

- Aka—demodulation.
- Conversion of echo voltages from radio frequency form to video form.
- Video form retains amplitudes of the echo voltages.
- Not operator controlled.

Compression

- Units—dB.
- Ratio of the largest to smallest amplitude or power that a system can handle.
- Changes the gray-scale characteristics of an image without losing the relationship between the largest and smallest amplitudes.
- Operator adjustable using the dynamic range or compression settings.
- Narrow or smaller dynamic range settings present a high-contrast image.
- Ultrasound amplifier uses a compression range of 100 to 120 dB.
- Echo dynamic range remaining after compensation is typically 50 to 100 dB.
- Imaging monitors display a compression range up to 30 dB.
- Human eye can appreciate approximately 20 dB.

IMAGE PROCESSOR

- Converts the digitized, filtered, and compressed serial scan line data into images that are stored in an image memory.
- Formats echo data into image form for image processing, storage, and display.
- Properly locates each series of echoes (depth) in individual scan lines for storage.
- Accomplished in a fraction of a second yielding one frame of information.
- Rapid sequence presentation of these frames yields real-time scanning.
- Three-dimensional images are acquired by assembling several two-dimensional scans into a 3-D volume of echo information in the image memory.
- Real-time presentation of 3-D images is called 4-D imaging.
- Functions include:
  - Preprocessing.
  - Persistence.
  - 3-D acquisition.
  - Storing image frames.
  - Cine loop.

- Postprocessing.
- Gray scale.
- Color scale.
- 3-D presentation.
- Digital-to-analog conversion.

Preprocessing

- Processes a signal or image before storing in memory.
- Operator adjustable.
- Accentuates boundaries.
- Examples of preprocessing include time gain compensation, dynamic range, write magnification, region of interest/expansion, persistence, pixel interpolation, spatial compounding, panoramic imaging, and 3-D acquisition.

Edge Enhancement

- Change in signal level along a particular scan line.
- Enhances boundaries.

Persistence

- Frame averaging.
- Reduces speckle and smoothes the image.
- Lower levels for following rapidly moving structures.
- Higher levels for slowly moving structures.

Region of Interest/Expansion

- Condenses the scan lines into a smaller image area.
- Increases detail resolution.

Write Magnification

- Rescans only in the area of interest.
- Acquires new data.
- Increases the number of pixels or scan lines.
- Improves spatial resolution.

Postprocessing (Contrast Variation)

- Assignments of display brightness before or after data are stored in memory.
- Examples of postprocessing include read magnification, measurement calipers, B-color, and 3-D presentation.
- Time gain compensation and overall gain may also be examples of postprocessing in modern ultrasound systems.

B-Color

- Presentation of different echo intensities in various colors.
- Improves contrast resolution.

Volume Presentation

- Surface rendering—popular in obstetrical imaging.
- 2-D slices through a 3-D volume—image plane orientation can be presented.
- Transparent views—allow a see-through image of anatomy similar to an x-ray film.

Read Magnification

- Displays only the original data.
- Number of pixels or scan lines is the same as in the original image.

IMAGE MEMORY

- Computer memory stores the echo amplitude and location in a binary (digital) format.
- Memory divides the image into numerous pixels (squares).
- Holding and displaying one frame out of the sequence is termed *freeze frame.*
- Holding and displaying the last several frames acquired before freezing is called cine loop, cine review, or image review feature.

Random-Access Memory (RAM)

- Stores echo amplitude and location.
- Information stored will be lost if the power is switched off.

Read-Only Memory (ROM)

- Data cannot be modified.

Bit

- Binary digit.
- Smallest amount of computer memory.
- Two levels of storage: 0 = Off; 1 = On.
- Determines the number of gray shades.
- Number of memory bits = 2^n shades of gray.
- 3-bit memory = $2^3 = 2 \times 2 \times 2 = 8$ shades of gray.
- 5-bit memory = 2^5 (to the 5th power) $2 \times 2 \times 2 \times 2 \times 2 = 32$ shades of gray.
- Multiple-bit memories allow for numerous shades of gray.
- Ultrasound systems typically employ 6-bit to 8-bit memories.

Binary Numbers

- Binary numbers in digital systems determine the number of gray shades.
- Off = 0; On = 1.

Shades of Gray Using Binary Numbers

BINARY NUMBER	64	32	16	8	4	2	1	DECIMAL NUMBER
0100101 =	0	1	0	0	1	0	1	= 32 + 4 + 1 = 37
1010010 =	1	0	1	0	0	1	0	= 64 + 16 + 2 = 82

DIGITAL-TO-ANALOG CONVERTER

- Converts the digital data received from the memory to analog voltages for display.
- Determines the brightness of the echoes on the display.

IMAGE DISPLAY

- Receives electrical impulses and translates them into a picture display.
- Each image is divided into multiple small squares similar to a checkerboard-termed matrix.
- Each square of the matrix is assigned either a number 0 = Off or 1 = On.
- The greater the number of rows and columns, the better the spatial resolution.

Pixel

- Smallest visible picture element of a display.
- Each pixel stores one shade of gray.

Pixel Density

- Number of picture elements per inch.
- Directly related to spatial and detail resolution.
- Inversely related to pixel size.

Voxel

- Smallest visible picture element of a three-dimensional display.
- Store length, width, and thickness.

LIQUID-CRYSTAL DISPLAY (LCD)

- Flat-panel display
- Thin, flat display device made up of any number of color or monochrome pixels arranged in front of a light source or reflector.
- Computer displays present image information in the form of horizontal lines from top to bottom and row by row (like reading a book).
- By controlling the voltage applied across the liquid-crystal layer in each pixel, light may pass through in varying amounts, forming different levels of gray.
- Generally, displayed in a 1024×768 rectangular matrix.

RECORDING TECHNIQUES

Hard Copy Imaging

X-ray Film

- Single emulsion x-ray film.
- Cellulose acetate sheet coated with a gelatin emulsion that contains silver bromide crystals.
- After exposure to light from the monitor, the film is chemically developed.

Thermal Processors

- Use of a paper medium to record the image.
- Small heat elements create the image.
- Decreased resolution and gray scale.
- Less stable than an x-ray film.
- Color thermal printers contain a ribbon of color inks.
- Colors include cyan, magenta, yellow, and black.

Laser Imaging

- Automated film handling and developing.
- 15 or more images per sheet of film.
- Higher resolution, better gray scale with less distortion.

Digital Recording Device

- Stores images on computer disks or memory.
- Allows viewing on monitors and film transfer.

ARCHIVE STORAGE

Magnetic-Optical Disk

- Safely stores information on an optical disk.
- Not susceptible to magnetic fields.
- Disk can be rewritten and erased.

Picture Archiving and Communication System (PACS)

- Also known as digital imaging network (DIN), information management archiving and communication stations (IMACS).
- Electronically communicates images and associated information to workstations external from the ultrasound system.
- Acquisition, display, hard copy, and computer components are interconnected using a local area network (LAN).
- Allows virtual access to archived studies of multiple imaging modalities.
- Ultrasound data are digitized and transferred to the network.
- Data do not deteriorate with passage of time.

STANDARDS FOR ARCHIVING MEDICAL FILES

American College of Radiology (ACR)

- Develops standards for encoding patient file information and interpretation.

Digital Imaging and Communications in Medicine (DICOM)

- Standardizes protocols for communicating image systems.
- Allows image interrogation by a wide variety of devices geographically.

National Electrical Manufacturers Association (NEMA)

- Develops standards for encoding patient file information and interpretation.

ARTIFACTS OF ULTRASOUND

- Incorrect representation of anatomy or function.
- An apparent echo for which distance, direction, or amplitude do not correspond to a real target.
- Include reflections that are not real, missing, improperly positioned, or of improper brightness, shape, or size.
- When corrective measures are taken, artifacts typically disappear.

Caused By

1. Ultrasound system assumptions.
2. Operator error.
3. Physics of ultrasound.
4. Equipment malfunction.
5. Improper use of equipment.

Assumptions in the Design of Ultrasound Systems

1. Image plane is thin.
2. Sound only travels in a straight line.
3. Echoes originate only from objects on the central axis.
4. Distance to a reflector is proportional to the time it takes for an echo to return.
5. Intensity of an echo corresponds to the strength of a reflector.
6. Sound travels directly to and from a reflector.
7. Sound travels in soft tissue at exactly 1.54 mm/μs.

Sonographic Artifacts

Propagation Group
- Comet tail
- Grating lobe
- Mirror image
- Range ambiguity
- Refraction
- Reverberation
- Ring-down
- Slice (section) thickness
- Speckle
- Speed error

Attenuation Group
- Enhancement
- Focal enhancement
- Refraction (edge) shadowing
- Shadowing

From Kremkau FW: *Sonography: principles and instruments*, ed 9, Philadelphia, 2016, Saunders/Elsevier.

Imaging Artifacts

ARTIFACT	DEFINITION	CAUSE	MANIFESTATION
Acoustic speckle	Low-intensity sound waves interfering with each other Constructive interference—echoes reinforce each other Destructive interference—echoes completely or partially cancel each other Instrument design may have a form of speckle reduction (e.g., SonoCT).	Interference of echoes from the distribution of scatterers in tissue Not a true artifact	Added objects Grainy image Interferes with the ability to detect low-contrast objects
Comet tail	Dense, tapering trail of echoes just distal to a strong reflector Located parallel to the sound beam	Reverberation Caused by two closely spaced strong reflectors in soft tissue Foreign body, calcium, or air	Added objects Appears as multiple small echogenic bands
Duplication	Redirection of the sound beam, passing through the medial edges of the abdominis rectus muscle	Refraction Unique to the abdominus rectus muscle	Added objects Incorrect object size
Edge shadowing	Redirection of the sound beam at the edge of round or oval structures Beam hits the edge of a structure larger than the beam width	Refraction Interference	Incorrect object brightness Missed objects
Enhancement	Increased brightness behind a weakly attenuating structure Sound beam passes through an area of low attenuation Reduced with spatial compounding Increased with increase in transducer frequency	Attenuation	Incorrect object brightness
Focal banding	Product of horizontal enhancement or banding at focal zone(s) Reduced by reducing number of focal zones and smoothing out the TGC curve.	Increase in the intensity of the sound beam in the focal zone(s)	Improper brightness
Grating lobes	Minor secondary (weaker) sound beams of an array transducer traveling in different directions than the primary beam Reduced by subdicing and apodization	Spacing of the active elements	Incorrect object location Duplicates structures lateral to the real structures

Imaging Artifacts —(cont'd)

ARTIFACT	DEFINITION	CAUSE	MANIFESTATION
Mirror image	Objects on one side of a strong reflector are duplicated on the other side of the reflector True and false images are equidistant from the strong reflector False image is placed deeper Reduced by decreasing gain settings and using a different acoustic window	Multiple reflections Diaphragm, pleura, and bowel Form of reverberation	Added objects
Multipath	Paths toward and away from the reflector are different Beam strikes an interface at an angle and is reflected from a second interface back toward the transducer	Reflection	Incorrect object location Improper brightness Degrades image quality and axial resolution
Propagation speed error	Reflectors appear in correct number but at improper locations Slow speeds place reflectors too deep	Speed error	Incorrect object location Displaces structures axially Incorrect object shape
Range ambiguity	All echoes are not received before the next pulse is emitted Reduced by decreasing imaging depth and PRF	Pulse repetition frequency is too high	Incorrect object location (closer than should be) Reduced frame rate
Refraction	Change in direction of the sound beam from one medium to the next	Bending of the transmitted beam Sound wave strikes a boundary at an oblique angle	Displaces structures laterally Incorrect object size Incorrect object shape Degrades lateral resolution
Resolution	Failure to distinguish two separate adjacent objects	Beam (pulse) width Spatial pulse length	Missing object Incorrect object size or shape
Reverberation	Equally spaced reflections of diminishing amplitude with increased imaging depth Two or more strong reflectors are encountered in the sound path; multiple reflections will occur More reflections than actually exist Reduced with harmonic imaging and decreasing gain settings	Multiple reflections between a structure and the transducer, between structures, or within a structure Created when a sound wave bounces back and forth between two strong reflectors	Added objects Appears in multiples Located parallel to the sound beam
Ring down	Appears as a series of parallel bands or a solid streak behind a reflector	Reverberation Resonance phenomenon associated with a gas bubble	Added objects
Shadowing	Reduction in reflection brightness from reflectors that lie behind a strongly attenuating structure or from the edges of reflecting structures Reduced with spatial compounding Increased with increase in transducer frequency	Attenuation Refraction	Incorrect object brightness
Side lobes	Minor secondary sound beams of a single-element transducer traveling in directions different from the primary beam	Transducer element changing thickness	Incorrect object location
Slice or section thickness Aka: Partial volume	Thickness of the scanned tissue volume Determined by the thickness of the imaging plane Imaging plane is not thin or uniform in thickness Reduced by harmonic imaging	Beam (pulse) width perpendicular to the scan plane is greater than the reflector's	Added objects True reflector lies lateral to the assumed imaging plane

Sonographic Terminology

Anechoic: without internal echoes

Echogenic: producing echoes of varying intensity

Heterogeneous: term used to describe a mixed echo texture

Homogeneous: term used to describe a uniform echo texture

Hyperechoic: comparative term used to describe an increase in echogenicity compared with another structure or the normal expected echo pattern of a structure

Hypoechoic: comparative term used to describe a decrease in echogenicity compared with another structure or the normal expected echo pattern of a structure

Isoechoic: echo texture equal to the surrounding structures

PULSE-ECHO INSTRUMENTATION REVIEW

1. The motion of moving structures in a 2-D image display describes:
   a. motion mode
   b. amplitude mode
   c. real-time imaging
   d. temporal resolution

2. In a brightness-mode display, the y-axis represents the:
   a. penetration depth
   b. compensation slope
   c. amplitude of the reflector
   d. right or left aspect of the body

3. The number of images per second defines the:
   a. frame rate
   b. line density
   c. pulse repetition period
   d. pulse repetition frequency

4. The frame rate in real-time imaging can be modified by adjusting the:
   a. output power
   b. dynamic range
   c. amplification
   d. imaging depth

Using Figure 4.2, answer question 5.

5. Which of the following changes would improve this sagittal sonogram of the left upper quadrant?
   a. decrease overall gain and place focus deeper
   b. place focus higher and increase overall gain
   c. increase gain in near zone and imaging depth
   d. decrease imaging depth and place focus higher

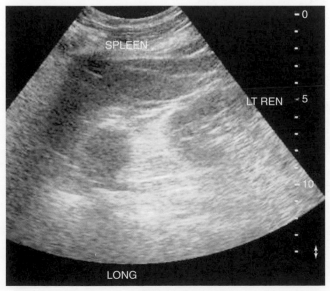

FIG. 4.2

6. Which of the following display modes demonstrates the strength of the reflections along the vertical axis?
   a. M-mode
   b. B-mode
   c. A-mode
   d. E-mode

7. Frame rate is determined by penetration depth and:
   a. temporal resolution
   b. operating frequency
   c. pulse repetition frequency
   d. propagation speed of the medium

8. If the line density is increased, which of the following is most likely to occur?
   a. frame rate will decrease
   b. spatial resolution will decrease
   c. temporal resolution will increase
   d. pulse repetition frequency will decrease

9. Propagation speed of a medium limits which of the following?
   a. penetration depth
   b. pixel interpolation
   c. harmonic frequencies
   d. spatial compounding

10. Which of the following is a function of the image processor?
    a. filtering
    b. detection
    c. persistence
    d. compression

11. Which of the following is a propagation speed artifact?
    a. shadowing
    b. focal banding
    c. edge shadowing
    d. mirror image

12. Which of the following is directly related to pulse repetition frequency?
    a. line density
    b. imaging depth
    c. spatial resolution
    d. operating frequency

13. Increasing the amplitude of the sound beam by 3 dB will:
    a. quadruple the acoustic intensity
    b. increase the signal-to-noise ratio
    c. increase the pulse repetition frequency
    d. increase the frequency of the transducer

14. Which of the following describes a function of the T/R switch?
    a. delivers electric voltage to the memory
    b. generates electric pulses to the crystal
    c. protects the amplifier components from the pulse voltage
    d. adjusts the pulse repetition frequency with imaging depth

15. Subdicing the elements in diagnostic ultrasound transducers is used to:
    a. reduce grating lobes
    b. narrow the bandwidth
    c. increase temporal resolution
    d. increase the near-zone length

Using Figure 4.3, answer question 16.

16. Which of the following imaging artifacts is demonstrated in this sonogram?
    a. focal banding
    b. range ambiguity
    c. mirror image
    d. slice thickness

17. Which of the following offsets for attenuation of the sound beam?
    a. filtering
    b. compression
    c. demodulation
    d. compensation

18. Which of the following describes a function of the transducer?
    a. delivers acoustic voltages to the display
    b. delivers electrical voltages to the memory
    c. controls the amplitude of the received signals
    d. adjusts the pulse repetition frequency for imaging depth

19. The knee of a time gain compensation curve represents the:
    a. area of minimum amplification
    b. area of maximum amplification
    c. depth at which variable compensation begins
    d. deepest region attenuation compensation can occur

20. Which component of the ultrasound system adjusts the pulse repetition frequency with changes in imaging depth?
    a. pulser
    b. T/R switch
    c. digitizer
    d. amplifier

21. The transmit and receiver switch is part of which of the following instruments?
    a. pulser
    b. digitizer
    c. beam former
    d. signal processor

22. Which of the following constitutes a transmission channel?
    a. an electrical voltage and an element
    b. an electrical voltage and firing delay
    c. a delay path and an individual element
    d. an independent pulse delay and an element

Using Figure 4.4, answer question 23.

23. The sonogram demonstrates which of the following artifacts?
    a. focal banding and edge shadowing
    b. acoustic speckle and duplication
    c. ringdown and posterior enhancement
    d. mirror image and posterior shadowing

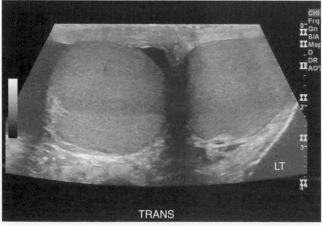

TRANS

FIG. 4.3

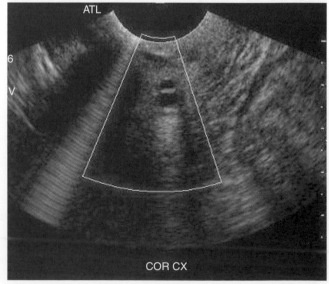

COR CX

FIG. 4.4

24. Slice thickness artifact may be reduced with:
    a. multifocal imaging
    b. harmonic imaging
    c. spatial compounding
    d. pixel interpolation

25. Which of the following allows for multiple focal zones and harmonic frequencies?
    a. channeling
    b. code excitation
    c. dynamic focusing
    d. constructive interference

26. Which of the following is a postprocessing feature?
    a. cine loop
    b. persistence
    c. write magnification
    d. 3-D acquisition

27. The binary number 0110010 corresponds to a decimal number of:
    a. 25
    b. 50
    c. 74
    d. 100

28. How many shades of gray are in a 6-bit memory?
    a. 32
    b. 48
    c. 64
    d. 96

29. What is the term used to describe a volume picture element?
    a. bit
    b. byte
    c. pixel
    d. voxel

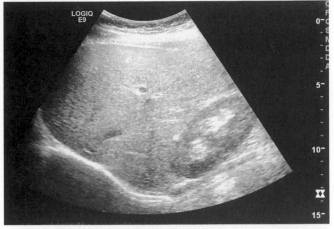

FIG. 4.5

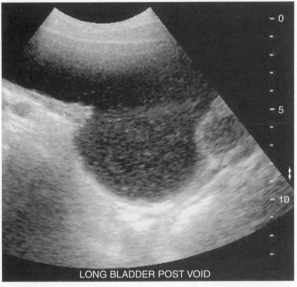

LONG BLADDER POST VOID

FIG. 4.6

Using Figure 4.5, answer question 30.

30. Which of the following modifications would improve this image?
    a. placing focus higher
    b. decreasing imaging depth
    c. decreasing overall gain
    d. decreasing transducer frequency

Using Figure 4.6, answer question 31.

31. Which of the following real-time imaging techniques is the most likely to improve this image of the urinary bladder?
    a. harmonic imaging
    b. pixel interpolation
    c. spatial compounding
    d. extended field of view

32. Which of the following is a characteristic of read magnification ?
    a. acquires new data
    b. displays only original data
    c. improves spatial resolution
    d. rescans only in the area of interest

33. An increase in echogenicity compared with an adjacent structure is termed:
    a. isoechoic
    b. heterogeneous
    c. hypoechoic
    d. hyperechoic

34. Which of the following is most likely related to pixel density?
    a. log compression
    b. spatial resolution
    c. lateral resolution
    d. temporal resolution

35. Storage of several preceding real-time frames describes:
    a. cine loop
    b. freeze frame
    c. video imaging
    d. frame averaging

36. Which of the following best describes a digital matrix?
    a. storage of picture elements
    b. smallest amount of computer memory
    c. number of picture elements in a digital image
    d. rows and columns of picture elements in a digital image

37. Which of the following improves contrast resolution?
    a. rejection
    b. B-color
    c. persistence
    d. compensation

38. Which of the following components increases the number of scan lines?
    a. read magnification
    b. B-color
    c. persistence
    d. write magnification

39. Which of the following artifacts improperly displays a true reflector's location?
    a. mirror image
    b. reverberation
    c. focal banding
    d. range ambiguity

40. When the Doppler gain setting is too high, which of the following artifacts is most likely to occur?
    a. aliasing
    b. mirror image
    c. range ambiguity
    d. acoustic speckle

41. Which of the following decreases the likelihood of range ambiguity artifact?
    a. perpendicular incidence
    b. decreasing the receiver gain
    c. decreasing the operating frequency
    d. decreasing the pulse repetition frequency

42. The design of ultrasound systems assumes:
    a. the thickness of the imaging plane is uniform
    b. sound travels at variable speeds in soft tissue
    c. sound travels directly to and from a reflector
    d. secondary beams travel lateral to the primary beam

43. Weakening of echoes distal to a strongly attenuating structure describes:
    a. refraction
    b. ring-down
    c. shadowing
    d. enhancement

Using Figure 4.7, answer question 44.

44. Which of the following adjustments will improve this image of the upper abdomen?
    a. increase overall gain
    b. decrease imaging depth
    c. increase gain in the far field
    d. increase gain in the near field

45. Enhancement of echo reflections occur distal to a:
    a. nonspecular reflector
    b. strongly reflecting structure
    c. weakly attenuating structure
    d. structure of high impedance

46. A change in direction of the ultrasound beam is more commonly a result of:
    a. the resonance phenomenon
    b. interference from multiple scatterers
    c. striking a boundary at an oblique angle
    d. secondary sound beams emitted from a phased array

47. Spaces between the active elements of a phased array transducer result in:
    a. multipath reflections
    b. the production of side lobes
    c. enhancement in the focal zone
    d. the production of grating lobes

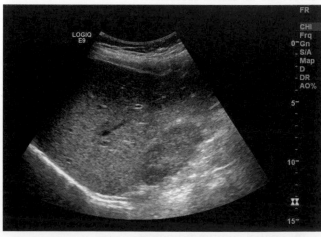

FIG. 4.7

48. The distance to a reflector is determined by the:
   a. intensity of the returning echo
   b. thickness of the imaging plane
   c. time it takes for an echo to return
   d. propagation speed of the medium

49. A surgical clip will most likely demonstrate which of the following artifacts?
   a. refraction
   b. multipath
   c. comet tail
   d. acoustic speckle

50. Shadowing and enhancement are a result of which type of imaging artifacts?
   a. reflection
   b. refraction
   c. attenuation
   d. propagation speed error

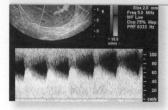

CHAPTER 5

Doppler Instrumentation and Hemodynamics

KEY TERMS

aliasing a misrepresentation of the Doppler shift in a negative direction occurring when the pulse repetition frequency is set too low; most common Doppler artifact.

arterioles smallest arteries in the circulatory system controlling the needs of organs and tissues.

Bernoulli effect pressure reduction in a region of high flow speed.

bruit auscultatory sound within an artery produced by turbulent blood flow.

capillaries the smallest of the body's blood vessels connecting the arterioles and venules and allowing the interchange of oxygen or carbon dioxide and nutrients to the tissue cells.

clutter noise in the Doppler signal caused by high-amplitude Doppler shifts.

Doppler effect observed frequency change of the reflected sound resulting from movement relative to the sound source or observer.

Doppler shift frequency shift created between the transmitted frequency and received frequency by an interface moving with velocity at an angle to the sound.

energy gradient energy difference between two points.

flow to move in a stream, continually changing position and direction.

gate electronic device controlling the transmission or reception of a Doppler signal; size of the gate is determined by the beam diameter, gate length, and emitted pulse.

helical flow twisting type of blood flow.

hemodynamics science or physical principles concerned with the study of blood circulation.

hue color map the perceived color; any one or a combination of primary colors.

hydrostatic pressure the pressure created in a fluid system, such as the circulatory system; when supine, the hydrostatic pressure is 0 mm Hg. When upright, the pressure is negative above the heart and positive below the heart.

incompetency weak or not properly performing valves allowing retrograde flow.

inertia the resistance to acceleration.

microcirculation consists of the arterioles, capillaries, and venules.

Nyquist limit the highest frequency in a sampled signal represented unambiguously; equal to one half the pulse repetition frequency.

packet positioning of multiple pulsed Doppler gates over the area of interest.

peak velocity maximum velocity at any given time.

plug flow speed is constant across the vessel.

Poiseuille's equation predicts volume flow in a cylindrical vessel.

pressure gradient difference in pressure required for flow to occur.

pulsatility index a parameter used to convey the pulsatility of a time-varying waveform.

Reynolds number predicts the onset of turbulent flow.

resistive index difference between the maximum and minimum Doppler frequency shifts divided by the maximum Doppler frequency shift; also known as Pourcelot index.

sample gate electronic device controlling the transmission or reception of a Doppler signal; size of the gate is determined by the beam diameter, gate length, and emitted pulse; sample volume.

saturation color map degree to which the original color is diluted with white; the paler the color (or the less saturated it is), the faster the flow velocity; the purer the color, the slower the flow velocity.

spectral broadening a vertical thickening of the spectral trace resulting from an increase range of Doppler shift frequencies; usually seen with turbulent flow.

stenosis a narrowing in the lumen of a vessel.

stroke volume amount of blood moving in a forward direction; blood being ejected.

Valsalva maneuver deep inspiration followed by bearing down results in abrupt cessation of venous blood flow in large to medium-sized veins.

variance mode the average velocity is calculated, with the colors placed side-to-side.

velocity rate of motion with respect to time; speed at which red blood cells are traveling in a particular direction.

velocity mode all measured velocities for each gate are averaged, then the colors are arranged up and down.

venules the smallest veins that receive blood from the capillaries and drain into larger-caliber veins.

volume flow rate the quantity of blood moving through the vessel per unit of time.

HEMODYNAMICS

- Force and motion of blood flow.
- A difference in pressure (pressure gradient) is required for flow to occur.
- Pressure difference can be generated by the heart or gravity.
- Blood flows from the higher pressure to the lower pressure.
- Equal pressure at both ends will result in no flow.
- The greater the pressure difference, the greater the volume of blood flow.

Cardiac Circulation

- Deoxygenated blood flows from the superior and inferior vena cava into the right atrium.
- From the right atrium, blood courses through the tricuspid valve to the right ventricle.
- Blood flows into the lungs through the pulmonary arteries from the right ventricle.
- Oxygenated blood flows into the left atrium through the pulmonary veins.
- Blood continues to flow through the mitral valve into the left ventricle.
- From the left ventricle, blood is pumped into the aorta and systemic circulation.
- Microcirculation consists of arterioles, capillaries, and venules.
- Valves are present in the heart to permit forward flow and to prevent reverse flow.
- Peripheral resistance is a primary regulatory control on cardiac output.
- Vasodilation of the lower extremity arteries decreases resistance, increasing the flow to the limbs.
- Vasoconstriction of the lower extremity arteries increases resistance, decreasing the flow to the limbs.
- Malfunctioning valves can restrict forward flow (stenosis) or allow reverse flow by not closing completely (insufficiency or regurgitation).

Blood Flow Variables

CONTRIBUTING FACTORS	DESCRIPTION
Density	Mass per unit volume
Fluids	Substances that flow and conform to the shape of their containers Gases and liquid
Kinetic energy	Proportional to its density and velocity squared
Mass	Measure of an object's resistance to acceleration Directly related to the inertia and force to accelerate
Pressure	Force per unit area Driving force behind blood flow Directly related to the blood flow volume With each cardiac contraction, the blood is pressure-waved into the arteriole system and microcirculation Equally distributed throughout a static fluid and is forced in all directions
Pressure gradient	Pressure difference required for flow to occur Proportional to the flow rate
Resistance	The resistance of the arterioles accounts for about one half of the total resistance in the systemic system The muscular walls of the arterioles can constrict or relax, producing dramatic changes in flow resistance Directly related to the length of the vessel and fluid viscosity Inversely related to the vessel radius
Velocity	Speed at which red blood cells (RBCs) travel in a vessel Not constant or uniform across a vessel Dependent on the left-ventricular output, resistance of the arterioles, cross-sectional area, and course of the vessel
Viscosity	A fluid's ability to resist a change in shape or flow Resistance to flow offered by a fluid in motion Directly related to the number of RBCs (varies with blood flow speed) Blood is 5 times more viscous than water Units—Poise or kg/m-s

VOLUMETRIC FLOW RATE

Volume Flow Rate = Average flow speed across the vessel × cross-section area of vessel.
- Volume of blood passing a point per unit time.
- Expressed in millimeter per minute or second.
- Adult cardiac flows at a rate of 5000 mL/min.
- Determined by the pressure difference and the resistance to flow.
- Depends on the pressure difference, length and diameter of the tube, and viscosity of the fluid.
- Cardiac Output = stroke volume × heart rate.
- Stroke Volume (mL) = end diastolic volume *minus* end systolic volume.

Continuity Rule

- Volumetric flow rate must be constant, because blood is neither created nor destroyed as it flows through a vessel.
- The average flow speed in a stenosis must be greater than that proximal and distal to it so that the volumetric flow rate is constant throughout the vessel.
- Concerns a short portion of a vessel.

Poiseuille's Equation

$$\text{Volume flow rate} = \frac{\text{Change in pressure} \times \pi \times \text{Vessel radius}^4}{8 \times \text{Viscosity of blood} \times \text{Length of the vessel}}$$

DEFINITION	RELATIONSHIP
Predicts flow volume in a long, straight cylindrical vessel	Directly related to the pressure difference and the size or radius of the vessel
	Inversely related to the vessel length, resistance, and fluid viscosity
	Relates to a steady flow in a long unobstructed tube

Bernoulli Effect

Pressure drop = 4(velocity in the jet)

DEFINITION	RELATIONSHIP
Region of decreased pressure in an area of high flow speed	If flow speed increases, pressure energy decreases
Pressure decreases before a stenosis to allow the fluid to accelerate into the stenosis and decelerate out of it	Relates to short obstructed vessel

Reynold's Number

$$\text{Reynold's number} = \frac{\text{velocity} \times \text{density of fluid} \times 2 \text{ radius of the vessel}}{\text{viscosity}}$$

DEFINITION	RELATIONSHIP
Predicts the onset of turbulence	Reynold's number meets or exceeds 2000

TYPES OF BLOOD FLOW

- Blood flow is not uniform or constant through a specific vessel or throughout the body.
- The muscular walls of the arterioles can constrict or relax, controlling blood flow to specific tissues and organs according to their needs.
- Low-resistance (low pulsatility) waveforms demonstrate a slow, broad upstroke in systole and a large amount of forward flow in diastole (e.g., internal carotid artery).
- High-resistance (high pulsatility) waveforms demonstrate a tall, sharp, and narrow upstroke in systole, and absent or low forward flow in diastole (e.g., external carotid artery, subclavian artery).

Types of Arterial Blood Flow

TYPE	DESCRIPTION
Laminar	Flow where layers of fluid slide over each other Straight and parallel flow Maximum flow velocity located in the center of the artery Minimum flow velocity located near the arterial wall Found in smaller arteries
Parabolic flow	Average flow velocity is equal to one-half the maximum flow speed at the center Uncommon form of laminar flow
Plug	Constant flow velocity across the vessel (moves as a unit) Found in large arteries (e.g., aorta)
Pulsatile	Alterations in the pressure of moving blood Nonsteady flow with acceleration and deceleration over the cardiac cycle Includes added forward flow and/or flow reversal throughout the cardiac cycle in some locations in the circulatory system *Biphasic flow*—low resistance waveform demonstrating peak forward flow in systole and forward flow during diastole *Triphasic flow*—high resistance waveform demonstrating peak forward flow in systole with a short flow reversal followed by low forward flow during diastole Arterial diastolic flow shows the state of downstream arterioles Flow reversal in diastole indicates high resistance distally
Disturbed	Altered or interrupted forward flow Found at bifurcations and mild obstructions May demonstrate spectral broadening Form of laminar flow
Turbulent	Random and chaotic flow pattern Characterized by eddies and multiple flow velocities (spectral broadening) Maintains a net forward flow Onset predicted by a Reynolds number greater than 2000 Caused by a curve in a vessel's course or a decrease in vessel diameter Nonlaminar flow

EFFECTS OF STENOSIS ON FLOW CHARACTERISTICS

- Increase in flow velocity is seen at the area of narrowing.
- Turbulence distal to the stenosis will be seen (poststenotic turbulence).
- Pressure downstream from stenosis is lower than the pressure upstream (Bernoulli effect).

VENOUS HEMODYNAMICS

- Veins offer little resistance to flow.
- The majority of the venous system demonstrates low-pressure, nonpulsatile flow.
- Greatest portion of the circulating blood is located in the venous system.
- Veins accommodate larger changes in blood volume with little change in pressure.
- Calf muscle (peripheral heart) contraction aids in venous return by increasing pressure to open valves for blood to flow toward the heart.

HYDROSTATIC PRESSURE

- Pressure exuded by a liquid.
- Pressure is lowest (zero) when the patient is lying flat.
- When patient is upright, the hydrostatic pressure will be negative above the heart and positive below the heart.

Venous Flow Characteristics

CHARACTERISTIC	DESCRIPTION
Augmentation	Increased flow velocity after one or more distal compression maneuvers
Continuous	Absence of normal respiratory variations Continuous monophasic flow Indicates obstruction proximally and sometimes distally to the site of Doppler sampling

Phasic	Flow variation during respiration
	Inspiration:
	    Increases abdominal pressure, decreasing venous flow from the lower extremities
	    Decreases thoracic pressure, increasing venous flow from the upper extremities
	Expiration:
	    Increases the thoracic pressure, decreasing venous flow from the upper extremities
	    Decreases the abdominal pressure, increasing venous flow from the lower extremities

Proximal pressure	Manual pressure or Valsalva maneuver impedes venous return Evaluates valvular competency
Spontaneous	Unprompted venous flow
Unidirectional	Flow in only one direction Exceptions include the hepatic veins and the proximal inferior vena cava
Valsalva response	Results in abrupt cessation of blood flow in large and medium-sized veins followed by a quick return of blood flood Documents patency of the venous system from the Doppler sample to the thorax

Doppler Shift

- The change in frequency caused by motion.
- Difference between the emitted frequency and the echo frequency returning from moving scatterers.
- Doppler shift is proportional to the flow speed and operating frequency.
- Doppler shift is dependent on the Doppler angle.
- Cosine values are inversely related to the Doppler angle.

DOPPLER EQUATION

- Relates the Doppler shift to the flow speed and operating frequency.

$$\text{Doppler shift} = \frac{2 \times \text{Transducer freq (MHz)} \times \text{Blood velocity (m/s)} \times \text{Cosine Doppler angle}}{\text{Propagation speed of the medium}}$$

- "2" in the equation is a result of a Doppler shift as a moving receiver and a Doppler shift as the moving emitter.
- Proportional to operating frequency.

DOPPLER EFFECT

- Units—Hz.
- Result of the motion of blood.
- Change in frequency caused by motion of a source, receiver, or reflector.
- Used to determine the flow velocity and direction of moving reflectors.

DETECTION OF DOPPLER SHIFT

- Difference between transmitted and received frequencies from a moving source.
- RBCs are smaller than the wavelength of the sound beam, resulting in Rayleigh scattering.

- If the received and transmitted frequencies are the same, there is no Doppler shift.
- A positive Doppler shift occurs when the received frequency is greater than the transmitted frequency.
- A negative Doppler shift occurs when the received frequency is lower than the transmitted frequency.
- Doppler shift occurs in the audible range.

FACTORS INFLUENCING THE DOPPLER SHIFT

- The angle between the source and reflector is inversely related to the Doppler shift.
- Error in the estimation of the Doppler angle is more critical at larger angles.
- Concentration of RBCs may directly affect the intensity of the Doppler shift.
- Operating frequency is directly related to the Doppler shift.
- A lower-frequency transducer may be necessary to achieve Doppler shifts at deeper depths.

Doppler Instrumentation

DOPPLER TYPE	INSTRUMENTATION	ADVANTAGES/DISADVANTAGES
Continuous wave Doppler	Uses two crystals—one to transmit and another to receive Doppler information Displays only a waveform Large sample volume in the region where the transmitting and receiving sound beams converge Sound is transmitted 100% of the time Phase quadrant detector separate forward and reverse channels which are sent to separate loudspeakers	**Advantages** Ability to measure high velocities (no aliasing) Ability to use high frequencies Highly sensitive to low-flow velocities Small probe size Simplest form of Doppler **Disadvantages** Lack of imaging ability Interrogates all vessels in the sampling area (range ambiguity)
Pulse wave Doppler	Uses a single crystal to transmit and receive Doppler information Displays a sonographic image of the vessel and Doppler information Sample volume or gate is placed within a specific vessel Width of the sample volume is equal to the beam width Minimum of 5 cycles per pulse and up to 30 cycles per pulse	**Advantages** Operator-adjusted placement of the sample volume (range resolution) Allows a smaller sample volume Duplex imaging capabilities **Disadvantages** Maximum detectable Doppler shift is determined by aliasing
Duplex imaging	Combination of 2-D gray-scale imaging and Doppler information Electronic scanning permits switching between imaging and Doppler functions (time-sharing) several times per s, giving the impression of simultaneous imaging Imaging frame rates are decreased to allow for interlaced acquisition of Doppler information	**Advantages** Ability to place sample volume in a specific vessel **Disadvantages** Decrease in gray-scale imaging frame rate
Spectral analysis	Allows visualization of the Doppler signal Provides quantitative data used for evaluating the Doppler shift Presents Doppler shift frequencies in frequency order Different flow conditions display information differently Vertical thickening to the spectral tracing is a result of an increase in range of Doppler shift frequencies Vertical axis represents frequency shift (velocity) Horizontal axis represents time Uses a fast Fourier transform (FFT) to convert Doppler shift information into a visual spectral analysis *FFT breaks down the complex signals of the Doppler shift into individual frequencies*	**Advantages** Allows measurement of peak, mean, and minimum flow velocities, flow direction, and characteristics of the blood flow Presents Doppler shift frequencies in frequency order **Disadvantages** Cannot accurately measure high velocities without aliasing

Continued

Doppler Instrumentation—(cont'd)

DOPPLER TYPE	INSTRUMENTATION	ADVANTAGES/DISADVANTAGES
Color flow Doppler	Presents 2-D color-coded information of motion imposed over a gray-scale image Displays color-coded flow velocity and direction Color is mapped in velocity or variance mode Faster velocities will display lighter colors or hues **Velocity Mode** Colors are arranged top to bottom Top color is assigned to velocities flowing toward the transducer Bottom color is assigned to velocities flowing away from the transducer Black signifies baseline and zero Doppler shift **Variance Mode** Colors are assigned side-to-side Side colors are used to demonstrate turbulent flow Color information is obtained in packets 3–32 pulses are used to obtain one scan line of color information Approximately 100–400 Doppler samples per scan line 4–60 frames per s are used depending on the size of the color box Increases in the length of the color box decreases the frame rate Changing the Doppler angle in an image produces various colors in different locations *Autocorrelation is necessary for rapid obtainment of Doppler shift frequencies*	**Advantages** Ability to detect blood flow quickly Aids in distinguishing low flow velocities Determines blood flow direction Demonstrates nonvascular motion (ureteral jets) Increasing packet size will increase sensitivity and accuracy **Disadvantages** Displays mean velocities Overgaining of the gray-scale image decreases color sensitivity Less accurate than spectral analysis Increasing packet size will decrease frame rate and temporal resolution Aliasing occurs at lower velocities compared with pulse or continuous wave Doppler
Power Doppler	A real-time image of the amplitude of the signal (z-axis) Displays a 2-D color image representing blood flow imposed over a gray-scale image	**Advantages** Increased sensitivity to Doppler shifts in slow low flow and within deep vessels Insensitive to Doppler angle effects and aliasing Better wall definition **Disadvantages** Does not demonstrate flow direction, speed, or character information

Doppler Controls

DOPPLER CONTROL	DESCRIPTION
Angle correction	Generally, demonstrates as a line that is placed parallel to the vessel walls Necessary to calculate flow velocity in spectral analysis (Doppler equation) Angle correction should range between 45 and 60 degrees Some institutions require a 60-degree angle to increase accuracy in serial examinations
Baseline	Zero velocity line between flow toward the transducer and flow away from the transducer Adjusting the baseline widens the range of flow towards or away from the transducer
Color box size	Adjusts the size of the sampled area Larger boxes decrease frame rate Depth of the color box is usually controlled by the trackball
Invert	Changes spectral and color Doppler flow from above baseline to below baseline and flow from below baseline to above baseline
Overall gain	Controls the overall amplification strength of Doppler shifts within the color box or sample gate
Priority	Adjusts gray scale echo strength below which color will be shown
Sample gate size	Controls size of sample volume during spectral analysis Depth of the sample gate is usually controlled by the trackball
Scale	Controls pulse repetition frequency (PRF) High flow velocities need a higher PRF to avoid aliasing

Doppler Controls—(cont'd)

DOPPLER CONTROL	DESCRIPTION
Steering	Adjusts direction of color box and sample gate Adjusts angle of color box and sample gate in modern systems
Sweep speed	Changes the speed of the spectral analysis
Wall filter	Rejects frequencies below an adjusted area Elimination of clutter caused by tissue and wall motion Improper adjustments alter detection of low flow velocities

Doppler Artifacts

ARTIFACT	DEFINITION	CAUSE	MANIFESTATION	METHODS OF OVERCOMING ARTIFACT
Aliasing	Misrepresenting the pulse wave Doppler shift in a negative direction Exceeding the Nyquist limit	Doppler shift exceeds one half of the pulse repetition frequency (Nyquist limit) Undersampling of the Doppler shift	Improper representation of the information sampled Wrap around of the pulse wave or color Doppler display Incorrect flow direction	Increase the pulse repetition frequency (PRF) (scale) Increase Doppler angle Adjust baseline to zero Decrease operating frequency Decrease depth of the sample volume Change to continuous wave
Color bleed	Aka: blossoming Extension of color Doppler beyond the region of blood flow	Overall color gain is too high	Extension of color Doppler beyond the region of blood flow	Decrease color gain
Flash	*Sudden burst* of color Doppler extending beyond the region of blood flow caused by tissue or transducer motion Aka: ghosting	Tissue motion Transducer motion	Extension of color Doppler beyond the region of blood flow	Increase the PRF Decrease the color gain Increase filtering of low flow velocities
Mirror imaging	Duplication of a vessel or Doppler shift on the opposite side of a strong reflector	Doppler gain is set too high	Added vessel or Doppler shift True vessel is located closest to transducer	Decrease color gain Use a different acoustic window
Range ambiguity	Doppler shifts received are not all from the same vessel	Improper placement of the sample volume	Improper representation of Doppler shift	Readjust placement of sample volume

SPECTRAL RATIOS

- Indexes are used to obtain information involving blood flow and vascular impedance that cannot be obtained by absolute velocity information alone.
- Indexes depend on ratios involving peak systole, end diastole, and mean velocity throughout the cardiac cycle, so angle correction is not necessary.

Pulsatility Index

- Most sensitive ratio.
- A parameter used to convey the pulsatility of a time-varying waveform.
- Equal to peak systole minus end diastole divided by the mean velocity.
- Used in abdominal and obstetrical imaging.

Resistive Index (Pourcelot Index)

- Index of pulsatility and opposition to flow.
- Low-resistance waveforms demonstrate broad systolic peaks and forward flow through diastole.
- High-resistance waveforms demonstrate tall, narrow, sharp systolic peaks and reversed or absent diastolic flow.

HEMODYNAMICS AND DOPPLER REVIEW

1. Blood flows from the pulmonary veins into the:
   a. left atrium
   b. right atrium
   c. left ventricle
   d. right ventricle

2. Which of the following is an auscultatory consequence of turbulent flow?
   a. bruit
   b. disturbed flow
   c. high resistance
   d. velocity increase

3. Which of the following is the most accurate definition of hemodynamics?
   a. The pressure created in a fluid system
   b. A fluid's ability to resist change in shape or flow
   c. The pressure difference required for blood to flow
   d. The physical principles concerned with the study of blood circulation

4. What type of arterial blood flow exhibits a constant velocity across the vessel?
   a. plug
   b. laminar
   c. pulsatile
   d. parabolic

5. The microcirculation consists of the:
   a. arteries and veins
   b. arterioles and venules
   c. arterioles, capillaries, and venules
   d. arteries, veins, venules, and capillaries

6. Zero Doppler shift is assigned the color:
   a. red
   b. blue
   c. white
   d. black

7. Which of the following will most likely resolve aliasing?
   a. decreasing the Doppler angle
   b. increasing the operating frequency
   c. increasing the pulse repetition period
   d. decreasing the depth of the sample volume

8. A positive Doppler shift occurs when the:
   a. spectral information is displayed below the baseline
   b. received frequency is less than the transmitted frequency
   c. received frequency is greater than the transmitted frequency
   d. transmitted frequency is equal to the received frequency

9. Which of the following will most likely increase the system's sensitivity of the Doppler shifts?
   a. increasing the Doppler angle
   b. repositioning the sample volume
   c. increasing the operating frequency
   d. decreasing the size of the sample gate

10. If the received and transmitted frequencies are identical, which of the following will occur?
    a. no Doppler shift
    b. positive Doppler shift
    c. negative Doppler shift
    d. proportional Doppler shift

11. A major advantage of continuous wave Doppler is the:
    a. ease of use
    b. small probe size
    c. ability to measure high velocities
    d. interrogation of multiple vessels simultaneously

12. The Doppler equation determines the:
    a. volume flow rate
    b. Reynolds number
    c. cosine of the Doppler angle
    d. change in the transmitted and received frequencies

13. Which of the following is the most consistent predictor of turbulent flow?
    a. Doppler shift
    b. resistive index
    c. pressure gradient
    d. Reynolds number

14. Which of the following is required for blood flow to occur?
    a. Doppler shift
    b. kinetic energy
    c. pressure gradient
    d. high cardiac output

15. Blood flow velocity is more likely dependent on which of the following?
    a. volume flow rate
    b. size of the capillaries
    c. left-ventricular output
    d. resistance of the venules

16. In which of the following positions is venous pressure the lowest?
    a. erect
    b. supine
    c. decubitus
    d. semierect

17. The greatest portion of circulating blood is located in the:
    a. brain
    b. heart
    c. venous system
    d. arterial system

18. What type of blood flow occurs if the average flow velocity is equal to one half the maximum flow speed in the center?
    a. plug flow
    b. laminar flow
    c. pulsatile flow
    d. parabolic flow

19. Normal respiratory variations in venous blood flow are termed:
    a. phasic
    b. pulsatile
    c. spontaneous
    d. bidirectional

20. Which of the following is a disadvantage of duplex imaging?
    a. decrease in imaging frame rate
    b. combines imaging and Doppler information
    c. allows measurement only of mean velocities
    d. inability to use high operating frequencies

21. Noise within the Doppler signal is known as:
    a. flash
    b. clutter
    c. aliasing
    d. blossoming

22. Which of the following is the driving force of blood flow?
    a. velocity
    b. pressure
    c. resistance
    d. volume flow rate

23. Observed frequency changes in moving structures most accurately defines:
    a. Doppler shift
    b. Nyquist limit
    c. Doppler effect
    d. pressure gradient

24. The Nyquist limit is equal to:
    a. the operating frequency
    b. the peak systolic velocity
    c. the pulse repetition frequency
    d. one half of the pulse repetition frequency

25. Which of the following blood flow types is most likely to demonstrate spectral broadening?
    a. plug
    b. laminar
    c. disturbed
    d. pulsatile

26. Thickening of the spectral trace is most likely a result of:
    a. the reverberation artifact
    b. low-amplitude Doppler shifts
    c. an increase in the range of Doppler shift frequencies
    d. the quantity of blood moving through the sample volume

27. This spectral thickening is termed:
    a. clutter
    b. aliasing
    c. saturation
    d. spectral broadening

28. The size of the sample volume is determined by the beam diameter, emitted pulse length, and:
    a. Doppler shift
    b. Doppler angle
    c. operating frequency
    d. gate length

29. Which of the following converts Doppler shift information into a visual spectral display?
    a. scan converter
    b. autocorrelation
    c. fast Fourier transform
    d. digital–analog converter

30. In color-flow Doppler, multiple sample gates positioned in the area of interest are termed:
    a. pixels
    b. voxels
    c. packets
    d. color volumes

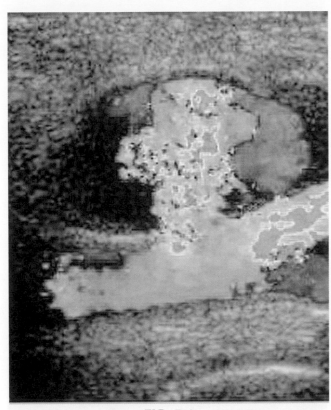

FIG. 5.1

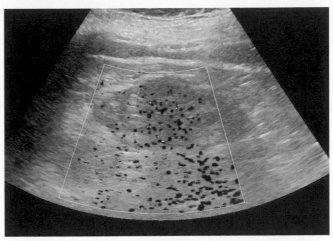

FIG. 5.2

Using Figure 5.1 and Color Plate 1, answer question 31.

31. Which of the following changes will improve this color Doppler image?
    a. raise color baseline
    b. decrease color gain
    c. increase color scale
    d. change acoustic window

32. Which of the following correctly describes the hemodynamics of blood flow?
    a. Blood only flows when pressures are equal
    b. Blood flows from low pressure to high pressure
    c. Blood flows from higher pressure to lower pressure
    d. Blood flows from higher velocity to lower velocity

33. Increasing the operating frequency will:
    a. overcome aliasing
    b. increase the packet size
    c. increase the Nyquist limit
    d. increase sensitivity to low Doppler shifts

Using Figure 5.2 and Color Plate 2, answer question 34.

34. Which of the following changes will improve this color Doppler image?
    a. decrease color scale
    b. decrease color gain
    c. decrease imaging depth
    d. decrease operating frequency

35. The greater the pressure gradient, the greater the:
    a. flow velocity
    b. flow resistance
    c. Reynolds number
    d. blood flow volume

36. Resistance to blood flow is proportional to the
    a. flow velocity
    b. Reynolds number
    c. blood flow volume
    d. length of the vessel

37. Which of the following occurs during inspiration?
    a. abdominal and thoracic pressure increase
    b. abdominal pressure decreases and thoracic pressure increases
    c. abdominal pressure increases and thoracic pressure decreases
    d. abdominal pressure decreases and thoracic pressure remains unchanged

38. Which of the following is the simplest form of Doppler?
    a. color
    b. amplitude
    c. pulse wave
    d. continuous wave

39. The vertical axis of a spectral analysis represents:
    a. time
    b. motion
    c. intensity
    d. frequency

40. Rate of motion with respect to time defines:
    a. energy
    b. inertia
    c. velocity
    d. acceleration

41. Poiseuille's equation predicts:
    a. the onset of aliasing
    b. the onset of turbulence
    c. resistance to acceleration
    d. flow volume in a cylindrical vessel

42. Pulse wave Doppler uses a maximum of:
    a. 5 cycles per pulse
    b. 15 cycles per pulse
    c. 20 cycles per pulse
    d. 30 cycles per pulse

43. Color Doppler frequency shifts are obtained using:
    a. beam profiler
    b. scan converter
    c. autocorrelation
    d. fast Fourier transfer

Using Figure 5.3, answer question 44.

44. In this spectral display, which of the following changes will most likely demonstrate the low-velocity blood flow?
    a. decrease wall filter
    b. increase spectral gain
    c. increase operating frequency
    d. decrease pulse repetition frequency

45. Demonstrating nonvascular motion is commonly accomplished using:
    a. color Doppler
    b. spectral analysis
    c. pulse wave Doppler
    d. continuous wave Doppler

46. Power Doppler imaging displays the signal's:
    a. energy
    b. velocity
    c. amplitude
    d. frequency shift

Using Figure 5.4, answer question 47.

47. Which of the following changes will improve this duplex image?
    a. increase wall filter
    b. decrease Doppler gain
    c. decrease pulse repetition frequency
    d. increase pulse repetition frequency

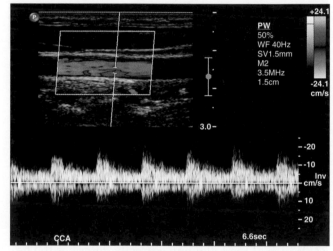

FIG. 5.4

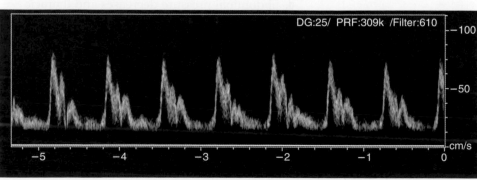

FIG. 5.3

48. Increasing the Doppler angle is a method of overcoming:
    a. flash
    b. aliasing
    c. mirror imaging
    d. range ambiguity

49. Smaller arteries commonly demonstrate:
    a. plug flow
    b. laminar flow
    c. parabolic flow
    d. turbulent flow

50. Increasing the packet size of color Doppler will decrease the:
    a. accuracy
    b. frame rate
    c. sensitivity
    d. Doppler shift

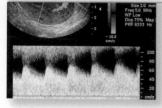

CHAPTER 6

Quality Assurance, Protocols, and New Technologies

KEY TERMS

beam profiler   a device that plots the reflection amplitudes received by the transducer.

dead zone   distance closest to the transducer in which imaging cannot be performed.

force-balance system   a device that measures the force (pressure) of the sound beam.

hydrophone   testing device that measures acoustic output.

phantom   tissue-equivalent testing device with characteristics that are representative of tissues.

preventive maintenance (PM) service   periodic internal cleaning and overall evaluation of the ultrasound system function; generally performed by the system manufacturer.

registration accuracy   ability to place echoes in proper position when imaging from different orientations.

system sensitivity   measure of how weak a reflection the system can display.

test objects   devices without tissue like properties designed to measure some characteristics of the imaging system.

QUALITY ASSURANCE (QA)

- Routine, periodic evaluation of data collected on the performance of the ultrasound system and transducers.
- Ensures diagnostic image quality and consistency.
- Reduces system breakdowns.
- Testing devices are available for determining whether sonographic or Doppler instruments are operating correctly and consistently.
- Usually performed with a tissue-equivalent phantom to assess image quality.
- American Institute of Ultrasound in Medicine (AIUM) require regular equipment maintenance and calibration.

QUALITY CONTROL (QC)

- Testing used to collect data on the operation and acoustic output of the ultrasound system.
- American College of Radiology (ACR) requires a minimum of semiannual quality control testing.

PERFORMANCE MEASUREMENTS

- Imaging performance is determined primarily by measuring the following:
  - Detail resolution.
  - Contrast resolution.
  - Penetration and dynamic range.
  - Time gain compensation.
  - Accuracy of depth and distance measurement.

METHODS OF EVALUATION

Operation Testing

- Takes into account the entire ultrasound instrument.
- Evaluates the ultrasound system as a diagnostic tool.
- Used by service professionals and instrument operators.

Acoustic Output Testing

- Considers only the beam former and the transducer acting together as a source of ultrasound.
- Evaluates the safety and biological effects of ultrasound and Doppler imaging.
- Requires specialized equipment and is generally performed by engineers and physicists.

Methods for Evaluating Operation

- Two categories:
  - Phantoms.
  - Test objects.

TESTING DEVICE	DESCRIPTION	PARAMETERS EVALUATED
AIUM 100 test object	A device without tissue properties designed to measure some system characteristics Provides measurement of system performance Uses 0.75-mm stainless steel rods placed in a mixture with a propagation speed of 1540 m/s	Dead zone Compensation Axial resolution Lateral resolution Vertical and horizontal calibration Registration accuracy System sensitivity *Cannot evaluate:* 　Gray scale 　Penetration 　Compression
Beam profiler/ slice thickness test object	Contains a thin, scattering layer in an echo-free material A device that plots 3-D reflection amplitudes received by the transducer	Beam width in the scan plane or perpendicular to it (section-thickness) Measures transducer characteristics
Tissue-equivalent phantom	Simulates tissue properties include soft tissue, cystic, and solid structures Attenuation similar to soft tissue Does not simulate tissue characteristics Small fibers are used to evaluate axial and lateral resolution	Dead zone Penetration Compression Compensation Axial resolution Lateral resolution Contrast resolution Slice thickness resolution Vertical and horizontal calibration System sensitivity Registration accuracy
Doppler test objects and tissue equivalent phantoms	A device using tissue and a blood-mimicking fluid Simulates clinical conditions Velocity, pulse rates, and durations are known Some may contain a stenosis, *or* moving string scatters the sound beam Calibrated by electromagnetic flow meter or by fluid volume collection over time Can produce pulsatile and retrograde motion	Penetration of the Doppler beam Flow direction Accuracy of gate location Accuracy of measured flow velocity Image congruency

AIUM, American Institute of Ultrasound in Medicine.

Methods for Evaluating Acoustic Output

- Normally used by engineers and physicists.

TESTING DEVICE	DESCRIPTION	PARAMETERS EVALUATED
Hydrophone Aka: microprobe	A small (<1mm) transducer element mounted on the end of a hollow needle *or* a large piezoelectric membrane with small metallic electrodes centered on each side Membrane is made of polyvinylidene fluoride (PVDF)	Relationship between the amount of acoustic pressure and the voltage produced Measures acoustic output Measures pressure and intensities across the sound beam Measures period, pulse repetition period, and pulse duration

RECORD KEEPING

- Helps detect gradual or sporadic system changes.
- Documents the need for replacement of existing equipment.
- Necessary for hospital and outpatient clinic accreditation.
- Files for each ultrasound unit should contain:
  - Original purchase order and warranty.
  - Equipment specifications.
  - Results of previous QA tests.
  - Documentation of problems.
  - Service and preventive maintenance reports or invoices.

STATISTICAL INDICES

- *Positive* means the test indicates disease.
- *Negative* means the test indicates disease-free.
- *True positive* (TP) means test matches gold standard—both are positive for disease.
- *True negative* (TN) means test matches gold standard—both are negative for disease.
- *False positive* (FP) means test does not match gold standard—the test says there is disease when there isn't.
- *False negative* (FN) means test does not match gold standard—the test says there is no disease when there is.

Chi square: comparison test versus gold standard.

Sensitivity: ability of a test to detect disease.

$$\frac{\text{True Positive}}{\text{True Positive} + \text{False Negative}}$$

Specificity: ability of a test to detect the absence of disease.

$$\frac{\text{True Negative}}{\text{True Negative} + \text{False Positive}}$$

Positive predictive value: measures how often the test is correct when positive for disease.

$$\frac{\text{True Positive}}{\text{True Positive} + \text{False Positive}}$$

Negative predictive value: measures how often the test is correct when negative for disease.

$$\frac{\text{True Negative}}{\text{True Negative} + \text{False Negative}}$$

Accuracy: measures the percentage of examinations that agree with the gold standard; quality of being near to the true value.

$$\frac{\text{True Positive} + \text{True Negative}}{\text{True Positive} + \text{True Negative} + \text{False Positive} + \text{False Negative}}$$

PROTOCOLS

- American Institute of Ultrasound Medicine (AIUM) and American College of Radiology (ACR) have adapted universal scanning protocols for medical sonography examinations.
- Extension of these protocols may be necessary when anomalies, abnormalities, and pathologies are discovered.
- Additional images should accurately represent findings and evaluate the surrounding structures, not just the area of interest.
- Images of abnormality(s) with and without measurements must be documented in two scanning planes.
- Images should include color Doppler and spectral analysis of abnormality.
- Abnormality(s) should be viewed with high- to low-gain settings in two scanning planes.
- Location, echo, and Doppler characteristics should be incorporated in sonographer technical reports.

NEW TECHNOLOGIES

Elastography

- Imaging version of palpation.
- Detects the relative tissue displacement precompression (nonstress) and compression (stress).
- The radiofrequency of each line of the signal is acquired before and after compression.
- The amount of time shift yields displacement for that segment of tissue.
- Depicts tissue stiffness—higher the elasticity of the medium, the less the stiffness, and the greater the deformity of response will be demonstrated.
- Commonly shown as an overlay on top of gray-scale image.
- Used to detect carcinoma of superficial anatomy, to assess viability of myocardium, and to monitor altered tissue therapies (e.g., ablation procedures).

Fusion Imaging

- Ultrasound images are paired with another imaging modality (MRI, CT) to enable a direct comparison.
- Optical or electromagnetic tracing systems are used to help align the ultrasound transducer producing the ultrasound image with the imported correlating imaging modality images.
- Biopsy or ablations can be performed using an interventional device with a tracing sensor displaying the needle in an overlay during real time imaging.

Parallel Processing

- Sophisticated processing technique that enables rapid image acquisition and very high frame rates (improves temporal resolution).
- Uses all elements in the transducer to send a broad, unfocused ultrasound beam exposing the entire width of the image.
- Uses a broad pulse.
- Transmitted pulse provides all of the echo information for all portions of the image, rather than just one scan line.
- Massive parallel processing sorts out the echoes from all portions of the exposed image plane, placing them in image memory.

QUALITY ASSURANCE, PROTOCOLS, AND NEW TECHNOLOGY REVIEW

1. The number of correct test results divided by the total number of tests defines:
   a. accuracy
   b. sensitivity
   c. specificity
   d. positive predictive value

2. The ability of a test to detect the absence of disease defines:
   a. sensitivity
   b. specificity
   c. accuracy
   d. negative predictive value

3. Which testing device measures acoustic output?
   a. test object
   b. hydrophone
   c. beam profiler
   d. tissue phantom

4. Which of the following most accurately describes quality assurance?
   a. routine evaluation of the ultrasound system
   b. periodic evaluation of the ultrasound transducers
   c. periodic internal cleaning of the ultrasound system
   d. routine evaluation of the transducers and ultrasound system

5. The beam profiler is a testing device that measures:
   a. acoustic output
   b. depth accuracy
   c. flow characteristics
   d. transducer characteristics

6. Which of the following is NOT a primary image performance measurement?
   a. contrast resolution
   b. temporal resolution
   c. time gain compensation
   d. accuracy of distance measurement

7. The ability to place reflections in proper positions regardless of the imaging orientation describes:
   a. accuracy
   b. quality assurance
   c. system specificity
   d. registration accuracy

8. Elastography depicts tissue:
   a. density
   b. stiffness
   c. temperature
   d. water content

9. A testing device with characteristics of specific soft tissue is termed a:
   a. phantom
   b. test object
   c. hydrophone
   d. tissue profiler

10. Protocols for medical sonography examinations have been adapted by the:
    a. American College of Radiology
    b. American Institute of Ultrasound Medicine
    c. American Registry of Diagnostic Medical Sonographers
    d. American College of Radiology and American Institute of Ultrasound Medicine

11. The American Institute of Ultrasound in Medicine (AIUM) 100 test object *cannot* evaluate:
    a. dead zone
    b. compression
    c. axial resolution
    d. system performance

12. Record keeping of each ultrasound unit is necessary for:
    a. service requests
    b. hospital and outpatient clinic accreditation
    c. detection of gradual or sporadic system changes
    d. scheduling the next preventive maintenance service

13. The American College of Radiology requires quality control testing:
    a. annually
    b. quarterly
    c. semiannually
    d. monthly

14. The positive predictive value is determined by the number of correct:
    a. true positive and true negative tests divided by the total number of tests
    b. true negative and false negative tests
    c. true positive tests divided by the sum of the true positive and true negative tests
    d. true positive tests divided by the sum of the true positive and false positive tests

15. The AIUM 100 test object evaluates which of the following?
    a. contrast resolution
    b. system sensitivity
    c. direction of blood flow
    d. gray-scale characteristics

16. Which testing device employs a small transducer element?
    a. hydrophone
    b. beam profiler
    c. AIUM test object
    d. tissue-equivalent phantom

17. Quality assurance programs provide assessment of:
    a. image quality
    b. sonographer accuracy
    c. examination protocols
    d. acoustic output of the ultrasound system

18. Which testing device will a quality assurance program most likely use?
    a. hydrophone
    b. Doppler phantom
    c. AIUM 100 test object
    d. tissue-equivalent phantom

19. System sensitivity measures:
    a. the ability to place echoes in the proper position
    b. the detail resolution of the ultrasound system
    c. how weak a reflection the system can display
    d. the ability of a test to detect disease

20. The hydrophone measures:
    a. temporal resolution
    b. registration accuracy
    c. blood flow direction
    d. pulse repetition period

21. The number of true positive test results divided by the sum of the true positive and false negative tests yields the:
    a. specificity
    b. accuracy
    c. sensitivity
    d. positive predictive value

22. Which of the following pair ultrasound images with another imaging modality for direct comparison?
    a. elastography
    b. contrast imaging
    c. fusion imaging
    d. parallel processing

23. Which of the following evaluates the operation of the ultrasound system?
    a. beam former
    b. force-balance system
    c. tissue-equivalent phantom
    d. preventive maintenance service

24. Which of the following evaluates the safety and biological effects of ultrasound imaging?
    a. operation testing
    b. transducer testing
    c. acoustic output testing
    d. system maintenance program

25. Negative predictive value is the ability of a diagnostic test to:
    a. predict normal findings
    b. predict abnormal findings
    c. predict the presence of actual disease
    d. identify the presence of actual disease

26. The output of the hydrophone evaluates the:
    a. likelihood of cavitation
    b. pressure of the sound beam
    c. likelihood of biological effects
    d. acoustic exposure to the patient

27. Very high frame rates are used in:
    a. elastography
    b. fusion imaging
    c. parallel processing
    d. code excitation

28. Which of the following testing devices measures the pulse repetition period?
    a. hydrophone
    b. beam profiler
    c. tissue phantom
    d. AIUM 100 test object

29. Which of the following is an imaging version of palpation?
    a. fusion imaging
    b. elastography
    c. parallel processing
    d. three-dimensional imaging

30. Tissue-mimicking phantoms are unable to evaluate:
    a. penetration
    b. compression
    c. direction of flow
    d. system sensitivity

31. Acoustic output testing considers only the:
    a. beam profiler
    b. digitizer and beam profiler
    c. beam profiler and transducer
    d. transducer and digitizer

32. Testing used to collect data on the operation and acoustic output of the ultrasound system describes:
    a. quality control
    b. registration accuracy
    c. quality assurance
    d. performance maintenance

33. Development of a quality assurance program ensures:
    a. laboratory accreditation
    b. image consistency
    c. increase in productivity
    d. teamwork among the staff

Using the following research, answer questions 34 to 37.

One hundred abdominal aorta examinations performed over a 6-month period correctly diagnosed 20 true positive, 5 false positive, 75 true negative, and 0 false negatives compared with the gold standard.

34. The positive predictive value of this study is:
    a. 20%
    b. 50%
    c. 75%
    d. 80%

35. The sensitivity of this study is:
    a. 21%
    b. 50%
    c. 80%
    d. 100%

36. The overall accuracy of this study is:
    a. 50%
    b. 75%
    c. 95%
    d. 100%

37. The negative predictive value of this study is:
    a. 50%
    b. 75%
    c. 95%
    d. 100%

38. Positive predictive value measures:
    a. the ability of a test to detect disease
    b. percentage of tests that agree with the gold standard
    c. how often the test is correct when positive for disease
    d. the ability of a test to detect absence of disease

39. The dead zone is located:
    a. near the transducer face
    b. adjacent to the focal zone
    c. superior to the focal zone
    d. farthest from the transducer face

40. The ability of a diagnostic technique to identify the presence of genuine disease is termed:
    a. specificity
    b. sensitivity
    c. positive predictive value
    d. negative predictive value

41. Use of a piezoelectric membrane is found in a:
    a. hydrophone
    b. beam profiler
    c. AIUM 100 test object
    d. moving-string phantom

42. Which of the following testing devices simulates clinical conditions?
    a. hydrophone
    b. Doppler phantom
    c. AIUM 100 test objects
    d. beam profiler

43. How often the test is correct when negative for disease describes:
    a. sensitivity
    b. specificity
    c. accuracy
    d. negative predictive value

44. The percentage of examinations that agree with the gold standard is termed:
    a. sensitivity
    b. accuracy
    c. specificity
    d. positive predictive value

45. Accuracy of a diagnostic test is most precisely defined as the:
    a. percentage of error
    b. identification of disease
    c. prediction of documenting disease
    d. quality of being near to the true value

46. Parallel processing uses a(n):
    a. narrow pulse
    b. broad pulse
    c. optical tracing system
    d. electromagnetic tracing system

47. A device that plots three-dimensional reflection amplitudes received by the transducer evaluates:
    a. acoustic output
    b. transducer characteristics
    c. intensity of the sound beam
    d. accuracy of the sample gate

48. Which of the following testing devices can simulate pulsatile or retrograde flow?
    a. hydrophone
    b. AIUM 100 test object
    c. moving-string phantom
    d. tissue-mimicking phantom

49. The relationship between the amount of acoustic pressure and the voltage produced is evaluated by the:
    a. hydrophone
    b. beam profiler
    c. force-balance system
    d. moving-string phantom

50. What is the accuracy of a diagnostic test if 2 examinations of 20 are misdiagnosed?
    a. 65%
    b. 75%
    c. 90%
    d. 95%

1. Reducing the likelihood of bioeffects from acoustic energy is the mission of the:
   a. Nyquist limit
   b. Reynolds number
   c. Huygens principle
   d. ALARA principle

2. The number of cycles in a pulse directly relates to the:
   a. duty factor
   b. spatial pulse length
   c. operating frequency
   d. pulse repetition frequency

3. The Doppler shift frequency is proportional to the:
   a. cosine values
   b. Doppler angle
   c. operating frequency
   d. velocity of the reflector

4. In the Fraunhofer zone, the beam:
   a. width diverges
   b. is conical in shape
   c. intensity is greatest
   d. intensity is inconsistent

5. Artifacts consisting of parallel equally spaced lines are characteristic of:
   a. multipath
   b. grating lobes
   c. reverberation
   d. range ambiguity

6. An increase in reflection amplitudes from reflectors behind a weakly attenuating structure is termed:
   a. comet-tail artifact
   b. acoustic shadowing
   c. slice thickness artifact
   d. acoustic enhancement

7. The ratio of the largest power to the smallest power the ultrasound system can handle describes:
   a. bandwidth
   b. compensation
   c. dynamic range
   d. contrast resolution

8. Axial resolution directly relates to the:
   a. spatial pulse length
   b. temporal resolution
   c. transducer diameter
   d. operating frequency

9. When voltage is applied to the piezoelectric crystal, the crystal will:
   a. vibrate
   b. increase in size
   c. decrease in size
   d. increase or decrease according to the polarity

10. The resistance of the arterioles accounts for approximately what percentage of the total systemic resistance?
    a. 25%
    b. 33%
    c. 50%
    d. 75%

11. Rayleigh scattering is mostly likely to occur when encountering the:
    a. liver
    b. pleura
    c. diaphragm
    d. red blood cells

12. Which color always represents the baseline in color Doppler imaging?
    a. red
    b. blue
    c. white
    d. black

13. Which of the following correctly defines acoustic frequency?
    a. length of one cycle
    b. number of pulses in a cycle
    c. number of cycles in a second
    d. strength of the compression wave

14. Pairing ultrasound images with another imaging modality for direct comparison describes:
    a. spatial compounding
    b. fusion imaging
    c. parallel processing
    d. multifocal imaging

15. Grating lobes are caused by:
    a. dynamic focusing
    b. reverberation artifact
    c. interference phenomenon
    d. spacing of the array elements

16. Clutter can be reduced using which of the following controls?
    a. wall filter
    b. smoothing
    c. dynamic range
    d. pulse repetition frequency

17. Regions of high density in an acoustic wave are termed:
    a. reflections
    b. rarefactions
    c. transmissions
    d. compressions

18. Decibel is the unit of measurement for:
    a. intensity
    b. pressure
    c. amplitude
    d. compression

19. Transmission of the sound wave from one medium to the next is determined by the media's:
    a. density
    b. stiffness
    c. impedance
    d. propagation speed

20. Focusing of the sound beam:
    a. decreases beam intensity
    b. improves lateral resolution
    c. increases specular reflections
    d. creates a spacious sound beam over a specified area

21. As the transducer diameter increases, the:
    a. near zone length decreases
    b. thickness of the element decreases
    c. intensity in the focal zone increases
    d. divergence in the far field decreases

22. Holding a single image of sonographic information for display is termed a:
    a. pixel
    b. scan line
    c. cine loop
    d. freeze frame

23. The binary number 0010011 converts to which decimal equivalent?
    a. 10
    b. 19
    c. 21
    d. 35

24. The thickness of the matching layer is equal to:
    a. the wavelength of the crystal
    b. twice the wavelength of the crystal
    c. one-half of the wavelength of the crystal
    d. one quarter of the wavelength of the crystal

25. What is the function of the Doppler priority control?
    a. control the size of the color box
    b. reject frequencies below an adjusted range
    c. control the active side of a dual imaging screen
    d. adjusts gray-scale echo strength below which color will be shown.

26. A high resistance waveform demonstrates a:
    a. slow upstroke
    b. broad upstroke
    c. sharp upstroke
    d. high flow velocity in diastole

27. Heat sterilization of ultrasound transducers is not recommended, because:
    a. the transducer's stability decreases
    b. heat will damage the electric cables
    c. the piezoelectric properties will be lost
    d. the transducer assembly cannot withstand the temperature

28. Intensity of the sound beam is:
    a. uniform within the pulse
    b. zero between pulses
    c. highest near the periphery
    d. uniform across the sound beam.

29. The Fresnel zone is another name for the:
    a. far zone
    b. dead zone
    c. near zone
    d. focal zone

30. Proximal to, at, and distal to a stenosis, which of the following must remain constant?
    a. velocity
    b. pressure
    c. resistance
    d. volumetric flow rate

31. The greater the impedance difference between two structures, the greater the:
    a. refraction
    b. reflection
    c. attenuation
    d. transmission

32. Which Doppler angle yields the greatest Doppler shift?
    a. 0 degrees
    b. 10 degrees
    c. 45 degrees
    d. 60 degrees

33. Increasing the transducer frequency will:
    a. decrease contrast resolution
    b. increase the penetration depth
    c. increase the amount of attenuation
    d. decrease sensitivity to Doppler shifts

34. Image quality is improved by:
    a. decreasing the output
    b. decreasing the frame rate
    c. increasing the beam width
    d. shortening the pulse length

35. What is the purpose of the damping material in the transducer assembly?
   a. increase in sensitivity
   b. reduction in pulse duration
   c. improvement in sound transmission into the body
   d. diminishment of reflections at the transducer surface

36. Which of the following instruments generates the pulse of sound?
   a. pulser
   b. transducer
   c. beam former
   d. master synchronizer

37. Firing delays found in array systems are determined by the:
   a. digitizer
   b. transducer
   c. beam former
   d. master synchronizer

38. The speed at which a wave travels through a medium is determined by the:
   a. distance from the sound source
   b. stiffness and density of the medium
   c. resistance and impedance of the medium
   d. amplitude and intensity of the sound beam

39. Which of the following is a method for overcoming aliasing?
   a. shift the baseline
   b. increase imaging depth
   c. decrease the Doppler angle
   d. increase the operating frequency

40. Brightening of echoes in the focal zone is a result of:
   a. acoustic speckle
   b. slice thickness artifact
   c. horizontal enhancement
   d. propagation speed error

41. A disadvantage of duplex imaging is a(n):
   a. decrease in gray-scale imaging frame rate
   b. inability to display peak velocities
   c. inability to demonstrate flow direction
   d. decrease in maximum penetration depth

42. Heat is dependent on which of the following intensities?
   a. SATP
   b. SPTA
   c. SATA
   d. SPTP

43. The duty factor in pulse ultrasound is proportional to the:
   a. pulse duration
   b. penetration depth
   c. operating frequency
   d. pulse repetition period

44. Depth gain compensation is necessary to:
   a. counteract attenuation
   b. increase axial resolution
   c. decrease contrast resolution
   d. store echo amplitudes and locations

45. The Reynolds number predicts the onset of:
   a. aliasing
   b. turbulent flow
   c. a Doppler shift
   d. biological effects

46. Which of the following types of resolution does the wavelength have the greatest effect on?
   a. axial
   b. lateral
   c. contrast
   d. temporal

47. The objective of the matching layer in the assembly of an ultrasound transducer is to reduce the:
   a. pulse duration
   b. spatial pulse length
   c. number of cycles in each pulse
   d. impedance difference between the element and skin

48. What is the minimum number of memory bits necessary to display 128 shades of gray?
   a. 2
   b. 5
   c. 7
   d. 10

49. Which of the following is a function of read magnification?
   a. frame averaging
   b. magnification and display of stored data
   c. acquisition and magnification of new information
   d. increase in the number of pixels per inch

50. Averaging the frame rate is operator adjustable using which of the following functions?
   a. read zoom
   b. persistence
   c. dynamic range
   d. contrast variation

51. At a stenosis, pressure will:
    a. double
    b. increase
    c. decrease
    d. remain unchanged

52. Reducing a 30-dB compensation gain by one-half would display a new gain setting of:
    a. 10 dB
    b. 15 dB
    c. 24 dB
    d. 27 dB

53. Reduction in the intensity of the sound wave is a result of:
    a. heat, reflection, and, transmission
    b. absorption, scattering, and reflection
    c. scattering, refraction, and absorption
    d. absorption, scattering, and transmission

54. Divergence of the sound beam is demonstrated in the:
    a. focal zone
    b. dead zone
    c. Fresnel zone
    d. Fraunhofer zone

55. The ability of a sonogram to identify the true absence of disease is a test's:
    a. accuracy
    b. specificity
    c. sensitivity
    d. positive predictive value

56. There is no confirmed significant biological effect in mammalian tissue for exposures:
    a. below 100 W/cm^2 with unfocused and 1 W/cm^2 with focused transducers
    b. above 100 W/cm^2 with unfocused and 1 W/cm^2 with focused transducers
    c. below 1 mW/cm^2 with unfocused and 1 mW/cm^2 with focused transducers
    d. below 100 mW/cm^2 with unfocused and 1 W/cm^2 with focused transducers

57. List the intensity ranges from smallest to highest:
    a. SPTP, SATP, SPTA, SATA
    b. SATA, SATP, SPTA, SPTP
    c. SATA, SPTA, SATP, SPTP
    d. SATA, SATP, SPTP, SPTA

58. Diagnostic ultrasound transducers operate on which of the following theories?
    a. Snell's law
    b. ALARA principle
    c. Piezoelectric effect
    d. Huygens principle

59. Uniform intensity of the sound beam is located in the:
    a. far field
    b. near field
    c. focal point
    d. center of the beam

60. The amplitude of the transmitted and received signals is the responsibility of the:
    a. pulser
    b. amplifier
    c. transducer
    d. system output

61. The formula to determine volume flow rate is: ?
    a. stroke volume × heart rate
    b. 4 × maximum peak velocity
    c. peak flow velocity × density of the fluid
    d. average speed across the vessel × cross-section area of the vessel

62. Line density is directly related to the:
    a. imaging depth
    b. temporal resolution
    c. pulse repetition period
    d. pulse repetition frequency

63. Which of the following are even harmonic frequencies of a 2-MHz transducer?
    a. 2, 4, 6
    b. 3, 5, 7
    c. 4, 6, 8
    d. 4, 8, 12

64. Which of the following will most likely occur if the pulse repetition frequency is set too high?
    a. flash
    b. aliasing
    c. acoustic speckle
    d. range ambiguity

Using Figure 1, answer question 65.

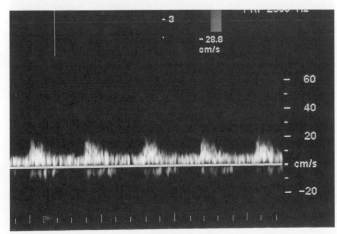

FIG. 1

65. Which of the following changes would improve evaluation of the spectral analysis waveform?
    a. raise the baseline; increase sweep speed and wall filter
    b. increase the pulse repetition frequency and priority control
    c. decrease the pulse repetition frequency and wall filter
    d. raise the baseline; decrease sweep speed; decrease the pulse repetition frequency if needed.

66. Mirror imaging artifact is a result of a(n):
    a. weak reflector
    b. strong reflector
    c. impedance difference
    d. strong attenuating structure

67. Approximately what percentage of the sound beam will reflect from a media boundary with perpendicular incidence, if the impedances are different?
    a. 1
    b. 10
    c. 50
    d. 99

68. Placement of an echo is determined by the reflector's round-trip time and:
    a. density of the medium
    b. stiffness of the medium
    c. amplitude of the reflectors
    d. propagation speed of the medium

Using Figure 2, answer question 69.

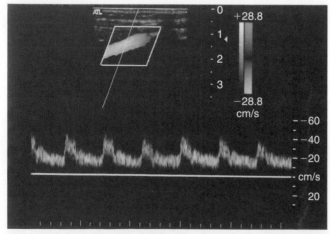

FIG. 2

69. Which of the following changes will improve this spectral display?
    a. decrease the wall filter; decrease the Doppler gain
    b. move baseline up; increase the Doppler gain
    c. decrease the focal zone; decrease the pulse repetition frequency
    d. decrease the wall filter; decrease the pulse repetition frequency

70. Which of the following determines the number of scan lines per frame?
    a. contrast resolution
    b. operating frequency
    c. temporal resolution
    d. pulse repetition frequency

71. When coursing from a medium of lower propagation speed to a medium of higher propagation speed, the frequency of the sound wave will:
    a. double
    b. increase
    c. decrease
    d. remain constant

72. Flow reversal in diastole indicates:
    a. a stenosis
    b. a proximal obstruction
    c. high resistance distally
    d. low resistance distally

73. How can the sonographer increase temporal resolution?
    a. increase beam width
    b. increase imaging depth
    c. decrease transducer frequency
    d. decrease the number of focal zones

74. How wide are the elements of a linear phased-array transducer?
    a. one wavelength
    b. one-half wavelength
    c. one tenth wavelength
    d. one quarter wavelength

75. Which of the following is a method to eliminate color blossoming?
    a. decrease imaging depth
    b. increase the wall filter
    c. decrease the color gain
    d. increase the pulse repetition frequency

76. The Nyquist limit predicts the onset of:
    a. aliasing
    b. turbulence
    c. helical flow
    d. range ambiguity

77. Specular reflections occur when the sound wave:
    a. strikes a rough surface
    b. encounters a strong reflector
    c. encounters a smaller reflector
    d. strikes a smooth, large reflector

78. The sonographer can improve lateral resolution by:
    a. increasing the frame rate
    b. increasing the imaging depth
    c. decreasing the spatial pulse length
    d. increasing the number of focal zones

Using Figure 3, answer question 79.

79. Which of the following changes will optimize this sonogram of the right upper quadrant?
    a. increase imaging depth; lower focal zone; increase overall gain
    b. decrease imaging depth; increase the time gain compensation in the far zone
    c. decrease imaging depth; lower focal zone; increase overall gain
    d. increase focal zone number; increase time gain compensation in the near zone

80. Operating frequency is determined by the:
    a. frequency of the active element
    b. thickness and diameter of the crystal
    c. diameter and propagation speed of the crystal
    d. propagation speed and thickness of the element

81. The portion of time the transducer is transmitting a pulse is termed:
    a. period
    b. duty factor
    c. pulse duration
    d. pulse repetition period

82. Unprompted venous flow is termed:
    a. phasic
    b. continuous
    c. pulsatile
    d. spontaneous

83. A large packet size in color-flow imaging will:
    a. increase the frame rate
    b. increase contrast resolution
    c. increase the volume flow rate
    d. decrease the temporal resolution

Using Figure 4, answer question 84.

84. The spectral display is demonstrating which of the following?
    a. aliasing
    b. bidirectional flow
    c. turbulent flow
    d. mirror image artifact

85. Which of the following controls adjusts the range of displayed signal amplitudes?
    a. rejection
    b. compression
    c. amplification
    d. compensation

86. Which adjustable system control affects the frame rate?
    a. image depth
    b. compression
    c. compensation
    d. transmit power

87. Varying the excitation voltage to each element in the array forming the ultrasound pulse is termed:
    a. subdicing
    b. apodization
    c. dynamic focusing
    d. spatial compounding

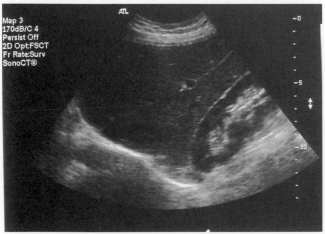

FIG. 3

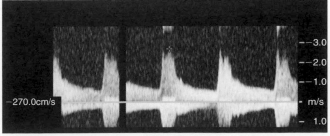

FIG. 4

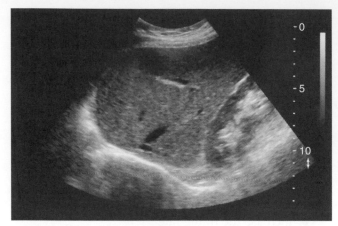

FIG. 5

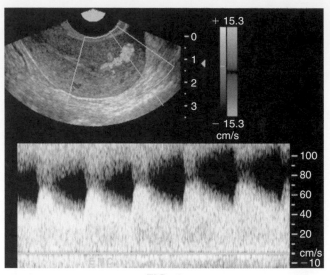

FIG. 6

Using Figure 5, answer question 88.

88. How would the sonographer improve this image using only one operator control?
    a. increase the transducer frequency
    b. decrease the imaging depth
    c. increase the number of focal zones
    d. increase the time gain compensation in the near field

89. The mechanical index is inversely proportional to the:
    a. beam width
    b. acoustic output
    c. acoustic pressure
    d. operating frequency

90. A linear phased array sweeps the ultrasound beam:
    a. electronically, by delayed activation of crystals in the array
    b. mechanically, by sequential activation of crystals in the array
    c. electronically, by sequential rotation of the crystals in the array
    d. electronically, by sequential activation of the crystals in the array

91. Which of the following is a technique most likely used in harmonic imaging?
    a. apodization
    b. pulse inversion
    c. pixel interpolation
    d. spatial compounding

92. Which of the following uses a variable receiving focus?
    a. subdicing
    b. apodization
    c. dynamic aperture
    d. dynamic focusing

Using Figure 6, answer question 93.

93. Which Doppler controls need adjustment in this spectral display?
    a. baseline; Doppler gain
    b. baseline shift; wall filter
    c. invert; baseline
    d. scale; wall filter

94. Which of the following is equal to one-half of the pulse repetition frequency?
    a. Nyquist limit
    b. pulsatility index
    c. Reynolds number
    d. attenuation coefficient

95. Equal intensity for all similar structures regardless of the depth is a function of:
    a. suppression
    b. rectification
    c. compression
    d. compensation

96. Which imaging technique is most likely to visualize structures beneath a highly attenuating structure?
    a. pulse inversion
    b. pixel interpolation
    c. spatial compounding
    d. harmonic frequencies

97. If flow speed increases, pressure energy:
    a. increases
    b. doubles
    c. decreases
    d. remains constant

98. Frequency is proportional to:
   a. period
   b. attenuation
   c. wavelength
   d. penetration depth

Using Figure 7, answer question 99.

99. Which of the following changes will optimize the diagnosis of this sonogram?
   a. increase overall gain
   b. increase imaging depth
   c. increase time gain compensation in the far zone
   d. increase time gain compensation in the near zone

100. What type of blood flow demonstrates a constant speed across the vessel?
   a. plug
   b. laminar
   c. pulsatile
   d. parabolic

101. If the amplitude of a wave doubles, the intensity will:
   a. double
   b. quadruple
   c. decrease by one-half
   d. decrease by one-tenth

102. Structures that have lower amplitude echoes than adjacent tissues are termed:
   a. anechoic
   b. isoechoic
   c. echogenic
   d. hypoechoic

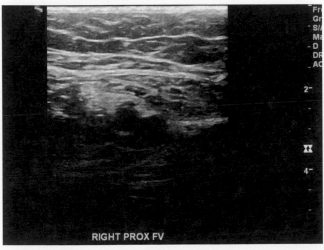

RIGHT PROX FV

FIG. 7

103. For refraction to occur, which of the following must take place?
   a. perpendicular incidence and a change of velocity
   b. perpendicular incidence and a change in impedance
   c. oblique incidence and a change of propagation speed
   d. oblique incidence and a change in the transmission angle

104. Power Doppler imaging displays flow:
   a. rate
   b. presence
   c. direction
   d. characteristics

105. The concentration of scan lines within the field of view directly relates to the:
   a. frame rate
   b. temporal resolution
   c. pulse repetition period
   d. pulse repetition frequency

106. A hydrophone is an instrument used to measure:
   a. cavitation
   b. thermal index
   c. acoustic output
   d. mechanical index

107. A rise in tissue temperature is significant when it exceeds:
   a. 1° C
   b. 2° C
   c. 5° C
   d. 9° C

108. Which of the following separates the received radiofrequencies into sub-bands?
   a. code excitation
   b. pulse inversion
   c. frequency compounding
   d. spatial compounding

109. What artifact displays a series of closely spaced echoes distal to a strong reflector?
   a. speckle
   b. multipath
   c. comet tail
   d. shadowing

110. Angling the color Doppler box to the right or left changes the:
   a. frame rate
   b. flow velocity
   c. Doppler shift
   d. pulse repetition frequency

111. Propagation speed less than that of soft tissue will place reflectors that are too:
    a. deep
    b. medial
    c. lateral
    d. superficial

112. To overcome range ambiguity, the:
    a. imaging depth should be increased
    b. Reynolds number should be reduced
    c. pulse repetition period should be reduced
    d. pulse repetition frequency should be reduced

113. Steering of the sound beam is accomplished by:
    a. reducing the pulse repetition frequency
    b. altering the frequency with increasing depth
    c. emitting pulses from different starting points
    d. altering the electronic excitation of the elements

114. Which of the following techniques provides quantitative data?
    a. amplitude mode
    b. duplex imaging
    c. spectral analysis
    d. color flow imaging

115. Which of the following structures demonstrates the highest attenuation coefficient?
    a. fat
    b. air
    c. liver
    d. muscle

116. The range of frequencies contained in a pulse is termed the:
    a. spectrum
    b. bandwidth
    c. harmonics
    d. resonant frequencies

117. Which of the following frequencies is in the infrasound range?
    a. 10 Hz
    b. 25 Hz
    c. 10 kHz
    d. 25 kHz

118. Which of the following techniques uses separate transmitter and receiver elements?
    a. duplex imaging
    b. motion mode
    c. real-time imaging
    d. continuous wave Doppler

119. The majority of imaging artifacts are likely a result of:
    a. operator error
    b. system assumptions
    c. weakly attenuating structures
    d. strongly attenuating structures

120. Structures within the focal zone may display an improper:
    a. size
    b. location
    c. brightness
    d. resolution

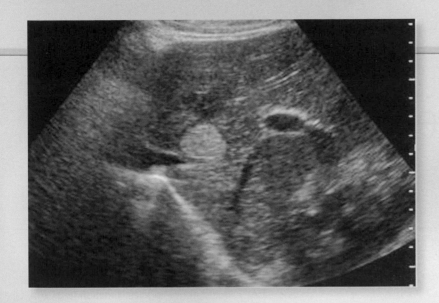

Abdomen

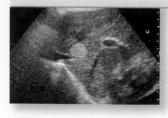

CHAPTER 7

Liver

KEY TERMS

bare area a large triangular area devoid of peritoneal covering located between the two layers of the coronary ligament.

Budd-Chiari syndrome thrombosis of the main hepatic veins.

cavernous hemangioma most common benign neoplasm of the liver consisting of large blood-filled cystic spaces.

cirrhosis irreversible and often progressive parenchymal fibrosis, scarring, and parenchymal necrosis with nodular regeneration.

collateral an accessory blood pathway developed through enlargement of secondary vessels.

Couinaud anatomy divides the liver into eight segments in an imaginary *H* pattern.

echinococcal cyst an infectious cystic disease associated with underdeveloped sheep-herding areas of the world.

fatty infiltration acquired and reversible condition resulting in accumulation of triglycerides in the hepatocytes.

functional lobar–segmental anatomy divides the liver into the right, left, and caudate lobes.

Glisson's capsule thin connective tissue layer covering the liver and portal veins.

hepatofugal blood flowing away from the liver.

hepatopetal blood flowing into the liver.

liver function tests (LFTs) generic term used for the laboratory values determining liver function (e.g., ALT, alkaline phosphatase).

porta hepatis region in the hepatic hilum containing the proper hepatic artery, common duct, and main portal vein.

portal hypertension increased venous pressure in the portal circulation associated with compression or occlusion of the portal or hepatic veins.

shunt a passageway between two natural channels.

stent a tube designed to be inserted in a passageway or vessel to keep it patent.

traditional lobar anatomy divides the liver into the right, left, caudate, and quadrate lobes.

true hepatic cyst congenital cyst formation associated with weakening of the bile duct wall.

varix an enlarged or tortuous vein, artery, or lymph vessel.

PHYSIOLOGY

Functions of the Liver

- Breaks down red blood cells, producing bile pigments.
- Secretes bile into the duodenum through the bile ducts.
- Converts excess amino acids into urea and glucose.
- Manufactures glycogen from glucose and stores it for future use.
- Releases glycogen as glucose.
- Manufactures heparin.
- Regulates blood volume.
- Detoxifies harmful substances absorbed by the intestines.
- Major source of body heat as a result of many hepatocellular chemical reactions.

ANATOMY (Figs. 7.1 and 7.2)

- The liver is the largest solid organ in the body, weighing up to 1800 grams in males and 1400 grams in females.
- It is covered by Glisson's capsule.

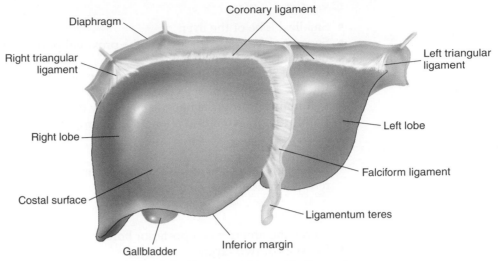

FIG. 7.1 Liver anatomy, anterior surface.

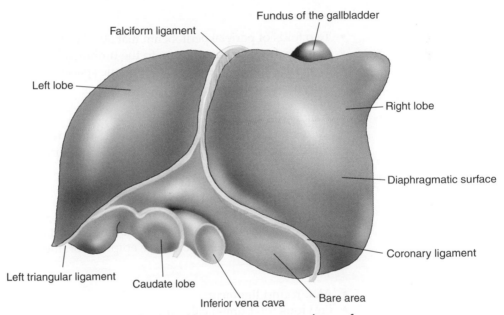

FIG. 7.2 Liver anatomy, posterior surface.

Liver Divisions

Left Lobe
- Divided into medial and lateral segments by the left hepatic vein and ligamentum teres.
- Size is variable.
- Separated from the caudate lobe by the ligamentum venosum.
- Separated from the right lobe by the middle hepatic vein superiorly and the main lobar fissure inferiorly.

Right Lobe
- Divided into the anterior and posterior segments by the right hepatic vein.
- Six times larger than the left lobe.
- Three posterior fossae: gallbladder, porta hepatis, and inferior vena cava.

Caudate Lobe

- Smallest lobe of the liver.
- Separated from the left lobe by the proximal portion of the left hepatic vein and the ligamentum venosum.
- Oxygen-rich blood supplied through the portal veins or hepatic arteries and drains directly into the inferior vena cava (IVC).
- Left margin forms the hepatic boundary of the superior recess of the lesser sac.
- Right margin extends in a tongue-like projection between the IVC and portal vein.

Liver Ligaments

- The liver is attached to the diaphragm, anterior abdominal wall, stomach, and retroperitoneum by ligaments.

Coronary

- Forms the anterior and posterior borders of the bare area.
- Consists of two layers.
- The right and left triangular ligaments are part of the coronary ligament.
- Connects the posterior liver to the diaphragm.

Falciform

- Two folds of parietal peritoneum that attaches the liver to the anterior abdominal wall.
- Extends from the diaphragm to the umbilicus.
- Separates the right and left subphrenic spaces.

Gastrohepatic

- Aka: lesser omentum.
- Connects the lesser curvature of the stomach to the liver.
- Continuous with the ligamentum venosum, first portion of the duodenum, and lesser curvature of the stomach.

Hepatoduodenal

- Connects the liver to the proximal duodenum.
- Surrounds portal triad just proximal to the porta hepatis.
- Forms the anterior border of the epiploic foramen.

Teres

- Aka: round ligament.
- Previous fetal umbilical vein.
- Originates at the umbilicus, connecting with the umbilical portion of the left portal vein.
- Lies within the falciform ligament.

Triangular

- The most lateral portion of the coronary ligament.
- Connects the liver to the body wall.

Venosum

- Separates the left lobe from the caudate lobe of the liver.
- Obliterated fetal ductus venosum.
- Extends from the base of the left portal vein to the IVC.
- Lesser omentum attaches to the liver in the fissure of the ligamentum venosum.

Liver Fissures

Left Intersegmental

- Divides the left lobe of the liver into medial and lateral segments.
- Contains the left hepatic vein, the ligamentum teres, the falciform ligament and the ascending segment of the left portal vein.

Main Lobar

- Divides the right and left lobes of the liver.
- Extends from the right portal vein to the gallbladder fossa.

Right Intersegmental

- Divides the right lobe into anterior and posterior segments.
- Contains the right hepatic vein.

Liver Spaces

Bare Space

- Triangular area located in the posterior aspect of the right lobe of the liver.
- Devoid of peritoneum.
- Attached to the right hemidiaphragm by firm areolar tissue.
- Bound by the coronary and triangular ligaments.

Morison Pouch (Hepatorenal Pouch)

- Located lateral to the right lobe of the liver and anterior to the right kidney.
- Communicates with the right paracolic space.

Subhepatic Space

- Space located between the inferior edge of the right lobe and anterior to the right kidney.

Subphrenic Space

- Space located between the diaphragm and the superior border of the liver.

VASCULAR ANATOMY

Hepatic Arteries

- Proper hepatic artery enters the liver at the porta hepatis and divides into the right and left hepatic arteries.
- Thirty percent of the liver's blood supply is through the hepatic artery.
- Lies medial to the common hepatic duct and anterior to the main portal vein.
- Normal diameter of the proper hepatic artery is 2 to 4 mm.

Hepatic Veins

- Right, middle, and left hepatic veins converge to empty into the inferior vena cava.
  - Left hepatic vein drains the left lobe of the liver.
  - Middle hepatic vein drains the right and medial left lobes of the liver.
  - Right hepatic vein drains the right lobe of the liver.
- Transport deoxygenated blood from the liver cells to the inferior vena cava.
- Course between lobes (interlobar) and between segments (intersegmental).
- Have a minimum amount of collagen in the walls.
- Follow a straight longitudinal course increasing in caliber closer to the diaphragm.

Portal Veins

- Main portal vein begins at the portal-splenic confluence.
- Main portal vein enters the porta hepatis, dividing into the right and left portal veins.
- Left portal vein provides blood to the left lobe and caudate lobe of the liver.
- Left portal vein subdivides into the left medial and left lateral portal veins.
- Right portal vein provides blood to the right lobe and caudate lobe of the liver.
- Right portal vein subdivides into the right anterior and right posterior portal veins.
- Provide approximately 70% to 75% of the liver's total blood volume.
- Portal vein blood is 80% saturated with oxygen, contributing up to one-half of the oxygen to the liver cells.

- Transport nutrient-rich blood from the digestive tract to the liver cells for metabolic processing and storage.
- Tributary veins include the splenic, superior and inferior mesenteric, coronary, pyloric, and paraumbilical veins.
- Are located within the lobes (intralobar) or within the segments (intrasegmental) of the liver.
- Walls contain fibrin.
- Normal diameter of the main portal vein should not exceed 13 mm.

LOCATION

- Liver is an intraperitoneal organ.
- Occupies the major portion of the right hypochondrium.
- Extends inferiorly into the epigastric and laterally into the left hypochondrium.
- Reaches the dome of the diaphragm superiorly.

Left Lobe

- Lies anterior to the porta hepatis, middle hepatic vein, body of the pancreas, splenic artery and vein.
- Located inferior to the diaphragm.
- May extend to the left upper quadrant.

Right Lobe

- Lies anterior to the right kidney.
- Located posterior to the middle hepatic vein.

Caudate Lobe

- Lies anterior to the inferior vena cava between the IVC and the ligamentum venosum.
- Located posterior to the ligamentum venosum and porta hepatis.
- Located lateral to the lesser sac.
- Right margin of the caudate lobe extends between the IVC and portal vein.

Normal Variants

ANOMALY	DESCRIPTION	SONOGRAPHIC FINDINGS	DIFFERENTIAL CONSIDERATIONS
Diaphragmatic slip	Diaphragmatic muscular bundles (slips) connect the central tendon of the diaphragm to the inner aspect of the lower thoracic cage. They cause hepatic invaginations	Linear hyperechoic indentations of the diaphragm that subdivide the liver parenchyma	Artifact
Left lobe variants	Extension into the left upper quadrant. Small left lobe	Extension of the left lobe into the sub-phrenic space or across midline. Left lobe does not extend across the midline. Small left lobe that does not extend across the midline. Echogenicity equal to the liver parenchyma	Splenomegaly Hepatomegaly Splenic neoplasm
Riedel lobe	Extension of the right lobe. Female prevalence	Extension of the right lobe inferior and anterior to the lower pole of the kidney. Echogenicity equal to the liver parenchyma. Left lobe rarely extends across the midline	Hepatomegaly Renal neoplasm

Size

SIZE	ETIOLOGY	CLINICAL FINDINGS	SONOGRAPHIC FINDINGS	DIFFERENTIAL CONSIDERATIONS
Normal adult			Midclavicular level 7–17 cm in length 10–21 cm in height 20–36 cm in width	
Hepatomegaly	Congestive heart failure Inflammatory processes Polycystic disease Fatty infiltration Biliary obstruction Neoplasm Budd-Chiari syndrome	Asymptomatic Right upper quadrant (RUQ) pain Palpable RUQ mass	Length exceeding 16–18 cm	Riedel lobe Left lobe variant Technical error

NORMAL SONOGRAPHIC APPEARANCE

Liver

- Medium shade of gray homogeneous liver parenchyma with moderately hyperechoic portal vein walls.
- Smooth contour.
- Isoechoic to slightly more echogenic than the normal renal cortex and hypoechoic to the normal renal sinus.
- The normal liver parenchyma is generally considered to be isoechoic to hyperechoic to the normal spleen, when in fact the normal adult liver is isoechoic to slightly hypoechoic to the normal spleen. This impression is due to the large number of vessels within the normal liver parenchyma.
- Anechoic tubular structures within the parenchyma representing blood vessels and biliary ducts.
- Main lobar fissure appears as a linear hyperechoic structure extending from the right portal vein to the gallbladder fossa.
- Falciform ligament appears as a hyperechoic sickle-shaped structure in the sagittal plane and a hyperechoic pyramidal structure in the transverse plane.

Bile Ducts

- Anechoic tubular structures coursing through the liver parenchyma.
- Smooth hyperechoic wall margins.
- No internal blood flow.

Hepatic Vein

- Anechoic tubular structures coursing toward the inferior vena cava.
- Caliber increases closer to the inferior vena cava.
- Smooth wall margins.
- Multiphasic hepatofugal blood flow pattern.
- Flow pattern is dependent on the activity of the right atrium of the heart.

Portal Vein

- Anechoic tubular structures coursing from the hepatic hilum through the liver parenchyma.
- Caliber increases closer to the porta hepatis.
- Anterior-posterior diameter approximately 11 mm at the porta hepatis in the adult patient.
- Prominent smooth hyperechoic wall margins.
- Mild phasic hepatopetal blood flow pattern.

- Abnormal pulsatile waveform may be observed in patients with right heart failure, tricuspid regurgitation, fistula between a hepatic and portal vein, and portal hypertension.

Hepatic Artery

- Anechoic tubular structure coursing through the liver parenchyma.
- Smooth wall margins.
- Low-resistance hepatopetal blood flow pattern, demonstrating continuous antegrade flow throughout diastole.
- Right hepatic artery lies between the right portal vein and common hepatic duct.
- Not typically visualized within the liver parenchyma.

EXAMINATION TECHNIQUES, PROTOCOLS, AND IMAGE OPTIMIZATION

Preparation

- No preparation is required before a liver ultrasound.
- If gallbladder and pancreas are to be evaluated patients should fast for:
  - Adult—6 to 8 hours.
  - Children—6 hours.
  - Infants—4 hours.

Transducer Selection

- Use the highest frequency possible to obtain optimal resolution for penetration depth:
  - Adults—3.0 to 5.0 MHz.
  - Children and small adults—5.0 to 7.0 MHz.
  - Obese patients—2.0 MHz may be required.
- Curvilinear transducers provide a wider field of view.
- Sector or vector transducers have a smaller footprint, great for intercostal imaging.
- Linear transducer may be used to demonstrate nodular surface changes of the liver.
- Higher frequency transducers can be used to demonstrate superficial liver lesions.

Patient Positioning

- Examination usually begins with the patient in a supine position.
- Left lateral decubitus, left posterior oblique, and upright positions may be helpful to evaluate the superior portion of the liver as well as alleviate overlying bowel gas.

Examination Protocol

- Systematic approach in the sagittal, coronal, and transverse planes carefully examining and imaging all portions of the liver including:
  - Left, right, and caudate lobes of the liver.
  - Falciform ligament, main lobar fissure.
  - Portal and hepatic venous structures.
  - Intra- and extrahepatic biliary tree.
  - Proper hepatic artery if possible.
- Length measurement of the liver at midclavicular level.
- Anterior-posterior intraluminal diameter measurement of the common ducts.
- Anterior-posterior diameter measurement of the main portal vein.
- Duplex imaging documenting flow type and direction of the main portal vein.
- Abnormalities should be documented and when applicable measured in two imaging planes. Color and/or spectral Doppler evaluation of the abnormality should be included.

Image Optimization

- Place gains settings to display normal liver parenchyma as a medium shade of gray with adjustments to reduce artifactually produce echoes within the hepatic vessels and biliary tree.

- Focal zone(s) should be placed at or below the area of interest. The use of multiple focal zones increases detail resolution and decreases temporal resolution.
- Sufficient imaging depth to visualize structures immediately posterior to the area of interest.
- Harmonic imaging should be used when documenting the biliary tree.
- Decreasing system compression (dynamic range) can be used to reduce artifactual echoes within normal anechoic structures.
- Spatial compounding can be used to improve visualization of structures posterior to highly attenuating structures.
- Doppler settings should be adjusted for the different flow states of the hepatic vasculature.
- Doppler angle should be 60 degrees or less, with a sample volume smaller than the vessel.
- The use of deep inspiration may improve visualization of the liver.
- The use of multiple patient positions may redistribute overlying bowel gas.

Examination Limitations

- Obesity.
- Dense liver parenchyma.
- Superior liver location (high under ribcage).

Helpful Hints

- Main lobar fissure is best visualized in the sagittal oblique plane.
- Hepatic veins are best visualized in the transverse plane with a slight cephalic angulation.
- The right portal vein and the junction of the right and left portal veins are best visualized in the transverse plane.
- The common hepatic artery is best visualized in the transverse plane at the celiac trunk.

Indications for Ultrasound Examination

- Abnormal liver function tests (LFTs).
- Hepatocellular disease.
- Biliary disease.
- Abdominal pain.
- Postprandial pain.
- Palpable liver or spleen.
- Pancreatitis.
- Evaluate mass documented on another imaging modality.

LABORATORY VALUES

Alkaline Phosphatase (ALP)

- Normal adult range 45 to 115 U/L.
- An enzyme produced primarily by the liver, biliary tract, bone, and placenta and in lower concentrations in the intestines and placenta.
- Excreted through the bile ducts.
- Most specific indicator of biliary obstruction.
- May signal bone and liver abnormalities.
- Moderate increase with hepatitis and cirrhosis.

Alpha-Fetoprotein

- A protein normally synthesized by the liver, yolk sac, and GI tract of the fetus.
- A nonspecific marker for malignancy.
- Elevation is associated with hepatocellular carcinoma.

Alanine Aminotransferase (ALT)

- Normal adult range 7 to 35 U/L.
- An enzyme found in high concentration in the liver and lower concentrations in the heart, muscle, and kidneys.
- Remains elevated longer than aspartate aminotransferase (AST).
- More specific than AST.
- Very specific indicator of liver cell destruction.
- Elevation associated with hepatocellular disease, biliary tract obstruction, pancreatitis, and fatty infiltration.
- Mild elevation associated with liver metastasis.

Aspartate Aminotransferase (AST)

- Normal adult 8 to 48 U/L.
- An enzyme present in many kinds of tissue that is released when cells are injured or damaged; levels will be proportional to the amount of damage and the time between cell injury and testing.
- Used to diagnose liver disease before jaundice occurs.
- Elevation associated with cirrhosis, hepatitis, mononucleosis, fatty infiltration, myocardial infarction, muscle disease, and cholestasis.

Bilirubin

- Normal adult total bilirubin ≤1.1 mg/dL.
- Normal adult direct bilirubin ≤0.5 mg/dL.
- A product from the breakdown of hemoglobin in old red blood cells; a disruption in the process may cause abnormal levels; leakage into tissues gives the skin a yellow appearance.
- Reflects the balance between production and excretion of bile.
- Elevated by:
  - An excessive amount of red blood cell destruction.
  - Malfunction of liver cells.
  - Blockage of ducts leading from cells.
- Elevation of direct or conjugated bilirubin is associated with biliary tract obstruction, hepatitis, cirrhosis, cholestasis, and liver metastasis.
- Elevation of indirect or nonconjugated bilirubin is associated with red blood cell destruction, and nonobstructive conditions.

Prothrombin Time

- Normal clotting time is 10 to 15 seconds.
- Enzyme produced by the liver.
- Production depends on amount of vitamin K.
- Elevation associated with cirrhosis, malignancy, malabsorption of vitamin K, and clotting failure.
- Decreases with subacute or acute cholecystitis, internal biliary fistula, carcinoma of the gallbladder, injury to biliary ducts, and prolonged extrahepatic biliary obstruction.

Serum Albumin

- Normal adult 3.5 to 5.0 g/dL.
- Assessment of depressed synthesis of proteins.
- Decrease suggests a decrease in protein synthesis and is associated with hepatocellular disease.

Hepatic Cysts

CYSTS	ETIOLOGY	CLINICAL FINDINGS	SONOGRAPHIC FINDINGS	DIFFERENTIAL CONSIDERATIONS
Cyst	Acquired secondary to parasitic infection, inflammation, or trauma True cyst is caused by a weakening of a bile ductile	Asymptomatic Dull right upper quadrant (RUQ) pain	Anechoic round- or oval-shaped mass Well-defined, smooth wall margins Posterior acoustic enhancement May contain septations or low-level internal echoes	Resolving hematoma Abscess Polycystic disease Cystadenoma Echinococcal cyst Necrotic tumor
Cystadenoma	Benign neoplasm containing cystic structures within the lesion Rare Middle-aged women	Hepatomegaly Palpable RUQ mass	Multiloculated cystic mass Well-defined margins Thin septations demonstrating thin wall margins Thick septations or mural nodules are suspicious for malignancy	Resolving hematoma Hemorrhagic cyst Echinococcal cyst Abscess Adenoma
Peribiliary cyst	Obstructed periductal glands Commonly found in patients with severe liver disease	Asymptomatic	Cluster of 0.2–2.5 mm cysts Cysts parallel bile ducts Located centrally near the junction of the right and left hepatic ducts Large clusters of cysts may obstruct biliary tract	Multiple hepatic cysts Caroli's disease
Polycystic disease (adult)	An inherited disorder Occurs in 1 of 500 Female prevalence Middle age	Asymptomatic Hepatomegaly Palpable RUQ mass RUQ pain Normal liver function tests	Multiple cystic structures within the liver tissue Difficult to distinguish normal liver parenchyma as disease progresses Posterior acoustic enhancement Multiple cysts may also be found in the kidneys (60%), pancreas, and spleen	Multiple simple cysts Necrotic metastasis Cystadenoma

Hepatic Inflammation and Infection

INFLAMMATION/ INFECTION	ETIOLOGY	CLINICAL FINDINGS	SONOGRAPHIC FINDINGS	DIFFERENTIAL CONSIDERATIONS
Abscess, includes: Amebic Fungal Pyogenic	Ascending cholangitis is most common (amebic) Biliary infection Appendicitis Diverticulitis Colitis Direct spread from another organ	Abdominal pain Fever and chills Leukocytosis Elevated alkaline phosphatase Jaundice Hepatomegaly Recent travel abroad	Hypoechoic or complex mass Right lobe is the most common location (80%) Oval or round shape Irregular wall margins Usually solitary Posterior acoustic enhancement	Resolving hematoma Complicated cyst Cavernous hemangioma Echinococcal cyst Metastases
Candidiasis	Fungal infection	Immune-suppressed patients Abdominal pain Fever and chills Palpable liver Leukocytosis	Uniformly hypoechoic lesions within the liver parenchyma Thick wall margins Hepatomegaly May demonstrate a target or "wheel within a wheel" appearance Hyperechoic lesions with posterior acoustic shadowing	Necrotic metastases Resolving hematoma Abscess Cystadenocarcinoma

Continued

Hepatic Inflammation and Infection—(cont'd)

INFLAMMATION/ INFECTION	ETIOLOGY	CLINICAL FINDINGS	SONOGRAPHIC FINDINGS	DIFFERENTIAL CONSIDERATIONS
Echinococcal cyst	Parasite *Echinococcus granulosum* History of sheep-farming exposure Recent travel to underdeveloped countries	Right upper quadrant (RUQ) pain Leukocytosis Fever Hepatomegaly Elevated alkaline phosphatase	Septated cystic mass (honeycomb) Mobile internal echoes (snowflakes) Cyst containing smaller cysts (daughter cysts) Collapsed cyst within a cyst (water lily sign) Round or oval shape Smooth wall margins Calcifications may occur	Complicated liver cyst Resolving abscess Resolving hematoma Cystadenoma
Hepatitis	**Type A** Viral infection Fecal–oral transmission Incubation of 30–40 days **Type B** Viral infection, transmitted by inoculation of infected blood or body fluids Increases risk of developing a hepatoma **Type C** Transmitted via blood to blood contact Increases risk of developing cirrhosis or hepatic neoplasm **Type D** Intravenous drug users Uncommon in North America	Fatigue Loss of appetite Fever and chills Nausea Nonobstructive jaundice Marked elevation in aspartate aminotransferase, alanine aminotransferase Elevated bilirubin Leukopenia	**Acute** Clinical recovery within 4 months Normal-appearing liver parenchyma Hypoechoic liver parenchyma Prominence of the portal veins (star effect) Increase in gallbladder wall thickness Hepatomegaly Associated splenomegaly **Chronic** Symptoms lasting longer than 6 months Coarse echogenic liver parenchyma Decrease in visualization of the portal vein walls Fibrosis may cause soft shadowing Nodular liver contour Associated splenomegaly	**Acute** Normal liver Biliary obstruction **Chronic** Fatty infiltration Cirrhosis
Peliosis hepatitis	Development of necrotic, blood-filled liver spaces communicating with the hepatic veins Rare disorder	Hepatomegaly Occurs in chronically ill patients	Focal or diffuse heterogenous liver masses Calcification	Necrotic metastases Abscess
Schistosomiasis	Parasite entering the skin or mucosa and traveling to the lung and then liver via the lymphatic and venous systems. Symptoms may take 4–6 weeks to appear May even take several years to develop Prevalence in Africa, Egypt, Brazil, and Venezuela	Rash Fever Diarrhea Lymphadenopathy RUQ pain	Increase in echogenicity of the portal walls Thick portal wall margins Atrophy of the right lobe Hypertrophy of the left lobe Thickening of the gallbladder wall Portosystemic collaterals	Hepatitis Cirrhosis Fatty infiltration

Benign Hepatic Conditions

CONDITION	ETIOLOGY	CLINICAL FINDINGS	SONOGRAPHIC FINDINGS	DIFFERENTIAL CONSIDERATIONS
Adenoma	Atypical hepatocytes frequently containing areas of biliary stasis Does not contain Kupffer cells or bile ducts Associated with Type 1 glycogen storage disease Confirmed by contrast enhanced ultrasound, CT or MRI	Asymptomatic Long history of use of oral contraceptives Normal labs Palpable mass Right upper quadrant (RUQ) pain	Solid hypoechoic mass Hypoechoic halo Echogenicity can vary with hemorrhage or necrosis Peripheral and central vascular flow	Cavernous hemangioma Focal nodular hyperplasia Hepatoma Abscess
Cavernous hemangioma	Benign congenital neoplasm consisting of large blood-filled cystic spaces Female prevalence Most common benign liver mass Typically located in the right lobe	Asymptomatic RUQ pain	Homogeneous hyperechoic mass Well-defined wall margins Round or oval in shape Enlarge slowly Complex echo pattern from hemorrhage or necrosis Internal blood flow is slow and not routinely demonstrated Larger hemangioma may demonstrate posterior acoustic enhancement	Focal nodular hyperplasia Adenoma Hepatoma Metastases
Cirrhosis	Alcoholism and chronic hepatitis C are the most common cause in the United States Hepatitis B most common worldwide Biliary obstruction Viral hepatitis Budd-Chiari syndrome Nutritional deficiencies Cardiac disease	Weakness and fatigue Weight loss Abdominal pain Ascites Elevated aspartate aminotransferase, alanine amino-transferase, and bilirubin Skin changes and hair loss Nonobstructive jaundice	Diffuse increase in parenchymal echogenicity Irregular nodular contour (nodules greater than 10 mm considered premalignant) Inability to distinguish portal vein wall margins Increase in sound attenuation Enlargement of the caudate lobe Splenomegaly Ascites Abnormal flow pattern in the hepatic veins	Fatty infiltration Diffuse metastases

Continued

Benign Hepatic Conditions—(cont'd)

CONDITION	ETIOLOGY	CLINICAL FINDINGS	SONOGRAPHIC FINDINGS	DIFFERENTIAL CONSIDERATIONS
Fatty infiltration Steatosis	Obesity Diabetes Cirrhosis Hepatitis Alcohol abuse Hyperlipidemia Corticosteroid therapy Metabolic disorder Ulcerative colitis	Asymptomatic Elevated liver function tests Hepatomegaly	**Mild** Minimal amount of diffuse increase in echogenicity of the liver parenchyma Normal visualization of the hepatic vessels and diaphragm **Moderate** Moderate amount of diffuse increase in echogenicity of the liver parenchyma Slight impaired visualization of the hepatic vessels and diaphragm **Severe** Marked increase in echogenicity of the liver parenchyma Poor penetration of the posterior portion of the liver Poor visualization of the hepatic vessels and diaphragm. **Fat Sparing** Areas of normal liver parenchyma appearing hypoechoic to the hyperechoic fatty liver. Most common areas of fat sparing are adjacent to the inferior vena cava (IVC), gallbladder fossa, anterior to the porta hepatis and along the liver margins	Cirrhosis Chronic hepatitis Metastases Glycogen storage disease
Focal nodular hyperplasia	Abnormal hepatocytes containing Kupffer cells and bile ducts. Hormone influence Congenital vascular malformation Second most common benign liver mass	Asymptomatic	Hyperechoic or isoechoic liver mass Well-defined wall margins Subcapsular location Hypoechoic central stellate scar Well-developed peripheral and central blood flow with larger arterial feeding vessels. Displacement of hepatic vessels Frequently found in the right lobe	Adenoma Cavernous hemangioma Metastases
Glycogen storage disease	Autosomal recessive disorder Usually found in infancy Excessive deposition of glycogen in the liver, kidneys, and GI tract Type I—Von Gierke disease is the most common and typically affects the liver Type II—Pompe disease typically affects the skeletal muscle and heart	Hepatomegaly Impaired growth Kidney failure Hypoglycemia Bruising Osteoporosis Cardiomegaly with congestive heart failure Muscle wasting	Marked diffuse increase in echogenicity of the liver parenchyma Increase in acoustic attenuation Hepatomegaly Solid liver masses Associated with nephromegaly, liver adenoma, and focal nodular hyperplasia	Fatty infiltration Cirrhosis Focal nodular hyperplasia

Benign Hepatic Conditions—(cont'd)

CONDITION	ETIOLOGY	CLINICAL FINDINGS	SONOGRAPHIC FINDINGS	DIFFERENTIAL CONSIDERATIONS

Hemangioendothelioma	Infantile hemangioma
	Most common symptomatic vascular tumor in infancy occurring before 6 months of age (85%)
	Female prevalence
	Complications:
	  Thrombocytopenia
	  Angiopathic anemia
	  Gastrointestinal bleeding
	  Intraabdominal rupture
		Abdominal mass
		Congestive heart failure
			Multiple hypoechoic lesions varying in size from 1–3 cm
			Echogenicity may vary
			Multiple peripheral vessels
			Usually grow rapidly and regress slowly
			Large draining veins with dilated proximal abdominal aorta with arteriovenous shunting
				Hepatoblastoma
				Abscess

Hemochromatosis	Rare disease characterized by excess iron deposits throughout the body May cause cirrhosis	Fatigue Shortness of breath Heart palpitations Chronic abdominal pain	Hepatomegaly Uniform increase in parenchymal echogenicity	Fatty infiltration Cirrhosis
Mesenchymal hamartoma	Rare lesion occurring in children less than 2 years of age Developmental unencapsulated cystic tumor Disordered arrangement of bile ducts, hepatic parenchyma, and primitive mesoderm	Diffuse abdominal distension Palpable abdominal mass	Well-defined large complex mass Predominantly anechoic Lacelike configuration If cysts are tiny, may appear as a solid mass	Hepatoblastoma Abscess

Malignant Hepatic Neoplasms

MALIGNANCY	ETIOLOGY	CLINICAL FINDINGS	SONOGRAPHIC FINDINGS	DIFFERENTIAL CONSIDERATIONS
Hemangiosarcoma	Exposure to arsenic, polyvinyl, and Thorotrast Adults between 60 and 70 years of age	Abdominal pain Loss of appetite Lethargy	Heterogeneous, hyperechoic mass Cystic mass with internal septation Metastatic lesions to the portal vein, spleen, lungs, lymph nodes, thyroid, and peritoneal cavity Internal blood flow	Hepatoblastoma Degenerating cavernous hemangioma Resolving hematoma Cystadenocarcinoma
Hepatoblastoma	Germ cell tumor Most common malignant tumor in children 3 years old or less Associated with Beckwith-Wiedemann syndrome, sporadic aniridia, hemihypertrophy, and precocious puberty	Abdominal distension Nausea/vomiting Weight loss Precocious puberty Marked elevation of alpha-fetoprotein	Heterogeneous, hyperechoic mass Cystic mass with internal septations High velocity, low resistance internal arterial blood flow	Metastases Focal nodular hyperplasia

Continued

Malignant Hepatic Neoplasms—(cont'd)

MALIGNANCY	ETIOLOGY	CLINICAL FINDINGS	SONOGRAPHIC FINDINGS	DIFFERENTIAL CONSIDERATIONS
Hepatocellular carcinoma (hepatoma)	Cirrhosis (80%) Chronic hepatitis B and C Exposure to carcinogens in food or environment Metabolic disorder Steatohepatitis Male prevalence	Palpable mass Abdominal pain Weight loss Unexplained fever Elevated alanine aminotransferase (ALT), aspartate aminotransferase (AST), and alkaline phosphatase Positive alpha-fetoprotein Jaundice	Solid mass with variable echogenicity May demonstrate a hypoechoic halo Multiple nodules or diffuse infiltrative masses may also be demonstrated Hepatomegaly Ascites High velocity blood flow May invade portal or hepatic veins	Metastases Abscess Cavernous hemangioma Adenoma Cirrhosis
Metastases	Gastrointestinal with the majority from colon Pancreas Breast Lung Renal cell carcinoma	Hepatomegaly Right upper quadrant (RUQ) pain Weight loss Loss of appetite Jaundice Increase in AST, ALT, and direct bilirubin Mild increase in alkaline phosphatase	Bull's-eye or target lesion Hypoechoic masses Hyperechoic masses Cystic masses with a hypoechoic halo Complex masses Diffuse heterogenous echogenicity Calcifications may occur	Nodular cirrhosis Fatty infiltration Multiple cavernous hemangiomas Hepatomas Complicated hepatic cysts

Hepatic Vascular Abnormalities

VASCULAR CONDITION	ETIOLOGY	CLINICAL FINDINGS	SONOGRAPHIC FINDINGS	DIFFERENTIAL CONSIDERATIONS
Budd-Chiari syndrome	Hepatoma Tumor extension (renal or liver) Hematologic disorder Congenital webbing of IVC or right atrium	Abdominal pain Abdominal distension Hepatomegaly Lower-extremity edema Mild increase in alkaline phosphatase Use of oral contraceptives	Hypoechoic intraluminal echoes in the hepatic veins (thrombus) Dilated hepatic veins Vein wall thickening Absence of or altered hepatic venous flow Hepatomegaly Enlarged caudate lobe Splenomegaly Ascites Hyperechoic liver parenchyma Thrombosis in the portal veins	Cirrhosis Portal vein thrombosis Technical error

Hepatic Vascular Abnormalities—(cont'd)

VASCULAR CONDITION	ETIOLOGY	CLINICAL FINDINGS	SONOGRAPHIC FINDINGS	DIFFERENTIAL CONSIDERATIONS
Cavernous transformation of the portal vein	Chronic portal vein thrombosis and occlusion with collateral formation	Abdominal distension Splenomegaly	Loss of normal extrahepatic portal vein Multiple anechoic tortuous collateral veins at a distorted porta hepatis Increase flow in proper hepatic artery	Tortuous gallbladder neck/cystic duct
Portal hypertension	**Presinusoidal** Tumor invasion Thrombosis of portal circulation **Intrahepatic** Cirrhosis (95%) Hepatitis Fatty infiltration Metabolic disorders **Posthepatic** Thrombosis of the hepatic veins or IVC	Splenomegaly Hepatomegaly Increase in liver function tests Hematemesis Jaundice Abdominal distension	Intrinsic liver disease Main portal vein diameter exceeding 13 mm Splenomegaly Ascites Splenic and superior mesenteric vein exceeding 10 mm Changes in portal venous blood flow a. hepatofugal b. pulsatile c. decrease in velocity Portosystemic collaterals Resistive index exceeding 0.8 in the hepatic artery implies portal hypertension	Cirrhosis Budd-Chiari syndrome Portal vein thrombosis
Portal vein thrombosis	Hepatoma or liver metastasis Sepsis Blood coagulation disorders Cirrhosis Idiopathic	Severe abdominal pain Loss of appetite Hematemesis Encephalopathy	**Acute** Hypoechoic intraluminal echoes in the portal vein(s) Increase in portal vein diameter Prominence of the intrahepatic arteries Absence or altered portal venous blood flow **Chronic** Numerous collateral vessels at the porta hepatis (cavernous transformation) Thrombosed vein may recanalize or remain chronically occluded	Budd-Chiari syndrome Cirrhosis Technical error

Continued

Hepatic Vascular Abnormalities—(cont'd)

VASCULAR CONDITION	ETIOLOGY	CLINICAL FINDINGS	SONOGRAPHIC FINDINGS	DIFFERENTIAL CONSIDERATIONS
Transjugular intrahepatic portosystemic shunt (TIPS)	A shunt is placed between a portal vein and a hepatic vein to reduce pressure in the portal system Commonly placed between the right portal vein and the right hepatic vein Complications include hepatic vein stenosis, stent occlusion, and stent stenosis	Asymptomatic Symptoms may vary with underlying liver disease	**Normal Gray Scale** Brightly echogenic, nonshadowing tubular structure Generally, connects the right portal vein to the right hepatic vein Stent should measure 8–12 mm in diameter throughout **Abnormal Gray Scale** Diameter less than 8 mm New onset of ascites **Normal Doppler** Turbulent hepatopetal flow in main portal vein at 20–60 cm/s Hepatofugal flow in right and left portal veins Peak flow velocity within stent ranges from 65–225 cm/s Velocity and flow direction should be evaluated and documented in three places along the stent. **Abnormal Doppler** Elevated velocity within the stent Velocity within the stent less than 60 cm/s Decrease in main portal vein velocity Retrograde flow within the stent	Technical error

Portal Hypertension Collaterals and Portal Caval Shunts

- In an effort to relieve the portal system pressure, collateral veins are formed that connect to the systemic veins.

COLLATERAL	DESCRIPTION
Coronary vein	Located in the midepigastric area superior to the portosplenic junction
Gastroesophageal	Located posterior to the left lobe of the liver near the gastroesophageal junction Tends to rupture and cause internal bleeding
Mesoenterocaval	Detection of retrograde flow in the superior mesenteric vein implies mesoenterocaval shunting Collaterals in the pelvis
Paraumbilical vein	Courses within the falciform ligament from the left portal vein to the umbilicus Hepatofugal flow
Splenorenal	Shunts blood from the splenic vein to the left renal vein Associated with enlargement of the left renal vein
Portal Caval Shunts Mesocaval	Surgical attachment of the mid to distal portion of the superior mesenteric vein to the inferior vena cava
Portacaval	Surgical attachment of the main portal vein at the portosplenic confluence to the anterior aspect of the inferior vena cava
Splenorenal	Surgical removal of the spleen with anastomosis of the splenic vein to the left renal vein

HEPATIC TRANSPLANT

- Hepatic artery provides the *only* blood supply to the biliary tree.
- Liver function tests are best indicators of rejection.

Preoperative Protocol

- Measure the diameter of the portal vein and hepatic artery.
- Document patency of the portal and hepatic veins, superior mesenteric vein, hepatic artery, and the inferior vena cava.
- Evaluate for portosystemic collaterals.
- Measure the length of the spleen.
- Evaluate liver and biliary tree for pathology.
- Evaluate abdominal cavity for ascites.

Postoperative Complications

- **Hepatic artery thrombosis**—most common and most serious complication in the first 6 weeks; increase in resistive index (RI).
- **Hepatic artery stenosis**—typically at anastomoses; normal peak systolic velocity may be as high as 250 cm/s; RI less than 0.5; prolonged systolic acceleration time.
- **Infection or fluid collections**—abscess, ascites, biloma, hematoma, lymphocele, and seroma.
- **Portal vein stenosis**—caused by folding or kinking at the anastomoses; peak systolic velocity greater than 100 cm/s.
- **Portal vein thrombosis**—associated with acute rejection; hepatic artery RI equal or less than 0.5.

Normal Sonographic Findings

- Homogeneous to slightly heterogeneous liver parenchyma.
- The hepatic artery should demonstrate a low resistance waveform with a rapid systolic upstroke.
- Resistive index of the proper hepatic artery should range between 0.5 and 0.7.

Abnormal Sonographic Findings

- Heterogeneous or hypoechoic liver parenchyma.
- Intrahepatic biliary dilatation.
- Prolonged systolic acceleration time of the hepatic artery.
- Resistive index of the proper hepatic artery should range less than 0.5.

LIVER REVIEW

1. In a post-liver transplant patient, the hepatic artery should demonstrate:
   a. a sharp systolic downstroke
   b. retrograde flow in early diastole
   c. a sharp systolic upstroke
   d. a high resistance waveform

2. Sonographic findings commonly associated with portal hypertension include which of the following?
   a. hypoechoic liver parenchyma and gastric varices
   b. splenomegaly and hepatofugal flow in the main portal vein
   c. hyperechoic liver parenchyma and hepatopetal flow in the main portal vein
   d. splenomegaly and decreased resistance in the proper hepatic artery.

3. Gain settings should be placed to demonstrate the normal liver:
   a. as a medium shade of gray
   b. hypoechoic to the spleen
   c. hyperechoic to the pancreas
   d. hyperechoic to the renal sinus

4. A hepatic cavernous hemangioma most commonly appears on ultrasound as a(n):
   a. complex mass
   b. hyperechoic mass
   c. isoechoic mass
   d. hypoechoic mass

5. Which of the following ligaments separates the left lobe from the caudate lobe of the liver?
   a. coronary
   b. falciform
   c. venosum
   d. hepatoduodenal

6. The most common cause of cirrhosis in the United States is:
   a. hepatitis B
   b. anorexia nervosa
   c. alcohol abuse
   d. biliary obstruction

7. Which of the following symptoms in not associated with hepatocellular carcinoma?
   a. weight loss
   b. abdominal pain
   c. unexplained fever
   d. elevated serum albumin

8. In the United States, a hepatic abscess is most likely to develop in which of the following conditions?
   a. acute pancreatitis
   b. biliary obstruction
   c. ascending cholangitis
   d. Budd-Chiari syndrome

9. Which of the following structures separate the left lobe of the liver from the right lobe?
   a. left hepatic vein and main lobar fissure
   b. middle hepatic vein and ligamentum venosum
   c. middle hepatic vein and main lobar fissure
   d. left hepatic vein and right intersegmental fissure

10. The right lobe of the liver is divided into anterior and posterior segments by the:
    a. main portal vein
    b. right portal vein
    c. right hepatic vein
    d. middle hepatic vein

11. An accumulation of triglycerides in the hepatocytes is found in which of the following?
    a. hepatic steatosis
    b. cavernous hemangioma
    c. glycogen storage disease
    d. focal nodular hyperplasia

12. Patients with a history of hepatitis B have a predisposing risk factor for developing:
    a. an adenoma
    b. a hepatoma
    c. focal nodular hyperplasia
    d. a cavernous hemangioma

13. "Daughter cysts" are associated with which of the following pathologies?
    a. adenoma
    b. fungal abscess
    c. cystadenoma
    d. echinococcal cyst

14. Which of the following hepatic structures is interlobar in location?
    a. hepatic artery
    b. portal vein
    c. hepatic vein
    d. biliary duct

15. The normal blood flow pattern in the main portal vein is described as:
    a. phasic
    b. pulsatile
    c. hepatofugal
    d. continuous

Using Figure 7.3, answer questions 16 and 17.

16. The hypoechoic area documented in the sonogram most likely represents:
    a. nodular fibrosis
    b. a lymph node
    c. a malignant lesion
    d. normal liver tissue

17. The hepatic pathology demonstrated in this sonogram most likely represents:
    a. cirrhosis
    b. lymphoma
    c. fatty infiltration
    d. liver metastasis

Using Figure 7.4, answer question 18.

18. The abnormality demonstrated in this sonogram most likely represents:
    a. an adenoma
    b. a hematoma
    c. a cavernous hemangioma
    d. focal nodular hyperplasia

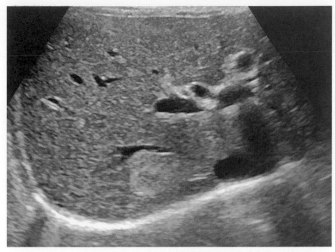

FIG. 7.4 Transverse liver.

Using Figure 7.5, answer question 19.

19. The finding in this duplex image of the porta hepatis is most commonly associated with which of the following conditions?
    a. hepatitis
    b. portal hypertension
    c. Budd-Chiari syndrome
    d. portal vein thrombosis

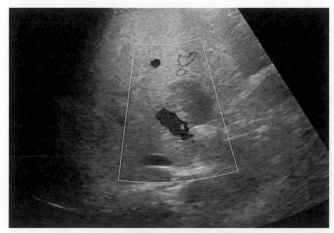

FIG. 7.3 Transverse liver.

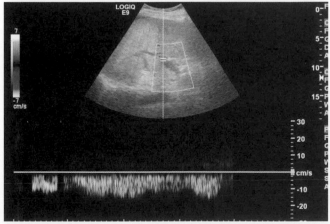

FIG. 7.5 Duplex sonogram of the main portal vein.

Using Figure 7.6, answer question 20.

20. The arrow identifies which of the following hepatic lobes?
    a. caudate lobe
    b. lateral left lobe
    c. medial left lobe
    d. anterior right lobe

Using Figure 7.7, answer question 21.

21. This sonogram of the right lobe of the liver is most likely demonstrating which of the following conditions?
    a. hepatitis
    b. cirrhosis
    c. Riedel lobe
    d. hepatomegaly

Using Figure 7.8, answer questions 22 and 23.

22. The mass identified in this sonogram is most consistent with a(n):
    a. biloma
    b. simple cyst
    c. resolving hematoma
    d. echinococcal cyst

23. Which of the following pathologies is also demonstrated in the sonogram?
    a. cholecystitis
    b. choledocholithiasis
    c. cholelithiasis
    d. cavernous hemangioma

24. Which of the following liver pathologies is associated with immune-suppressed patients?
    a. adenoma
    b. candidiasis
    c. echinococcal cyst
    d. polycystic disease

25. Metastatic lesions involving the liver most commonly originate from a primary malignancy of the:
    a. pancreas
    b. colon
    c. stomach
    d. gallbladder

26. Which of the following ligaments serves as a barrier between the subphrenic space and Morison pouch?
    a. falciform
    b. coronary
    c. gastrohepatic
    d. hepatoduodenal

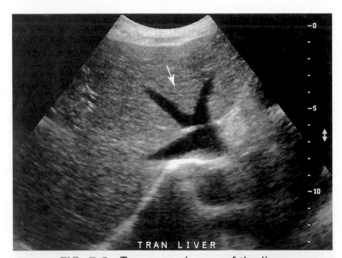

FIG. 7.6 Transverse image of the liver.

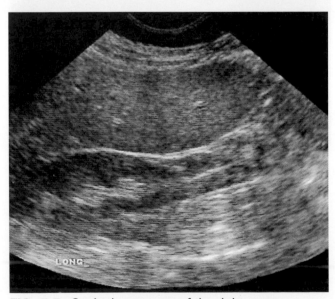

FIG. 7.7 Sagittal sonogram of the right upper quadrant.

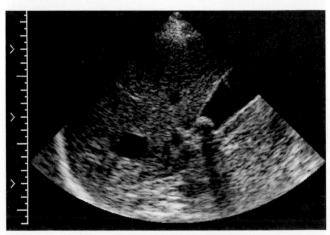

FIG. 7.8 Right upper quadrant.

27. An abnormally enlarged or dilated vein is most commonly termed a(n):
    a. shunt
    b. varix
    c. aneurysm
    d. perforator

28. Traditional lobar anatomy divides the liver into:
    a. three lobes
    b. four lobes
    c. six lobes
    d. eight lobes

29. Severe insult to the liver cells leading to subsequent necrosis describes:
    a. cirrhosis
    b. portal hypertension
    c. Budd-Chiari syndrome
    d. focal nodular hyperplasia

30. Von Gierke disease is most commonly associated with:
    a. cirrhosis
    b. schistosomiasis
    c. glycogen storage disease
    d. focal nodular hyperplasia

31. Prominence of the portal veins is most commonly associated with which of the following pathologies?
    a. cirrhosis
    b. hepatitis
    c. polycystic disease
    d. glycogen storage disease

32. A transjugular intrahepatic portosystemic shunt (TIPS) is commonly placed between the:
    a. right hepatic vein and the right portal vein
    b. middle hepatic vein and the inferior vena cava
    c. right portal vein and the inferior vena cava
    d. left portal vein and the inferior vena cava

33. The paraumbilical vein courses from the umbilicus to the:
    a. left hepatic vein
    b. superior mesenteric vein
    c. middle hepatic vein
    d. left portal vein

34. The right hepatic artery lies between the:
    a. main portal vein and common bile duct
    b. right portal vein and common hepatic duct
    c. left portal vein and common hepatic duct
    d. right portal vein and common bile duct

35. Which of the following spaces is located superior to the liver and inferior to the diaphragm?
    a. pleura
    b. lesser sac
    c. subhepatic space
    d. subphrenic space

36. Enlargement of the caudate lobe is most commonly associated with which of the following pathologies?
    a. cirrhosis
    b. candidiasis
    c. fatty infiltration
    d. portal hypertension

37. On spectral Doppler, the hepatic veins are characterized by which of the following flow types?
    a. laminar
    b. parabolic
    c. multiphasic
    d. turbulent

38. Which of the following ligaments attaches the liver to the anterior abdominal wall?
    a. venosum
    b. falciform
    c. triangular
    d. right coronary ligament

Using Figure 7.9 and Color Plate 3, answer question 39.

39. A transverse duplex image of the liver displays:
    a. normal portal venous flow
    b. normal hepatic venous flow
    c. normal and abnormal portal venous flow
    d. normal and abnormal hepatic venous flow

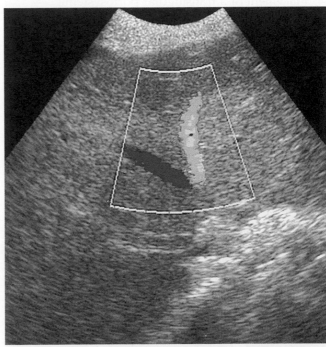

FIG. 7.9   Sagittal image of the liver (see Color Plate 3).

40. Which of the following most accurately describes the location of the caudate lobe?
   a. medial to the lesser sac
   b. posterior to the inferior vena cava
   c. posterior to the porta hepatis
   d. lateral to the inferior vena cava

Using Figure 7.10 and Color Plate 4, answer question 41.

41. This color Doppler image of the left upper quadrant is most suspicious for:
   a. flash artifact
   b. gastric varices
   c. bowel peristalsis
   d. abdominal aortic aneurysm

42. Decreases in prothrombin time are associated with which of the following?
   a. cirrhosis
   b. clotting failure
   c. acute cholecystitis
   d. malabsorption of vitamin K

43. The most common symptom associated with acute thrombosis of the portal veins is:
   a. weight loss
   b. tachycardia
   c. severe abdominal pain
   d. lower-extremity edema

44. Placement of a transjugular portosystemic shunt (TIPS) will normally result in which of the following?
   a. phasic flow in the main portal vein
   b. hepatopetal flow in the right portal vein
   c. hepatofugal flow in the left portal vein
   d. slow flow velocities with the shunt

Using Figure 7.11, answer question 45.

45. A 30-year-old female patient presents to the ultrasound department with postprandial pain. The patient has been taking oral contraceptives for 10 years. Based on this clinical history and sonogram, the mass is most suspicious for:
   a. an adenoma
   b. a hepatoma
   c. a cavernous hemangioma
   d. focal nodular hyperplasia

Using Figure 7.12, answer questions 46 and 47.

46. The sonographic findings are most consistent with which of the following pathologies?
   a. cirrhosis
   b. fatty infiltration
   c. candidiasis
   d. liver metastasis

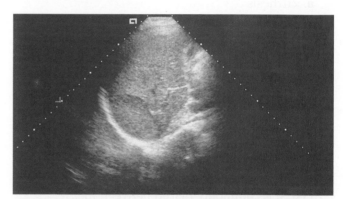

FIG. 7.11   Transverse sonogram of the liver.

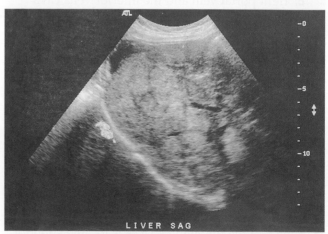

FIG. 7.12   Sagittal sonogram of the liver.

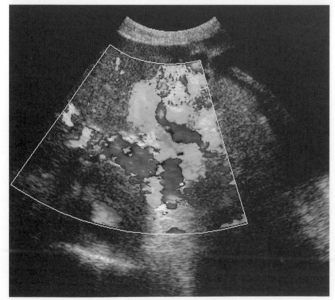

FIG. 7.10   Doppler image of the left upper quadrant (see Color Plate 4).

47. The fluid collection identified in this image is located in which of the following spaces?
    a. right pleura
    b. subhepatic space
    c. right paracolic gutter
    d. right subphrenic space

Using Figure 7.13, answer question 48.

48. What pathology is identified is this sonogram?
    a. choledochal cyst
    b. simple hepatic cyst
    c. abnormal lymph node
    d. hepatic artery aneurysm

Using Figure 7.14, answer question 49.

49. Which of the following ligaments is demonstrated in this transverse image of the liver?
    a. coronary
    b. venosum
    c. falciform
    d. triangular

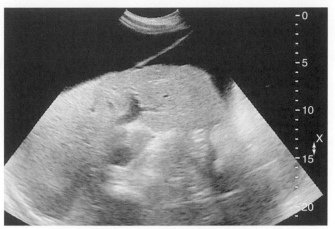

FIG. 7.14 Transverse liver.

Using Figure 7.15, answer question 50.

50. The sonogram is most suspicious for which of the following pathologies?
    a. candidiasis
    b. acute hepatitis
    c. fatty infiltration
    d. portal vein thrombosis

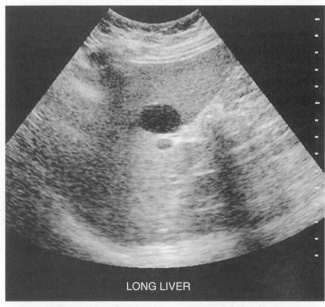

FIG. 7.13 Sagittal sonogram of the liver.

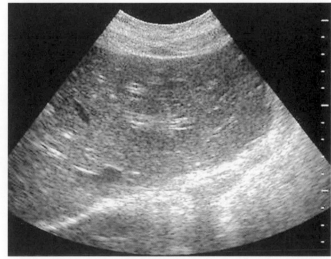

FIG. 7.15 Transverse liver.

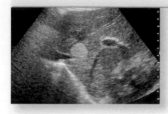

CHAPTER 8

Biliary System

KEY TERMS

adenoma   a benign epithelial tumor; histologically similar to a bowel wall polyp; most common benign neoplasm.

adenomyomatosis   hyperplasia of epithelial and muscle layers in the gallbladder wall; a small polypoid mass of the gallbladder wall; diverticulosis of the gallbladder.

ampulla of Vater   opening in the duodenum for the entrance of the common bile duct.

ascariasis   infection by a roundworm that may result in abdominal cramping or obstruction.

bile   a fluid secreted by the liver, concentrated in the gallbladder, and poured into the small intestine via the bile ducts; plays a role in emulsification, absorption, and digestion of fats.

bilirubin   yellow pigment in bile formed by the breakdown of red blood cells.

biliary atresia   partial or complete absence of the biliary system.

biliary colic   visceral pain associated with passing of stone(s) through the bile ducts; also called cholecystalgia.

biloma   an extrahepatic collection of extravasated bile from trauma, surgery, or gallbladder disease.

Bouveret syndrome   gastric outlet obstruction caused by duodenal impaction of a large stone that has migrated through a cholecystoduodenal fistula.

Caroli disease   a segmental, saccular, or beaded appearance to the intrahepatic biliary ducts.

Charcot triad   fever, chills, and jaundice.

cholangitis   inflammation of a bile duct.

cholangiocarcinoma   carcinoma of a bile duct.

cholecystitis   inflammation of the gallbladder.

cholecystokinin   a hormone secreted in the small intestine that stimulates gallbladder contraction and secretion of pancreatic enzymes; stimulation occurs after food reaches the duodenum.

choledochal cyst   cystic dilatation of the common bile duct.

choledocholithiasis   calculus in the common duct; stones contain bile pigments, bile calcium salts, and cholesterol.

cholelithiasis   the presence or formation of gallstones; stones contain cholesterol, calcium bilirubinate, and calcium carbonate.

cholesterolosis   a form of hyperplastic cholecystosis caused by the accumulation of triglycerides and esterified sterols in the macrophage of the gallbladder wall.

cholesterosis   type of cholesterolosis associated with a strawberry appearance to the gallbladder.

chronic cholecystitis   recurrent attacks of acute cholecystitis.

clonorchiasis   parasite that typically resides in the intrahepatic ducts; the gallbladder and pancreas may also be affected.

common duct   term used to include the extrahepatic common hepatic duct and common bile duct.

Courvoisier sign   painless jaundice associated with an enlarged gallbladder caused by the obstruction of the distal common bile duct by an external mass (typically adenocarcinoma of the pancreatic head).

cystic duct   small duct that drains the gallbladder.

emphysematous cholecystitis   gas in the gallbladder wall or lumen.

empyema   pus in the gallbladder.

hematobilia   bleeding into the biliary tree associated with liver biopsy, blunt trauma, or rupture of a hepatic artery aneurysm.

Hartmann pouch   small posterior pouch near the gallbladder neck.

jaundice   yellowish discoloration of the skin or sclera related to an increased level of bilirubin in the blood. Obstructive jaundice is caused by an obstruction along the biliary tree. Nonobstructive jaundice is cuased by hepatic dysfunction, or hematologic or metabolic abnormalities.

junctional fold   fold or septation of the gallbladder at the junction of the neck and body.

Klatskin tumor   carcinoma located at the junction of the right and left hepatic ducts.

main lobar fissure   a hyperechoic line extending from the right portal vein to the gallbladder fossa; a boundary between the left and right lobes of the liver.

Mirizzi syndrome   impacted stone in the cystic duct causing compression on the common hepatic duct resulting in jaundice, recurrent cholangitis, formation of biliary fistulas, or cholangitis cirrhosis.

parallel channeling   condition in biliary obstruction representing imaging of the dilated hepatic duct and adjacent portal vein.

phrygian cap   fold in the gallbladder fundus.

pneumobilia   air in the biliary tree.

polyp   a soft tissue mass protruding from the gallbladder wall.

KEY TERMS—cont'd

porcelain gallbladder   complete or partial calcification of the gallbladder wall.

positive Murphy sign   Severe pain when pressure is increased over the gallbladder.

sludge   echogenic viscous bile associated with biliary stasis.

sludgeball   mobile, echogenic, nonshadowing mass in the dependent portion of the gallbladder.

tumefactive sludge   echogenic bile that does not layer evenly; resembles a polypoid mass.

WES sign   wall-echo-shadow sign; "double arc" sign; seen with a stone-filled gallbladder.

BILIARY SYSTEM

Functions of the Biliary System

- Transport bile to the gallbladder through the bile ducts.
- Store and concentrate bile in the gallbladder.
- Transport bile through the bile ducts to the duodenum.

BILIARY ANATOMY (Fig. 8.1)

Bile Ducts

- The biliary system originates in the liver as a series of ductules coursing between the liver cells.
- Biliary ducts are subdivided into intrahepatic and extrahepatic ducts.
- Intrahepatic ducts follow the course of the portal veins and hepatic arterial branches.
- The main right and left hepatic ducts lie anterior to the corresponding portal venous trunk.
- Extrahepatic ducts include the cystic and common ducts.
- Bile from the liver reaches the gallbladder through the hepatic and cystic ducts.
- Bile flows if intraductal pressure is lower than the hepatic secretory pressure. Pressure differences are affected by the activity of the sphincter of Oddi, filling and resorption of the bile in the gallbladder, and the bile flow from the liver.

Common Hepatic Duct

- The right and left hepatic ducts join near the level of the porta hepatis, forming the common hepatic duct (CHD).
- Located anterior to the proper hepatic artery, portal vein, and inferior vena cava
- Located inferior to the right and left hepatic ducts.

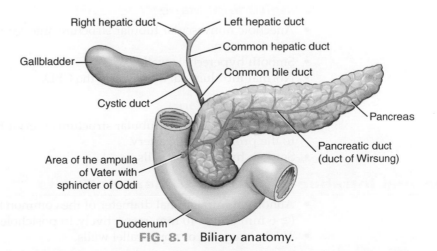

FIG. 8.1   Biliary anatomy.

Cystic Duct

- Drains the gallbladder.
- Variable configuration and length. An average length of 4 cm has been reported at surgery.
- Postcholecystectomy, the cystic duct remnant is variable and may measure up 1 to 2 cm in length.
- Contains the spiral valves of Heister.
- Courses posterior and inferiorly merging with the CHD to form the common bile duct (CBD).
- Located anterior to the main portal vein and inferior to the common hepatic duct.
- Difficult to visualized on ultrasound.

Common Bile Duct

- The CHD is joined by the cystic duct to form the CBD.
- Courses posterior and inferiorly, joining the main pancreatic duct at the ampulla of Vater to enter the descending portion (second portion) of the duodenum.
- Lies anterior to the main portal vein and lateral to the proper hepatic artery.

Size of the Normal Bile Duct

- Average intraluminal diameter of the CHD is less than 5 mm and should not exceed 6 mm in adults.
- Average intraluminal diameter of the CBD is 6 mm in diameter or less in adults.
- Starting at age 60, the CBD may increase in diameter by 1 mm per decade.
- Postcholecystectomy patients may demonstrate a slight increase in diameter but should not exceed 10 mm.
- Average intraluminal diameter of the CBD is less than 4 mm in children, less than 2 mm in infants up to 1 year, and less than 1 mm in neonates.
- The CBD will decrease in size or remain unchanged after a fatty meal.

SONOGRAPHIC APPEARANCE

Normal Intrahepatic Bile Ducts

- Anechoic nonvascular tubular structures coursing within the hepatic parenchyma.
- Smooth hyperechoic walls.
- Normal intraluminal diameter of the CHD.
- The right and left hepatic bile ducts generally lie anterior to the corresponding portal vein.
- Intrahepatic bile ducts are not routinely visualized on ultrasound.

Normal Extrahepatic Bile Ducts

Longitudinal Plane

- Anechoic nonvascular tubular structure anterior to the main portal vein and proper hepatic artery.
- Smooth hyperechoic walls.
- Normal intraluminal diameter of the CBD.

Transverse Plane

- Anechoic nonvascular tubular structure anterior to the main portal vein and lateral to the proper hepatic artery.
- Smooth hyperechoic walls.

Abnormal Intrahepatic and Extrahepatic Ducts

- Abnormal intraluminal diameter of the common hepatic or common bile ducts ($\geq$ 6 mm and $\geq$ 10 mm, respectively, in postcholecystectomy adult patients).
- Thick, irregular, or nonparallel walls.

GALLBLADDER PHYSIOLOGY AND ANATOMY

Functions of the Gallbladder

- Concentrates bile through the gallbladder epithelium.
- Stores concentrated bile.
- Contracts to release bile when the hormone cholecystokinin is released into the bloodstream.

Gallbladder Divisions

- *Fundus* most inferior and anterior portion; blind end.
- *Body* midportion between the neck and fundus.
- *Neck* narrow, tapering tube-like structure connected to the cystic duct; most superior portion; smallest transverse diameter; fixed anatomical relationship to the main lobar fissure and right portal vein.

Layers of the Gallbladder Wall

1. Outer serosal layer—visceral peritoneum.
2. Subserous layer—connective tissue.
3. Muscular layer—contracts in response to cholecystokinin.
4. Inner epithelial layer—mucosal layer.

Gallbladder Location

- An intraperitoneal organ.
- Located in the gallbladder fossa on the posteroinferior portion of the right lobe of the liver.
- Lies lateral to the inferior vena cava and anterior and medial to the right kidney.
- Lies posterior and inferior to the main lobar fissure.
- Gallbladder neck lies most superior.
- Fundus is posterior to the peritoneum and transverse colon.

GALLBLADDER ANATOMICAL VARIANTS

- *Hartmann pouch*—small posterior pouch between the neck and junctional fold.
- *Junctional fold*—fold or septation of the gallbladder at the junction of the neck and body (most common).
- *Phrygian cap*—fold in the gallbladder fundus.

CONGENITAL ANOMALIES

- Agenesis—rare.
- Duplication—partial or complete.
- Hypoplasia—associated with cystic fibrosis.
- Intrahepatic or ectopic location—gallbladder completely or almost completely is surrounded by liver parenchyma. May herniate into the lesser sac.
- Multiseptated—congenital malformation. Mimics ischemic pathology.

GALLBLADDER SIZE

- The normal fasting adult gallbladder measures approximately 8 to 12 cm in length and 3 to 4 cm in diameter.
- The normal fasting pediatric gallbladder measures approximately 1.5 to 3.0 cm in length and 1.2 cm in width in infants less than 1 year of age, and 3 to 7 cm in length and 1 to 3 cm in diameter in children between 2 and 16 years of age.

SONOGRAPHIC APPEARANCE

Normal Fasting Gallbladder

- An ellipsoid anechoic structure located in the gallbladder fossa demonstrating posterior acoustic enhancement.
- Demonstrates smooth hyperechoic walls measuring 3 mm or less in thickness in both adult and pediatric patients.
- Located in the posterior inferior medial aspect of the liver.

Abnormal Fasting Gallbladder

- Transverse diameter less than 2 cm or exceeding 5 cm.
- Thick or edematous wall exceeding 3 mm in thickness.
- Irregular wall contour.
- Intraluminal focus or echoes.
- Acoustic shadowing posterior to the gallbladder fossa.

Reasons for Nonvisualization of the Gallbladder

- Nonfasting patient.
- Surgically absent.
- Obliteration of the gallbladder lumen by intestinal air or gallstones.
- Patient body habitus.
- Ectopic location.
- Agenesis.

Noninflammatory Causes of Gallbladder Wall Thickening

- Nonfasting patient.
- Ascites.
- Cirrhosis.
- Congestive heart failure.
- Hypoalbuminemia.
- Acute hepatitis.
- Sepsis.
- Renal disease.

EXAMINATION TECHNIQUES, PROTOCOLS, AND IMAGE OPTIMIZATION

Preparation

- To obtain an optimal evaluation of the gallbladder the patient should fast before the ultrasound examination.
  - Adult – 6 to 8 hours.
  - Children – 6 hours.
  - Infants – 4 hours.
- There is no preparation necessary in postcholecystectomy patients, although fasting is still recommended to decrease the amount of bowel gas in the gastrointestinal tract.
- In cases of emergency, a gallbladder study can still be performed satisfactorily. Be sure to label the images "nonfasting" gallbladder and indicate the amount of time since ingestion of food.

Transducer Selection

- Use the highest frequency possible to obtain optimal resolution for penetration depth.
  - Adults – 3.0 to 5.0 MHz.
  - Children and small adults – 5.0 to 7.0 MHz.
  - Obese patients – 2.0 MHz may be required.

- Curvilinear transducers provide a wider field of view.
- Sector or vector transducers have a smaller footprint aiding in intercostal imaging.
- Linear transducers may help eliminate acoustic artifacts with superficial gallbladders in thin patients.
- Higher frequency transducers can help demonstrate posterior acoustic enhancement of gallstones.

Patient Positioning

- Examination usually begins with the patient in a supine position.
- Left lateral decubitus, left posterior oblique and upright positions may be helpful to evaluate the mobility of gallstones as well as alleviate overlying bowel gas.
- Ingestion of 16 ounces of water and placing the patient in a reverse Trendelenburg can aid in visualization of the distal common bile duct and the head of the pancreas

Examination Protocol

- Systematic approach in the sagittal and transverse planes carefully examining and imaging all portions of the gallbladder and biliary tree including:
  - Neck, body, and fundus of the gallbladder.
  - Intra- and extrahepatic biliary tree to include distal common bile duct.
- Measurement of the thickness of the gallbladder wall.
- Measure the anterior-posterior intraluminal diameter of the common hepatic and common bile ducts.
- When encountered, document mobility of echogenic focus(i) in the lumen of the gallbladder with changes in patient positions.
- Abnormalities should be documented and when applicable measured in two imaging planes. Color and/or spectral Doppler evaluation of the abnormality should be included and documented.
- Due to the association of the pancreas and liver with the biliary tree, sagittal and transverse images of these structures should be included in the gallbladder examination along with flow type and direction of the main portal vein.

Image Optimization

- Place gains settings to display normal liver parenchyma as a medium shade of gray and the normal gallbladder as an anechoic ovoid structure.
- Focal zone(s) should be placed at or below the area of interest. The use of multiple focal zones increases detail resolution and decreases temporal resolution.
- Sufficient imaging depth to visualize structures immediately posterior to the area of interest.
- Harmonic imaging should be used to evaluate and document the biliary tree.
- Decreasing system compression (dynamic range) can be used to reduce artifactual echoes within the gallbladder lumen, main portal vein, and biliary ducts.
- Spatial compounding can be used to improve visualization of structures posterior to highly attenuating structures.
- Doppler settings should be adjusted for a slow flow rate.
- The use of deep inspiration may improve visualization of the gallbladder and common ducts.
- The use of multiple patient positions may relocate overlying bowel gas.

Examination Limitations

- Incomplete patient preparation.
- Gastrointestinal gas.
- Obesity.

Helpful Hints

- Main lobar fissure is best visualized in the sagittal oblique plane.
- Trendelenburg and right posterior oblique positions may aid in visualization of the cystic duct.
- The common hepatic and common bile ducts are usually visualized best in a sagittal oblique plane.
- The length of the main right and left hepatic ducts is best visualized in a sagittal oblique plane.
- Higher frequency transducers and the use of harmonics imaging can help demonstrate posterior acoustic enhancement of gallstones.
- The distal common bile duct is visualized best in the transverse plane.
- The use of spatial compound imaging may obscure posterior shadowing.

Indications for Ultrasound Examination

- RUQ pain—may radiate to the upper back and chest.
- Increase in liver function tests.
- Nausea/vomiting.
- Intolerance to fatty foods.
- Postprandial pain.
- Positive Murphy sign.
- Jaundice.

LABORATORY VALUES

Alkaline Phosphatase (ALP)

- Normal adult range 45 to 115 U/L.
- An enzyme produced primarily by the liver, biliary tract, bone, and in lower concentrations in the intestines and placenta.
- Excreted through the bile ducts.
- Most specific indicator of biliary obstruction.
- May signal bone and liver abnormalities.
- Moderate increase with hepatitis and cirrhosis.

Alanine Aminotransferase (ALT)

- Normal adult range 7 to 55 U/L.
- An enzyme found in high concentration in the liver and lower concentrations in the heart, muscle, and kidneys.
- Remains elevated longer than aspartate aminotransferase (AST).
- More specific than AST.
- Very specific indicator of liver cell destruction.
- Elevation associated with hepatocellular disease, biliary tract obstruction, pancreatitis, and fatty infiltration.
- Mild elevation associated with liver metastasis.

Aspartate Aminotransferase (AST)

- Normal adult 8 to 48 U/L.
- An enzyme present in many kinds of tissue that is released when cells are injured or damaged; levels will be proportional to the amount of damage and the time between cell injury and testing.
- Used to diagnose liver disease before jaundice occurs.
- Elevation associated with cirrhosis, hepatitis, mononucleosis, fatty infiltration, myocardial infarction, muscle disease, and cholestasis.

Bilirubin

- Normal adult total bilirubin $\leq$ 1.1 mg/dL.
- Normal adult direct bilirubin $\leq$ 0.5 mg/dL.
- A product from the breakdown of hemoglobin in old red blood cells; a disruption in the process may cause abnormal levels; leakage into tissues gives the skin a yellow appearance.
- Reflects the balance between production and excretion of bile.
- Elevated by:
  - An excessive amount of red blood cell destruction.
  - Malfunction of liver cells.
  - Blockage of ducts leading from cells.
- Elevation of direct or conjugated bilirubin is associated with subacute cholecystitis, choledocholithiasis, retained bile duct stones, gallbladder carcinoma, injury to the bile ducts, and internal biliary fistula.
- Elevation of indirect or nonconjugated bilirubin is demonstrated in a prehepatic or hepatic abnormality.

Leukocyte Count (WBC)

- Normal serum levels: 4500 to 11,000 mm^3.
- Reflects the severity of inflammation.
- Associated with:
  - Acute cholecystitis.
  - Chronic cholecystitis.
  - Injury to bile ducts.

Intrahepatic Pathology

PATHOLOGY	ETIOLOGY	CLINICAL FINDINGS	SONOGRAPHIC FINDINGS	DIFFERENTIAL CONSIDERATIONS
Biliary dilatation	Biliary obstruction	Asymptomatic Right upper quadrant (RUQ) pain Jaundice Elevated direct bilirubin and alkaline phosphatase	Dilated intrahepatic and/or extrahepatic bile ducts Parallel channeling (shotgun) Portal vein may appear flattened with progressive dilatation Peripheral anechoic area(s) in the liver that demonstrate posterior enhancement Increase in bile duct size following a fatty meal	Normal biliary tree Portal hypertension

Biliary atresia	Congenital anomaly
	Viral infection
	Male prevalence
	Complications:
	  Death
	  Cirrhosis
	  Cholangitis
	  Portal hypertension
	  Malabsorption
		Persistent jaundice	Absent hepatic biliary radicles
			Small or absent gallbladder
			Absent common hepatic duct (CHD)
			Hepatomegaly
				Normal biliary tree
				Hepatitis

Hemobilia	Liver biopsy Trauma Vascular malformation	Abdominal pain Hematemesis	Low-level echoes within the bile ducts Gravity dependent	Technical error Cholangitis

Continued

Intrahepatic Pathology—(cont'd)

PATHOLOGY	ETIOLOGY	CLINICAL FINDINGS	SONOGRAPHIC FINDINGS	DIFFERENTIAL CONSIDERATIONS
Pneumobilia	Surgical procedure Trauma Infection Incompetent sphincter of Oddi	Asymptomatic RUQ pain	Hyperechoic focus(i) in the intrahepatic bile ducts Comet-tail reverberation artifact Often centrally located	Foreign body Biliary calculus Arterial calcification
Caroli disease	Congenital disorder	Abdominal pain Abdominal cramping Fever Intermittent jaundice	Segmental, saccular, or beaded appearance of the intrahepatic bile ducts Multiple cystic structures in the liver that communicate with the biliary tree	Polycystic liver disease Biliary obstruction
Clonorchiasis	Ingestion of raw freshwater fish contaminated with a parasitical worm	RUQ pain Fever Leukocytosis	Dilatation of the intrahepatic bile ducts Diffuse thickening of the bile duct walls Echogenic focus within the bile duct	Cholangitis Cholangiocarcinoma
Klatskin tumor	Idiopathic Primary sclerosing cholangitis Caroli disease Choledochal cyst	Jaundice Acute onset of abdominal pain Biliary colic Weight loss Elevated bilirubin and alkaline phosphatase levels Mild increase in aspartate aminotransferase (AST) and alanine aminotransferase (ALT) levels	Small echogenic mass near the hepatic hilum Dilatation of the intrahepatic bile ducts Normal extrahepatic bile ducts	Artifact Portal vein thrombosis Hepatic tumor Lymphadenopathy

Extrahepatic Pathology

PATHOLOGY	ETIOLOGY	CLINICAL FINDINGS	SONOGRAPHIC FINDINGS	DIFFERENTIAL CONSIDERATIONS
Biloma	Surgery Trauma Gallbladder disease	Right upper quadrant (RUQ) pain	Anechoic fluid collection near the porta hepatis Fluid may demonstrate mobility with changes in patient position Check pelvis and paracolic gutters for free fluid	Seroma Fluid in the stomach or intestines Ascites
Cholangitis	Congenital or acquired stricture Infection Parasitical infestation (ansariasis most common in U.S.) Biliary stasis Ulcerative colitis Autoimmune deficiency syndrome (AIDS)	Abdominal pain Fever Leukocytosis Recurrent episodes of sepsis with right upper quadrant pain Jaundice Charcot triad Mild elevation in aspartate aminotransferase (AST) and alanine aminotransferase (ALT) levels Marked elevation in bilirubin and alkaline phosphatase levels	Biliary dilatation Thickening of the bile duct walls Pneumobilia Gallbladder hydrops (30%) Thickened gallbladder wall Brightly echogenic portal triad	Biliary obstruction Caroli disease

Extrahepatic Pathology—(cont'd)

PATHOLOGY	ETIOLOGY	CLINICAL FINDINGS	SONOGRAPHIC FINDINGS	DIFFERENTIAL CONSIDERATIONS
Cholangiocarcinoma	**Risk Factors:** Ulcerative colitis Cholangitis Choledochal cyst Chronic biliary stasis Caroli disease Male prevalence	Jaundice Acute onset of abdominal pain Biliary colic Weight loss Fatigue Elevated bilirubin and alkaline phosphatase levels Mild increase in AST and ALT	Echogenic mass within a bile duct Dilatation of the intrahepatic and extrahepatic bile ducts Gallbladder hydrops Hepatomegaly Gallstones (30% of cases) Ascites	Artifact Portal vein thrombosis Lymphadenopathy Choledocholithiasis Pancreatic mass
Choledocholithiasis Complications: Biliary obstruction Cholangitis Pancreatitis	Stone within the common duct Majority have migrated from the gallbladder	Biliary colic Elevated direct bilirubin and alkaline phosphatase Mild increase in AST and ALT levels Jaundice	Echogenic focus(i) within the common duct Posterior acoustic shadowing (60%-80% of cases) Biliary dilatation Hydropic gallbladder	Surgical clip Tortuous bile duct Cystic duct remnant Intestinal air Intraductal tumor
Choledochal cyst	Congenital weakness of the ductile wall Reflux of pancreatic juices into the bile duct Most common in East Asian populations Female prevalence	Asymptomatic Jaundice RUQ mass RUQ colicky pain Failure to thrive Weight loss Recurrent fever and chills	Nonvascular cystic mass in the porta hepatis separate from the gallbladder Dilated common hepatic duct (CHD), common bile duct (CBD), or cystic duct entering the cystic mass Dilated intrahepatic bile ducts	Hepatic cyst Pancreas cyst Normal junction of the common hepatic and cystic ducts Gallbladder duplication Biloma
Ascariasis	Ingestion of contaminated water or food More prevalent in Southern gulf states of the U.S., Africa, Asia, and South America	Asymptomatic RUQ pain Biliary colic Fever Leukocytosis	Spaghetti-like echogenic structure within a bile duct Nonshadowing Posterior acoustic enhancement Acalculous cholecystitis	Stent Cholangitis Cholangiocarcinoma Choledocholithiasis

Gallbladder Pathology

PATHOLOGY	ETIOLOGY	CLINICAL FINDINGS	SONOGRAPHIC FINDINGS	DIFFERENTIAL CONSIDERATIONS
Adenoma (polyp)	Benign epithelial tumor	Asymptomatic Dull right upper quadrant (RUQ) pain Intolerance to fatty foods	Echogenic intraluminal focus(i) Immobile Nonshadowing Thickening of the gallbladder wall	Cholelithiasis Fold in the gallbladder Carcinoma
Adenomyomatosis	Hyperplasia of the epithelial and muscle layers of the gallbladder wall	Asymptomatic Dull RUQ pain Intolerance to fatty foods	Echogenic intraluminal focus(i) Diffuse comet-tail reverberation artifact Twinkling artifact on color Doppler Immobile	Cholelithiasis Fold in the gallbladder Carcinoma

Continued

Gallbladder Pathology—(cont'd)

PATHOLOGY	ETIOLOGY	CLINICAL FINDINGS	SONOGRAPHIC FINDINGS	DIFFERENTIAL CONSIDERATIONS
Cholesterolosis	Local disturbance in cholesterol metabolism Not associated with serum cholesterol levels Two types—cholesterosis and cholesterol polyps	Asymptomatic Abdominal pain	Echogenic intraluminal foci Nonshadowing Normal gallbladder in the majority of cases Strawberry appearance with cholesterosis	Cholelithiasis Carcinoma Fold in the gallbladder
Cholelithiasis	Abnormal bile composition Bile stasis Infection **Risk Factors:** Family history Fair complexion Female prevalence (4:1) Obesity Pregnancy Diabetes Estrogen replacement therapy Prolong fasting Abnormal hemolysis Alcohol cirrhosis	Asymptomatic RUQ pain Epigastric pain Chest or shoulder pain Elevated liver function tests Nausea/vomiting Postprandial pain Fatty food intolerance	Hyperechoic intraluminal focus(i) Round or triangular in shape Posterior acoustic shadowing Mobile Immobile when lodged in the neck or cystic duct Wall-echo-shadow (WES) Floating hyperechoic focus(i) caused by thick bile or air in stone	Intestinal air Adenomyomatosis Polyp Fold in the gallbladder Surgical clip Refraction artifact
Porcelain gallbladder	Decrease in vascular supply to the gallbladder Cystic duct obstruction causing bile stasis Chronic low-grade infection **Risk Factors:** Female prevalence	Asymptomatic Vague RUQ pain	Gallstones (95%) Complete or partial hyperechoic wall Marked posterior acoustic shadowing	Contracted gallbladder with stones (WES) Intestinal air Adenomyomatosis
Mirizzi syndrome	Impacted stone in the cystic duct or gallbladder neck causing obstruction of the CHD superior to the obstruction and jaundice	RUQ pain Recurrent cholangitis Jaundice Elevated bilirubin and alkaline phosphatase Increase in aspartate aminotransferase (AST) and alanine aminotransferase (ALT) levels	Immobile calculus in the cystic duct or neck of the gallbladder Dilatation of the intrahepatic and CHDs Normal common bile duct (CBD) Dilated CHD superior to the obstruction	Choledocholithiasis Portal triad lymph node compressing the CHD
Sludge	Prolonged fasting Biliary stasis Biliary obstruction Cholecystitis Sickle cell anemia Pregnancy Rapid weight loss Long term total parenteral nutrition	Asymptomatic RUQ pain Nausea/vomiting	Nonshadowing low-amplitude echoes layering in the dependent portion of the gallbladder Echoes move slowly with position change May fill entire gallbladder with internal echoes May demonstrate fluid-fluid levels May form sludge balls	Technical factors Intestinal air Carcinoma Hematobilia

Gallbladder Pathology—(cont'd)

PATHOLOGY	ETIOLOGY	CLINICAL FINDINGS	SONOGRAPHIC FINDINGS	DIFFERENTIAL CONSIDERATIONS
Gallbladder carcinoma	Most common biliary malignancy and fifth most common malignancy Adenocarcinoma in greater than 95% of cases **Risk Factors:** Cholelithiasis Porcelain gallbladder Cholecystitis Female prevalence (3:1) ≥ 50 yrs of age	Asymptomatic RUQ pain Palpable mass Jaundice Anorexia Nausea/vomiting Elevated alkaline phosphatase and direct bilirubin Mild increase in AST and ALT levels	Thick, irregular gallbladder wall Irregular intraluminal mass Immobile mass Demonstrate internal blood flow on Color and spectral Doppler Cholelithiasis (90% of cases) Lymphadenopathy Metastatic liver lesions	Adenoma Sludge Cholecystitis Adenomyomatosis Metastases
Metastatic gallbladder disease	**Direct Extension:** Pancreas Stomach Bile duct **Indirect Extension:** Melanoma—most common Lung Kidney Esophagus	Asymptomatic RUQ pain Jaundice Nausea/vomiting Elevated alkaline phosphatase	Focal gallbladder wall thickening Irregular intraluminal mass Nonshadowing Demonstrate internal blood flow on Color and spectral Doppler Absence of gallstones	Cholecystitis Adenoma Primary carcinoma

Gallbladder Inflammation

INFLAMMATION	ETIOLOGY	CLINICAL FINDINGS	SONOGRAPHIC FINDINGS	DIFFERENTIAL CONSIDERATIONS
Acalculous cholecystitis	Recent surgery Infection Diabetes Congestive heart failure Total parenteral nutrition Extrinsic obstruction of the cystic duct	Acute RUQ pain Nausea/vomiting Fever/chills Positive Murphy sign	Diffuse gallbladder wall thickening greater than 3 mm in diameter Absence of gallstone(s) Gallbladder hydrops Sludge Positive Murphy sign Pericholecystic fluid	Acute cholecystitis Technical factors Gallbladder perforation
Acute cholecystitis **Complications:** Ascending cholangitis Empyema Perforation Pericholecystic or liver abscess Septicemia Bouveret syndrome	Obstruction of the cystic duct Infection Idiopathic **Risk Factors:** Female prevalence (3:1) Cholelithiasis 40-50 yrs of age	Severe epigastric or right upper quadrant (RUQ) pain Biliary colic Positive Murphy sign Nausea/vomiting Fever and chills Elevated aspartate aminotransferase (AST), and alkaline Phosphatase Mild elevation of total bilirubin Leukocytosis	Thick, edematous gallbladder wall; "halo sign" Impacted stone in the cystic duct or gallbladder neck Cholelithiasis (90% of cases) Pericholecystic fluid Positive Murphy sign Peripheral hyperemia on color Doppler Sludge	Liver abscess Ascites Nonfasting patient

Continued

Gallbladder Inflammation—(cont'd)

INFLAMMATION	ETIOLOGY	CLINICAL FINDINGS	SONOGRAPHIC FINDINGS	DIFFERENTIAL CONSIDERATIONS
Emphysematous cholecystitis	Cholelithiasis Idiopathic	RUQ pain Nausea/vomiting Fever Leukocytosis	Echogenic focus(i) within the gallbladder wall or lumen Ill-defined posterior acoustic shadowing Cholelithiasis Pericholecystic fluid	Acute cholecystitis Porcelain gallbladder Large gallstone Intestinal air

Gangrenous cholecystitis	**Risk Factors:**
	  Diabetes
	  Older adult
	  Male prevalence
		RUQ pain radiating to the back
		Positive Murphy sign
		Fever
		Leukocytosis
		Elevated AST, total bilirubin, and alkaline phosphatase
			Diffuse echogenic focus within the lumen
			Immobile
			Nonshadowing
			Nonlayering
				Acute cholecystitis
				Emphysematous cholecystitis
				Adenoma
				Carcinoma

Gallbladder perforation	**Risk Factors:**
	  Diabetes
	  Older adult
	  Infection
	  Cholelithiasis
	  Trauma
		RUQ mass
		Severe RUQ or epigastric pain
		Positive Murphy sign
		Nausea/vomiting
		Leukocytosis
			Edematous, thick gallbladder wall
			Pericholecystic fluid
			Cholelithiasis
				Ascites
				Hepatic abscess
				Perforated peptic ulcer

Chronic cholecystitis	Recurrent inflammation secondary to infection, obstruction, or metabolic disorders	Asymptomatic Vague RUQ pain Heartburn Fatty food intolerance Intermittent nausea/vomiting Mild increase in AST and alanine aminotransferase (ALT) levels Possible increase in alkaline phosphatase and direct bilirubin	Small or contracted gallbladder Thick, hyperechoic walls Cholelithiasis (90% of cases) Posterior acoustic shadowing Sludge	Nonfasting patient Cholelithiasis Porcelain gallbladder Carcinoma
Hydrops	Obstruction of the cystic duct Prolonged biliary stasis Surgery Hepatitis Gastroenteritis Diabetes	Asymptomatic RUQ or epigastric pain Nausea/vomiting Palpable mass	Enlargement Gallbladder transverse diameter exceeding 4 cm Thin, hyperechoic walls Evaluate for Mirizzi syndrome	Normal gallbladder Hepatic cyst Phrygian cap
Gallbladder varices	Portal hypertension Portal vein thrombosis Cholecystitis	Dependent on etiology	Multiple tortuous tubular structures in the gallbladder periphery Vascular flow	Intestinal fluid Normal vessels

BILIARY REVIEW

1. Cholangiocarcinoma located at the junction of the right and left hepatic ducts is termed a(n):
   a. biloma
   b. phlegmon
   c. Caroli disease
   d. Klatskin tumor

2. Which of the following patient positions may aid in visualization of the cystic duct?
   a. supine
   b. prone
   c. left posterior oblique
   d. Trendelenburg

3. A small septation located between the neck and body of the gallbladder *best* describes:
   a. a junctional fold
   b. a phrygian cap
   c. Hartmann pouch
   d. diverticulosis of the gallbladder

4. A hyperechoic focus with marked posterior acoustic shadowing is demonstrated in the anterior wall of the gallbladder. This is most consistent with which of the following pathologies?
   a. emphysematous cholecystitis
   b. porcelain gallbladder
   c. cholelithiasis
   d. Mirizzi syndrome

5. Nonshadowing, low-amplitude echoes located in the dependent portion of the gallbladder *best* describes:
   a. cholecystitis
   b. cholelithiasis
   c. biliary sludge
   d. adenomyomatosis

6. Which of the following is associated with cholesterolosis?
   a. increase in serum cholesterol levels
   b. intolerance to fatty foods
   c. decrease in serum cholesterol levels
   d. local disturbance in cholesterol metabolism

7. The spiral valves of Heister are located in which of the following structures?
   a. cystic duct
   b. duct of Wirsung
   c. common bile duct
   d. common hepatic duct

8. A patient presents with a sudden onset of abdominal pain and extreme tenderness over the gallbladder fossa. Localized gallbladder wall thickening is visualized on ultrasound. This most likely represents:
   a. cholelithiasis
   b. acute cholecystitis
   c. adenomyomatosis
   d. gallbladder carcinoma

Using Figure 8.2, answer questions 9 and 10.

9. Which of the following findings is identified in this sonogram?
   a. cholangitis
   b. cholecystitis
   c. cholangiocarcinoma
   d. choledocholithiasis

10. Complications with this abnormality would most likely include:
    a. biliary obstruction
    b. cholecystitis
    c. lymphadenopathy
    d. portal hypertension

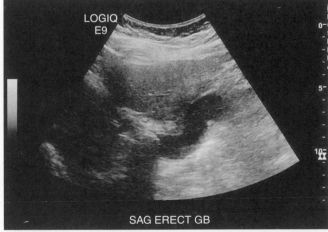

FIG. 8.2 Sagittal sonogram of the porta hepatis.

Using Figure 8.3, answer question 11.

11. A sagittal sonogram in a neonate demonstrates a small contracted gallbladder (arrow) and a large anechoic, nonvascular tubular structure in the region of the porta hepatis. The anechoic structure is most suspicious for:
   a. a hepatic cyst
   b. a hepatic artery aneurysm
   c. a choledochal cyst
   d. gallbladder duplication

Using Figure 8.4, answer questions 12 and 13.

12. The gallbladder in this sonogram is demonstrating:
   a. a phrygian cap
   b. Hartmann pouch
   c. a junctional fold
   d. a gallbladder diverticulum

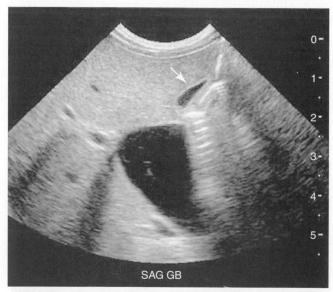

SAG GB

FIG. 8.3 Transverse image of the gallbladder *(arrow)*.

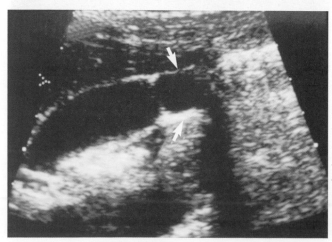

FIG. 8.4 Transverse image of the gallbladder.

13. Which type of sonographic artifact is demonstrated adjacent to this structure?
   a. grating lobe
   b. refraction
   c. reverberation
   d. slice thickness

14. The biliary system has three main functions. Which of the following describes one of these functions?
   a. produces bile
   b. stores enzymes
   c. stores fats
   d. stores bile

15. Which of the following conditions is most likely to occur with an episode of prolonged fasting?
   a. cholangitis
   b. biliary sludge
   c. cholelithiasis
   d. gallbladder carcinoma

16. The gallbladder wall is composed of which of the following layers?
   a. serosal, subserosal, muscular, and epithelial
   b. serosal, endothelial, muscular, and epithelial
   c. serosal, subserosal, muscular, and endothelial
   d. serosal, subserosal, endothelial, and epithelial

17. The distal portion of the common bile duct terminates in which of the following structures?
   a. pylorus
   b. pancreas
   c. duodenum
   d. hepatic hilum

18. In the portal hepatis, the common hepatic duct is located:
   a. posterior to the main portal vein
   b. lateral to the proper hepatic artery
   c. medial to the proper hepatic artery
   d. anterior to the common hepatic artery

19. Which of the following is an indication for a gallbladder ultrasound?
   a. elevated creatinine
   b. left upper quadrant pain
   c. positive McBurney sign
   d. intolerance to fatty foods

20. Which of the following hormones stimulates gallbladder contraction and the secretion of pancreatic enzymes?
   a. amylase
   b. gastrin
   c. bilirubin
   d. cholecystokinin

21. The diameter of a normal fasting adult gallbladder should *not* exceed:
    a. 2 cm
    b. 4 cm
    c. 6 cm
    d. 10 cm

Using Figure 8.5, answer question 22.

22. The findings demonstrated in this sonogram most likely represent:
    a. an abscess
    b. empyema
    c. biliary sludge
    d. gallbladder carcinoma

Using Figure 8.6, answer questions 23 and 24.

23. The hyperechoic linear structure identified by the arrow is the:
    a. ligamentum venosum
    b. intrasegmental fissure
    c. main lobar fissure
    d. falciform ligament

24. This hyperechoic structure is routinely used as a sonographic landmark to locate which of the following structures?
    a. caudate lobe
    b. gallbladder
    c. left lobe of the liver
    d. common hepatic duct

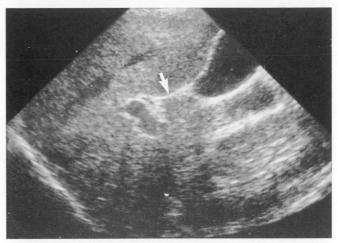

FIG. 8.6   Sagittal sonogram near the porta hepatis.

Using Figure 8.7, answer questions 25 and 26.

25. This sonogram of the gallbladder shows which of the following pathologies?
    a. cholelithiasis
    b. adenomyomatosis
    c. acute cholecystitis
    d. tumefactive sludge

26. Which of the following technical factors would aid in the diagnosis of this pathology?
    a. deep inspiration
    b. drinking 12 oz of water
    c. an intercostal approach
    d. patient position change

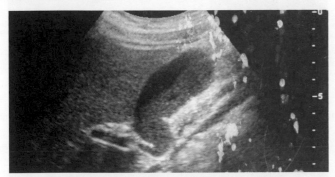

FIG. 8.5   Supine sagittal image of the gallbladder.

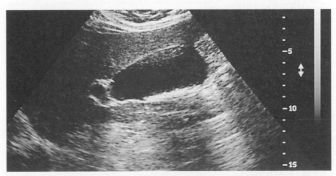

FIG. 8.7   Sagittal image of the gallbladder.

27. Gravity dependent low-level echoes within the bile ducts describe:
    a. hemobilia
    b. cholangitis
    c. pneumobilia
    d. Klatskin tumor

28. Which of the following enzymes is produced primarily by the liver, bone, and placenta?
    a. alanine aminotransferase (ALT)
    b. alkaline phosphatase
    c. aspartate aminotransferase (AST)
    d. prothrombin

29. A decrease in diameter of the common bile duct after ingestion of a fatty meal is associated with:
    a. normal findings
    b. cholecystitis
    c. distal pathology
    d. obstructive jaundice

30. Thickness of the gallbladder wall in a normal fasting patient should *not* exceed:
    a. 3 mm
    b. 6 mm
    c. 8 mm
    d. 10 mm

31. Dilatation of the intrahepatic ducts with normal extrahepatic ducts is characteristic of:
    a. cholangitis
    b. a Klatskin tumor
    c. choledocholithiasis
    d. a pancreatic neoplasm

32. Which of the following complications associated with acute cholecystitis is more prevalent in older diabetic patients?
    a. hepatic abscess
    b. ascending cholangitis
    c. gangrenous cholecystitis
    d. emphysematous cholecystitis

33. As dilatation of the intrahepatic biliary tree progresses, the portal system becomes:
    a. rounded
    b. fusiform
    c. beaded
    d. flattened

Using Figure 8.8, answer question 34.

34. The sonogram is most likely demonstrating:
    a. acute cholecystitis
    b. gallbladder hydrops
    c. chronic cholecystitis
    d. ectopic gallbladder

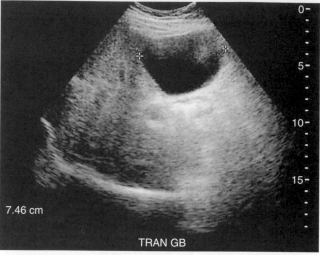

FIG. 8.8 Transverse image of the gallbladder.

Using Figure 8.9, answer question 35.

35. The gallbladder in this sonogram is demonstrating a:
    a. WES sign
    b. target sign
    c. Murphy sign
    d. comet-tail artifact

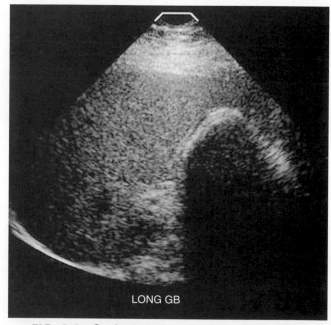

FIG. 8.9 Sagittal sonogram of the gallbladder.

Using Figure 8.10, answer question 36.

36. The sonographic findings are most consistent with:
   a. adenomyomatosis
   b. tumefactive sludge
   c. multiple adenomas
   d. metastatic lesions

Using Figure 8.11, answer question 37.

37. An asymptomatic patient with a history of chole-cystectomy 3 years earlier presents for an abdominal ultrasound. Based on the clinical history, the abnormality documented in this sonogram most likely represents:
   a. surgical clips
   b. pneumobilia
   c. arterial calcifications
   d. choledocholithiasis

Using Figure 8.12, answer questions 38 and 39.

38. The sonographic findings are most consistent with:
   a. cholelithiasis
   b. acute cholecystitis
   c. chronic cholecystitis
   d. adenomyomatosis

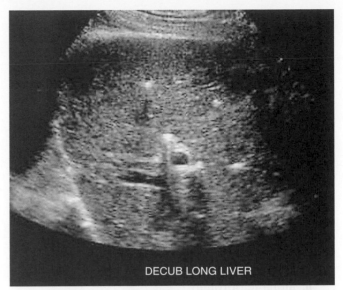

DECUB LONG LIVER

FIG. 8.11   Sagittal sonogram of the liver.

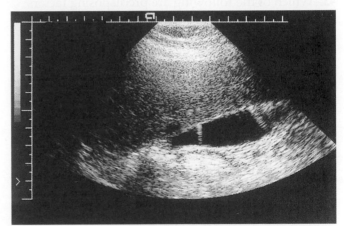

FIG. 8.12   Sagittal sonogram of the right upper quadrant.

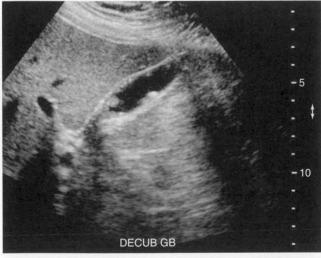

DECUB GB

FIG. 8.10   Sagittal sonogram of the gallbladder.

39. Which of the following acoustic artifacts is associated with this finding?
   a. comet-tail artifact
   b. edge artifact
   c. mirror image
   d. posterior acoustic shadowing

40. A small protrusion near the neck of the gallbladder describes:
   a. a junctional fold
   b. Hartmann pouch
   c. a choledochal cyst
   d. Morison pouch

41. In biliary obstruction, identifying multiple anechoic tubular structures in the left lobe of the liver is termed:
   a. parallel channeling
   b. star effect
   c. Murphy sign
   d. twinkle sign

42. Which of the following liver function tests is produced from the breakdown of hemoglobin?
   a. bilirubin
   b. alpha fetoprotein
   c. alpha phosphatase
   d. alanine aminotransferase

43. Which of the following are predisposing factors linked to the development of cholelithiasis?
   a. family history, pregnancy, obesity, and pancreatitis
   b. female gender, family history, progesterone replacement therapy, and hepatitis
   c. diabetes mellitus, fair complexion, male gender, and cirrhosis
   d. obesity, fair complexion, pregnancy, and diabetes mellitus

44. Which of the following technical factors would most likely aid in demonstrating shadowing posterior to small-caliber gallstones?
   a. decreased image depth
   b. decreased overall gain
   c. increased transducer frequency
   d. fewer focal zones

45. Which of the following is the most likely cause of ascariasis?
   a. bile stasis
   b. surgical procedure
   c. ingestion of contaminated water
   d. hyperplasia of the gallbladder wall

46. All of the following are potential differential considerations in cases of pneumobilia *except:*
   a. stent
   b. surgical clip
   c. biliary calculus
   d. cavernous hemangioma

Using Figure 8.13, answer questions 47 and 48.

47. Differential considerations for the findings in this ultrasound may include all of the following *except:*
   a. adenoma
   b. tumefactive sludge
   c. gallbladder carcinoma
   d. metastatic gallbladder disease

48. Additional clinical history of pancreatic carcinoma is documented in the patient's chart. Multiple target-shaped lesions are demonstrated within the liver. Given this additional information, the echogenic mass is most suspicious for:
   a. adenoma
   b. tumefactive sludge
   c. gallbladder carcinoma
   d. metastatic gallbladder disease

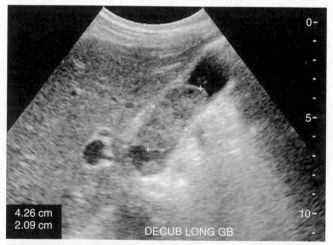

FIG. 8.13 Left lateral decubitus image of the gallbladder.

Using Figure 8.14, answer question 49.

49. Which of the following congenital gallbladder anomalies is *most likely* demonstrated in this sonogram of the gallbladder?
    a. phrygian cap
    b. gallbladder duplication
    c. multiseptated gallbladder
    d. strawberry gallbladder

Using Figure 8.15, answer question 50.

50. A patient presents with an acute onset of right upper quadrant pain. Based on this clinical history, the sonogram is most suspicious for:
    a. Wall-echo-shadow (WES)
    b. acute cholecystitis
    c. cholangiocarcinoma
    d. gallbladder carcinoma

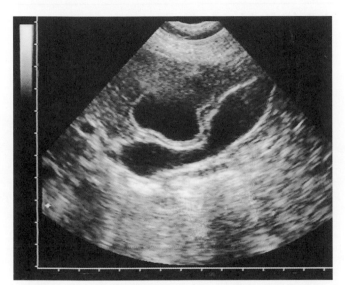

FIG. 8.14   Sagittal image of the gallbladder fossa.

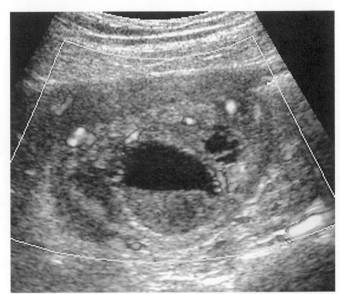

FIG. 8.15   Transverse power Doppler image.

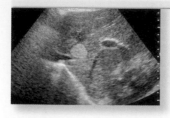

CHAPTER 9

Pancreas

KEY TERMS

acini cells produce pancreatic enzymes to help digest fats, proteins, carbohydrates, and nucleic acids.

acute pancreatitis acute inflammation causing escape of pancreatic enzymes from the acinar cells into the surrounding tissue. Most commonly caused by biliary disease followed by alcohol abuse.

amylase digestive enzyme produced in the pancreas that aids in converting starches to sugars; also produced in the salivary glands, liver, and fallopian tubes.

ampulla of Vater opening in the duodenum for the entrance of the common bile duct.

chronic pancreatitis multiple, persistent, or prolonged episodes of pancreatitis.

Courvoisier sign painless jaundice associated with a hydropic gallbladder caused by the obstruction of the distal common bile duct by an external mass usually in the head of the pancreas.

cystic fibrosis autosomal recessive exocrine gland disorder where organs become clogged with mucus secreted by the exocrine glands.

endocrine pertaining to a process in which a group of cells secrete into the blood or lymph circulation a substance (e.g., hormone) that has a specific effect on tissues in another part of the body Mosby's Medical Dictionary 2017.

exocrine the process of secreting outwardly through a duct to the surface of an organ.

duct of Santorini secondary secretory duct of the pancreas.

duct of Wirsung primary secretory duct of the pancreas.

glucose controls the blood sugar level in the body.

lipase enzyme produced primarily by the pancreas that changes fats to fatty acids and glycerol; increases after damage has occurred to the pancreas.

pancreaticoduodenal pertaining to the pancreas and duodenum.

pancreatoduodenectomy also known as Whipple procedure; a surgical resection of the pancreatic head or periampullary area; relieves obstruction of the biliary tree that is often caused by a malignant tumor. The remaining normal pancreatic tissue is attached to the duodenum.

phlegmon an extension of pancreatic inflammation into the peripancreatic tissues, resulting in an enlarged solid inflammatory mass with retroperitoneal fat necrosis.

portosplenic confluence the joining of the portal, splenic, and superior mesenteric veins.

pseudocyst a space or cavity, without a lining membrane, containing gas or liquid; caused by a leakage of pancreatic enzymes into surrounding tissues.

sphincter of Oddi a sheath of muscle fibers surrounding the distal common bile and pancreatic ducts as they cross the wall of the duodenum.

Whipple procedure see pancreatoduodenectomy.

PANCREAS PHYSIOLOGY

Functions of the Pancreas

Exocrine

- Highly digestive enzymes are secreted by the acinar cells and drain into the duodenum through the pancreatic ducts.
  a. amylase—breaks down complex carbohydrates.
  b. lipase—breaks down fats.
  c. trypsin—breaks down proteins into amino acids.
- Chyme from the duodenum stimulates release of hormones that act on the pancreatic juices.
  a. cholecystokinin—produced in the duodenum to stimulate secretion of pancreatic enzymes and contraction of the gallbladder.

b. gastrin—secreted by the stomach to stimulate secretion of gastric acids; stimulates growth of mucosa of the exocrine pancreas. Controlled by the vagus nerve.

c. secretin—produced in the duodenum to stimulate secretion of sodium bicarbonate.

Endocrine

- Islet cells of Langerhans secrete hormones directly into the bloodstream.
    a. alpha cells secrete glucagon (increases blood glucose).
    b. beta cells secrete insulin which stimulates the release of glucose, amino and fatty acids out of the bloodstream into the tissue cells (decreases blood glucose).
    c. delta cells secrete somatostatin which regulates the secretion of glucose and glycagon (autoregulator).
- Failure to produce sufficient amount of insulin leads to diabetes mellitus.

PANCREAS ANATOMY (FIG. 9.1)

- An elongated organ lying transverse and obliquely in the epigastric and hypochondriac regions of the body.
- Retroperitoneal organ located in the anterior pararenal space, posterior to the lesser sac.
- Lies anterior to the great vessels.

Pancreas Divisions and Location

- Overall size depends on age and body habitus.
- Divided into the tail, body, neck, head, and uncinate process.

Tail

- Most superior portion of the pancreas lying anterior and parallel with the splenic vein.
- Lies medial to the spleen and anterior- medial to the upper pole of the left kidney.
- Located posterior to the stomach, and lateral to the spine.
- Generally, extends toward the splenic hilum (occasionally left renal hilum).

Body

- Largest and most anterior aspect of the pancreas.
- Lies anterior to the aorta, superior mesenteric artery, superior mesenteric vein, splenic vein, left renal vein, and spine.
- Lies posterior to the antrum of the stomach.

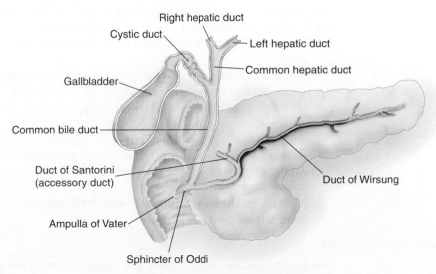

FIG. 9.1 Pancreas anatomy.

Neck

- Separates the head from the body of the pancreas.
- Lies directly anterior to the superior mesenteric vein and portosplenic confluence.
- Lies posterior to the pylorus of the stomach.

Head

- Lies medial to the descending (second) portion of the duodenum and gallbladder.
- Located right lateral to the superior mesenteric vein, uncinate process, splenic vein, aorta, and neck of the pancreas.
- Lies inferior to the main portal vein and hepatic artery.
- Located anterior to the inferior vena cava and left lobe of the liver in some patients.
- Gastroduodenal artery lies in the anterolateral portion of the pancreatic head.
- Distal common bile duct is situated in the posterolateral and inferior portion of the pancreatic head.

Uncinate Process

- Portion of the pancreatic head directly posterior to the superior mesenteric vein and anterior to the aorta and inferior vena cava.
- Variable in size.

Ducts of the Pancreas

- Contain smooth muscles that aid in transportation of the pancreatic enzymes.

Duct of Wirsung

- Primary secretory duct extending the entire length of the pancreas.
- Joins the distal common bile duct entering the descending portion of the duodenum through the ampulla of Vater.
- Frequently visualized in the body of the pancreas.

Duct of Santorini

- Secondary secretory duct draining the upper anterior portion of the pancreas.
- Enters the duodenum at the minor papilla approximately 2 cm proximal to the ampulla of Vater.

CONGENITAL ANOMALIES

Pancreatic Divisum

- Most common variant occurring in 10% of the population.
- Failure of the normal fusion of the ducts of Wirsung and Santorini.
- Duct of Wirsung is small and only drains the inferior portion of the pancreatic head.
- Duct of Santorini drains the majority of the pancreas.
- Associated with a higher incidence of pancreatitis.
- Difficult to evaluate with sonography.

Annular Pancreas

- Rare anomaly caused by the failure of a normal regression of the left ventral bud.
- The head of the pancreas surrounds the duodenum, resulting in obstruction of the biliary tree or duodenum.
- May cause partial or complete duodenal atresia.
- Male prevalence.

Ectopic Pancreatic Tissue

- Eighty percent (80%) of ectopic tissue occurs in the greater curvature of the stomach antra, pylorus, duodenal bulb, and proximal jejunum.

- May also be found in the ileum and in a coexisting Meckel diverticulum.
- Small, polypoid-appearing mass.
- Solitary or multiple implants.
- Male prevalence.

Cystic Fibrosis

- Autosomal recessive exocrine gland disorder in which organs become clogged with mucus secreted by the exocrine glands.
- Pancreas becomes hyperechoic as a result of fibrosis or fatty replacement.
- Small cysts may be present.

Pancreas Size

- The size of the pancreas varies with age and body habitus.

	HEAD	NECK	BODY	TAIL
Adult	≤ 3.0 cm	≤ 2.5 cm	≤ 2.5 cm	≤ 2.0 cm

SONOGRAPHIC APPEARANCE

Normal Pancreas

- Smooth or coarse homogeneous parenchyma.
- Adult pancreas is either isoechoic or hyperechoic compared with the normal liver.
- May appear hypoechoic in young children and hyperechoic in older adults.
- May demonstrate a cobblestone appearance.
- Variable shape:
  - sausage.
  - dumbbell.
  - tadpole.

Abnormal Pancreas

- Irregular or heterogeneous parenchyma.
- Calcifications.

Normal Pancreatic Duct

- Anechoic nonvascular tubular structure.
- Smooth parallel hyperechoic walls measuring ≤ 3 mm in the head/neck and ≤ 2 mm in the body.
- Most commonly visualized in the body of the pancreas.

Abnormal Pancreatic Duct

- Anechoic nonvascular tubular structure.
- Irregular or nonparallel hyperechoic walls.
- Measurement exceeding 3 mm in the head/neck or 2 mm in the body.

EXAMINATION TECHNIQUES, PROTOCOLS, AND IMAGE OPTIMIZATION

Preparation

- To obtain an optimal evaluation of the pancreas the patient should fast before the ultrasound examination.
  - Adult – 6 to 8 hours.
  - Children – 6 hours.
  - Infants – 4 hours.

- Purpose of fasting:
  1. Biliary system is usually included in an ultrasound examination of the pancreas.
  2. Fasting ensures an empty stomach.
  3. Fasting reduces bowel gas.
- In cases of emergency, an ultrasound examination of the pancreas can still be performed satisfactorily without preparation.

Transducer Selection

- Use the highest frequency possible to obtain optimal resolution for penetration depth.
  - Adults – 3.0 to 5.0 MHz.
  - Children and small adults - 5.0 to 7.0 MHz.
  - Obese patients – 2.0 MHz may be required.
- Curvilinear transducers provide a wider field of view.
- Linear transducers may be used in thin patients.

Patient Positioning

- Examination usually begins with the patient in a supine position.
- Left lateral decubitus, left posterior oblique and upright positions may be helpful to alleviate overlying bowel gas.
- Ingestion of 16 ounces of water and placing the patient in a reverse Trendelenburg (semi-Fowler) or right posterior oblique position can aid in visualization of the pancreas.
- Right lateral decubitus position may aid in visualizing the tail of the pancreas.

Examination Protocol

- Systematic approach in the transverse oblique plane to carefully examine and image the entire pancreas including:
  - Head, neck, body, tail, and uncinate process including surrounding vascular landmarks.
- Measure the anterior-posterior intraluminal diameter of the distal common bile duct.
- Sagittal images of the pancreas should be included.
- Abnormalities should be documented and when applicable measured in two imaging planes. Color and/or spectral Doppler evaluation of the abnormality should be included and documented.
- Due to the association of the liver and biliary tree with the pancreas, sagittal and transverse images of these structures should be included in an ultrasound examination of the pancreas.

Image Optimization

- Place gains settings to display normal liver parenchyma as a medium shade of gray and the normal gallbladder as an anechoic ovoid structure.
- Focal zone(s) should be placed at or below the area of interest. The use of multiple focal zones increases detail resolution and decreases temporal resolution.
- Sufficient imaging depth to visualize structures immediately posterior to the area of interest.
- Spatial compounding can be used to improve visualization of structures posterior to highly attenuating structures.
- Doppler settings should be adjusted for a slow flow rate.
- The use of deep inspiration or the Valsalva maneuver may improve visualization of the pancreas.
- The use of multiple patient positions may relocate overlying bowel gas.

Examination Limitations

- Body habitus.
- Gastrointestinal gas.
- Small left lobe of the liver.

Helpful Hints

- Structures that will mimic the pancreatic duct include:
  - Splenic vein.
  - Splenic artery.
  - Posterior wall of the stomach.
  - Retroperitoneal fat.
- With the patient in a left lateral decubitus position, angle caudally through the left lobe of the liver to visualize the pancreas.
- Using a right posterior oblique position, the tail of the pancreas may be seen using the spleen as an acoustic window.
- Valsalva maneuver may reposition bowel gas and aid in visualization of the pancreas.
- Using a larger curvilinear transducer compress over the transverse colon to reposition bowel gas.
- The splenic vein courses along the posterior inferior aspect of the pancreas.
- The distal common bile duct is visualized best in the transverse plane.

Indications for Ultrasound Examination

- Severe epigastric pain.
- Abdominal pain radiating to the back.
- Elevated pancreatic enzymes.
- Biliary disease.
- Abnormal liver enzymes.
- Abdominal distention with hypoactive bowel sounds.
- Pancreatitis.
- Weight loss.
- Anorexia.
- Pancreas neoplasm.
- Evaluate mass from previous imaging study (e.g., CT).

LABORATORY VALUES

Serum Amylase

- Normal range is 23 to 85 U/L.
- Increases with acute pancreatitis, pancreatic pseudocyst, intestinal obstruction, peptic ulcer disease, ectopic pregnancy, and other diseases of the salivary glands or ducts.
- Decreases with hepatitis and cirrhosis.
- Remains elevated for approximately 24 hours in episodes of acute pancreatitis.

Urine Amylase

- Remains increased longer than serum amylase in episodes of acute pancreatitis.

Serum Lipase

- Normal range less than 160 U/L.
- Remains elevated for a longer period (up to 14 days).
- Increases with pancreatitis, obstruction of the pancreatic duct, pancreatic carcinoma, acute cholecystitis, cirrhosis, and severe renal disease.

Glucose

- Normal range ≤ 100 mg/dL (fasting), ≤ 145 mg/dL (2 hours postprandial).
- Increases with severe diabetes mellitus, chronic liver disease, and overactivity of several of the endocrine glands.
- Decreases with tumors of the islets of Langerhans in the pancreas.

Pancreas Inflammation

PANCREAS INFLAMMATION	ETIOLOGY	CLINICAL FINDINGS	SONOGRAPHIC FINDINGS	DIFFERENTIAL CONSIDERATIONS
Acute pancreatitis	Biliary disease (most common) Alcohol abuse Trauma Peptic ulcer disease Idiopathic	Abrupt onset of epigastric pain Nausea/vomiting Elevated lipase and amylase Leukocytosis Paralytic ileus	Normal findings (30%) Decrease in parenchymal echogenicity Smooth borders Diffuse enlargement **Fluid collections:** Lesser sac Anterior pararenal space Posterior pararenal space Around the left lobe of the liver	Normal pancreas Neoplasm
Chronic pancreatitis	Repeated, prolonged, or persistent attacks of pancreatitis Hypocalcemia Hyperlipidemia	Chronic right upper quadrant (RUQ) or epigastric pain Nausea/vomiting Weight loss Abnormal glucose tolerance test Normal amylase and lipase values	Increase in parenchymal echogenicity Increased sound attenuation Irregular borders Calcifications Pseudocyst formation Atrophy Prominent pancreatic duct	Fatty replacement Neoplasm
Cystic fibrosis	Exocrine gland disorder Occurs almost exclusively in Caucasians	Abdominal pain Bloating Flatulence Diabetes Failure to thrive	Increase in parenchymal echogenicity (due to multiple small cysts) Small cysts May appear inhomogeneous Nonvisualization of the gallbladder Biliary sludge Thick, irregular folds in the GI tract ("donut sign") Fatty infiltration of the liver Portal hypertension	Chronic pancreatitis Fatty replacement Polycystic disease

Complications of Pancreatitis

COMPLICATIONS	DESCRIPTION	CLINICAL FINDINGS	SONOGRAPHIC FINDINGS
Abscess	Develops as a result of infection of the necrotic pancreas Occurs 2-4 weeks following an episode of acute pancreatitis	Abdominal pain Leukocytosis Nausea/vomiting Fever	Thick walled anechoic/hypoechoic complex mass Irregular or smooth borders Fluid-debris levels
Duodenal obstruction	High protein concentration in the pancreas enzymes can irritate the duodenum	Abdominal pain Abdominal distention Nausea/vomiting Constipation	Limited bowel peristalsis

Complications of Pancreatitis—(cont'd)

COMPLICATIONS	DESCRIPTION	CLINICAL FINDINGS	SONOGRAPHIC FINDINGS
Hemorrhage	Rapid development of inflammation causing necrosis and hemorrhage	Severe abdominal pain Nausea/vomiting Abdominal distention Elevated amylase and lipase Decrease in hematocrit level and serum calcium levels	Well-defined homogeneous mass Cystic mass with debris Fluid-debris levels
Phlegmon	Extension of pancreatic inflammation into the peripancreatic tissues Enlarged solid inflammation with retroperitoneal fat necrosis	Severe abdominal pain Nausea/vomiting Elevated amylase and lipase	Hypoechoic solid mass adjacent to the pancreas Posterior acoustic enhancement Irregular borders Usually involves the lesser sac, transverse mesocolon, and anterior pararenal space
Pseudocyst	Focal collection of inflammatory necrotic tissue, blood, and pancreas secretions Most often located in the lesser sac followed by the anterior pararenal space Most commonly associated with alcoholic or biliary disease **Complications** Rupture causing sudden shock and peritonitis (50% mortality rate)	Abdominal pain Palpable mass Solitary or multiple Persistent elevated amylase	Anechoic or complex mass Well-defined borders Variable shape

Cysts of the Pancreas

PATHOLOGY	ETIOLOGY	CLINICAL FINDINGS	SONOGRAPHIC FINDINGS	DIFFERENTIAL CONSIDERATIONS
Cyst	Congenital anomalous development of the pancreatic duct **Acquired:** Retention cyst Parasitical cyst Neoplastic cyst	Asymptomatic Dyspepsia Jaundice	Anechoic mass Smooth borders Posterior acoustic enhancement	Fluid-filled stomach Pseudocyst Polycystic disease
Cystadenoma	**Microcystic:** Accounts for 50% of cystic neoplasms involving the pancreas **Macrocystic:** Arise from the ducts Malignant potential	Asymptomatic Abdominal pain Palpable mass Weight loss Female prevalence (4:1)	Majority are located in the body and tail **Microcystic:** Echogenic or complex mass **Macrocystic:** Multiloculated cystic mass Irregular margins Solid nodules Displacement of the common bile duct, pancreatic duct, and splenic vein may occur	Pseudocyst Polycystic disease Abscess Fluid-filled stomach
Polycystic disease	Associated with polycystic liver or kidney disease	Asymptomatic Abdominal pain	Multiple cysts Associated with multiple cysts in the liver, kidney, or spleen	True cyst Fluid-filled loops of bowel Cystadenoma
Pseudocyst	Inflammation of the pancreas	Abdominal pain Palpable mass Elevated amylase	Anechoic or complex mass Thick, irregular borders Variable in size and shape Solitary or multiple	Fluid-filled stomach Neoplasm Dilated pancreatic duct Left renal vein Omental cyst Cystadenoma

Pancreas Neoplasms

NEOPLASM	ETIOLOGY	CLINICAL FINDINGS	SONOGRAPHIC FINDINGS	DIFFERENTIAL CONSIDERATIONS
Carcinoma Fourth most common malignancy	Adenocarcinoma in 90% of cases 70% involve the head of the pancreas 20% involve the body	Abdominal pain Severe back pain Weight loss Painless jaundice Anorexia New onset of diabetes Thrombophlebitis of the lower extremities	Hypoechoic mass in the pancreas Irregular borders Dilated biliary tree Hydropic gallbladder Liver metastasis Ascites	Focal pancreatitis Adenoma Caudate lobe of the liver
Islet cell tumor	**Functional:** Insulinoma Gastrinoma **Nonfunctional:** 90% are malignant Comprise one third of all islet cell tumors	**Insulinoma:** Increase in insulin levels Hypoglycemia Headaches Obesity Confusion **Gastrinoma:** Gastric hyperstimulation associated with peptic ulcer disease	Small, well-defined hypoechoic mass Large tumors are more echogenic Typically located in the body or tail Calcifications Necrotic cystic areas are more likely malignant Majority are hypervascular	Adenoma Carcinoma Complex cyst

PANCREATODUODENECTOMY (Whipple Procedure) (FIG. 9.2)

Preoperative Criteria

- Absence of extrapancreatic metastasis.
- Portal, splenic, and superior mesenteric veins are evaluated for patency and absence of tumor or thrombus.
- Celiac axis and superior mesenteric arteries are evaluated for patency.

Basic Procedure

- Gallbladder is removed.
- Common duct is ligated superior to the cystic duct and anastomosed to the duodenum distal to the pancreas.
- Remaining pancreas tissue is attached to the duodenum.
- Stomach is anastomosed distal to the bile duct.

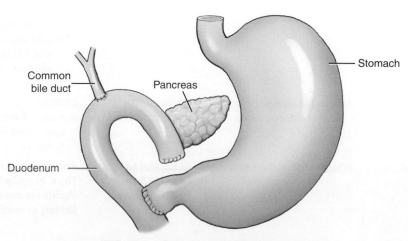

FIG. 9.2 Pancreatoduodenectomy.

PANCREAS REVIEW

1. Demonstration of the pancreatic head surrounding the duodenum is consistent with:
   a. a phlegmon
   b. ectopic pancreas tissue
   c. pancreas divisum
   d. an annular pancreas

2. Common clinical findings associated with acute pancreatitis include:
   a. left upper quadrant pain, flank pain, elevated glucose levels
   b. severe epigastric pain, nausea/vomiting, elevated bilirubin
   c. paralytic ileus, severe epigastric pain, elevated serum lipase
   d. right upper quadrant pain, nausea/vomiting, elevated alkaline phosphatase

3. Which of the following enzymes is responsible for the breakdown of proteins into amino acids?
   a. amylase
   b. gastrin
   c. lipase
   d. trypsin

4. The location of the uncinate process is described as:
   a. superior to the aorta
   b. anterior to the main portal vein
   c. posterior to the superior mesenteric vein
   d. lateral to the gastroduodenal artery

5. The most common complication associated with acute pancreatitis is a(n):
   a. abscess
   b. phlegmon
   c. pseudocyst
   d. bowel obstruction

6. Islet cells of Langerhans secrete hormones directly into the:
   a. duodenum
   b. bloodstream
   c. lymphatic circulation
   d. main pancreatic duct

7. In a Whipple procedure, normal pancreatic tissue is attached to the:
   a. liver
   b. stomach
   c. duodenum
   d. common bile duct

8. Extension of pancreatic inflammation into the peripancreatic tissues is called a(n):
   a. abscess
   b. pseudocyst
   c. phlegmon
   d. annular pancreas

9. The most *common cause* of acute pancreatitis is:
   a. alcohol abuse
   b. biliary disease
   c. hyperlipidemia
   d. peptic ulcer disease

Using Figure 9.3, answer question 10.

10. A 59-year-old male inpatient presents with a history of acute pancreatitis. Based on this clinical history, the calipers in this sonogram are *most likely* measuring a:
    a. biloma
    b. phlegmon
    c. pseudocyst
    d. duodenal obstruction

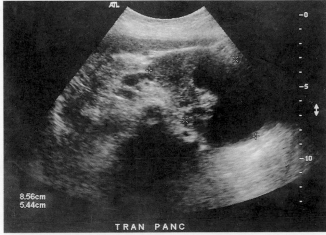

FIG. 9.3 Transverse image of the pancreas.

Using Figure 9.4, answer question 11.

11. Which of the following structures is demonstrated directly anterior to the splenic vein?
    a. splenic artery
    b. pancreatic duct
    c. common bile duct
    d. gastroduodenal artery

Using Figure 9.5, answer question 12.

12. Which of the following vascular structures does the arrow identify?
    a. abdominal aorta
    b. splenic artery
    c. left renal vein
    d. superior mesenteric artery

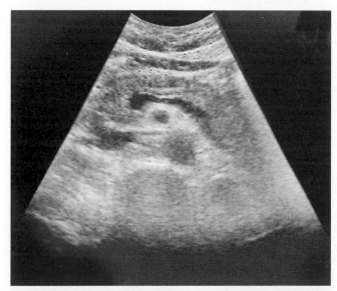

FIG. 9.4 Transverse image of the pancreas.

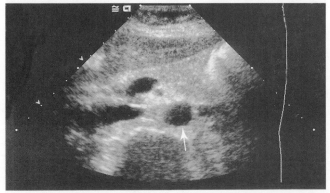

FIG. 9.5 Transverse image of the pancreas.

Using Figure 9.6, answer questions 13 and 14.

13. The findings in this sonogram are most suspicious for a(n):
    a. abscess
    b. pseudocyst
    c. malignant neoplasm
    d. islet cell tumor

14. The anechoic tubular structure demonstrated anterior to the splenic vein is most likely a(n):
    a. gastric varix
    b. dilated pancreatic duct
    c. tortuous splenic artery
    d. enlarged superior mesenteric vein

15. Pseudocyst formation is most commonly located in which of the following abdominal recesses?
    a. lesser sac
    b. perirenal space
    c. anterior pararenal space
    d. subhepatic space

16. Which of the following enzymes changes fats into fatty acids and glycerol?
    a. amylase
    b. gastrin
    c. lipase
    d. trypsin

17. Which region of the pancreas is located most superiorly?
    a. head
    b. body
    c. neck
    d. tail

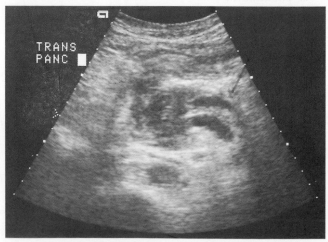

FIG. 9.6 Transverse image of the pancreas.

18. Ectopic pancreatic tissue is most commonly located in which of the following organs?
    a. liver
    b. spleen
    c. kidney
    d. stomach

19. The pancreas and surrounding vascular landmarks should be examined from the level of the:
    a. celiac axis to below the renal veins
    b. superior mesenteric artery to below the renal arteries
    c. main portal vein to below the renal veins
    d. splenic artery to below the superior mesenteric vein

20. Which of the following pathologies accounts for half of the cystic neoplasms involving the pancreas?
    a. retention cyst
    b. cystic fibrosis
    c. polycystic disease
    d. microcystic cystadenoma

21. In acute pancreatitis, which of the following laboratory tests remains elevated longest?
    a. lipase
    b. amylase
    c. bilirubin
    d. glucose

22. The main pancreatic duct is most commonly visualized in which section of the pancreas?
    a. head
    b. body
    c. neck
    d. tail

23. The majority of nonfunctioning islet cell tumors are:
    a. malignant
    b. hyperechoic in echo texture
    c. located in the head of the pancreas
    d. dependent on insulin levels

24. Chronic pancreatitis is most likely to appear on ultrasound as a(n):
    a. enlarged hypoechoic pancreas with multiple parenchymal calcifications
    b. hyperechoic enlarged pancreas with associated pseudocyst formation
    c. hypoechoic irregular pancreas with multiple parenchymal calcifications
    d. hyperechoic pancreas with a prominent pancreatic duct and multiple parenchymal calcifications

25. Clinical findings commonly associated with pancreatic carcinoma may include:
    a. chest pain
    b. weight gain
    c. new onset of diabetes
    d. intolerance to fatty foods

Using Figure 9.7, answer question 26.

26. A patient presents with a history of elevating insulin levels. Based on this history, the sonographic finding is most suspicious for a(n):
    a. adenoma
    b. focal pancreatitis
    c. islet cell tumor
    d. adenocarcinoma

Using Figure 9.8, answer question 27.

27. The sonographic appearance of the pancreas in this asymptomatic patient is most suspicious for:
    a. a phlegmon
    b. microlithiasis
    c. chronic pancreatitis
    d. normal pancreas parenchyma

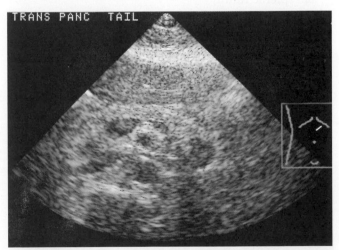

FIG. 9.7   Transverse image of the pancreas.

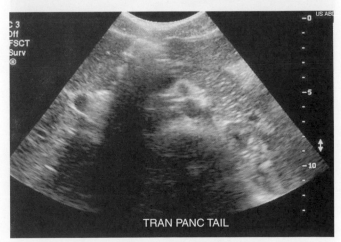

FIG. 9.8   Transverse image of the pancreas.

Using Figure 9.9, answer question 28.

28. The anechoic structure located in the lateral portion of the pancreatic head is the:
    a. common bile duct
    b. gastroduodenal artery
    c. common hepatic duct
    d. superior mesenteric vein

29. An endocrine function of the pancreas includes secretion of:
    a. gastrin
    b. lipase
    c. insulin
    d. trypsin

30. Which of the following vascular landmarks is located superior to the pancreas?
    a. splenic vein
    b. celiac axis
    c. main portal vein
    d. superior mesenteric artery

31. The tail of the pancreas generally extends toward the:
    a. stomach
    b. splenic hilum
    c. pararenal space
    d. left renal hilum

32. Which of the following vascular structures is used as a sonographic landmark in locating the tail of the pancreas?
    a. splenic artery
    b. left renal vein
    c. splenic vein
    d. portosplenic confluence

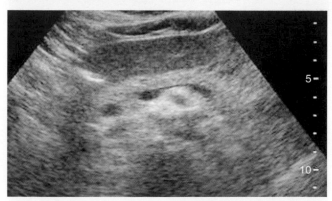

FIG. 9.9   Transverse image of the pancreas.

33. The diameter of the pancreatic duct in the head/neck region should not exceed:
    a. 2 mm
    b. 3 mm
    c. 6 mm
    d. 10 mm

34. Which of the following structures is responsible for the secretion of pancreatic enzymes?
    a. beta cells
    b. acinar cells
    c. alpha cells
    d. islet cells of Langerhans

35. Which of the following best describes the location of the pancreatic neck?
    a. posterior to the superior mesenteric vein
    b. superior to the celiac axis
    c. anterior to the portosplenic confluence
    d. posterior to the superior mesenteric artery

36. The majority of pancreatic malignancies involve which portion of the pancreas?
    a. head
    b. neck
    c. body
    d. tail

37. In which section of the pancreas are islet cell tumors most commonly located?
    a. body and tail
    b. head and body
    c. neck and body
    d. head and tail

38. The secondary secretory duct of the pancreas is termed the duct of:
    a. Vater
    b. Langerhans
    c. Santorini
    d. Wirsung

39. Gain settings should be in place to demonstrate the normal adult pancreas as:
    a. hypoechoic compared with the normal liver
    b. hypoechoic compared with the normal renal cortex
    c. hyperechoic compared with the normal spleen
    d. isoechoic compared with the normal liver

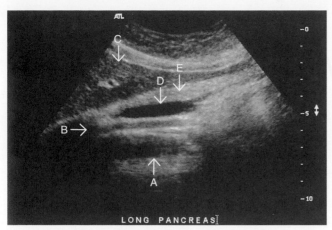

FIG. 9.10 Sagittal image of the pancreas.

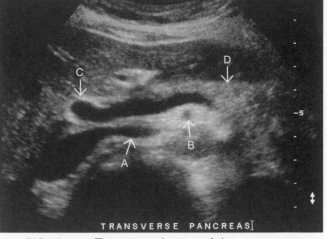

FIG. 9.11 Transverse image of the pancreas.

Using Figure 9.10, answer questions 40 through 42.

40. The superior mesenteric vein corresponds to which of the following letters?
a. A
b. B
c. D
d. E

41. The abdominal aorta corresponds to which of the following letters?
a. A
b. B
c. D
d. E

42. The superior mesenteric artery corresponds to which of the following letters?
a. A
b. B
c. D
d. E

Using Figure 9.11, answer questions 43 and 44.

43. Letter *B* corresponds to which of the following vascular structures?
a. splenic artery
b. celiac axis
c. right renal artery
d. superior mesenteric artery

44. Letter *C* corresponds to which of the following vascular structures?
a. splenic vein
b. coronary vein
c. main portal vein
d. superior mesenteric vein

45. The majority of cystadenomas involving the pancreas are located in the:
a. body and tail
b. head and neck
c. head and body
d. uncinate process

46. The section of the pancreas lying most anterior is the:
a. head
b. neck
c. body
d. tail

47. Which of the following structures should be evaluated when multiple cysts are discovered in the pancreas?
a. kidneys, liver, spleen
b. kidneys, liver, adrenal glands
c. spleen, kidneys, ovaries/testes
d. liver, spleen, abdominal aorta

48. Rapid progression of pancreatic inflammation is a complication associated with:
a. acute cholecystitis
b. cystic fibrosis
c. acute pancreatitis
d. biliary obstruction

49. A sheath of muscle fibers surrounding the distal common bile duct describes the:
a. ampulla of Vater
b. minor papilla
c. sphincter of Oddi
d. major papilla

50. The leakage of pancreatic enzymes into the surrounding peritoneal space describes a(n):
a. abscess
b. seroma
c. pseudocyst
d. phlegmon

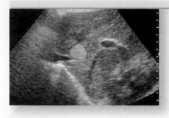

CHAPTER 10

Urinary System

KEY TERMS

acute tubular necrosis (ATN)   ischemic necrosis of tubular cells; most common cause of renal failure.

afferent arteriole   carries blood entering the glomerulus.

angiomyolipoma   benign tumor composed of blood vessels, smooth muscle, and fat.

angiotensin   polypoid in the blood that causes vasoconstriction, increase in blood pressure, and the release of aldosterone.

Bowman's capsule   cup-like structure surrounding the glomerulus.

efferent arteriole   carries the blood away from the glomerulus.

fascia   fibrous connective membrane of the body that may be separate from other structures.

Gerota's fascia   protective covering of tissue surrounding each kidney.

glomerulonephritis   inflammation of the glomerulus of the kidney.

glomerulus   structure composed of blood vessels or nerve fibers.

hypertrophied column of Bertin   enlargement of a column of Bertin that extends into the renal pyramid.

infundibulum   portion of the collecting system composed of the minor and major calyces.

medullary pyramid   renal pyramid.

papilla   blunt apex of the renal pyramid.

parapelvic cyst   fluid-filled mass of lymphatic origin located within the renal sinus.

pelviectasis   dilation of the renal pelvis.

renal colic   sharp, severe flank pain radiating to the groin.

renal failure   the inability of the kidneys to excrete waste, concentrate urine, and conserve electrolytes.

renal insufficiency   partial kidney function failure characterized by less than normal urine output.

renal lobe   portion of the kidney consisting of a single pyramid, bordered on both sides by the interlobar arteries, with cortical tissue at its base.

renal parenchyma   the functional tissue of the kidney consisting of the nephrons.

renal sinus lipomatosis   excessive accumulation of fat in the renal sinus.

renin   renal enzyme that affects blood pressure.

staghorn calculus   large stone forming in the renal pelvis and extending into some or all of the calyces.

twinkle artifact   quick fluctuating color Doppler signal from a rough surface or highly reflective object.

urachus   epithelial tube connecting the apex of the urinary bladder to the umbilicus.

ureterocele   prolapse of the distal ureter into the urinary bladder.

PHYSIOLOGY

- The nephron is the basic functional unit of the kidney.
- Nephron is composed of:
  a. Renal corpuscle.
    - glomerulus.
    - Bowman's capsule.
    - afferent arteriole.
    - efferent arteriole.
  b. Renal tubule.
    - proximal convoluted tubule.
    - loop of Henle.
    - distal convoluted tubule.
- Each kidney contains more than one million nephrons.

Functions of the Urinary System

- Produces urine and erythropoietin.
- Influences blood pressure, blood volume, and intake or excretion of salt and water through the renin–angiotensin system.
- Regulates serum electrolytes.
- Regulates acid–base balance.

ANATOMY

Renal Anatomy (Fig. 10.1)

ANATOMY	DESCRIPTION
Renal capsule	Fibrous capsule (true capsule) surrounding the cortex
Renal cortex	Outer portion of the kidney Bound by the renal capsule and arcuate vessels Contains glomerular capsules and convoluted tubules
Medulla	Inner portion of the renal parenchyma Within the medulla lie the renal pyramids **Renal pyramids:** • Triangular structure with a narrow tip (apex) that sits within the minor calyx and the wider base that abuts the renal cortex • Contain tubules and the loops of Henle
Collecting system	Consists of the infundibulum and renal pelvis
Column of Bertin	Inward extension of the renal cortex between the renal pyramids
Renal sinus	Central portion of the kidney Contains the major and minor calyces, peripelvic fat, fibrous tissues, arteries, veins, lymphatics, and part of the renal pelvis
Renal hilum	Contains the renal artery, renal vein, and ureter

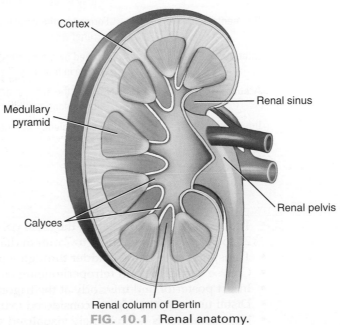

FIG. 10.1 Renal anatomy.

Renal Vasculature

RENAL VESSEL	DESCRIPTION
Main renal artery(s)	The right renal artery arises from the anterolateral aspect of the aorta; the left renal artery arises from the posterolateral aspect of the aorta May have multiple ipsilateral arteries A single ipsilateral artery may divide into multiple renal arteries at the hilum Courses posterior to the renal vein and anterior to the ureter Main renal artery arises 1.0–1.5 cm inferior to the origin of the superior mesenteric artery Right renal artery is longer than the left renal artery Demonstrates low-resistance blood flow with a sharp systolic peak Supplies the kidney, ureter, and adrenal gland
Segmental arteries	After entering the renal hilum, the main renal artery(s) divides into 4–5 segmental arteries Demonstrates low-resistance blood flow
Interlobar arteries	Branch of the segmental artery Course alongside the renal pyramids Demonstrates low-resistance blood flow Resistive index (RI) less than 0.7
Arcuate arteries	Boundary between the cortex and medulla Branch of the interlobar artery located at the base of the medulla Arcuate arteries give rise to the interlobular arteries Demonstrates low-resistance blood flow RI less than 0.7
Interlobular arteries	Give rise to the afferent arteries to enter the glomerulus
Main renal vein	Formed from the junction of tributaries in the renal hilum Courses anterior to the renal artery Left renal vein receives the left suprarenal and left gonadal vein Left renal vein is longer than the right renal vein Dilatation of the left renal vein, caused by mesenteric compression as it courses between the superior mesenteric artery and abdominal aorta may be demonstrated (Pincer effect)
Segmental veins	Formed by the convergence of the interlobar veins forming the main renal vein
Interlobar veins	Formed by the convergence of the arcuate veins Course in between the medullary pyramids
Arcuate veins	Parallel the arcuate arteries Course along the base of the medullary pyramids
Interlobar veins	Receive blood from the efferent veins

Ureter Anatomy

- Tubular structure connecting the renal pelvis to the urinary bladder measuring 25 to 34 cm in length and 4 to 7 mm in diameter.
- Transport urine to the bladder through a peristaltic action.
- Course vertically with retroperitoneum along the psoas muscles.
- Insert posterior and inferiorly at the trigone of the bladder.
- Distal ureter at the trigone considered extraperitoneal.
- Normal ureter is not routinely visualized with ultrasound.

Arterial Supply to the Ureter

- Renal artery.
- Testicular or ovarian artery.
- Superior vesical artery.
- Hypogastric artery.

Urethra Anatomy

- A small tubular structure that drains urine from the bladder.
- 20 cm in length in males and 3.5 cm in length in females.
- Internal sphincters control urine flow from the bladder.
- Urethral orifice indicates the neck of the bladder.

Support Structure of the Kidneys	
Psoas muscle	Major groin muscle Primary flexor of the hip joint Lies posterior to the inferior pole of each kidney
Quadratus lumborum muscle	Muscle of the posterior abdominal wall Lies posterior and medial to each kidney
Transversus abdominis muscle	Deepest layer of flat muscles of the anterolateral wall Lies lateral to each kidney
Gerota's fascia	Fibrous covering of tissue surrounding each kidney Also known as Gerota's capsule; renal fascia
Perinephric fat	Fatty tissue surrounding each kidney
Renal capsule	Protective connective tissue capsule surrounding each kidney

Location

- Paired bean-shaped structures lying in a sagittal oblique plane in the retroperitoneal cavity.
- Located between the first and third lumbar vertebrae.
- Superior poles lie more posterior and medial.
- Inferior poles lie more anterior and lateral.
- Left kidney lies superior to the right kidney.

Left Kidney Is Located

- Posterior to the tail of the pancreas, spleen, jejunum, stomach, and the splenic flexure.

Right Kidney Is Located

- Posterior to the right lobe of the liver, second portion of the duodenum, hepatic flexure, jejunum, ileum, and Morison's pouch.

Each Kidney Is Located

- Anterior to the diaphragm, psoas, transversus, and quadratus lumborum muscles.
- Medial to the transverse abdominis muscle.
- Lateral to the quadratus lumborum muscle.
- Inferior and slightly lateral to the adrenal gland.

Renal Anatomic Variants

VARIANT	DESCRIPTIONS	CLINICAL FINDINGS	SONOGRAPHIC FINDINGS	DIFFERENTIAL CONSIDERATIONS
Dromedary hump	Cortical bulge on the lateral aspect of the kidney Demonstrated most often on the left	Asymptomatic	Lateral outward cortical bulge Echogenicity equal to the cortex	Carcinoma Hematoma Complex renal cyst Hypertrophied column of Bertin
Extrarenal pelvis	Renal pelvis extrudes from the renal hilum	Asymptomatic	Anechoic oval-shaped structure medial to the renal hilum No vascular flow	Hydroureter Renal cyst Renal vein
Fetal lobulation	Immature renal development	Asymptomatic	Scalloped or lobulated appearance in the renal contour	Junctional parenchymal defect Dromedary hump
Hypertrophied column of Bertin	Enlarged column of Bertin	Asymptomatic	Mass extending from the cortex into the renal pyramids Echogenicity similar to cortex Demonstrates arcuate arteries within the extension	Carcinoma Renal duplication Abscess
Junctional parenchymal defect	Embryonic remnant of the fusion site between the upper and lower portions of the kidney	Asymptomatic	Triangular echogenic area in the superior anterior aspect of the kidney Courses obliquely toward the renal sinus	Technical factors Calcified artery Angiomyolipoma Fetal lobulation

Congenital Anomalies

ANOMALY	DESCRIPTION	CLINICAL FINDINGS	SONOGRAPHIC FINDINGS	DIFFERENTIAL CONSIDERATIONS
Agenesis	Absence of the kidney(s) Unilateral or bilateral	Asymptomatic when unilateral Fatal when bilateral Associated with genital anomalies	Empty renal fossa(e) Large, contralateral kidney Ipsilateral gonad is frequently absent	Pelvic kidney Surgical removal Crossed fused ectopia
Cake kidney	Variant of a horseshoe kidney Found in the pelvis	Asymptomatic Pelvic mass	Fusion of entire medial aspect of both kidneys Anterior rotation of the renal pelvis	Crossed fused ectopia Renal mass
Crossed fused ectopia	Both kidneys are fused in the same quadrant Two separate collecting systems Two normally located adrenal glands	Asymptomatic Abdominal mass	One single, large kidney Irregular contour Inferior pole is directed medially	Renal mass Cake kidney Sigmoid kidney
Duplication	Two distinct collecting systems May involve kidney, ureter, and/or renal pelvis May be partial or complete	Asymptomatic Flank pain	Increase in renal length Two distinct collecting systems The superior system is most likely to obstruct	Hypertrophied column of Bertin Renal mass

Congenital Anomalies—(cont'd)

ANOMALY	DESCRIPTION	CLINICAL FINDINGS	SONOGRAPHIC FINDINGS	DIFFERENTIAL CONSIDERATIONS
Horseshoe kidney	Fusion of the kidneys usually at the inferior poles Connected by an isthmus of functioning parenchyma or nonfunctioning fibrotic tissue Anterior rotation of the renal pelves and ureters Separate collecting systems Most common form of renal fusion	Asymptomatic Pulsatile abdominal mass	Bilateral low-lying medially placed kidneys with partial or complete fusion of the inferior poles "Dipping effect" of both inferior poles Isthmus of tissue demonstrated anterior to the abdominal aorta Isthmus echo texture is similar to the renal cortex	Renal mass Lymphadenopathy Bowel Retroperitoneal tumor
Pelvic kidney	Failure to ascend with development Associated with a short ureter Renal artery and vein are located more inferior Renal vein drains directly into the inferior vena cava (IVC)	Asymptomatic Pelvic pain	Elongated core of echogenic tissue surrounded by less echogenic parenchyma Located in the lower abdomen or pelvis Empty ipsilateral renal fossa Lies in an oblique plane	Bowel Pelvic mass
Renal ptosis	Unusual mobile kidney that descends from the normal position toward the pelvis Poor support structures	Asymptomatic	Abnormal mobility of a kidney	Pelvic kidney Horseshoe kidney
Sigmoid kidney	Variant of the horseshoe kidney	Asymptomatic Abdominal mass	Superior pole of one kidney is fused with the inferior pole of the contralateral kidney S-shaped	Bowel Abdominal mass
Thoracic kidney	Kidney migrates into the chest through a herniation in the diaphragm Rare finding	Chest mass	Elongated core of echogenic tissue surrounded by less echogenic parenchyma Located in the chest Not easily demonstrated on ultrasound	Chest mass

SIZE

- Left kidney is generally longer than the right kidney.
- The left pediatric kidney is approximately the size of the adjacent spleen.

Adult

- 9.0 to 12.0 cm in length.
- 4.0 to 5.0 cm in width.
- 2.5 to 3.0 cm in height.
- Minimum of 1 cm in cortical thickness.
- Abnormal if length of one kidney exceeds 1.5 cm compared with the length of the contralateral kidney.

Child

- 7.0 to 8.0 cm in length.
- Formula: (© SDMS National Certification Examination Review: Abdominal Sonography: 2010).
  - Renal length (cm) = 6.79 + [0.22 × age (years)].

Infant

- 5.0 to 6.0 cm in length.
- Formula: (© SDMS National Certification Examination Review: Abdominal Sonography: 2010).
  - Renal length (cm) = 4.98 + [0.155 × age (months)].

Neonate

- 3.3 to 5.0 cm in length.
- 2.0 to 3.0 cm in width.
- 1.5 to 2.5 cm in height.

SONOGRAPHIC APPEARANCE

Normal Sonographic Appearance—Adult Kidney

DIVISION	SONOGRAPHIC APPEARANCE
Renal capsule	Well-defined echogenic line surrounding the kidney
Renal cortex	Homogeneous, fine, moderate, to low-level echogenicity Less echogenic compared with the normal liver parenchyma
Medulla	Hypoechoic triangular structures between the renal cortex and sinus; may appear anechoic
Columns of Bertin	Moderate to low-level echogenicity
Renal sinus	Hyperechoic; most echogenic
Arcuate vessels	Small echogenic foci at the corticomedullary junction
Cortical thickness	Minimum 1 cm

Normal Sonographic Appearance—Infant Kidney

DIVISION	SONOGRAPHIC APPEARANCE
Renal capsule	Sparse amount of perinephric fat makes it difficult to distinguish the capsule
Renal cortex	Isoechoic to slightly hyperechoic compared with the liver or spleen parenchyma
Medulla	Commonly anechoic but may appear hypoechoic Larger in size compared with the adult medulla Do not mistake for hydronephrosis
Renal sinus	Barely visible in infants

EXAMINATION TECHNIQUES, PROTOCOLS, AND IMAGE OPTIMIZATION

Preparation

- No preparation is required before an ultrasound of the urinary system.
- Suggested preparation:
  - Kidneys—patient should be hydrated.
  - Bladder:
    - Adults should drink 8 to 16 ounces of water 1 hour before the examination.
    - Children—8 ounces of water 1 hour before the examination.
    - Infants—no preparation is necessary.
  - Renal vessels—nothing by mouth for 6 to 8 hours before the examination.

Transducer Selection

- Use the highest frequency possible to obtain optimal resolution for penetration depth.
  - Adults—3.0 to 5.0 MHz.
  - Children and small adults—5.0 to 7.0 MHz.
  - Obese patients—2.0 MHz may be required.
- Curvilinear transducers provide a wider field of view.
- Sector or vector transducers have a smaller footprint, great for intercostal imaging.
- Subcostal or prone imaging in some patients may be helpful.
- Higher frequency transducers can be used in thin adult patients.

Patient Positioning

- Examination usually begins with the:
  - Adult patient in a supine, posterior oblique or lateral decubitus position.
  - Pediatric patient in a prone position.

PATIENT POSITION	DEMONSTRATES/BENEFITS
Supine	Right superior pole with intercostal approach Right inferior pole with subcostal approach
Left posterior oblique (LPO)	Allows bowel to move away from right kidney Subcostal or intercostal approach
Left lateral decubitus	Liver and kidney "fall" from the rib cage Aids in obese or gassy patients
Right posterior oblique (RPO)	Left superior pole with intercostal approach Posterior subcostal approach for left inferior pole
Right lateral decubitus	Left posterior approach with deep inspiration
Prone	Demonstrates mid and inferior poles of both kidneys Great for infants and small children Superior poles may be visualized Used in renal biopsies

Examination Protocol

- Systematic approach in the sagittal, coronal, and transverse planes carefully examining:
  - Superior pole, renal hilum, and inferior pole of each kidney.
  - Medial and lateral border of each kidney.
- Length, height, and width measurement of each kidney.
- Cortical thickness measurement of each kidney.
- Image of the liver/right kidney and the spleen/left kidney relationship for comparison of parenchymal echogenicity.
- Color Doppler imaging of the renal vasculature and perfusion.
- Evaluation and documentation of the bladder wall.
- Prevoid and postvoid volumes may be included.
- Color Doppler imaging of ureteral jets should be included when urinary obstruction is encountered.
- Abnormalities should be documented and when applicable measured in two imaging planes. Color and/or spectral Doppler evaluation of the abnormality should be included.

Image Optimization

- Place gains settings to display the normal renal cortex hypoechoic to the normal liver and splenic parenchyma.

- Focal zone(s) should be placed at or below the area of interest. The use of multiple focal zones increases detail resolution and decreases temporal resolution.
- Sufficient imaging depth to visualize structures immediately posterior to the area of interest (immediately anterior when patient is prone).
- Harmonic imaging and decreasing system compression (dynamic range) can be used to reduce artifactual echoes within normal anechoic structures.
- Spatial compounding can be used to improve visualization of structures posterior to highly attenuating structures.
- Doppler settings should be adjusted for a slow flow rate.
- The use of deep inspiration may improve visualization of the kidneys.
- The use of multiple patient positions may redistribute overlying bowel gas.

Examination Limitations

- Superior location of the kidneys (high under ribcage).
- Gastrointestinal gas.
- Obesity.

Helpful Hints

- Multiple imaging windows may be necessary to evaluate each kidney in its entirety.
- In the lateral decubitus position have the patient rest their arm above their head to increase the space between the inferior rib cage and superior portion of the pelvis.
- In the posterior oblique or lateral decubitus positions, using the subcostal approach, angle up under the ribcage to aid in visualization of the kidney.
- High-frequency transducers and turning off compound scanning can increase appreciation of acoustic shadowing posterior to renal calculus(i).
- Prone imaging in adults can aid in visualizing the inferior pole of the kidneys.
- The use of harmonics improves imaging of obese patients.
- The origin of the right renal artery is around 10:00 and the origin of the left renal artery is around 4:00.
- The renal artery lies directly posterior to the renal vein.
- Left lateral decubitus position using a coronal plane can demonstrate both renal artery origins (banana peel), with the right renal artery coursing up toward the transducer and the left renal artery coursing away from the transducer.

Indications for Examination

- Increase in creatinine or blood to nitrogen (BUN) levels.
- Urinary tract infection.
- Flank pain.
- Hematuria.
- Hypertension.
- Decrease in urine output.
- Trauma.
- Evaluate mass from previous medical imaging study (e.g., computed tomography [CT]).

LABORATORY VALUES

Creatinine

- Normal 0.6 to 1.2 mg/dL.
- A waste product produced from meat protein and normal wear and tear on the muscles in the body.
- More specific in determining renal dysfunction than BUN levels.
- Elevated in renal failure, chronic nephritis, or urinary obstruction.

Blood Urea Nitrogen

- Normal 11 to 23 mg/dL.
- Produced from the breakdown of food proteins.
- Elevated in acute or chronic renal disease, renal damage, renal failure, dehydration, and urinary stasis. May also be due to gastrointestinal bleeding, congestive heart failure, shock, and starvation.
- Decreased levels associated with overhydration, pregnancy, liver failure, decrease in protein intake, and smoking.

Hematuria

- Visible or microscopic red blood cells in the urine.
- Associated with early renal disease.

Proteinuria

- Abnormal amount of proteins in the urine.
- Associated with nephritis, nephrolithiasis, carcinoma, polycystic disease, hypertension, and diabetes mellitus.
- Increases risk of developing progressive renal dysfunction.

Concentration–Dilution Urinalysis

- Used to detect chronic renal disease.

Cystic Pathology of the Kidneys

PATHOLOGY	ETIOLOGY	CLINICAL FINDINGS	SONOGRAPHIC FINDINGS	DIFFERENTIAL CONSIDERATIONS

Cortical cyst	Acquired condition
	Found in 50% of patients over the age of 55
		Asymptomatic
		Palpable mass
		Abdominal pain
			Simple Cyst
			Anechoic mass
			Hyperechoic thin walls
			Smooth margins
			Posterior acoustic enhancement
			Complex Cyst
			May contain:
			  Septations
			  Fluid levels
			  Calcifications
			Smooth wall margins
			Posterior acoustic enhancement
			Calcifications may demonstrate posterior acoustic shadowing
			Complex cysts require a 3-month follow up
				Liver cyst
				Adrenal cyst

Parapelvic cyst	Lymphatic in origin	Asymptomatic Hypertension Hematuria	Anechoic mass(es) located within the renal calyces (renal sinus) Does not communicate with the collecting system Smooth, thin wall margins Posterior acoustic enhancement	Hydronephrosis Renal vein Extrarenal pelvis Renal artery aneurysm

Continued

Cystic Pathology of the Kidneys—(cont'd)

PATHOLOGY	ETIOLOGY	CLINICAL FINDINGS	SONOGRAPHIC FINDINGS	DIFFERENTIAL CONSIDERATIONS
Adult polycystic kidney disease Third most common cause of renal failure	Autosomal dominant inherited disorder Normal renal parenchyma is replaced with cysts Increased incidence of renal calculi and infection	Asymptomatic Palpable abdominal mass Hypertension Hematuria Colicky pain Elevated blood urea nitrogen (BUN) and creatinine Renal failure	Bilateral disease Multiple cysts Irregular margins Normal renal parenchyma may not be visualized Associated cysts in liver (80%), pancreas, and spleen	Multicystic dysplasia Multiple simple cysts Hydronephrosis
Childhood polycystic kidney disease	Autosomal recessive inherited disorder Normal renal parenchyma is replaced with cysts	Palpable abdominal mass Hypertension Hematuria Colicky pain Renal failure	Bilateral disease Hyperechoic enlarged kidneys	Chronic renal failure Renal sinus lipomatosis
Medullary cystic disease	Adult onset—autosomal dominant Juvenile onset—autosomal recessive	Polyuria Polydipsia Hypertension Anemia Azotemia Increase in BUN and creatinine in late stages	Involves both kidneys Increased echogenicity of the medullary pyramids Thin cortex Loss of corticomedullary differentiation	Medullary sponge kidney Nephrocalcinosis Acute tubular necrosis
Multicystic dysplasia Most common renal cystic disease in infants	Affects the left kidney more frequently Noninherited disorder Urinary obstruction in early embryology Male prevalence (2:1) Infants of diabetic mothers	Asymptomatic Palpable abdominal mass Flank pain Hypertension	Unilateral disease (90%) Numerous cysts of variable shape and size Associated with ureteropelvic junction obstruction and malrotation Normal renal parenchyma may not be visualized Decreases in size in late stages Hypertrophy of contralateral kidney	Multiple simple cysts Hydronephrosis

Inflammatory Conditions

INFLAMMATORY CONDITION	ETIOLOGY	CLINICAL FINDINGS	SONOGRAPHIC FINDINGS	DIFFERENTIAL CONSIDERATIONS
Renal abscess **Risk Factor:** Diabetes	Infection	Flank pain Fever or chills Leukocytosis Pyuria Hematuria Bacteremia Normal laboratory values in 20% of cases.	Hypoechoic or complex mass Thick irregular wall margins May demonstrate posterior acoustic enhancement Shadowing associated with gas formation	Neoplasm Focal pyelonephritis Complicated cyst Resolving hematoma
Acute tubular necrosis (ATN)	Toxic drug exposure Hypotension Trauma Surgery of the heart or aorta Jaundice Sepsis	Asymptomatic Renal failure Oliguria Uremia Electrolyte imbalance	Bilateral enlarged kidneys Hyperechoic renal pyramids Normal renal cortex (89%) Elevated resistive index	Renal sinus lipomatosis Chronic pyelonephritis Renal failure Nephrocalcinosis

Inflammatory Conditions—(cont'd)

INFLAMMATORY CONDITION	ETIOLOGY	CLINICAL FINDINGS	SONOGRAPHIC FINDINGS	DIFFERENTIAL CONSIDERATIONS

Chronic renal failure	Glomerulonephritis
	Hypertension
	Vascular disease
	Diabetes mellitus
	Chronic hydrone-
	  phrosis
		Elevated BUN and
		  creatinine
		Proteinuria
		Oliguria
		Headaches
		Fatigue
		Weakness
		Anemia
		Nausea/vomiting
			Renal atrophy
			Hyperechoic parenchyma
			Thin renal cortex
			Calyceal clubbing with dilation
			Difficult to distinguish the
			  kidney from surrounding
			  structures
				Renal sinus lipomatosis
				Hypoplastic kidney

Glomerulonephritis	Immune diseases Infection Strep throat Lupus Chronic hepatitis C Vasculitis	Asymptomatic Proteinuria Oliguria Hypertension Hematuria Fatigue Edema Azotemia Elevated potassium	Hyperechoic renal cortex Normal medulla Enlarged kidney(s)	Renal sinus lipomatosis

Pyelonephritis
 	
Risk Factors:
  Vesicoureteral reflux
  Obstruction
  Diabetes
	Bacteria ascends
	  from the bladder
		Flank pain
		Fever or chills
		Dysuria
		Pyuria
		Leukocytosis
		Microscopic
		  hematuria
		Bacteremia
			Kidneys may appear normal
			Generalized or focal swelling
			  of the kidney(s)
			Well-defined renal pyramids
			Loss of corticomedullary
			  definition
				Renal abscess
				Neoplasm

Obstruction and Calculus of the Kidney

OBSTRUCTION	ETIOLOGY	CLINICAL FINDINGS	SONOGRAPHIC FINDINGS	DIFFERENTIAL CONSIDERATIONS

Hydronephrosis	Obstruction of
	  the urinary tract
		Flank pain
		Hematuria
		Fever
		Leukocytosis
			Grade 1
			Splaying of only the renal sinus
			  with a small amount of fluid
			Grade 2
			Dilation of the renal sinus and some
			  but not all calyces
			Grade 3
			Marked dilation of renal sinus, pel-
			  vis and all calyces
			Echogenic line separating the col-
			  lecting system from the paren-
			  chyma can be demonstrated
			Grade 4
			Prominent dilatation of renal sinus,
			  renal pelvis and all calyces
			Cortical thinning
			Unable to separate collecting
			  system and renal parenchyma
			Regardless of the grade evaluate
			  bladder for ureteral jets using
			  color Doppler
			Resistive index of the interlobar and
			  arcuate arteries greater than 0.7
			  is associated with acute renal
			  obstruction
				Extrarenal pelvis
				Parapelvic cyst(s)
				Polycystic disease
				Reflux
				Overdistended urinary
				  bladder

Continued

Obstruction and Calculus of the Kidney—(cont'd)

OBSTRUCTION	ETIOLOGY	CLINICAL FINDINGS	SONOGRAPHIC FINDINGS	DIFFERENTIAL CONSIDERATIONS
Hydroureter	Obstruction of the ureteropelvic junction (UPJ), ureterovesical junction (UVJ), or region where the ureter crosses the pelvic brim	Asymptomatic Flank pain	Anechoic tubular structure connecting the renal pelvis to the urinary bladder No internal blood flow Evaluate bladder for ureteral jet(s)	Fluid filled bowel
Nephrolithiasis	Urinary stasis Hypercalcemia Dehydration High protein diet Male prevalence 4:1	Asymptomatic Renal colic Flank pain Hematuria	Hyperechoic focus(i) within the kidney parenchyma or collecting system Occurs in the corticomedullary junction Posterior acoustic shadowing Color Doppler Twinkle artifact Hydronephrosis if obstructive	Calcified vessel Angiomyolipoma
Staghorn calculus **Risk Factors:** Chronic history of kidney stones Recurrent urinary tract infections	Abnormal concentration, usually of mineral salts	Asymptomatic Flank pain Hematuria Urinary tract infection	Calcified mass filling the renal pelvis and collecting system Calcified mass conforms to the renal pelvis and calyces Posterior acoustic shadowing May demonstrate hydronephrosis	Nephrocalcinosis Medullary sponge kidney Multiple renal stones

Benign Pathology of the Kidney

BENIGN PATHOLOGY	ETIOLOGY	CLINICAL FINDINGS	SONOGRAPHIC FINDINGS	DIFFERENTIAL CONSIDERATIONS
Adenoma **Risk Factors:** Male prevalence (3:1) Tobacco use Long-term dialysis	Benign tumor derived of glandular epithelium tissue Most common cortical tumor	Asymptomatic Painless hematuria Flank pain	Well-defined subcapsular hypoechoic cortical mass Generally small Majority solitary (75%)	Abscess Complicated cyst Renal cell carcinoma
Angiomyolipoma Aka: renal hamartoma	Composed of fat, blood vessels, and muscle Tends to hemorrhage Female prevalence	Asymptomatic Flank pain Gross hematuria	Well-defined hyperechoic parenchymal or exophytic mass May distort renal architecture	Carcinoma Junctional parenchymal defect Lipoma
Lipoma	Composed of fat	Asymptomatic	Well-defined hyperechoic mass	Angiomyolipoma Junctional parenchymal defect
Medullary sponge kidney	Benign congenital condition Medullary nephrocalcinosis (80%)	Asymptomatic	Hyperechoic medullary pyramids Widening of the distal collecting system Unilateral (25%) Solitary affected pyramid (25%)	Nephrolithiasis Acute tubular necrosis
Mesoblastic nephroma Most common solid renal tumor in infants	Pediatric parenchymal tumor 90% occur in first year of life Benign version of the Wilm's tumor Male prevalence	Palpable flank mass Hematuria Hypertension	Homogeneous hypoechoic mass Large solid parenchymal mass Typically involves the renal sinus Frequently grow through the renal capsule Does not invade the renal vein	Wilms' tumor Neuroblastoma

Benign Pathology of the Kidney—(cont'd)

BENIGN PATHOLOGY	ETIOLOGY	CLINICAL FINDINGS	SONOGRAPHIC FINDINGS	DIFFERENTIAL CONSIDERATIONS
Nephrocalcinosis **Risk Factors:** Endocrine abnormalities Prolonged immobilization Urinary stasis Medullary sponge kidney Excessive vitamin D	Formation of aggregates of calcium in the distal tubules and loops of Henle	Asymptomatic Hyperparathyroidism Hypercalcemia Hypercalciuria	Hyperechoic medullary pyramids Normal renal size and cortex echogenicity Calcifications within medullary pyramids May demonstrate shadowing	Acute tubular necrosis Nephrolithiasis Medullary sponge kidney Staghorn calculus
Renal sinus lipomatosis	Obesity Previous urinary obstruction Chronic renal infection Steroid therapy	Asymptomatic Elevated creatinine	Increase in echogenicity of the renal sinus Thinning of the renal cortex Normal renal contour	Chronic renal failure

Malignant Pathology of the Kidney

MALIGNANT PATHOLOGY	ETIOLOGY	CLINICAL FINDINGS	SONOGRAPHIC FINDINGS	DIFFERENTIAL CONSIDERATIONS
Renal cell carcinoma **Stages:** 1. Confined to the kidney 2. Spread to perinephric fat 3. Extension to the renal vein, inferior vena cava (IVC), or lymph nodes 4. Extension to near or distant structures	Cortex carcinoma consisting of tubular cells Adenocarcinoma most common	Painless gross hematuria Uncontrolled hypertension Palpable mass Flank pain	Irregular mass with echogenicity ranging from hypoechoic (larger mass) to hyperechoic (smaller mass) Focal bulge in renal contour Indistinct borders Hypervascular mass Metastasis to the lung, liver, and long bones Extension into the renal vein and IVC	Adrenal tumor Abscess Focal pyelonephritis Adenoma Angiomyolipoma
Wilms' tumor (nephroblastoma) **Risk Factors:** Beckwith-Wiedemann syndrome Hemihypertrophy Sporadic aniridia Male prevalence Omphalocele 5 years of age or less	Malignant mixed tumor composed of embryonal elements	Palpable mass Abdominal pain Nausea/vomiting Gross or microscopic hematuria Hypertension	Predominately solid, well-defined renal mass Variable echo pattern Echogenic rim Occasional calcification (10%) Intramural vascular flow Displacement of the IVC and aorta Metastasis to the renal vein, IVC, liver, contralateral kidney, and lymph nodes	Neuroblastoma Renal cell carcinoma Mesoblastic nephroma
Metastases	Primary malignancy of the bronchus, breast, gastrointestinal tract, contralateral kidney, non-Hodgkin's lymphoma, and neuroblastoma	Asymptomatic	Multiple small bilateral masses of variable echogenicity	Angiomyolipomas Renal cell carcinoma
Transitional cell carcinoma	Primary malignant epithelial tumor originating in the renal sinus, ureters, and bladder	Painless hematuria Dull flank pain Urinary frequency Dysuria	**Kidney** Discrete solid mass separating the renal sinus **Ureter** Eccentric or circumferential wall thickening	Hypertrophied column of Bertin Complex pararenal cyst

Vascular Disorders of the Kidneys

VASCULAR DISORDER	ETIOLOGY	CLINICAL FINDINGS	SONOGRAPHIC AND DOPPLER FINDINGS	DIFFERENTIAL CONSIDERATIONS
Infarction **Risk Factors:** Trauma Emboli Arterial or venous thrombosis Vasculitis	Necrosis of tissue caused by occlusion of the arterial blood supply	Asymptomatic Acute flank pain Hematuria Proteinuria Elevated white blood count	Focal-wedge-shaped hypoechoic (acute) or hyperechoic (chronic) renal defect	Complex renal cyst Angiomyolipomas Junctional parenchymal defect Calcified artery
Renal artery stenosis	Atherosclerosis (60%) Fibromuscular hyperplasia (35%)	Uncontrolled hypertension Renal insufficiency Abdominal bruit Decrease in urine sodium concentration Hematuria	Peak systolic velocity greater than 180 cm/s Spectral broadening Absence of diastolic flow Delayed acceleration time Renal artery/aorta ratio greater than 3.5 Visual narrowing of the renal artery by atherosclerosis or thickening of the arterial wall Kidney atrophy Kidney infarct	Tortuous artery Poor Doppler angle
Renal artery aneurysm **Risk Factor:** Pregnancy	Fibromuscular dysplasia Blunt trauma Kawasaki disease Intraluminal catheter-induced injury Atherosclerosis	Asymptomatic Hypertension Flank pain Hematuria	Doubling of size of the normal artery Artery diameter of 1.5 cm or greater Risk of rupture when the diameter exceeds 2 cm	Tortuous renal artery Bifurcation of the renal artery Renal vein
Arteriovenous fistula	Congenital malformation Trauma Renal biopsy complication	Asymptomatic	High-peak systolic velocity associated with high diastolic velocity Extremely turbulent flow	Renal artery stenosis
Renal vein thrombosis **Risk Factors:** Malignancy Primary renal disease IVC obstruction Systemic lupus erythematosus Sickle cell anemia Amyloidosis Hypercoagulable state	Renal disease Surgery Trauma Dehydration	Asymptomatic Flank pain Gross hematuria Hypertension Proteinuria Azotemia Anuria	Increase in vein diameter Hypoechoic or complex echoes within the renal vein Continuous, minimal, or absent intraluminal venous flow May demonstrate flow reversal during diastole. Enlarged kidney (acute) Atrophic hyperechoic kidney (chronic)	Renal vein tumor extension Improper gain or focal zone settings Improper Doppler settings or angle
Renal vein tumor extension	Renal carcinoma Renal lymphoma Nephroblastoma	Depends on the underlying cause	Increase in vein diameter Echogenic mass within the renal vein Vascular flow within the mass Continuous, minimal, or absent intraluminal venous flow	Renal vein thrombosis Improper gain or focal zone settings Improper Doppler settings or angle

RENAL DIALYSIS

- Renal dialysis is a process of diffusing blood across a membrane to remove substances a normal kidney would eliminate.
- Renal dialysis may restore electrolytes and acid–base balance.
- Renal dialysis patients have an increased incidence of developing a renal:
  a. cyst.
  b. adenoma.
  c. carcinoma.

RENAL TRANSPLANT

- Transplanted kidney is usually placed in the anterior right iliac fossa.
- Renal artery is anastomosed to the ipsilateral internal iliac artery.
- Renal vein is anastomosed to the ipsilateral external iliac vein.
- Ureter is implanted into the superior portion of the urinary bladder.
- Fat from around the bladder is placed over the ureter to act as a valve.

Renal Transplant Complications

TRANSPLANT COMPLICATION	DESCRIPTION
Renal artery stenosis	Occurs months to years posttransplant
Renal artery thrombosis	Occurs in the first few days
Primary renal vein thrombosis	Originates in the renal vein
Secondary renal vein thrombosis	Extends into the iliac vein Can result from iliac compression
Hematoma	Hypoechoic when acute Complex when subacute Anechoic when chronic
Urinoma	Develops in the first few weeks Rapid increase in size on serial examinations Anechoic fluid collection
Lymphocele	Usually found medial to the transplant Anechoic fluid collection frequently containing septations
Abscess	Usually develops in the first few weeks Variable sonographic appearance

Normal Sonographic Appearance of the Renal Transplant

- Renal sinus appears hyperechoic.
- Renal cortex appears hypoechoic.
- Prominent renal pyramids.
- Arcuate vessels may be demonstrated.
- May demonstrate mild hydronephrosis.

Abnormal Sonographic Appearance of the Renal Transplant

- Increase in renal size (circular in appearance).
- Increase in size of the renal pyramids.

- Increase in echogenicity of the renal cortex.
- Decrease in echogenicity of the renal sinus.
- Loss of corticomedullary definition.
- Hypoechoic areas within the renal parenchyma.

Normal Doppler Appearance of the Renal Transplant

- Low-resistance vascular flow in the renal, segmental, and arcuate arteries.
- Resistive index (RI) of 0.7 or less.
- Peak systolic velocity may be as high as 250 cm/s.

Abnormal Doppler Appearance of the Renal Transplant

- Absence of diastolic flow or demonstration of flow reversal in the renal, segmental or arcuate arteries.
- RI of greater than 0.7 suggests acute rejection.
- Pulsatility index (PI) less than 1.5 or greater than 1.8.

URINARY BLADDER ANATOMY

- Extraperitoneal elastic muscle reservoir for urine.
- Bladder wall contains three layers; serosa, muscle, mucosa.
- Only superior portion is covered by an extension of peritoneum.
- Anchored to the pelvis by the pubvesical (female) or pubprostate (male) ligaments.
- Normal bladder wall thickness is 3 mm when distended.
- Normal bladder wall thickness is 5 mm when empty.
- Normal bladder wall is thicker in infants than in adults.
- Ureters enter the bladder wall at an oblique angle approximately 5 cm above the bladder outlet (trigone).
- Postvoid residual normally should not exceed 20 mL in the adult patient.

Apex

- Superior portion of the bladder.

Neck

- Inferior portion of the bladder continuous with the urethra.

Trigone

- Inflexible region between the apex and neck of the bladder.
- Area where ureters enter the bladder.

Arterial Supply to the Bladder

- Superior, mid, and inferior vesicle arteries.

NORMAL SONOGRAPHIC APPEARANCE

- Anechoic fluid-filled structure located in the pelvic midline.
- Ureteric orifices appear as small echogenic protuberances on the posterior aspect of the bladder.
- Bladder wall thickness is dependent on distention of urinary bladder but should not exceed 5 mm.

Congenital Anomalies of the Urinary Bladder

CONGENITAL ANOMALIES	ETIOLOGY	CLINICAL FINDINGS	SONOGRAPHIC FINDINGS	DIFFERENTIAL CONSIDERATIONS
Bladder exstrophy	Failure of the mesoderm to form over the lower abdomen Associated with epispadia	Typically discovered in utero	Lower anterior abdominal wall defect Mass protruding from this defect Normal bladder not identified	Omphalocele Inguinal hernia Umbilical hernia
Bladder diverticulum	Bladder wall muscle weakness causing herniation of the mucosa through muscular wall May be associated with bladder obstruction or chronic inflammation	Asymptomatic Urinary tract infection (UTI) Pelvic pain	Anechoic pedunculation of the urinary bladder Neck of diverticulum is small May enlarge when bladder contracts	Ovarian cyst Fluid-filled bowel Ascites
Bladder ureterocele	Herniation of the ureter into the bladder resulting in recurrent UTI Congenital obstruction of the ureteric orifice	Asymptomatic UTI	Hyperechoic septation seen within the bladder at the ureteric orifice Demonstrated when urine enters the bladder Uni- or bilateral	Artifact Bladder tumor Catheter balloon
Urachal anomaly	Epithelial tube connecting the apex of the bladder with the umbilicus	Asymptomatic Fluid draining from the umbilicus	**Patent Urachal Sinus** Anechoic linear tubular structure extending from the apex of the urinary bladder to the umbilicus **Urachal Cyst** Anechoic urine trapped between two fused ends of the urachus **Urachal Diverticulum** Closed umbilical end of urachus and patent bladder end allowing urine to fill patent area	Rectus abdominis hematoma Subcutaneous fat

Pathology of the Urinary Bladder

BLADDER PATHOLOGY	ETIOLOGY	CLINICAL FINDINGS	SONOGRAPHIC FINDINGS	DIFFERENTIAL CONSIDERATIONS
Bladder adenoma	Papilloma	Asymptomatic Frequent urination Painless hematuria	Echogenic intraluminal mass Smooth wall margins Immobile with patient position change Internal vascular flow	Malignant tumor Bladder sludge Ureterocele Metastatic tumor
Bladder calculus	Urinary stasis Migrates from the kidney(s)	Asymptomatic Hematuria Urinary frequency and urgency Recurrent urinary tract infections	Hyperechoic focus(i) within the urinary bladder Posterior acoustic shadowing Mobile with patient position change	Intestinal air Calcified vessel

Continued

Pathology of the Urinary Bladder—(cont'd)

BLADDER PATHOLOGY	ETIOLOGY	CLINICAL FINDINGS	SONOGRAPHIC FINDINGS	DIFFERENTIAL CONSIDERATIONS
Cystitis	Infection Female prevalence	Dysuria Urinary frequency Leukocytosis Hematuria	Focal or diffuse increase in bladder wall thickness Mobile internal echoes	Bladder sludge Hematuria
Bladder sludge	Debris in the bladder	Asymptomatic	Homogeneous low-level echoes Mobile with patient position change	Cystitis Hematuria
Bladder malignancy **Risk Factors:** Analgesic abuse Tobacco use Excessive coffee consumption Recurrent UTI Elderly and male prevalence	Transitional cell carcinoma	Painless hematuria Frequent urination Dysuria	Polypoid echogenic bladder mass Irregular margins Immobile with patient position change Internal vascular blood flow May demonstrate irregular bladder wall thickening	Benign tumor Bladder sludge Ureterocele Metastatic tumor

URINARY SYSTEM REVIEW

1. Which of the following terms describes the typical sonographic appearance of the medullary pyramids in the neonate?
   a. anechoic
   b. hypoechoic
   c. hyperechoic
   d. isoechoic

2. Which of the following conditions is associated with a decrease in blood urea nitrogen (BUN)?
   a. dehydration
   b. hydronephrosis
   c. liver failure
   d. renal failure

3. The renal arteries arise from which aspect of the abdominal aorta?
   a. medial
   b. lateral
   c. anterior
   d. inferior

4. Which of the following structures is considered the basic functional unit of the kidney?
   a. nephron
   b. glomerulus
   c. loop of Henle
   d. collecting tubule

5. The quadratus lumborum is a muscle located in the:
   a. medial abdominal wall
   b. lateral abdominal wall
   c. anterior abdominal wall
   d. posterior abdominal wall

6. Fusion of the entire medial aspect of both kidneys is a congenital anomaly termed:
   a. crossed fused ectopia
   b. cake kidney
   c. sigmoid kidney
   d. junctional parenchymal defect

7. Which of the following conditions is most likely to mimic a duplicated urinary system?
   a. junctional parenchymal defect
   b. fetal lobulation
   c. dromedary hump
   d. hypertrophied column of Bertin

8. Dialysis patients are at increased risk for developing:
   a. nephrocalcinosis
   b. renal carcinoma
   c. nephrolithiasis
   d. renal vein thrombosis

9. The most common renal neoplasm identified in patients over the age of 55 years is a(n):
   a. simple cyst
   b. renal calculus
   c. angiomyolipoma
   d. renal cell carcinoma

10. A staghorn calculus begins forming in the:
    a. calyces
    b. renal cortex
    c. renal pelvis
    d. medullary pyramid

Using Figure 10.2, answer question 11.

11. This sagittal image of the urinary bladder demonstrates a:
    a. ureterocele
    b. bladder diverticulum
    c. catheter balloon
    d. small amount of residual urine

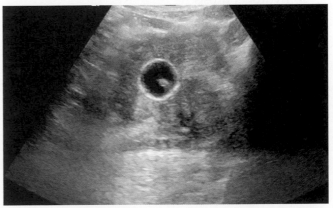

FIG. 10.2   Longitudinal image of the urinary bladder.

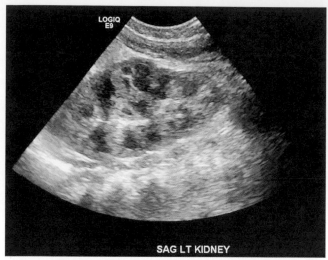

FIG. 10.3 Longitudinal image of the kidney.

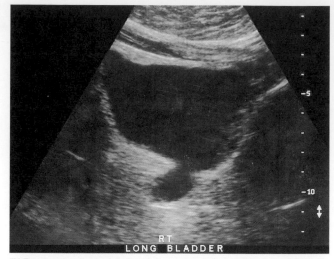

FIG. 10.5 Longitudinal image of the right side of the urinary bladder.

Using Figure 10.3, answer question 12.

12. An infant presents to the ultrasound department with a history of a single urinary tract infection. The sonogram of the kidney most likely demonstrates:
    a. hydronephrosis
    b. infantile polycystic disease
    c. normal medullary pyramids
    d. multicystic dysplastic kidney

Using Figure 10.4, answer questions 13 and 14.

13. Which of the following conditions is most likely demonstrated in this sonogram of the kidney
    a. pelviectasis
    b. pyelonephritis
    c. nephrolithiasis
    d. hydronephrosis

14. The most common etiology for this pathology is:
    a. bladder infection
    b. kidney infection
    c. urinary stasis
    d. urinary tract obstruction

Using Figure 10.5, answer question 15.

15. The pathology identified in this sonogram is most suspicious for a:
    a. ureterocele
    b. malignant tumor
    c. dilated urethra
    d. bladder diverticulum

16. Which of the following renal structures is composed of blood vessels or nerve fibers?
    a. glomerulus
    b. loop of Henle
    c. renal pyramid
    d. renal tubule

17. A patient complaining of sharp, severe flank pain radiating to the groin is describing:
    a. renal colic
    b. dysuria
    c. Mittelschmerz
    d. dyspareunia

18. Which of the following structures are contained in the renal sinus?
    a. renal artery, renal vein, ureter
    b. lymphatics, perinephric fat, minor calyces
    c. major calyces, renal pelvis, ureter
    d. lymphatics, peripelvic fat, major calyces

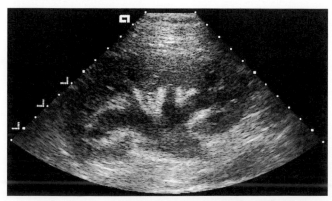

FIG. 10.4 Longitudinal image of the kidney.

19. Which of the following muscles is located lateral to each kidney?
    a. psoas
    b. quadratus lumborum
    c. internal oblique
    d. transversus abdominis

20. A triangular shaped hyperechoic focus located in the anterior renal cortex in an asymptomatic patient most likely represents:
    a. adenoma
    b. ischemic necrosis
    c. renal calculus
    d. a junctional parenchymal defect

21. Normal postvoid residual urine volume in an adult patient should not exceed:
    a. 5 mL
    b. 20 mL
    c. 50 mL
    d. 100 mL

22. A 43-year-old female patient presents to the ultrasound department complaining of right flank pain and dysuria. A generalized swelling of the kidney is demonstrated. The medullary pyramids appear well defined. This is most suspicious for:
    a. pyelonephritis
    b. metastatic disease
    c. hydronephrosis
    d. acute tubular necrosis

23. Which of the following patient positions is typically used for renal biopsy procedures?
    a. supine
    b. prone
    c. Trendelenburg
    d. Reverse Trendelenburg

24. Small echogenic protuberances identified on the posterior wall of the urinary bladder most likely represent:
    a. arcuate vessels
    b. ureteric orifices
    c. hydroureters
    d. bladder diverticulums

25. Patients with adult polycystic renal disease have an increased incidence of developing:
    a. nephrocalcinosis
    b. renal calculi
    c. renal carcinoma
    d. an adrenal adenoma

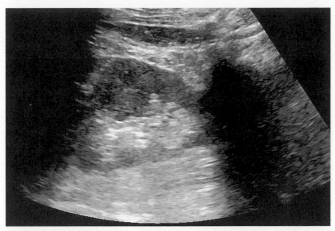

FIG. 10.6 Sagittal image of the right upper quadrant.

Using Figure 10.6, answer question 26.

26. Which of the following anatomic variants is most likely identified in this sonogram?
    a. renal duplication
    b. crossed fused ectopia
    c. junctional parenchymal defect
    d. hypertrophied column of Bertin

Using Figure 10.7, answer question 27.

27. The arrow in this sonogram most likely identifies:
    a. perinephric fat
    b. a renal abscess
    c. pyelonephritis
    d. thrombosis in the inferior vena cava

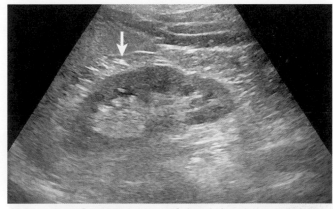

FIG. 10.7 Sagittal image of the right upper quadrant.

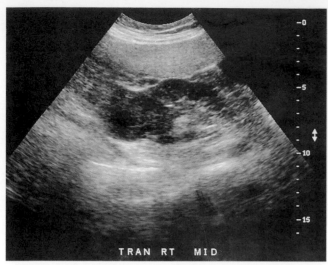

FIG. 10.8 Transverse image of the right kidney.

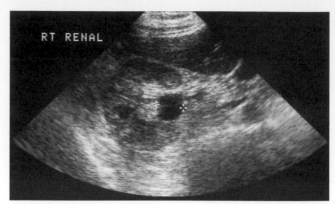

FIG. 10.10 Transverse image of the right kidney.

Using Figure 10.8, answer question 28.

28. A mass is identified in the mid portion of the right kidney that demonstrates internal blood flow. The mass identified in the sonogram is most suspicious for a:
   a. hematoma
   b. dromedary hump
   c. renal cell carcinoma
   d. hemorrhagic cyst

Using Figure 10.9, answer question 29.

29. This image of the female pelvis is demonstrating a:
   a. bladder diverticulum
   b. ureterocele
   c. catheter balloon
   d. dilated distal ureter

Using Figure 10.10, answer question 30.

30. The anechoic area demonstrated in the sonogram is most consistent with a(n):
   a. extrarenal pelvis
   b. pelviectasis
   c. parapelvic cyst
   d. hydroureter

31. Mesoblastic nephromas are more likely to occur in patients under:
   a. 1 year of age
   b. 5 years of age
   c. 10 years of age
   d. 18 years of age

32. A benign tumor composed of fat, blood vessels, and muscle describes a(n):
   a. adenoma
   b. lipoma
   c. fibroma
   d. angiomyolipoma

33. Fibromuscular hyperplasia is most commonly associated with stenosis in which of the following renal arteries?
   a. main renal artery
   b. arcuate artery
   c. interlobar artery
   d. segmental artery

34. Renal artery stenosis is suggested after the peak systolic velocity exceeds:
   a. 90 cm/s
   b. 135 cm/s
   c. 180 cm/s
   d. 230 cm/s

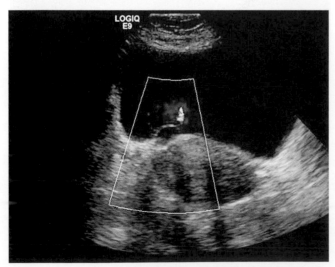

FIG. 10.9 Transverse image of the female pelvis.

35. Which of the following conditions is most likely associated with painless hematuria?
    a. hydronephrosis
    b. pyelonephritis
    c. angiomyolipoma
    d. renal cell carcinoma

36. Which of the following conditions is frequently associated with urinary stasis?
    a. parapelvic cyst
    b. nephrolithiasis
    c. renal carcinoma
    d. chronic renal failure

37. Fusion of the superior pole of one kidney to the inferior pole of the contralateral kidney is most consistent with which of the following congenital anomalies?
    a. cake kidney
    b. crossed fused ectopia
    c. sigmoid kidney
    d. duplicated kidney

38. The normal adult renal cortex should measure a minimum of
    a. 0.5 cm
    b. 1.0 cm
    c. 1.5 cm
    d. 2.0 cm

39. The complete inability of the kidneys to excrete waste, concentrate urine, and converse electrolytes is termed renal:
    a. colic
    b. failure
    c. obstruction
    d. insufficiency

Using Figure 10.11, answer question 40.

40. This sonogram is most likely identifying which of the following conditions?
    a. angiomyolipomas
    b. nephrocalcinosis
    c. glomerulonephritis
    d. metastatic lesions

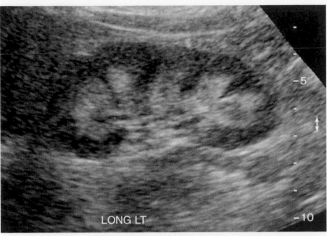

FIG. 10.11 Sagittal sonogram of the left kidney.

Using Figure 10.12, answer question 41.

41. Which of the following congenital anomalies is most likely demonstrated in this sonogram?
    a. lump kidney
    b. cake kidney
    c. renal duplication
    d. sigmoid kidney

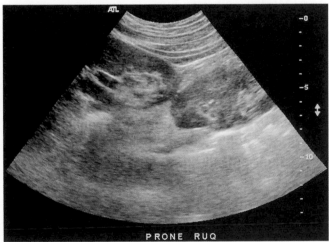

FIG. 10.12 Prone image of the right flank.

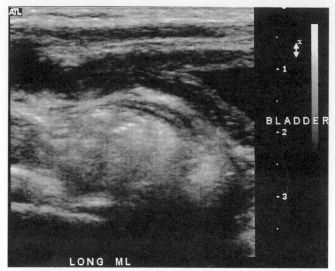

FIG. 10.13 Sagittal sonogram of the pelvis.

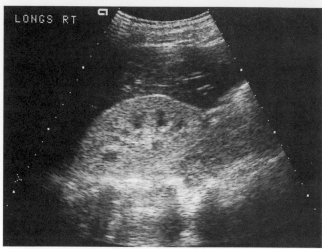

FIG. 10.14 Longitudinal image of the kidney.

Using Figure 10.13, answer question 42.

42. A patient presents with a history of intermittent umbilical discharge. Based on the clinical history, the sonogram is most likely demonstrating which of the following conditions?
   a. rectus abdominis hematoma
   b. umbilical abscess
   c. Meckel's diverticulum
   d. patent urachal sinus

Using Figure 10.14, answer question 43.

43. A patient hospitalized with malaria presents with a history of proteinuria. Based on this clinical history, the sonogram is most suspicious for which of the following conditions?
   a. pyelonephritis
   b. acute tubular necrosis
   c. glomerulonephritis
   d. renal sinus lipomatosis

Using Figure 10.15, answer question 44.

44. A 40-year-old patient presents with a history of elevated creatinine levels. Based on the clinical and sonographic findings, the masses are most suspicious for:
   a. a nephroblastoma
   b. renal sinus lipomatosis
   c. polycystic kidney disease
   d. a medullary sponge kidney

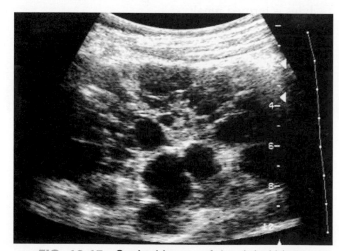

FIG. 10.15 Sagittal image of the right kidney.

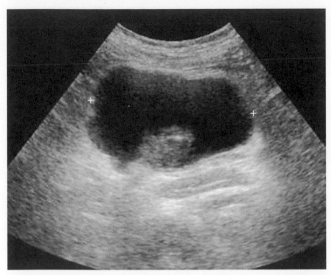

FIG. 10.16 Transverse image of the urinary bladder.

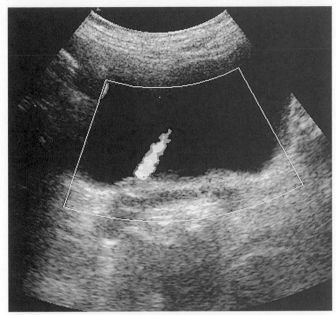

FIG. 10.17 Transverse Doppler sonogram (see Color Plate 5).

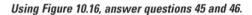

Using Figure 10.16, answer questions 45 and 46.

45. An incidental mass was discovered in the urinary bladder. Blood flow was demonstrated within the mass using color Doppler imaging. This incidental finding is most suspicious for a bladder:
    a. diverticulum
    b. adenoma
    c. carcinoma
    d. sludge ball

46. When encountering this type of pathology, which of the following questions in most important for the sonographer to ask the patient?
    a. Do you have high blood pressure?
    b. How often do you urinate each day?
    c. Have you noticed any blood in your urine?
    d. How much water do you drink each day?

Using Figure 10.17 and Color Plate 5, answer question 47.

47. This image of the urinary bladder is most likely demonstrating which of the following?
    a. ureterocele
    b. ureteral jet
    c. flash artifact
    d. external iliac artery

Using Figure 10.18, answer question 48.

48. This sonogram is most likely demonstrating:
    a. pyelonephritis
    b. fetal lobulation
    c. renal carcinoma
    d. hypertrophied column of Bertin

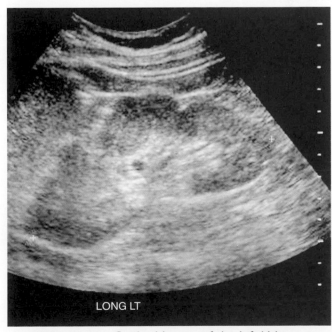

FIG. 10.18 Sagittal image of the left kidney.

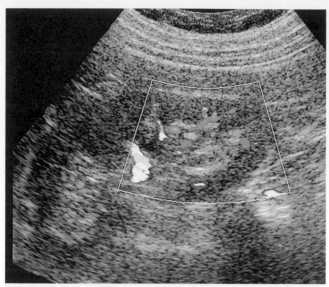

FIG. 10.19 Sagittal Doppler image (see Color Plate 6).

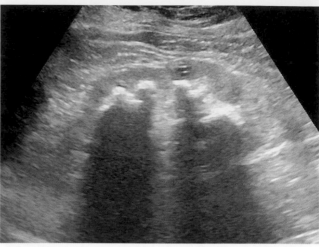

FIG. 10.20 Sagittal image of the left kidney.

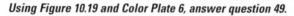

Using Figure 10.19 and Color Plate 6, answer question 49.

49. Duplex imaging of the lower pole of the left kidney most likely demonstrates which of the following?
    a. renal veins
    b. renal arteries
    c. Bertin vessels
    d. arcuate vessels

Using Figure 10.20, answer question 50.

50. Which of the following pathologies is most likely demonstrated in this sonogram?
    a. nephrocalcinosis
    b. hydronephrosis
    c. staghorn calculus
    d. medullary sponge kidney

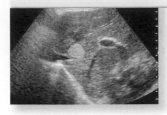

CHAPTER 11

Spleen

KEY TERMS

accessory spleen   a nodule of normal splenic tissue commonly located near the splenic hilum.

anemia   a decrease in hemoglobin levels in the blood.

asplenia syndrome   absence of the spleen associated with two right lungs, a midline liver, and gastrointestinal and urinary anomalies.

bilateral left-sidedness   a syndrome in which normally unpaired organs develop more symmetrically in mirror image; two spleens, one on each side, are usually present, and cardiovascular anomalies are common.

hamartoma   a rare benign neoplasm composed of lymphoid tissue. Also known as splenoma.

hematocrit   the percentage of red blood cells in the blood.

hemoglobin   carries oxygen from the lungs to the cells and returns carbon dioxide back to the lungs.

intraparenchymal hematoma   hematoma located within the splenic parenchyma.

leukemia   proliferation of white blood cells.

leukocytosis   white blood cell count above 20,000 mm³.

leukopenia   white blood cell count below 4000 mm³.

lymphoma   malignant disorder involving the lymphoreticular system.

polycythemia vera   a slow-growing cancer in which your blood marrow makes too many red blood cells (RBC). This increase in RBC thickens the blood, slowing its flow, which may cause blood clots.

polysplenia   multiple small spleens associated with two left lungs and gastrointestinal, cardiovascular, and biliary anomalies.

sickle cell anemia   genetic mutation in African Americans resulting in altered shape and phasicity of red blood cells. Leads to increased blood viscosity, stasis, small vessel occlusion, infarction, and necrosis

splenic artery aneurysm   a localized dilatation of the splenic artery.

splenic infarction   occlusion of the main splenic artery or one of its branches.

subcapsular hematoma   hematoma located between the splenic capsule and parenchyma.

wandering spleen   refers to an abnormal location of the spleen.

PHYSIOLOGY

Function of the Spleen

- Removes foreign material from the blood.
- Initiates an immune reaction, resulting in production of antibodies and lymphocytes.
- Major destruction site of old red blood cells; red blood cells are removed and hemoglobin is recycled.
- Reservoir for blood.
- Erythropoiesis in the fetus.

ANATOMY (Fig. 11.1)

- Predominant organ in the left upper quadrant.
- Except at the hilum, the spleen is covered by the peritoneum.
- The spleen is divided into the:
  1. Superior and medial portion.
  2. Inferior and lateral portion.
  3. Splenic hilum.

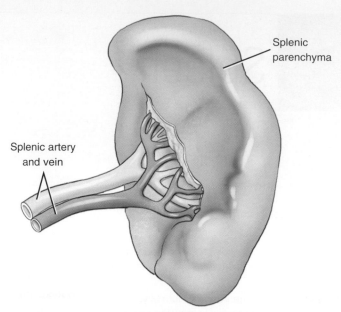

Splenic parenchyma

Splenic artery and vein

FIG. 11.1   Splenic anatomy.

Splenic Vasculature

- The splenic artery arises from the celiac axis, courses along superior pancreatic borders, dividing into six branches after entering the splenic hilum.
- The splenic arterial and venous systems do not tend to anastomose within the spleen. There is no collateral circulation in cases of splenic ischemia.
- The splenic vein joins the superior mesenteric vein, forming the main portal vein.
- The inferior mesenteric vein may confluence with the splenic vein.
- In cases of portal hypertension, the splenic vein may shunt blood directly into the left renal vein.

Location

- Intraperitoneal organ.
- Predominantly located in the left hypochondriac region with the superior aspect extending into the epigastric region.
- Located inferior to the diaphragm and anterior to the left kidney.
- Lies posterior and lateral to the stomach.
- Located lateral to the pancreas.
- Located inferior and posterior to the body of the pancreas.

Congenital Anomalies

VARIANT	DESCRIPTION	CLINICAL FINDINGS	SONOGRAPHIC FINDINGS	DIFFERENTIAL CONSIDERATIONS
Accessory spleen Aka: splenuculi	Improper splenic fusion Common variant incidentally found in 30% of the population May enlarge after splenectomy	Asymptomatic	Homogeneous mass typically located medial to the splenic hilum Echogenicity similar to spleen Round or oval in shape Variable size	Lymphadenopathy Pancreatic mass Adrenal mass Renal mass
Aplasia	Failure of the spleen to develop	Asymptomatic	Absence of the spleen	Splenectomy Wandering spleen

Congenital Anomalies—(cont'd)

VARIANT	DESCRIPTION	CLINICAL FINDINGS	SONOGRAPHIC FINDINGS	DIFFERENTIAL CONSIDERATIONS
Polysplenia	Rare Multiple small spleens May have bilateral left sidedness	Asymptomatic Varies with associated congenital anomalies Male prevalence	Multiple small spleens Located along the greater curvature of the stomach Associated with gastrointestinal, cardiovascular, genitourinary, and biliary anomalies	Lymphadenopathy Retroperitoneal masses
Wandering spleen	Improper fusion of the dorsal mesentery with the posterior peritoneum May undergo torsion	Asymptomatic Severe abdominal pain with acute torsion	Abnormal location of the spleen	Asplenia Splenic rupture

Splenic Size

SIZE	ETIOLOGY	CLINICAL FINDINGS	SONOGRAPHIC FINDINGS	DIFFERENTIAL CONSIDERATIONS
Normal adult spleen			Length: ≤12 cm Width: <4 cm Anteroposterior <8 cm	
Normal pediatric spleen			**Infant ≤3 months** <6 cm in length **Children >3 months** 5.7 + 0.31 × age in years for normal length in cm	
Splenomegaly	Congestive heart failure Cirrhosis Portal hypertension Portal vein thrombosis Infection Diabetes mellitus Hypertension Hepatitis Trauma Lymphoma Cystic fibrosis Hemolytic anemia	Asymptomatic Dyspepsia Fatigue Left upper quadrant (LUQ) pain Palpable LUQ mass Lower extremity edema	Enlargement of the spleen Length exceeding 13 cm in the adult patient Hypoechoic parenchyma Prominent splenic vasculature near the hilum Evaluate liver for pathology Evaluate abdominal cavity for ascites	Technical error Splenic rupture

NORMAL SONOGRAPHIC APPEARANCE

- Moderately echogenic homogeneous parenchyma.
- Isoechoic to slightly hyperechoic compared with the normal liver parenchyma.
- The normal splenic parenchyma is generally considered to be equal to or less echogenic than the normal liver, when in fact the normal adult spleen is actually iso- to slightly hyperechoic compared with the normal liver parenchyma. This impression is due to the large number of vessels within the normal liver parenchyma.

EXAMINATION TECHNIQUES, PROTOCOLS, AND IMAGE OPTIMIZATION

Preparation

- No preparation is required before an ultrasound of the spleen.
- The liver and biliary tree including the gallbladder may be included in the examination, which would require a fasting preparation for optimal evaluation of the gallbladder.
  - Adult—6 to 8 hours.
  - Children—6 hours.
  - Infants—4 hours.

Transducer Selection

- Use the highest frequency possible to obtain optimal resolution for penetration depth.
  - Adults—3.0 to 5.0 MHz.
  - Children and small adults—5.0 to 7.0 MHz.
  - Obese patients—2.0 MHz may be required.
- Curvilinear transducers provide a wider field of view.
- Sector or vector transducers have a smaller footprint great for intercostal imaging.
- Subcostal imaging in some patients may be helpful.
- Higher frequency transducers can be used to demonstrate superficial lesions of the spleen.

Patient Positioning

- Examination usually begins with the patient in a supine or right lateral decubitus.
- Right posterior oblique position may reposition overlying bowel gas.

Examination Protocol

- Systematic approach in the coronal and transverse planes carefully examining and imaging all portions of the spleen including:
  - Superior-medial and inferior-lateral segments of the spleen.
  - Splenic hilum with and without color Doppler.
- Superior-inferior measurement of the spleen.
- Coronal and transverse images of the left kidney and left pleural space.
- Abnormalities should be documented and when applicable measured in two imaging planes. Color and/or spectral Doppler evaluation of the abnormality should be included.

Image Optimization

- Place gains settings to display normal splenic parenchyma as a medium shade of gray, isoechoic to slightly hyperechoic to normal liver parenchyma.
- Focal zone(s) should be placed at or below the area of interest. The use of multiple focal zones increases detail resolution and decreases temporal resolution.
- Sufficient imaging depth to visualize structures immediately posterior to the area of interest.
- Harmonic imaging and decreasing system compression (dynamic range) can be used to reduce artifactual echoes within normal anechoic structures.
- Spatial compounding can be used to improve visualization of structures posterior to highly attenuating structures.
- Doppler settings should be adjusted for a slow flow rate.
- The use of deep inspiration may improve visualization of the spleen.
- The use of multiple patient positions may redistribute overlying bowel gas.

Examination Limitations

- Left lobe of the liver may extend into the left upper quadrant mimicking an enlarged spleen or superior splenic mass.
- Superior location of the spleen (high under ribcage).
- Gastrointestinal gas.
- Obesity.

Helpful Hints

- In the right lateral decubitus position have the patient rest their left arm above their head to increase the space between the inferior rib cage and superior left pelvis.
- In the right posterior oblique or right lateral decubitus positions, using the left subcostal approach, angle up under the ribcage to aid in visualization of the spleen.

Indications for Examination

- Chronic liver disease.
- Infection.
- Leukocytosis.
- Leukopenia.
- Palpable mass.
- Abdominal pain.
- Fatigue.
- Trauma.

LABORATORY VALUES

Erythrocyte

- Normal serum levels:
  - Male—4.6 to 6.2 million/mm^3.
  - Female—4.2 to 5.4 million/mm^3.
- Red blood cell.
- Carries oxygen from the lungs to the tissues in the body.
- Carries carbon dioxide back to the lungs.
- Develops in the bone marrow and has a life span of 120 days.
- Spleen stores red blood cells and destroys old red blood cells.
- Contains hemoglobin.
- Elevation associated with polycythemia vera and severe diarrhea.
- Decreases associated with internal bleeding, hemolytic anemia, Hodgkin's disease, and hemangiosarcomas.

Leukocyte

- Normal serum levels: 4500 to 11,000 mm^3.
- White blood cell.
- Defends the body from infection.
- Elevation associated with acute inflammation, infection, leukemia, polycythemia vera, and malignancy.
- Decreases associated with viral infection, leukemia, hypersplenia, aplastic anemia, and diabetes mellitus.

Hematocrit

- Normal serum levels:
  - Male—40 to 54 mL/dL.
  - Female—37 to 47 mL/dL.
- Percentage of red blood cells in the blood.

- Elevation associated with severe dehydration, shock, polycythemia vera, chronic obstructive pulmonary disease (COPD), and infection.
- Decreases associated with hemorrhage, anemia, leukemia, and cirrhosis.

Hemoglobin

- Normal serum levels:
  - Male—13 to 18 g/dL.
  - Female—12 to 16 g/dL.
- Oxygen-carrying pigment of the red blood cell.
- Carries oxygen from the lungs to the cells and carbon dioxide from the cells back to the lungs.
- Developed in the bone marrow inside the red blood cell.
- Recycled by the spleen into iron.
- Basis of bilirubin.

Blood Disorders

BLOOD DISORDER	ETIOLOGY	CLINICAL FINDINGS	SONOGRAPHIC FINDINGS
Polycythemia Vera	Mutation in a gene causes a problem with blood cell production Bone marrow makes too many red blood cells (RBCs), white blood cells (WBCs), and platelets Increases blood viscosity leading to poor profusion More common in adults older than 60 years Not inherited	Asymptomatic Increase in RBC count, hematocrit, and hemoglobin Left upper quadrant (LUQ) pain or fullness Fatigue Unexplained weight loss Itchiness May have increase in platelet and WBC counts	Normal findings Splenomegaly Hepatomegaly May also demonstrate splenic thrombosis and/or splenic infarct Deep vein thrombosis
Sickle cell anemia	Sickled shaped RBC that are unable to carry enough oxygen throughout the body Can obstruct small vessels, which can slow or block flow to parts of the body Autosomal recessive inheritance in the African American population	Episodes of pain (crisis) Painful swelling of hands and feet Frequent infections Delayed growth Vision disturbances	Normal findings Splenomegaly in children with splenic atrophy later in life Possible infarct and/or thrombosis Kidney or liver damage Gallstones

Splenic Pathology

PATHOLOGY	ETIOLOGY	CLINICAL FINDINGS	SONOGRAPHIC FINDINGS	DIFFERENTIAL CONSIDERATIONS
Abscess	Infective endocarditis—most common Infection Trauma	Fever Left upper quadrant (LUQ) pain Leukocytosis	Hypoechoic or complex splenic mass Ill-defined, thick wall margins May demonstrate posterior acoustic enhancement May demonstrate posterior acoustic shadowing with intraluminal gas	Hematoma Splenic infarction Cavernous lymphangioma
Calcifications	Granulomatosis Splenic infarction Calcified cyst Abscess	Asymptomatic Abdominal pain	Hyperechoic focus(i) disperse within the splenic parenchyma May demonstrate posterior acoustic shadowing	Calcified vessel(s)
Cavernous hemangioma Most common benign splenic neoplasm	Consists of large blood-filled cystic spaces Male prevalence 20–50 years of age	Asymptomatic LUQ pain	Well-defined hyperechoic splenic mass Homogeneous or complex echo texture Typically, less than 4 cm in diameter	Splenic infarction Hemangiosarcoma Metastases

Splenic Pathology—(cont'd)

PATHOLOGY	ETIOLOGY	CLINICAL FINDINGS	SONOGRAPHIC FINDINGS	DIFFERENTIAL CONSIDERATIONS
Cavernous lymphangioma	Malformation of the lymph system	Asymptomatic	Hypoechoic solid splenic mass	Abscess Hematoma
Cyst	Rare finding Congenital Infective Neoplastic Parasitic Previous trauma	Asymptomatic	Well-defined anechoic mass Smooth wall margins Posterior acoustic enhancement May demonstrate septations or debris Usually solitary	Hematoma Abscess Cystic lymphangiomyomatosis
Cystic lymphangiomyomatosis	Rare neoplasm Proliferation of the smooth muscle cells in the lymph node	Asymptomatic Abdominal mass	Diffuse or focal multiloculated cystic mass	Splenic cyst
Hamartoma Aka: splenoma	Rare benign neoplasm Composed of lymphatic tissue	Asymptomatic	Hyperechoic parenchymal mass Well-defined borders Solitary or multiple in number	Cavernous hemangioma Metastases Hemangiosarcoma
Splenic artery aneurysm **Risk Factors:** Atherosclerosis Portal hypertension Pregnancy Trauma Female prevalence	Localized dilatation of the splenic artery	Asymptomatic LUQ pain Nausea/vomiting Shoulder pain	Anechoic dilatation of the splenic artery Strong association with calcifications High risk of rupture when diameter exceeds 1.5 cm	Tortuous artery Splenic vein
Splenic candidiasis	Multiple splenic infections Associated with patients with autoimmune disorders	Fever Splenomegaly	Target lesion or "wheel within a wheel" appearance	Metastases
Splenic infarction	Emboli from the heart Associated with subacute bacterial endocarditis, leukemia, sickle cell anemia, atherosclerosis, metastasis, and pancreatitis	Usually asymptomatic LUQ pain	**Acute Stage:** Peripheral hypoechoic wedge-like mass Well-defined margins May demonstrate variable shape and irregular wall margins **Chronic Stage:** Hyperechoic mass (fibrosis) Well-defined margins Splenic atrophy	Hematoma Cavernous hemangioma Small spleen

Splenic Trauma

TRAUMA	ETIOLOGY	CLINICAL FINDINGS	SONOGRAPHIC FINDINGS	DIFFERENTIAL CONSIDERATIONS
Splenic rupture	Blunt abdominal trauma Splenomegaly Infectious disorder	Asymptomatic Left upper quadrant pain Tachycardia Palpable mass Abdominal pain Decrease in hematocrit Hypovolemic shock	Hypoechoic or complex mass May demonstrate posterior acoustic enhancement Subcapsular rupture appears as a crescent-shaped fluid collection Evaluate abdominal cavity for free fluid	Recent splenic infarction Abscess Cyst Pleural effusion

Malignancy of the Spleen

MALIGNANCY	ETIOLOGY	CLINICAL FINDINGS	SONOGRAPHIC FINDINGS	DIFFERENTIAL CONSIDERATIONS
Hemangiosarcoma Aka: splenic angiosarcoma	Rare splenic malignancy 50–60 years of age	Anemia is most common Left upper quadrant (LUQ) pain Weight loss Fatigue Fever Leukocytosis Thrombocytopenia GI bleeding	Hyperechoic or complex mass Splenomegaly Frequently metastasizes to the liver	Abscess Hematoma Cavernous hemangioma
Leukemia	Proliferation of white blood cells Male prevalence	Lymphadenopathy Palpable spleen Joint pain Weakness Fever Easy bruising Recurrent infections Elevated white blood cells (WBC) Anemia	Splenomegaly Diffuse increase in parenchyma echogenicity Hypoechoic or hyperechoic nodules	Hematoma Lymphoma Metastases
Lymphoma	Malignant disorder involving the lymphoreticular system Divided into Hodgkin's and non-Hodgkin's Male prevalence	Lymphadenopathy Low-grade fever Weight loss Fatigue Night sweats Anemia Elevated WBC (lymphocytes)	Hypoechoic splenic mass(es) Ill-defined margins May demonstrate splenomegaly	Metastatic lesion Hematoma
Metastases	Melanoma is the most common Breast Lung Ovary Leukemia Lymphoma	Asymptomatic	Typically, multiple hypoechoic or target lesions	Multiple abscesses Lymphoma Splenic candidiasis Leukemia

SPLEEN REVIEW

1. The most common location of an accessory spleen is near the:
   a. left renal hilum
   b. left adrenal gland
   c. splenic hilum
   d. lesser curvature of the stomach

2. Gain settings should be placed to demonstrate the normal spleen as:
   a. isoechoic to the normal pancreas
   b. hyperechoic to the normal liver
   c. hypoechoic to the normal renal cortex
   d. isoechoic to the normal liver

3. The spleen is predominantly located in which of the following quadrants?
   a. left lumbar
   b. epigastrium
   c. hypogastrium
   d. left hypochondrium

4. The most common benign neoplasm of the spleen is a(n):
   a. cyst
   b. accessory spleen
   c. cystadenoma
   d. cavernous hemangioma

5. Hematocrit is defined as the percentage of:
   a. platelets in the red blood cell
   b. oxygen in the red blood cell
   c. red blood cells in the blood
   d. platelets in the blood

6. The most common clinical finding associated with a hemangiosarcoma is:
   a. anemia
   b. weight loss
   c. leukopenia
   d. abdominal pain

7. Metastasis to the spleen most commonly originates from which of the following malignancies?
   a. hepatoma
   b. melanoma
   c. nephroblastoma
   d. adrenocortical carcinoma

8. Multiple splenic infection is a predisposing factor for which of the following conditions?
   a. infarction
   b. candidiasis
   c. arterial calcification
   d. cavernous hemangioma

9. In patients with a history of polycythemia vera, the spleen will mostly demonstrate:
   a. atrophy
   b. enlargement
   c. calcifications
   d. multiple cysts

10. Hemangiosarcoma involving the spleen frequently metastasizes to which of the following organs?
    a. liver
    b. colon
    c. lung
    d. kidney

Using Figure 11.2, answer questions 11 and 12.

11. This sonogram of the left upper quadrant is most consistent with which of the following conditions?
    a. lymphoma
    b. splenomegaly
    c. splenic rupture
    d. splenic infarction

12. Based on this sonographic finding the sonographer should also evaluate for which of the following pathologies?
    a. pancreatitis
    b. portal hypertension
    c. lymphadenopathy
    d. abdominal aortic aneurysm

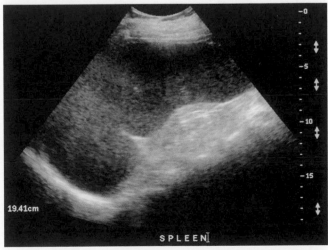

19.41cm

SPLEEN

FIG. 11.2 Coronal sonogram of the left upper quadrant.

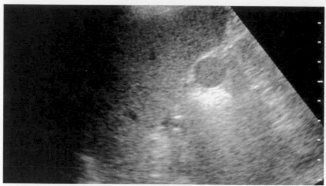

FIG. 11.3 Coronal sonogram of the left upper quadrant.

Using Figure 11.3, answer question 13.

13. The sonogram is most likely demonstrating a(n):
    a. pancreatic mass
    b. enlarged lymph node
    c. accessory spleen
    d. adrenal adenoma

Using Figure 11.4, answer question 14.

14. What abnormality is documented in this sonogram?
    a. splenic cyst
    b. hematoma
    c. fluid-filled stomach
    d. cystic lymphangioma

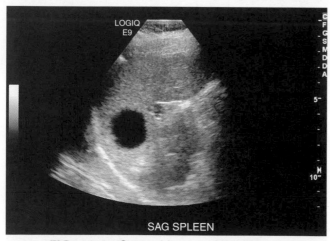

FIG. 11.4 Coronal image of the spleen.

15. Which of the following splenic abnormalities is most commonly linked to infective endocarditis?
    a. hematoma
    b. abscess
    c. infarction
    d. hamartoma

16. The location of the spleen is best described as:
    a. anterior to the stomach
    b. posterior to the left kidney
    c. lateral to the stomach
    d. medial to the left adrenal gland

17. Patients with a history of portal hypertension have an increased risk of developing a splenic:
    a. cyst
    b. infarction
    c. hamartoma
    d. artery aneurysm

18. A congenital anomaly of the spleen associated with gastrointestinal, cardiovascular, genitourinary, and biliary anomalies is most consistent with:
    a. asplenia syndrome
    b. a wandering spleen
    c. polysplenia syndrome
    d. an accessory spleen

19. The splenic artery is a branch of which of the following vascular structures?
    a. abdominal aorta
    b. celiac axis
    c. gastric artery
    d. superior mesenteric artery

20. A clinical finding associated with splenic infarction may include:
    a. hypertension
    b. leukocytosis
    c. no symptoms
    d. epigastric pain

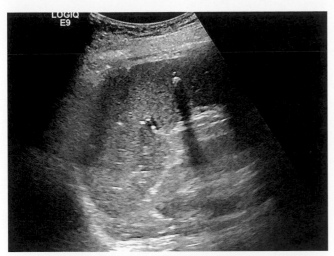

FIG. 11.5 Coronal sonogram of the left upper quadrant.

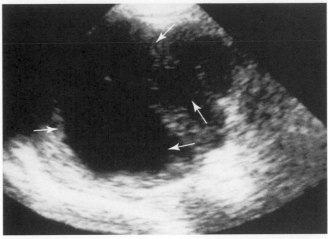

FIG. 11.6 Coronal sonogram of the left upper quadrant.

Using Figure 11.5, answer questions 21 and 22.

21. The hyperechoic foci identified in the splenic parenchyma are most suspicious for:
  a. candidiasis
  b. pneumobilia
  c. splenic calcifications
  d. multiple small hemangiomas

22. These sonographic findings are most likely considered:
  a. life threatening
  b. incidental findings
  c. postsurgical changes
  d. hypervascular lesions

Using Figure 11.6, answer question 23.

23. A female patient presents to the ultrasound department complaining of vague left upper quadrant pain. She admits to "wrestling" with her brother a week earlier. Based on this clinical history, the sonographic findings are most suspicious for which of the following conditions?
  a. hematoma
  b. polycystic disease
  c. loculated abscess
  d. pseudocyst

Using Figure 11.7, answer question 24.

24. The mass identified by the arrow most likely represents a(n):
  a. abscess
  b. lipoma
  c. cavernous hemangioma
  d. primary malignant tumor

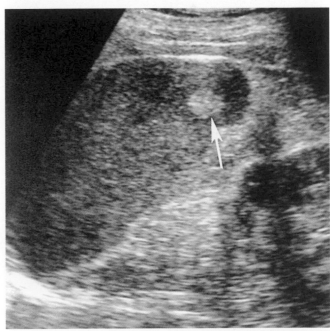

FIG. 11.7 Coronal sonogram of the spleen.

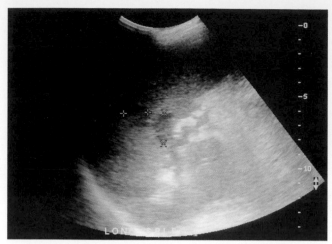

FIG. 11.8 Coronal sonogram of the spleen.

Using Figure 11.8, answer question 25.

25. An afebrile patient with a history of leukemia presents to the ultrasound department complaining of left upper quadrant pain. This sonogram of the spleen most likely documents:
    a. candidiasis
    b. primary malignant tumors
    c. multiple splenic abscesses
    d. metastatic disease

26. Which of the following structures carries carbon dioxide back to the lungs?
    a. platelet
    b. lymphocyte
    c. hematocrit
    d. hemoglobin

27. A hemangiosarcoma located in the spleen on ultrasound would appear as a(n):
    a. anechoic or hypoechoic mass
    b. hyperechoic or complex mass
    c. hypoechoic or complex mass
    d. isoechoic or hyperechoic mass

28. Which of the following is an indication for an ultrasound of the spleen?
    a. fatigue
    b. hypotension
    c. weight gain
    d. elevated serum amylase

29. Which of the following splenic pathologies is associated with granulomatosis?
    a. cysts
    b. calcifications
    c. cavernous hemangioma
    d. cavernous lymphangioma

30. A patient presents with a history of portal hypertension. The spleen is expected to demonstrate:
    a. atrophy
    b. enlargement
    c. intraparenchymal calcifications
    d. reversal of flow in the splenic vein

31. Leukocytosis is defined as a white blood cell count:
    a. below 4000
    b. below 11,000
    c. above 12,000
    d. above 20,000

32. A hematoma located below the splenic capsule most commonly appears on ultrasound as a:
    a. lateral anechoic mass
    b. hypoechoic parenchymal mass
    c. crescent-shaped fluid collection inferior to the diaphragm
    d. loculated mass anterior to the left kidney

33. Which of the following pathologies is associated with a "wheel within a wheel" appearance on ultrasound?
    a. candidiasis
    b. infarction
    c. hemangiosarcoma
    d. cystic lymphangiomatosis

34. Splenic infarction is most commonly associated with an embolism originating from which of the following structures?
    a. heart
    b. liver
    c. spleen
    d. pancreas

35. Which of the following conditions is most likely to demonstrate an elevated hematocrit?
    a. infection
    b. leukemia
    c. hemorrhage
    d. overhydration

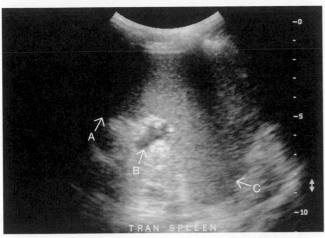

FIG. 11.9   Transverse sonogram of the spleen.

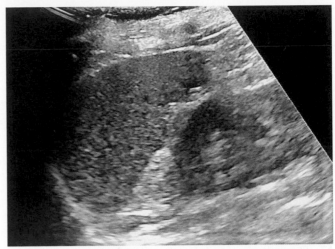

FIG. 11.10   Sonogram of the left upper quadrant.

Using Figure 11.9, answer questions 36 through 38.

36. Which of the following splenic regions is identified by arrow *A*?
   a. superior portion
   b. inferior portion
   c. splenic hilum
   d. anterior portion

37. Which of the following splenic regions is identified by arrow *B*?
   a. superior portion
   b. inferior portion
   c. splenic hilum
   d. anterior portion

38. Which of the following splenic regions is identified by arrow *C*?
   a. superior portion
   b. inferior portion
   c. splenic hilum
   d. posterior portion

Using Figure 11.10, answer question 39.

39. Which of the following scanning planes is most likely demonstrated in this sonogram?
   a. anterior
   b. subcostal
   c. transverse
   d. coronal

Using Figure 11.11, answer question 40.

40. Which of the following findings is most likely demonstrated in this sonogram of the left upper quadrant?
   a. ascites
   b. phlegmon
   c. pleural effusion
   d. hemoperitoneum

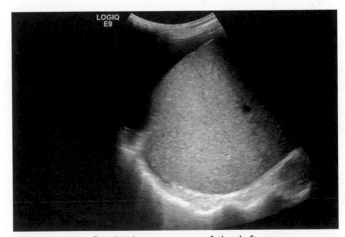

FIG. 11.11   Sagittal sonogram of the left upper quadrant.

41. A patient arrives at the emergency department following a motor vehicle accident. An abdominal ultrasound is most likely ordered to evaluate for which of the following conditions?
    a. pancreatitis
    b. biliary obstruction
    c. urinary obstruction
    d. hemoperitoneum

42. In which of the following conditions is the spleen enlarged as a child and atrophic as an adult?
    a. lymphoma
    b. sickle cell anemia
    c. leukemia
    d. polycythemia vera

43. The splenic vein joins the superior mesenteric vein to form the:
    a. coronary vein
    b. hepatic vein
    c. portal vein
    d. gastric vein

44. Leukopenia is defined as a white blood cell count:
    a. below 4000
    b. below 11,000
    c. above 12,000
    d. above 20,000

45. Which of the following structures is recycled into iron by the spleen?
    a. erythrocytes
    b. platelets
    c. leukocytes
    d. hemoglobin

46. Which of the following conditions is most likely associated with a decrease in leukocytes?
    a. anemia
    b. lymphoma
    c. leukemia
    d. malignancy

47. Normal hemoglobin levels should not exceed:
    a. 5 g/dL
    b. 10 g/dL
    c. 20 g/dL
    d. 50 g/dL

48. In a 40-year-old patient, splenomegaly is suggested after the length of the spleen exceeds:
    a. 7 cm
    b. 11 cm
    c. 13 cm
    d. 18 cm

49. A patient with an accessory spleen will most likely present with which of the following symptoms?
    a. dyspepsia
    b. no symptoms
    c. left upper quadrant pain
    d. palpable abdominal mass

50. Which of the following benign neoplasms is composed of lymphoid tissue?
    a. lipoma
    b. adenoma
    c. hamartoma
    d. cavernous hemangioma

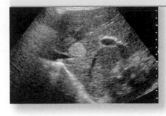

CHAPTER 12

Retroperitoneum

KEY TERMS

Addison disease life-threatening condition caused by partial or complete failure of the adrenocortical function. Also known as adrenocortical insufficiency.

adrenogenital syndrome congenital disorder causing an increase in production of androgens.

Conn syndrome uncommon condition resulting from excessive aldosterone secretions.

Cushing syndrome a metabolic disorder resulting from chronic and excessive production of cortisol by the adrenal cortex. Results in the inability of the body to regulate secretions of cortisol or adrenocorticotrophic hormone (ACTH). Also known as hyperadrenalism.

diaphragmatic crura fibers that connect the vertebral column and diaphragm. They are identified as hypoechoic linear structures superior to the celiac axis and lie anterior to the aorta and posterior to the inferior vena cava.

floating aorta enlarged lymph nodes posterior to the aorta giving the impression that the aorta is floating above the spine.

hyperaldosteronism excessive production of aldosterone.

lymphadenopathy focal or generalized enlargement of the lymph nodes.

neuroblastoma malignant tumor of the adrenal gland found in young children.

pheochromocytoma rare vascular tumor of the adrenal medulla.

retroperitoneal pertaining to organs closely attached to the posterior abdominal wall.

retroperitoneal fibrosis dense fibrous tissue proliferation typically confined to the paravertebral and central retroperitoneum areas.

suprarenal glands adrenal glands.

PHYSIOLOGY

Adrenal Glands (Fig. 12.1)

- A pair of endocrine glands located in the retroperitoneum.

Function of the Adrenal Glands

- Produce hormones.
- The medulla and cortex function independently.

Cortex Secretes Steroids

- Mineralocoids.
  - Main steroid production is aldosterone.
  - Aldosterone helps maintain the body's fluid and electrolyte balance by promoting sodium reabsorption and potassium excretion within the kidneys.
  - Aids in controlling the amount of water in the body.
- Glucocorticoids.
  - Production of cortisol (hydrocortisone).
  - Aids in the body's response to stress.
  - Modifies the body's response to infection, surgery, or trauma.
  - Regulates the metabolism of proteins, carbohydrates, and lipids.
  - Increases with stress and decreases with inflammation.
- Gonadal hormones.
  - Produce androgens, estrogens, and progesterone.

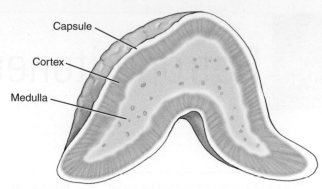

FIG. 12.1   Adrenal anatomy.

Medulla Secretes

- Catecholamines.
  - Epinephrine (adrenaline).
    - Increases in times of excitement or emotional stress.
    - "Fight or flight" response.
  - Norepinephrine.
    - Aids to increase blood pressure by vasoconstriction without affecting cardiac output.

ANATOMY

- Consists of two regions.
- **Medulla.**
  - Inner portion, which comprises 10% of the gland.
  - Regulates blood pressure and heart rate.
  - Secretes epinephrine and norepinephrine.
- **Cortex.**
  - Outer portion, which comprises 90% of the gland.
  - Beneath the adrenal capsule are three layers, from outer to inner as follows:
    - Zona glomerulosa.
      - Produces mineralocorticoids.
    - Zona fasciculate.
      - Produces glucocorticoids.
    - Zona reticularis.
      - Stimulates production of testosterone and estrogen.

LOCATION

- Retroperitoneal structures located in Gerota's fascia within the perinephric space.
- Located anterior, medial, and superior to each kidney.
- Lie lateral to the diaphragmatic crura.
- Right adrenal gland lies posterior and lateral to the inferior vena cava.
- Left adrenal gland lies lateral to the aorta and posterior to the stomach, lesser sac, splenic artery, and tail of the pancreas.

SIZE

- Adult adrenal gland measures approximately 3 to 5 cm in length, 2 to 3 cm in width, and 1 cm in height.
- Adult—adrenal gland is approximately 1/13 of renal length.
- Infant—adrenal gland is approximately 1/3 of renal length.

VASCULAR ANATOMY

- The superior, middle, and inferior suprarenal arteries supply the adrenal glands.
- Superior suprarenal artery arises from the inferior phrenic artery.
- Middle suprarenal artery arises from the lateral aspect of the abdominal aorta.
- Inferior suprarenal artery arises from the renal artery.
- Right suprarenal vein drains directly into the inferior vena cava.
- Left suprarenal vein drains into the left renal vein.

NORMAL SONOGRAPHIC APPEARANCE OF ADRENAL GLANDS

- The right adrenal gland is shaped like a triangule or pyramid similar to a "Y" or "V" (Fig. 12.2).
- The left adrenal gland demonstrates a semilunar or crescent shape (Fig. 12.3).
- Solid structures with a hyperechoic medulla (center) surrounded by a hypoechoic cortex.
- Hypoechoic cortex is generally surrounded by hyperechoic retroperitoneal fat.
- Prominent in the neonate and young children.
- Difficult to visualize in the adult.

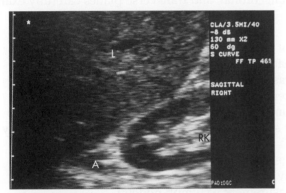

FIG. 12.2   Right adrenal gland.

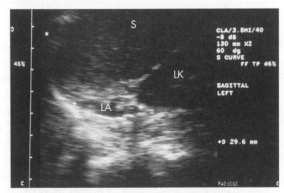

FIG. 12.3   Left adrenal gland.

EXAMINATION TECHNIQUES, PROTOCOLS, AND IMAGE OPTIMIZATION

Preparation

- No preparation is required before an ultrasound of the adrenal glands or retroperitoneum.
- Fasting may improve visualization of the retroperitoneum.
  - Adult—6 to 8 hours.
  - Children—6 hours.
  - Infants—4 hours.

Transducer Selection

- Use the highest frequency possible to obtain optimal resolution for penetration depth.
  - Adults—3.0 to 5.0 MHz.
  - Children and small adults—5.0 to 7.0 MHz.
  - Obese patients—2.0 MHz may be required.
- Curvilinear transducers provide a wider field of view.
- Sector or vector transducers have a smaller footprint great for intercostal imaging.
- Subcostal or prone imaging in some patients may be helpful.
- Higher frequency transducers can be used in thin adult patients.

Patient Positioning

Right Adrenal Gland

- Supine, left posterior oblique, or left lateral decubitus.
  - Intercostal approach at the midaxillary or anterior axillary line.
  - Imaging using the right lobe of the liver as an acoustic window perpendicular to the crus of the diaphragm.

Left Adrenal Gland

- Supine, right anterior oblique, or right lateral decubitus.
  - Intercostal approach at the midaxillary or posterior axillary line.
  - Have patient drink 16 ounces of water to fill stomach. Place patient in a supine semirecumbent position with the head elevated 30 degrees. Angle down through the fluid-filled stomach may aid in visualizing the left adrenal gland.

Retroperitoneum

- Supine, prone, right and left lateral decubitus.
- Right and left posterior oblique may aid in moving overlying bowel gas.

Examination Protocol

- Systematic approach in the sagittal, coronal, and transverse planes carefully examining and imaging:
- **Adrenal glands.**
  - Superior and inferior border of each adrenal gland.
  - Medial and lateral border of each adrenal gland.
  - Length, height, and width measurement of each adrenal gland.
  - Color Doppler imaging of adrenal vasculature.
  - Abnormalities should be documented and when applicable measured in two imaging planes. Color and/or spectral Doppler evaluation of the abnormality should be included.
- **Retroperitoneum.**
  - Orthogonal images of anatomy or area of interest.
  - Length, height, and width measurement of lymph node(s).
  - Color Doppler of lymph node vasculature.
  - Abnormalities should be documented and when applicable measured in two imaging planes. Color and/or spectral Doppler evaluation of the abnormality should be included.

Image Optimization

- Place gains settings to display the normal renal cortex hypoechoic to the normal liver and splenic parenchyma with adjustments to reduce artifactually produced echoes within the lumen of the abdominal vessels.
- Focal zone(s) should be placed at or below the area of interest. The use of multiple focal zones increases detail resolution and decreases temporal resolution.
- Sufficient imaging depth to visualize structures immediately posterior to the area of interest.
- Harmonic imaging and decreasing system compression (dynamic range) can be used to reduce artifactual echoes within normal anechoic structures.
- Spatial compounding can be used to improve visualization of structures posterior to highly attenuating structures.
- Doppler settings should be adjusted for a slow flow rate.
- The use of deep inspiration may improve visualization of the adrenal glands.
- The use of multiple patient positions may redistribute overlying bowel gas.

Examination Limitations

- Superior location of the adrenal glands (high under ribcage).
- Gastrointestinal gas.
- Obesity.

Helpful Hints

- Adrenal glands are best visualized in the transverse plane.
- The echogenicity of the normal liver and spleen is similar to the echogenicity of the adrenal cortex.
- Multiple imaging windows may be necessary to evaluate each adrenal gland in its entirety.
- The right adrenal gland is easier to visualize than the left adrenal gland.
- Altering intercostal spaces may aid in visualizing the adrenal gland in its entirety.
- In the left posterior oblique or left lateral decubitus position using a subcostal oblique approach parallel with the rib cage may aid in visualizing the right adrenal gland.
- A round adrenal gland is abnormal.
- Crura of the diaphragm are best demonstrated in the transverse plane.

Indications for Examination

- Hypertension.
- Abdominal distension.
- Severe anxiety.
- Sweating.
- Tachycardia.
- Weight loss.
- Diabetes mellitus.
- Evaluate mass from previous medical imaging study (e.g., CT).

LABORATORY VALUES

Adrenocorticotrophic Hormone (ACTH)

- Normal range: 10 to 80 pg/mL.
- Regulates cortisol production.
- Produced in the pituitary gland.
- Elevation associated with adrenal tumor, Cushing disease, and lung tumor.

Aldosterone

- Normal range:
  - Recumbent 3 to 10 ng/dL.
  - Erect 5 to 30 ng/dL.
- Steroid secreted by the cortex.
- A measure of adrenal function.
- Regulates sodium and water levels, which affects blood volume and pressure.
- Elevation associated with hyperaldosteronism.
- Decreases associated with hypoaldosteronism and Addison disease.

Potassium

- Normal range: serum 3.5 to 5.0 mEq/L.
- Essential to the normal function of every organ system.
- Maintains necessary concentration of nutrients inside and outside of the cell.
- Elevation associated with Addison disease.
- Decreases associated with Cushing disease and hyperaldosteronism.

Sodium

- Normal range: serum 135 to 145 mEq/L.
- Major component in determining blood volume.
- Decreases associated with Addison disease.

Serum Cortisol

- Normal range: 7 to 25 mcg/dL.
- Measures adrenal hormonal levels.
- Blood tests are taken at 8 AM and 4 PM. Ideally the 8 AM should be halved at the 4 PM reading.

Benign Adrenal Pathology

PATHOLOGY	ETIOLOGY	CLINICAL FINDINGS	SONOGRAPHIC FINDINGS	DIFFERENTIAL CONSIDERATIONS
Adenoma	Benign cortical mass of epithelial origin Functioning or non-functioning **Risk Factors:** Diabetes mellitus Obesity Hypertension Elderly population	Asymptomatic Elevated adrenal hormones Cushing's syndrome Conn's disease	Hypoechoic, homogeneous mass Smooth wall margins May demonstrate necrosis or hemorrhage	Adrenal hyperplasia Adrenocortical carcinoma Renal or liver mass Adrenal hemorrhage
Adrenal cyst	Rare **Type** Endothelial Pseudocyst Epithelial Parasitic	Asymptomatic Hypertension	Anechoic mass Well-defined wall margins Posterior acoustic enhancement Wall calcifications may be seen with pseudocysts and parasitic cysts. Unilateral	Cyst of the liver, spleen, or kidney Adrenal hemorrhage Hydronephrosis
Adrenal hemorrhage	Adrenal mass Hypoxia Traumatic delivery Septicemia Infant of diabetic mother	Asymptomatic Palpable abdominal mass Decrease in hematocrit	Dependent on the age of hemorrhage Anechoic mass in early stages. May appear as a homogeneously echogenic or complex mass Residual calcification may be present following reabsorption Frequently located on the right	Cyst or neoplasm of the liver, spleen, or kidney Adenoma Adrenocortical carcinoma
Adrenal hyperplasia	Proliferation in adrenal cells Typically, bilateral	Asymptomatic Hypertension Elevated adrenocortico-trophic hormone (ACTH) level	Enlargement of the adrenal gland(s) Change in the normal triangular shape	Adenoma Adrenocortical carcinoma
Pheochromocytoma	Rare vascular tumor of the medulla Small percentage are malignant Right-side prevalence	Hypertension Sweating Tachycardia Chest or epigastric pain Headache Palpitations Severe anxiety Elevation in epinephrine and norepinephrine	Highly vascular solid mass Homogeneous texture May appear complex because of necrosis or hemorrhage May calcify Metastasis to liver, lymph nodes, lung, and bone if malignant	Renal mass Adrenocortical carcinoma Adrenal adenoma Adrenal hemorrhage

Malignant Adrenal Pathology

PATHOLOGY	ETIOLOGY	CLINICAL FINDINGS	SONOGRAPHIC FINDINGS	DIFFERENTIAL CONSIDERATIONS
Adrenocortical carcinoma	Epithelial neoplasm of the adrenal cortex Functioning or nonfunctioning	Hypertension Weakness Abdominal pain Weight loss Weakening of the bones	Complex or echogenic mass Irregular wall margins Tends to invade the inferior vena cava Metastasis to the lungs and bone	Renal mass Adrenal hemorrhage Pheochromocytoma Metastases
Metastases	Lung most common Breast Stomach	Hypertension Abdominal pain Addison's disease	Focal mass Variable in appearance	Renal mass Adrenal hemorrhage Pheochromocytoma Adrenocortical carcinoma
Neuroblastoma Third most common malignancy in infancy	Sarcoma of the adrenal medulla or autonomic nervous system Common in young children Half occur before 2 years of age More common on the left	Asymptomatic Palpable mass Abdominal distension Sweating Weight loss Fatigue Tachycardia Hypertension Pallor Fever Elevation of epinephrine and norepinephrine	Heterogeneous mass Poorly defined wall margins Pinpoint calcifications (30%) Lymphadenopathy Mass encases the aorta, inferior vena cava, superior mesenteric artery, and vein No invasion of the renal vein Metastasis to the bone and lymph nodes (most frequent) May also metastasize to liver, brain, lung, and orbit	Nephroblastoma Lymphoma Adrenal hemorrhage

Conditions Associated with the Adrenal Glands

CONDITION	DESCRIPTION	ETIOLOGY	CLINICAL FINDINGS
Addison disease	Life-threatening condition caused by partial or complete failure of adrenocortical function (hypofunction) Destruction of the adrenal cortex Loss of cortisol and aldosterone secretions Increased incidence in females Diagnosis is established if the amount of cortisol in the plasma and steroid in the urine do not increase after stimulation with adrenocorticotrophic hormone (ACTH)	Autoimmune reaction Tuberculosis Adrenal hemorrhage Chronic infection Surgical removal of both adrenal glands	Anorexia Bronze skin pigmentation Chronic fatigue Dehydration Emotional changes GI disorders Hypotension Weakness Salt cravings Elevated serum potassium Decreases in serum sodium and glucose
Adrenogenital syndrome	Congenital disorder causing excessive secretion of sexual hormones and adrenal androgens	Congenital disorder Adrenal tumor or hyperplasia	Increased androgen production Increases in body hair Deepening of the voice Atrophy of the uterus Acne
Conn syndrome	Excessive production of aldosterone	Adrenal adenoma is the most common (70% with female prevalence) Adrenal hyperplasia (male prevalence) Adrenal carcinoma (rare)	Hypertension Elevated aldosterone levels Muscular weakness Abnormal electrocardiogram

Continued

Conditions Associated with the Adrenal Glands—(cont'd)

CONDITION	DESCRIPTION	ETIOLOGY	CLINICAL FINDINGS
Cushing disease	Rare and serious disorder resulting from excessive production of cortisol Excessive use of cortical hormones	Results in accumulation of fat on the abdomen, face, upper back, and upper chest Pituitary mass is the most common cause Adrenal mass Polycystic ovarian disease Excessive amount of glucocorticoid hormone	Fatigue Purplish striae on the skin Decrease in immunity to infection Emotional changes Increase in thirst and urination Muscle weakness New onset of diabetes mellitus Osteoporosis Elevation in ACTH, white blood cells, and blood glucose levels Decrease in serum potassium

RETROPERITONEUM

- Area of the body behind the peritoneum.

Borders of the Retroperitoneum

- Superior border—diaphragm.
- Inferior border—pelvic rim.
- Anterior border—posterior parietal peritoneum.
- Posterior border—posterior abdominal wall muscles and spine.
- Lateral border—transversalis fascia and peritoneal portions of the mesentery.

Spaces in the Retroperitoneum

Anterior Pararenal

- Fat area between the posterior peritoneum and Gerota's fascia.
- Includes: pancreas, descending portion of the duodenum, ascending and descending colon, superior mesenteric vessels, and inferior portion of the common bile duct.

Posterior Pararenal

- Space between Gerota's fascia and the posterior abdominal wall muscles.
- Includes: iliopsoas and quadratus lumborum muscles and the posterior abdominal wall.
- Contains fat and nerves.

Perirenal

- Space separated from the pararenal space by Gerota's fascia.
- Includes: kidneys, adrenal glands, perinephric fat, ureters, renal vessels, aorta, inferior vena cava, and lymph nodes.

LYMPH NODES

Functions of Lymph Nodes

- Filter the lymph of debris and organisms.
- Form lymphocytes and antibodies to fight infection.

Divisions of Lymph Nodes

Parietal Nodes

- Located in the retroperitoneum and course along the prevertebral vessels.
- Surround the aorta.
- Kidney, adrenal gland, ovarian/testicular nodes drain into the paraaortic nodes.
- Subdivided into:
  - Common iliac.
  - Epigastric.
  - External iliac.
  - Iliac circumflex.
  - Internal iliac.
  - Lumbar.
  - Sacral.

Visceral Nodes

- Located in the peritoneum and follow the course along the vessels supplying the major organs.
- Generally located at hilum of the organ.

SONOGRAPHIC APPEARANCE OF THE NORMAL LYMPH NODE

- Hypoechoic solid mass.
- Hyperechoic fatty center.
- Smooth margins.
- Oval shape.
- Internal vascular blood flow especially at the hilum.
- Usually measures less than 1 cm.

SONOGRAPHIC APPEARANCE OF THE ABNORMAL LYMPH NODE

- Enlarged hypoechoic mass exceeding 1 cm in size.
- Loss of hyperechoic fatty center.
- Smooth wall margins and oval shape typically caused by infection.
- Irregular margins and round shape suspicious for malignancy.
- Displacement of adjacent structures.
  - Anterior displacement of the aorta—floating aorta sign.
  - Enlarged mantle of nodes surround aorta and possibly inferior vena cava— "Donut-ring."
  - Enlarged nodes at the hepatic hilum may produce intrahepatic biliary dilatation.
- Assess abdomen and pelvis for primary tumor or inflammatory disease.

SONOGRAPHIC APPEARANCE OF RETROPERITONEAL MASSES

- Hyperechoic to hypoechoic mass(es).
- Irregular wall margins.
- Anterior displacement of the kidneys, inferior vena cava, aorta, and mesenteric vessels.
- Deformity of the inferior vena cava and urinary bladder.
- Obstruction of the urinary tract or biliary system.
- Loss of organ definition.

Lymphadenopathy Patterns

NODE REGION	LOCATION	ASSOCIATED PATHOLOGY
Gastrohepatic	Region of the gastrohepatic ligament	Stomach, esophageal, and pancreatic carcinoma Lymphoma Metastatic disease
Mesenteric	Along the mesentery	Inflammatory bowel Small bowel carcinoma
Pancreaticoduodenal	Anterior to the inferior vena cava Between the duodenum and head of the pancreas	Colon and stomach carcinoma Carcinoma of the pancreatic head Lymphoma Metastatic disease
Pelvic	Along the iliac vessels	Carcinoma of the pelvis
Perisplenic	Splenic hilum	Leukemia Non-Hodgkin's lymphoma Small bowel and colon carcinoma Metastatic disease
Porta hepatis	Anterior and posterior to the portal vein	Gallbladder, biliary, liver, stomach, and pancreatic carcinoma Lymphoma Metastatic disease
Retrocrural	Inferior posterior mediastinum	Lung carcinoma Lymphoma
Retroperitoneal	Periaortic, pericaval, and intraaortocaval	Lymphoma Renal carcinoma Metastatic disease from testicular, cervical, and prostatic carcinoma
Superior mesenteric and celiac arteries	Periaortic	Intraabdominal neoplasms

Benign Pathology of the Retroperitoneum

PATHOLOGY	DESCRIPTION	SONOGRAPHIC FINDINGS	DIFFERENTIAL CONSIDERATIONS
Lymphadenopathy	Any disorder characterized by a localized or generalized enlargement of the lymph nodes or lymph vessels	Hypoechoic mass May appear complex Smooth or irregular margins Exceeds 1 cm in size Internal vascular flow especially at the hilum	Lipoma Retroperitoneal fibrosis Retroperitoneal hemorrhage Horseshoe kidney
Lymphocele	A fluid collection containing lymph from an injured lymph vessel Commonly associated with organ transplant and lymph node removal	Anechoic encapsulated fluid collection Round or oval in shape Well-defined borders Frequently contain septations Posterior acoustic enhancement	Hematoma Urinoma Ascites Abscess
Retroperitoneal abscess	A collection of pus between the peritoneum and the posterior abdominal wall	Hypoechoic or complex mass Irregular margins May demonstrate posterior acoustic shadowing Mass takes on the shape of the space	Hemorrhage Lymphadenopathy Retroperitoneal fibrosis Horseshoe kidney
Retroperitoneal fibrosis	A chronic inflammatory process in which fibrotic tissue surrounds the large blood vessels located in the lumbar area Usually idiopathic	Hypoechoic bulky midline mass Rarely extends above the second lumbar vertebra May extend inferiorly to the dome of the bladder May demonstrate associated hydronephrosis	Lymphadenopathy Retroperitoneal hemorrhage Retroperitoneal abscess Horseshoe kidney

Benign Pathology of the Retroperitoneum—(cont'd)

PATHOLOGY	DESCRIPTION	SONOGRAPHIC FINDINGS	DIFFERENTIAL CONSIDERATIONS
Retroperitoneal hemorrhage	Associated with trauma, surgery, bleeding disorders, or anticoagulants therapy	Hypoechoic fluid collections (early) May demonstrate echogenic clot or calcifications (late) Shape conforms to the space	Ascites Retroperitoneal fibrosis Lymphadenopathy Horseshoe kidney
Urinoma	A cyst filled with urine Adjacent or within the urinary tract Typically located in the perinephric space	Elliptical anechoic fluid collection Smooth, thin walls Frequently contain septations Rapid increase in size on serial examinations	Lymphocele Hematoma Cyst Abscess

Benign Neoplasms of the Retroperitoneum

PATHOLOGY	DESCRIPTION	SONOGRAPHIC FINDINGS	DIFFERENTIAL CONSIDERATIONS
Fibroma	A neoplasm consisting largely of fibrous connective tissue	Hyperechoic mass Well-defined wall margins	Lipoma Mesothelioma Myxoma
Lipoma	A neoplasm consisting of fatty tissue	Hyperechoic mass Well-defined wall margins	Fibroma Liposarcoma Mesothelioma Myxoma
Mesothelioma	Abnormal growth of the epithelial cells	Localized echogenic mass Irregular wall margins Similar appearance to the fetal placenta	Liposarcoma Lymphadenopathy Lipoma Myxoma Horseshoe kidney
Myxoma	A neoplasm consisting of connective tissue Subcutaneous, retroperitoneal, cardiac, and urinary in location May be extremely large	Complex or echogenic mass Lobulated or smooth wall margins	Fibroma Lipoma Mesothelioma Lymphadenopathy Horseshoe kidney
Teratoma	A neoplasm composed of different types of tissues that do not occur together or at the site of the tumor	Complex mass	Leiomyosarcoma Abscess Myxoma

Malignant Neoplasms of the Retroperitoneum

PATHOLOGY	DESCRIPTION	SONOGRAPHIC FINDINGS	DIFFERENTIAL CONSIDERATIONS
Fibrosarcoma	A sarcoma containing fibrous connective tissues	Hypoechoic or complex mass May infiltrate surrounding structures	Lymphadenopathy Retroperitoneal fibrosis Retroperitoneal hemorrhage Horseshoe kidney
Leiomyosarcoma	A sarcoma containing large spindle cells of smooth muscle	Echogenic or complex mass Cystic areas of necrosis may be demonstrated	Teratoma Rhabdomyosarcoma Retroperitoneal abscess
Liposarcoma	A malignant growth of fat cells Most common retroperitoneal neoplasm	Hyperechoic mass Thick wall margins May infiltrate surrounding tissues	Lipoma Fibroma Rhabdomyosarcoma Mesothelioma
Rhabdomyosarcoma	A highly malignant tumor derived from striated muscle	Hyperechoic or complex mass	Teratoma Liposarcoma Fibrosarcoma Leiomyosarcoma

RETROPERITONEUM REVIEW

1. Which of the following hormones modifies the body's response to inflammation?
   a. aldosterone
   b. norepinephrine
   c. glucocorticoids
   d. epinephrine

2. A malignant neoplasm derived from striated muscle describes a:
   a. myxoma
   b. leiomyosarcoma
   c. rhabdomyosarcoma
   d. pheochromocytoma

3. Gastrohepatic lymphadenopathy is associated with:
   a. lymphoma
   b. renal cell carcinoma
   c. uterine carcinoma
   d. inflammatory bowel

4. Which of the following adrenal pathologies is typically demonstrated bilaterally?
   a. adrenal cyst
   b. pheochromocytoma
   c. adrenal adenoma
   d. adrenal hyperplasia

5. Which of the following is considered a function of the lymph node?
   a. modify the body's response to inflammation
   b. maintain the water and sodium balance
   c. form antibodies to fight infection
   d. maintain normal blood circulation

6. Which of the following is a symptom associated with adrenocortical carcinoma?
   a. severe anxiety
   b. weight loss
   c. muscle cramps
   d. hypotension

7. Which of the following is the most common cause of Conn syndrome?
   a. adrenal adenoma
   b. adrenal carcinoma
   c. adrenal hemorrhage
   d. adrenal hyperplasia

8. Which of the following adrenal neoplasms is most likely to infiltrate surrounding structures?
   a. teratoma
   b. liposarcoma
   c. mesothelioma
   d. leiomyosarcoma

9. A urinoma is most likely to develop in which of the following regions?
   a. lesser sac
   b. paracolic gutter
   c. perinephric space
   d. subhepatic space

10. The most common neoplasm to develop in the retroperitoneum is a:
    a. liposarcoma
    b. myxoma
    c. fibrosarcoma
    d. mesothelioma

11. Which of the following statements correctly describes the adrenal glands?
    a. The medulla comprises 25% of the gland.
    b. Gonadal hormones are secreted by the medulla.
    c. Norepinephrine is secreted by the cortex.
    d. The arteries supplying the adrenal glands arise from the aorta, renal, and inferior phrenic arteries.

12. The anterior pararenal space is most accurately defined as the area between the:
    a. perirenal space and the posterior pararenal space
    b. posterior peritoneum and Gerota's fascia
    c. anterior abdominal wall and the psoas muscle
    d. anterior peritoneum and Gerota's fascia

13. Young children have a predisposing factor for developing which of the following adrenal neoplasms?
    a. nephroblastoma
    b. Wilms' tumor
    c. neuroblastoma
    d. liposarcoma

14. Which of the following structures form the anterior border of the retroperitoneum?
    a. diaphragm
    b. pelvic rim
    c. posterior parietal peritoneum
    d. posterior abdominal wall muscles

15. An enlarged irregular lymph node demonstrating a round appearance is most consistent with an underlying:
    a. malignancy
    b. hemorrhage
    c. infection
    d. obstruction

16. Which of the following structures is located in the anterior pararenal space?
    a. kidneys
    b. pancreas
    c. adrenal glands
    d. inferior vena cava

17. Benign adrenal pathology associated with hypertension, tachycardia, and palpitations is most consistent with which of the following pathologies?
    a. hyperplasia
    b. pheochromocytoma
    c. hemorrhage
    d. adenoma

18. Visceral lymph nodes are located:
    a. around the aorta
    b. along the prevertebral vessels
    c. in the peritoneum
    d. near the adrenal glands

19. The location of the right adrenal gland most accurately correlates to which of the following regions?
    a. lateral to the right kidney
    b. posterior to the inferior vena cava
    c. medial to the diaphragmatic crura
    d. medial to the inferior vena cava

20. Elevation in which of the following laboratory tests is a clinical finding in Addison disease?
    a. cortisol
    b. aldosterone
    c. serum sodium
    d. serum potassium

21. Which of the following conditions is a predisposing factor for development of an adrenal adenoma?
    a. anorexia
    b. hypotension
    c. diabetes mellitus
    d. polycythemia vera

22. The "floating aorta" sign is caused by lymphadenopathy in which of the following regions?
    a. perinephric space
    b. anterior to the aorta
    c. surrounding the aorta
    d. posterior to the aorta

23. How would an adrenal mass displace the upper pole of the kidney?
    a. cephalad and laterally
    b. inferior and medially
    c. cephalad and medially
    d. lateral and caudally

24. Which of the following hormones is secreted by the adrenal medulla?
    a. cortisol
    b. epinephrine
    c. estrogen
    d. aldosterone

25. A condition caused by complete or partial failure of the adrenocortical function describes:
    a. Conn syndrome
    b. Addison disease
    c. Cushing disease
    d. Graves disease

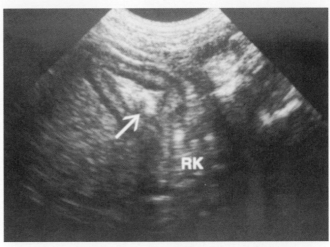

FIG. 12.4 Transverse sonogram of the right upper quadrant

Using Figure 12.4, answer question 26.

26. The arrow identifies which of the following?
    a. angiomyolipoma
    b. normal adrenal cortex
    c. an adrenal hemorrhage
    d. normal adrenal medulla

Using Figure 12.5, answer questions 27 and 28.

27. A 35-year-old man presents with a history of a sudden onset of hypertension. The sonogram is most suspicious for a(n):
    a. adrenal cyst
    b. liver cyst
    c. pheochromocytoma
    d. retroperitoneal hemorrhage

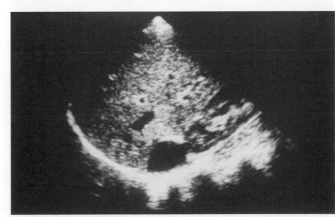

FIG. 12.5 Sagittal image of the right upper quadrant.

28. The pathology identified in this sonogram is considered a:
    a. result of trauma
    b. rare finding
    c. common incidental finding
    d. rare vascular tumor

Using Figure 12.6, answer question 29.

29. Which of the following is demonstrated in this transverse sonogram?
    a. horseshoe kidney
    b. lymphadenopathy
    c. mesenteric cysts
    d. retroperitoneal fibrosis

30. Which of the following abnormalities is the most likely complication of retroperitoneal fibrosis?
    a. pancreatitis
    b. cholecystitis
    c. hydronephrosis
    d. portal hypertension

31. An enlarged lymph node demonstrating an oval shape and smooth wall margins is most consistent with an underlying:
    a. malignancy
    b. hemorrhage
    c. infection
    d. obstruction

32. Which of the following fluid collections is most likely to demonstrate a rapid increase in size following renal transplant surgery?
    a. seroma
    b. hematoma
    c. urinoma
    d. lymphocele

33. An abnormal growth of epithelial cells is demonstrated in which of the following neoplasms?
    a. myxoma
    b. teratoma
    c. lipoma
    d. mesothelioma

34. Which of the following malignant neoplasms contains cells of smooth muscle?
    a. fibrosarcoma
    b. liposarcoma
    c. leiomyosarcoma
    d. mesothelioma

35. The sonographic appearance of a liposarcoma is most likely described as a:
    a. hypoechoic mass with thin wall margins
    b. hyperechoic mass with thick wall margins
    c. complex mass with irregular wall margins
    d. hyperechoic mass with irregular wall margins

Using Figure 12.7, answer question 36.

36. In a neonatal patient, this sonogram of the right upper quadrant is most likely demonstrating a(n):
    a. neuroblastoma
    b. adrenal adenoma
    c. adrenal hemorrhage
    d. normal adrenal gland

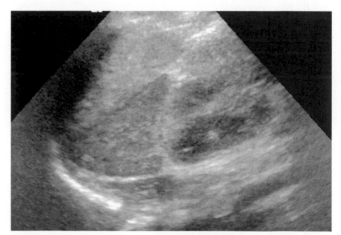

FIG. 12.7   Sagittal sonogram of the right upper quadrant.

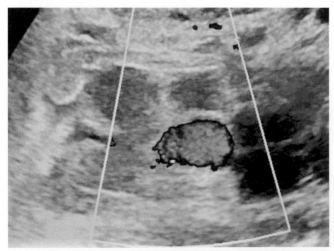

FIG. 12.6   Transverse sonogram of the aorta.

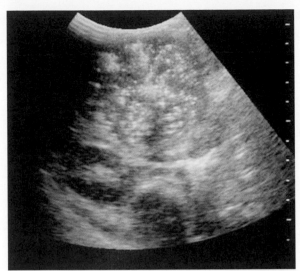

FIG. 12.8 Transverse sonogram of the right upper quadrant.

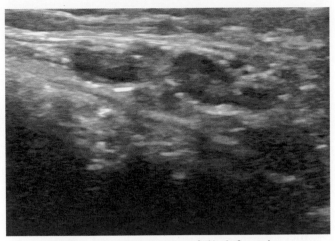

FIG. 12.9 Sonogram of the left groin.

Using Figure 12.8, answer question 37.

37. A hypervascular mass is identified in the right upper quadrant of a 15-month-old toddler. This is most suspicious for which of the following pathologies?
    a. nephroblastoma
    b. intussusception
    c. neuroblastoma
    d. adrenal hemorrhage

Using Figure 12.9, answer question 38.

38. A sonogram of the left groin demonstrates oval-shaped masses. These masses are most likely:
    a. lipomas
    b. hematomas
    c. lymph nodes
    d. liposarcomas

39. The outer portion of the adrenal gland comprises:
    a. 10% of the gland
    b. 25% of the gland
    c. 75% of the gland
    d. 90% of the gland

40. The adrenal glands are also known as the:
    a. cortisol glands
    b. adrenaline glands
    c. suprarenal glands
    d. retroperitoneal glands

41. The right suprarenal vein empties into which of the following vascular structures?
    a. splenic vein
    b. right renal vein
    c. inferior vena cava
    d. right gonadal vein

42. Which of the following hormones increases during times of excitement or stress?
    a. cortisol
    b. aldosterone
    c. epinephrine
    d. norepinephrine

43. Which of the following components is a major factor in determining blood volume?
    a. sodium
    b. vitamin K
    c. potassium
    d. calcium

44. Obesity is most likely a predisposing factor in developing which of the following adrenal neoplasms?
    a. cyst
    b. hemorrhage
    c. adenoma
    d. pheochromocytoma

45. Which of the following hormones is produced by the pituitary gland?
    a. trypsin
    b. epinephrine
    c. aldosterone
    d. adrenocorticotrophic hormone

46. Which of the following is considered a function of the adrenal glands?
    a. produce hormones
    b. release secretin hormones
    c. regulate serum electrolytes
    d. release glycogen as glucose

47. A rare vascular tumor of the adrenal gland defines a:
    a. teratoma
    b. neuroblastoma
    c. rhabdomyosarcoma
    d. pheochromocytoma

48. The inner portion of the adrenal gland is termed the:
    a. hilum
    b. cortex
    c. intima
    d. medulla

49. The location of the left adrenal gland most accurately correlates to which of the following regions?
    a. anterior to the stomach
    b. medial to the aorta
    c. anterior to the tail of the pancreas
    d. posterior to the splenic artery

50. Cushing disease is most commonly caused by which of the following pathologies?
    a. adrenal hyperplasia
    b. pituitary mass
    c. adrenal mass
    d. polycystic ovarian disease

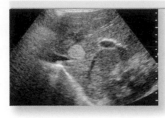

CHAPTER 13

Abdominal Vasculature

KEY TERMS

abdominal aortic aneurysm dilatation of the aorta equal to or exceeding 3 cm in diameter; also known as AAA.

aneurysm a localized widening or dilatation of a blood vessel.

aortic dissection spontaneous longitudinal separation of the intima and media layers creating a false lumen.

arterial stenosis narrowing or constriction of an artery usually caused by atherosclerosis, arteriosclerosis, or fibrointimal hyperplasia.

arteriosclerosis pathological thickening, hardening, and loss of elasticity of the arterial walls.

arteriovenous fistula an abnormal connection between an artery and vein; also known as arteriovenous shunting.

atherosclerosis disorder characterized by yellowish plaques of lipids and cellular debris in the medial and intimal layers of the arterial walls.

berry aneurysm small saccular aneurysm primarily affecting the cerebral arteries.

ectatic aneurysm dilatation of an artery compared with a more proximal segment. In the abdominal aorta, the ectatic dilatation does not exceed 3.0 cm.

fusiform aneurysm characterized by a uniform dilatation of the arterial walls; most common type of abdominal aortic aneurysm.

mesenteric ischemia decrease in arterial supply to the intestinal system.

mycotic aneurysm a saccular dilatation of a blood vessel caused by a bacterial infection.

pseudoaneurysm dilatation of an artery as a result of damage to one or more layers of the arterial wall caused by trauma or aneurysm rupture; also known as pulsatile hematoma.

saccular aneurysm dilatation of an artery characterized by a focal outpouching of one arterial wall; most often caused by trauma or infection.

PHYSIOLOGY AND ANATOMY

Functions of the Vascular System

- Arteries and arterioles carry blood away from the heart to organs and tissues to ensure oxygenation and metabolism.
  - Two exceptions: pulmonary artery and umbilical arteries in the fetus.
- Arterioles are the main controllers of blood pressure and blood flow.
- Arterioles are responsible for waveform morphology.
- Capillaries connect the arterial and venous systems.
- Capillaries exchange nutrients and waste.
- Veins and venules carry oxygen depleted blood toward the heart.
  - Two exceptions: pulmonary vein and umbilical vein of the fetus.
- Lower extremity veins contain valves to counteract gravity preventing retrograde flow during cardiac diastole.
- Valves extend inward toward the intima.

Vessel Wall Layers

- Venous walls are thinner and less elastic compared with arterial walls.

Tunica Adventitia

- Outer layer.
- Comprised of elastic tissue surrounded by a thin fibrous layer.
- Lends greater elasticity to the arteries.

Tunica Media

- Middle muscle layer.
- Comprised of collagenous fiber and smooth muscle.
- Helps regulate blood flow by controlling the vessel-wall diameter.

Tunica Intima

- Inner layer.
- Composed of three layers giving it a smooth surface.
- Layers: endothelial cells; connective tissue; internal elastic membrane.

ARTERIAL ANATOMY (Fig. 13.1)

Abdominal Aorta

- Originates at the diaphragm and courses inferiorly until it bifurcates into the right and left common iliac arteries.
- Tapers in size as it courses anterior and inferior in the abdomen.
- Common iliac arteries are the terminal branches of the abdominal aorta.
- Common iliac artery bifurcates into the external and internal (hypogastric) iliac arteries.
- External iliac artery becomes the common femoral artery after passing beneath the inguinal ligament.
- Internal iliac artery bifurcates into anterior and posterior divisions.

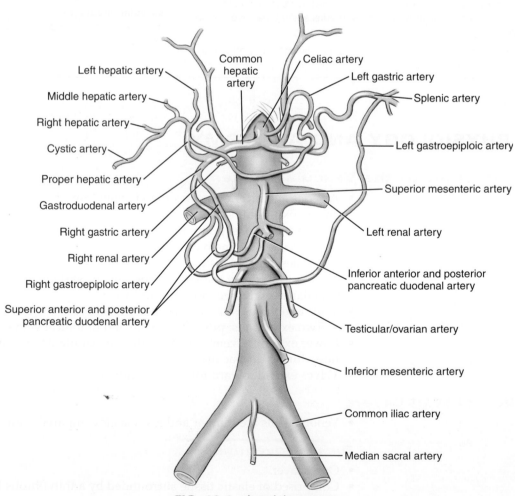

FIG. 13.1 Arterial anatomy.

Main Visceral Branches of the Abdominal Aorta

Celiac Axis (CA)

- First major branch of the abdominal aorta.
- Arises from the anterior aspect of the aorta.
- Branches into the splenic, left gastric, and common hepatic arteries.
- 1 to 3 cm in length.
- Low-resistance blood flow, with continuous forward flow in diastole.
- Peak systolic velocity should not exceed 200 cm/s.
- Peak systolic velocity remains unchanged after a meal.
- Located:
  - Anterior to the aorta.
  - Posterior to the left gastric vein.
  - Superior to the superior mesenteric artery, splenic vein, and body of the pancreas.
  - Inferior to the gastroesophageal junction.

Superior Mesenteric Artery (SMA)

- Second major branch of the abdominal aorta.
- Arises from the anterior surface of the aorta, inferior to the celiac axis.
- Courses inferiorly and parallel to the aorta.
- Branches supply the jejunum, ileum, cecum, ascending colon, portions of the transverse colon, and the head of the pancreas.
- Preprandial—high-resistance waveform with a sharp systolic peak and absent late diastolic flow. Should not exceed 280 cm/s.
- Postprandial—low-resistance waveform with continuous flow throughout diastole. Normal flow velocities may increase.
- Distance from the anterior wall of the aorta to the posterior wall of the SMA should not exceed 11 mm.
- Located:
  - Anterior to the aorta and left renal vein.
  - Posterior to the splenic vein, superior mesenteric vein, and body of the pancreas.
  - Superior to the renal arteries and veins.

Middle Suprarenal Arteries

- Arise from the lateral aspect of the abdominal aorta.
- Course laterally and slightly superior over the crura of the diaphragm to the adrenal glands.

Main Renal Arteries

- Right renal artery arises from the anterior lateral aspect of the abdominal aorta.
- Left renal artery arises from the posterior lateral aspect of the abdominal aorta.
- Located 1.0 to 1.5 cm inferior to the origin of the superior mesenteric artery.
- Right side arises superior to the contralateral left.
- Renal artery bifurcates into segmental arteries at the renal hilum.
- Renal artery gives rise to the inferior suprarenal artery.
- Low-resistance blood flow, with continuous forward flow in diastole.
- Duplicated arteries are found in 33% of the population.
- Right renal artery is located:
  - Anterior to the crus of the diaphragm.
  - Posterior to the inferior vena cava, right renal vein, portosplenic confluence, and the head/uncinate process of the pancreas.
  - Inferior to the right adrenal gland.

- Left renal artery is located:
  - Anterior to the crus of the diaphragm.
  - Posterior to the left renal vein, splenic vein, and tail of the pancreas.
  - Inferior to the left adrenal gland.

Gonadal Arteries

- Arise from the anterior aspect of the abdominal aorta inferior to the renal arteries.
- Course parallel to the psoas muscle into the pelvis.
- Low-resistance blood flow, with continuous flow through diastole.
- Not routinely visualized with ultrasound.

Inferior Mesenteric Artery (IMA)

- Last major branch of the abdominal aorta superior to the aortic bifurcation.
- Arises from the anterior aorta.
- Courses inferior and to the left of midline.
- Supplies the left transverse colon, descending colon, upper rectum, and sigmoid.
- Source of collateral flow to the lower extremities.
- Located:
  - Slightly to the left of midline and approximately 1 cm superior to the aortic bifurcation.
- Low-resistance blood flow, with continuous flow through diastole.

Main Parietal Branches of the Abdominal Aorta

Inferior Phrenic Artery

- Arises from the anterior aspect of the abdominal aorta branching into the right and left inferior phrenic arteries just below the diaphragm near the level of the 12th thoracic vertebrae.
- Supplies the inferior portion of the diaphragm.
- Gives rise to the superior suprarenal artery.

Lumbar Arteries

- Four arteries arise on each side of the abdominal aorta.
- Supplies the abdominal wall and spinal cord.
- Located inferior to the gonadal arteries and superior to the inferior mesenteric artery.

Median Sacral Artery

- Located inferior to the inferior mesenteric artery and superior to the aortic bifurcation.
- Source of collateral flow to the lower extremities.

Additional Abdominal Arteries

Gastroduodenal Artery (GDA)

- Branch of the common hepatic artery.
- Lies between the superior portion of the duodenum and the anterior surface of the pancreatic head.
- Visualized on ultrasound in the anterolateral portion of the head of the pancreas.
- Located:
  - Anterior to the inferior vena cava, common bile duct, and the head/neck of the pancreas.
  - Inferior to the proper hepatic artery.

Hepatic Artery

- Common hepatic artery is a branch of the celiac axis.
- Gives rise to the gastroduodenal artery and is now termed the proper hepatic artery.

- Proper hepatic artery gives rise to the right gastric artery.
- Horizontal rightward course toward the porta hepatis.
- The proper hepatic artery bifurcates into the right and left hepatic arteries at the hepatic hilum.
- The right hepatic artery gives rise to the cystic artery to supply the gallbladder.
- Low-resistance blood flow, with continuous flow through diastole.
- Increased flow velocity is associated with jaundice, cirrhosis, lymphoma, and metastases.
- Common hepatic artery located:
  - Anterior to the inferior vena cava, celiac axis.
  - Posterior to the left gastric artery.
  - Superior to the head of the pancreas and superior mesenteric artery.
- Proper hepatic artery located:
  - Anterior to the main portal vein.
  - Posterior to the common duct.
  - Superior to the gastroduodenal artery.

Left Gastric Artery

- Branch of the celiac axis.
- Courses superiorly to the left then toward the right to anastomose with the right gastric artery.
- Supplies the left side of the lesser curvature of the stomach.
- Often originates from the splenic artery.
- Not routinely visualized on ultrasound.
- Located:
  Anterior to the celiac axis, splenic artery and common hepatic artery.

Splenic Artery

- Tortuous branch of the celiac axis.
- Gives rise to the left gastroepiploic artery and additional branches to the pancreas and stomach.
- Courses along the superior margin of the pancreatic body and tail toward the splenic hilum.
- Low-resistance blood flow, with continuous flow through diastole.
- May be mistaken for a dilated pancreatic duct.
- Located:
  - Anterior to the celiac axis, and tail of the pancreas, superior pole of the left kidney.
  - Posterior to the left gastric artery and stomach.
  - Superior to the splenic vein, superior mesenteric artery, and the body of the pancreas.

VENOUS ANATOMY (Fig. 13.2)

Inferior Vena Cava (IVC)

- Formed at the junction of the right and left common iliac veins.
- Carries oxygen-depleted blood from the body superiorly terminating in the right atrium of the heart.
- Major abdominal branches include lumbar veins, right gonadal vein, renal veins, right suprarenal vein, inferior phrenic vein, and hepatic veins.
- Demonstrates respiratory variation.

Main Venous Tributaries

Common Iliac Veins

- Drain blood from the lower extremities and pelvis.
- Formed by the junction of the external and internal iliac veins.

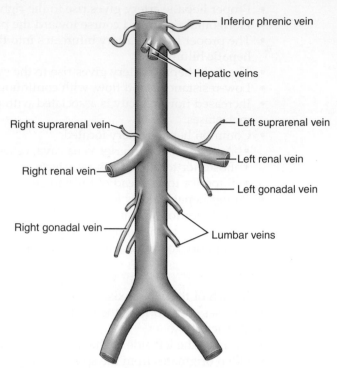

FIG. 13.2 Venous anatomy.

- Located:
  - Anterior to the psoas muscle.
  - Posterior to the common iliac arteries.

Renal Veins

- Course anterior to the renal arteries.
- Left renal vein courses posterior to the superior mesenteric artery and anterior to the abdominal aorta.
- Left renal vein receives the left suprarenal and left gonadal veins.
- Left renal vein may appear dilated because of compression from the mesentery.
- Right renal vein has a short course to drain into the lateral aspect of the IVC.
- Demonstrates spontaneous phasic blood flow.
- Right renal vein is located:
  - Anterior to the right renal artery.
  - Posterior to the head of the pancreas.
  - Inferior to the right adrenal gland.
- Left renal vein is located:
  - Anterior to the left renal artery and aorta.
  - Posterior to the body/tail of the pancreas.
  - Inferior to the left adrenal gland.

Hepatic Veins

- Lie at the boundaries of the hepatic segments (intersegmental) and course toward the IVC.
- Three major branches: left, middle, and right hepatic veins.
- Right hepatic vein courses coronally within the intersegmental fissure between the anterior and posterior segments of the right hepatic lobe.
- Middle hepatic vein follows an oblique course within the main lobar fissure between the left and right hepatic lobes.
- Left hepatic vein courses posterior within the intersegmental fissure between the medial and lateral segments of the left hepatic lobe.

- Doppler demonstrates spontaneous, multiphasic, and pulsatile blood flow toward the IVC (hepatofugal).
- Increase in blood flow with inspiration and diminished flow with Valsalva maneuver.
- Located:
  - Anterior to the inferior vena cava.

Additional Abdominal Veins

Main Portal Vein

- Drains the gastrointestinal tract, pancreas, spleen, and gallbladder.
- Provides approximately 70% to 75% of the liver's blood supply.
- Formed by the junction of the splenic and superior mesenteric veins.
- Bifurcates into the right and left portal veins just beyond the porta hepatis.
- Should not exceed:
  - 1.3 cm in diameter in adults greater than 20 years of age.
  - 1.0 cm in diameter between 10 and 20 years of age.
  - 0.85 cm in diameter less than 10 years of age.
- Demonstrates phasic low-flow velocities toward the liver (hepatopetal).
- Pulsatile waveform may be observed in patients with right heart failure, tricuspid regurgitation, fistula between a hepatic and portal vein, and portal hypertension.
- Blood flow will decrease with inspiration and increase with expiration.
- Diameter will increase after a meal.
- Located:
  - Anterior to the inferior vena cava and uncinate process of the pancreas.
  - Posterior to the common and proper hepatic arteries., common duct, and neck of the pancreas.
  - Superior to the head of the pancreas.
- Additional tributaries include:
  a. Coronary vein—
    - enters at the superior border of the portosplenic confluence.
    - drains the left gastric vein.
    - common anastomotic route between esophageal and gastric veins in some cases of portal hypertension.
  b. Inferior mesenteric vein—
    - usually drains into the splenic vein but may enter at the inferior border of the portosplenic confluence.
    - drains the descending and sigmoid colon and rectum.

Splenic Vein

- Joins the superior mesenteric vein to form the main portal vein.
- Courses posterior to the pancreas and crosses anterior to the superior mesenteric artery.
- Demonstrates spontaneous phasic flow away from the spleen and toward the liver.
- Normal adult diameter is 10 mm or less.
- Increase in caliber with inspiration.
- Drains the spleen, pancreas, and a portion of the stomach.
- Located:
  - Anterior to the left kidney, left renal artery and vein.
  - Posterior to the neck/body of the pancreas.

Superior Mesenteric Vein

- Courses parallel to the superior mesenteric artery.
- Joins the splenic vein to form the main portal vein.
- Demonstrates spontaneous phasic flow toward the liver.
- Normal adult diameter is 10 mm or less.
- Caliber will increase with inspiration and following a meal.
- Drains the small intestines, ascending and transverse colon.

- Located:
  - Anterior to the inferior vena cava and inferior head of the pancreas.
  - Posterior to the neck of the pancreas.

Gonadal Veins

- Right gonadal vein empties directly into the inferior vena cava.
- Left gonadal vein empties into the left renal vein and occasionally into the left suprarenal vein.

Lumbar Veins

- Branches of the common iliac veins.
- Course lateral to the spine and posterior to the psoas muscles.

LOCATION

Abdominal Aorta

- Lies to the left of midline adjacent to the inferior vena cava.
- Courses inferior and anterior in the abdomen to the level of the fourth lumbar vertebra (umbilicus), where it bifurcates into the right and left common iliac arteries.
- Lies anterior to the spine and psoas muscle.
- Lies posterior to the splenic and left renal veins, celiac axis and branches, superior mesenteric artery, stomach, and the body/tail of the pancreas.
- Separated from the spine by 0.5 to 1.0 cm of soft tissue.

Inferior Vena Cava

- Lies to the right of midline parallel to the abdominal aorta.
- Formed at the level of the fifth lumbar vertebra at the junction of the right and left common iliac veins coursing superiorly in the abdomen to the right atrium of the heart.
- Lies anterior to the spine, psoas muscle, crus of the diaphragm, and right adrenal gland.
- Lies posterior to the head of the pancreas, main portal vein, common bile duct, posterior surface of the liver and hepatic veins.

SIZE

Abdominal Aorta

- The size of the normal abdominal aorta should not exceed 3 cm in diameter.
- The aorta tapers as it courses inferiorly and measures approximately:
  - Suprarenal: 2.5 cm.
  - Renal: 2.0 cm.
  - Infrarenal: 1.5 cm.
  - Common iliac: 1.0 cm.

Inferior Vena Cava

- Usually measures less than 2.5 cm in diameter.
- Should not exceed 3.7 cm in diameter.
- Decrease in caliber is demonstrated in expiration and an increase in size is demonstrated with suspended inspiration.

SONOGRAPHIC APPEARANCE

- Anechoic tubular structure.
- Thin hyperechoic wall margins.

- Internal vascular flow.
- Aorta demonstrates a high-resistance laminar waveform with a low diastolic component proximal to the renal arteries (suprarenal) and a triphasic waveform inferior to the origin of the main renal arteries (infrarenal).
- Inferior vena cava demonstrates spontaneous phasic flow and multiphasic pulsatile flow as it nears the diaphragm.

EXAMINATION TECHNIQUES, PROTOCOLS, AND IMAGE OPTIMIZATION

Preparation

- No preparation is required before an ultrasound of the great vessels.
- Fasting is recommended when examining the renal arteries and mesenteric arteries to limit flash artifact from gastrointestinal peristalsis.
- Fasting may also reduce gastrointestinal gas.
  - Adult—6 to 8 hours.
  - Children—6 hours.
  - Infants—4 hours.

Transducer Selection

- Use the highest frequency possible to obtain optimal resolution for penetration depth.
  - Adults—3.0 to 5.0 MHz.
  - Children and small adults—5.0 to 7.0 MHz.
  - Obese patients—2.0 MHz may be required.
- Curvilinear transducers provide a wider field of view.
- Sector or vector transducers have a smaller footprint great for intercostal imaging.
- Higher frequency transducers can be used in thinner patients.

Patient Positioning

- Examination usually begins with the patient in a supine position.
- Lateral decubitus, posterior oblique, semierect, and erect positions may be helpful to alleviate overlying bowel gas.

Examination Protocol

Aorta

- Systematic approach in the sagittal and transverse planes carefully evaluating and imaging the entire length of the abdominal aorta including proximal common iliac arteries.
- Measure the maximum outer edge to outer edge anterior posterior diameter of the proximal, mid, and distal portions of the abdominal aorta and proximal iliac arteries in the sagittal plane.
- Measure the maximum outer edge to outer edge transverse diameter of the proximal, mid, and distal portions of the abdominal aorta including proximal common iliac arteries.
- Spectral analysis of a minimum of two areas along the abdominal aorta to demonstrate normal arterial flow.
  - High-resistance waveform with a low diastolic component proximal to the renal arteries.
  - High-resistance triphasic waveform distal to renal arteries.
- Color Doppler may be used to assess patency and aortic thrombus/plaque formation.
- Aneurysms should be documented and measured from outer edge to outer edge in the anterior posterior and transverse planes.
- Document level of aneurysm in reference to the renal arteries (e.g., infrarenal).
- If intraluminal thrombus is present, measurement of the vessel lumen should be included.

Inferior Vena Cava

- Systematic approach in the sagittal and transverse planes carefully evaluating and imaging the cephalic segment.
- Duplex imaging of proximal segment demonstrating normal phasic pulsatile flow.
- Abnormalities should be documented and when applicable measured in two imaging planes. Color and/or spectral Doppler evaluation of the abnormality should be included.

Image Optimization

- Place gains settings to display normal liver parenchyma as a medium shade of gray with adjustments to reduce artifactually produced echoes within the lumen of the abdominal aorta and inferior vena cava.
- Focal zone(s) should be placed at or below the area of interest. The use of multiple focal zones increases detail resolution and decreases temporal resolution.
- Sufficient imaging depth to visualize structures immediately posterior to the area of interest.
- Harmonic imaging or decreasing system compression (dynamic range) can be used to reduce artifactual intraluminal echoes.
- Spatial compounding can be used to improve visualization of structures posterior to highly attenuating structures.
- Doppler settings should be adjusted for the different flow states of the great vessels and branches/tributaries.
- Doppler angle should be 60 degrees or less with a sample volume smaller than the vessel.

Examination Limitations

- Obesity.
- Gastrointestinal gas.

Helpful Hints

- When measuring the transverse diameter, make sure you are 90 degrees to the sagittal course of the abdominal aorta.
- Sagittal plane perpendicular to the long axis of the aorta is most accurate for anterior posterior diameter measurement.
- The use of deep inspiration may improve visualization of the proximal aorta and inferior vena cava.
- The use of multiple patient positions may redistribute overlying bowel gas.
- Origin of the common hepatic, main renal and splenic arteries is best visualized in the transverse plane.
- Left lateral decubitus position using a coronal plane can demonstrate the origin of both renal arteries (banana peel). With the right renal artery coursing up toward the transducer and the left renal artery coursing away from the transducer.
- The IMA is best visualized in a sagittal oblique plane, to the left of midline, approximately 1 cm superior to the aortic bifurcation.
- Hepatic veins are best visualized in the transverse plane.
- The junction of the right and left portal veins is best visualized in the transverse plane just inferior to the junction of the hepatic veins and IVC.

Indications for Examination

- Pulsatile abdominal mass.
- Abdominal bruit.
- Family history of abdominal aortic aneurysm.
- Hypertension.
- Abdominal or lower back pain.

- History of arteriosclerosis.
- Severe postprandial pain.
- Pulmonary embolism.
- Liver disease.
- Evaluate mass from previous medical imaging study (e.g., CT).

Aneurysms of the Abdominal Aorta

- Weakening of the arterial wall.
- All layers of the artery are stretched but intact.
- Rare in patients under 50 years of age.
- Male prevalence (5:1)
- Growth rate of 2 mm/yr. is average and considered normal up to 5 mm/yr.
- Abdominal aortic aneurysm measures 3.0 cm or greater in diameter.
- Common iliac aneurysm measures greater than 1.5 cm in diameter.
  - Coexisting AAA in 90% of cases.
- Popliteal aneurysm measures greater than 1.0 cm in diameter.
  - Coexisting AAA in 25% of cases.

ANEURYSM	ETIOLOGY	CLINICAL FINDINGS	SONOGRAPHIC FINDINGS	DIFFERENTIAL CONSIDERATIONS
Abdominal aortic aneurysm Aka: 　True abdominal aortic aneurysm	Arteriosclerosis most common Infection Hypertension Family history	Asymptomatic Pulsatile abdominal mass Back and/or leg pain Abdominal pain Abdominal bruit	Typically, fusiform-shaped dilatation of the aorta Saccular dilatation of the aorta may be demonstrated Diameter of 3 cm or greater Vessel becomes tortuous Wall calcifications Intramural thrombus Risk of rupture within 5 years.: 　5 cm = 5% 　6 cm = 16% 　7 cm = 75%	Lymphadenopathy Retroperitoneal tumor Dissection
Ectatic aneurysm	Weakening of the arterial wall	Asymptomatic	Dilatation of the aorta compared with a more proximal segment Dilatation measures less than 3 cm in diameter	Tortuous artery Technical error
Mycotic aneurysm	Bacterial infection	Asymptomatic Abdominal pain Pulsatile abdominal mass	Typically, saccular-shaped dilatation of the aorta Asymmetrical wall thickening	Lymphadenopathy Retroperitoneal tumor Intramural thrombus
Pseudoaneurysm	Trauma to the arterial wall permits the escape of blood into the surrounding tissues Most common complication of an aortic graft	Pulsatile mass Focal pain Bruising	Fluid collection communicating with an artery Doppler will demonstrate turbulent swirling blood flow within the fluid collection To and fro blood flow pattern is demonstrated in the neck of the aneurysm	Hematoma Lymphadenopathy Aneurysm Arteriovenous fistula

Continued

ANEURYSM	ETIOLOGY	CLINICAL FINDINGS	SONOGRAPHIC FINDINGS	DIFFERENTIAL CONSIDERATIONS
Ruptured aneurysm	Tear in all three layers of the aortic wall with leakage of blood	Severe abdominal pain Severe groin pain Hypotension Loss of consciousness Hypovolemic shock	Normal aortic size Aneurysm may still be visualized Asymmetrical or unilateral paraaortic hypoechoic mass "Veil appearance" over the aorta and surrounding structures Free fluid in the peritoneal cavities	Lymphadenopathy Chronic intraluminal thrombus
Surgical repair	Previous history of aneurysm	Asymptomatic Abdominal or lower back pain	Anechoic space between the graft and repaired aorta Hyperechoic parallel echoes along the arterial walls	Dissection Rupture aneurysm Chronic intraluminal clot Retroperitoneal pathology

Abdominal Aorta Pathology

PATHOLOGY	ETIOLOGY	CLINICAL FINDINGS	SONOGRAPHIC FINDINGS	DIFFERENTIAL CONSIDERATIONS
Abdominal aortic dissection **Risk Factors** AAA 40–70 years of age Hypertension Smoking Pregnancy Drug abuse	Extension of thoracic dissection Iatrogenic Marfan and Ehlers syndromes Trauma Atherosclerosis Uncontrolled hypertension Fibromuscular dysplasia	Sharp chest or abdominal pain Audible bruit Headache Shock	Thin hyperechoic membrane within the aorta Membrane flaps with arterial pulsations Doppler demonstrates opposite flow directions between the membrane during diastole	Chronic intraluminal thrombus Postsurgical repair Artifact
Arteriomegaly/ Aortic ectasia	Degenerative changes to the media layer of the arterial wall Typically, found in the elderly	Asymptomatic	Diffuse enlargement of the abdominal aorta without distal tapering	Technical error Aneurysm
Mesenteric ischemia	Embolus Thrombus Atherosclerosis Prolonged vessel constriction	Acute abdominal pain Postprandial pain Weight loss	Diagnosis is made when a minimum of two mesenteric vessels demonstrate stenosis CA peak systolic velocity greater than 200 cm/s SMA peak systolic velocity greater than 280 cm/s SMA high resistive index without an increase in diastolic flow postprandial IMA evaluate for turbulence or vessel narrowing	Tortuous artery Technical error

Abdominal Venous Pathology

VENOUS PATHOLOGY	ETIOLOGY	CLINICAL FINDINGS	SONOGRAPHIC FINDINGS	DIFFERENTIAL CONSIDERATIONS
Arteriovenous shunts (AV fistula)	Trauma Congenital Surgery Inflammation Neoplasm	Presence of a bruit or "thrill" Lower back or abdominal pain Edema Hypertension	Doppler demonstrates: Pulsatile flow within the vein Increase in arterial flow proximal to site of shunting Decrease in arterial flow distal to site of shunting Turbulent waveform with high velocities in both the artery and the vein	Tortuous vessel Stenotic vessel
Enlargement	Congestive heart failure Thrombosis Infiltrating neoplasm	Asymptomatic Edema	Inferior vena cava exceeding 3.7 cm in diameter Main portal vein exceeding 1.3 cm in diameter Splenic or superior mesenteric vein exceeding 1.0 cm Intraluminal medium-level to low-level echoes seen with neoplasms or thrombus	Extrinsic compression Arteriovenous shunting Portal hypertension Technical error
Infiltrating neoplasm of the IVC	Renal carcinoma (most common) Metastases from lymphoma, hepatocellular, and breast carcinoma	Asymptomatic Edema	Intraluminal medium-level to low-level echoes Vascular flow within intraluminal mass	Venous thrombosis Primary caval tumor Technical error
Primary caval neoplasm of the IVC	Leiomyosarcoma is most common	Asymptomatic Edema	Intraluminal medium-level to low-level echoes Vascular flow within intraluminal mass	Infiltrating tumor Venous thrombosis Technical error
Thrombosis of the IVC	Extension of thrombus from femoral (most common), iliac, renal, hepatic, or gonadal veins	Asymptomatic Edema/ swelling of the lower extremities Pulmonary embolism (PE) History of lower extremity DVT	Vessel enlargement Intraluminal medium-level to low-level echoes May result in complete or partial occlusion Spectral analysis may demonstrate continuous nonphasic flow	Infiltrating tumor Primary caval tumor Technical error

ABDOMINAL VASCULATURE REVIEW

1. A true aortic aneurysm is defined as a dilatation of the abdominal aorta:
   a. compared with a more proximal segment
   b. measuring 3.0 cm or greater
   c. compared with a previous imaging study
   d. measuring 2.5 cm or greater

2. A fusiform aneurysm is best described as:
   a. a focal outpouching of one arterial wall
   b. a uniform dilatation of the arterial walls
   c. asymmetrical thrombus formation
   d. an increase in size compared with a more proximal segment

3. The first visceral branch of the abdominal aorta is the:
   a. gastric artery
   b. celiac axis
   c. inferior phrenic artery
   d. middle suprarenal artery

4. The left renal vein receives tributaries from which of the following veins?
   a. inferior mesenteric and coronary veins
   b. left suprarenal and inferior mesenteric veins
   c. coronary and left suprarenal veins
   d. left suprarenal and left gonadal veins

5. The main portal vein bifurcates at the hepatic hilum into the:
   a. anterior and posterior portal veins
   b. medial and lateral portal veins
   c. left and right portal veins
   d. superior and inferior portal veins

6. Which of the following statements most accurately describes the left renal vein?
   a. The left renal vein demonstrates a pulsatile flow pattern.
   b. The left renal artery is located anterior to the left renal vein.
   c. The superior mesenteric artery courses posterior to the left renal vein.
   d. The left renal vein may appear dilated because of compression from the mesentery.

7. Which of the following structures is located anterior to the inferior vena cava?
   a. psoas muscle
   b. right adrenal gland
   c. diaphragmatic crura
   d. head of the pancreas

8. The abdominal aorta usually bifurcates into the right and left common iliac arteries at the level of the:
   a. 12th thoracic vertebra
   b. 2nd lumbar vertebra
   c. 4th lumbar vertebra
   d. 5th lumbar vertebra

9. The celiac axis branches into which of the following arteries?
   a. proper hepatic, left gastric, and splenic arteries
   b. common hepatic, right gastric, and splenic arteries
   c. proper hepatic, gastroduodenal, and splenic arteries
   d. common hepatic, left gastric, and splenic arteries

10. The presence of a palpable "thrill" within an artery is suspicious for a(n):
    a. aneurysm
    b. occlusion
    c. stenosis
    d. arteriovenous fistula

11. The contour of a mycotic aneurysm is most commonly described as:
    a. berry-shaped
    b. saccular-shaped
    c. fusiform-shaped
    d. teardrop-shaped

12. The gonadal arteries arise from the:
    a. renal arteries
    b. abdominal aorta
    c. lumbar arteries
    d. internal iliac arteries

13. Which of the following arteries gives rise to the gastroepiploic artery?
    a. gastric artery
    b. splenic artery
    c. gastroduodenal artery
    d. superior mesenteric artery

14. Which of the following veins courses in an oblique plane between the right and left lobes of the liver?
    a. right hepatic vein
    b. right portal vein
    c. main portal vein
    d. middle hepatic vein

15. The normal diameter of the main portal vein in a middle age patient should not exceed:
    a. 0.8 cm
    b. 1.0 cm
    c. 1.3 cm
    d. 1.8 cm

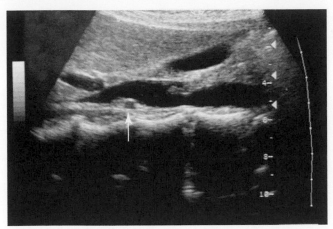

FIG. 13.3 Sagittal sonogram of the right upper quadrant.

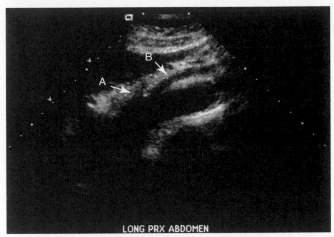

LONG PRX ABDOMEN

FIG. 13.4 Sonogram of the abdominal aorta.

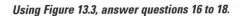

Using Figure 13.3, answer questions 16 to 18.

16. A patient presents with a history of pulmonary embolism. On the basis of the clinical history, the mass is most suspicious for a(n):
    a. neoplasm
    b. thrombus
    c. incompetent valve
    d. ulcerative plaque

17. The arrow is demonstrating which of the following vascular structures?
    a. hepatic artery
    b. portal vein
    c. hepatic vein
    d. right renal artery

18. The anechoic structure lying anterior to the inferior vena cava and posterior to the liver most likely represents the:
    a. main portal vein
    b. gallbladder
    c. right hepatic vein
    d. superior mesenteric vein

Using Figure 13.4, answer questions 19 and 20.

19. Which of the following visceral branches of the abdominal aorta is identified by arrow *A*?
    a. renal artery
    b. celiac axis
    c. inferior phrenic artery
    d. superior mesenteric artery

20. Which of the following branches of the abdominal aorta is identified by arrow *B*?
    a. celiac axis
    b. renal artery
    c. superior mesenteric artery
    d. inferior suprarenal artery

21. Which of the following conditions most commonly coexists with a popliteal aneurysm?
    a. carotid stenosis
    b. venous insufficiency
    c. abdominal aortic aneurysm
    d. dissection of the thoracic aorta

22. Development of an abdominal aortic aneurysm is most commonly caused by:
    a. trauma
    b. infection
    c. arteriosclerosis
    d. fibrointimal hyperplasia

23. Which of the following aneurysms is associated with a recent history of bacterial infection?
    a. ectatic
    b. dissecting
    c. mycotic
    d. ruptured

24. The inferior vena cava is considered enlarged after the diameter exceeds:
    a. 2.0 cm
    b. 2.5 cm
    c. 3.0 cm
    d. 3.7 cm

25. Development of an arteriovenous fistula may be caused by:
    a. neoplasm
    b. hypertension
    c. venous thrombosis
    d. congestive heart failure

26. An infiltrating neoplasm within the inferior vena cava most commonly originates from which of the following structures?
    a. liver
    b. spleen
    c. kidney
    d. adrenal gland

27. Direct extension of thrombus into the inferior vena cava is most likely caused by thrombus originating in the:
    a. renal vein
    b. femoral vein
    c. hepatic vein
    d. right gonadal vein

28. Berry-shaped aneurysms primarily affect which of the following arteries?
    a. splenic
    b. cerebral
    c. extracranial
    d. abdominal aorta

29. Diagnosis of mesenteric ischemia is made when:
    a. one of the mesenteric vessels demonstrates stenosis
    b. the superior mesenteric artery demonstrates stenosis
    c. a minimum of two mesenteric vessels demonstrate stenosis
    d. all three mesenteric vessels demonstrate stenosis

30. Hypovolemic shock is a clinical finding in patients with a history of:
    a. Marfan syndrome
    b. a ruptured aortic aneurysm
    c. a mycotic aortic aneurysm
    d. an arteriovenous shunt

Using Figure 13.5, answer question 31.

31. A 65-year-old local farmer presents with a history of leukocytosis and an enlarging, pulsatile abdominal mass. The anterior, posterior, and lateral borders of the distal aorta are outlined by the calibers. On the basis of the clinical history, the sonogram is most likely demonstrating which of the following pathologies?
    a. lymphadenopathy
    b. arterial dissection
    c. retroperitoneal fibrosis
    d. mycotic abdominal aortic aneurysm

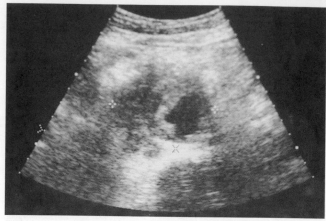

FIG. 13.5 Transverse sonogram of the distal abdominal aorta.

Using Figure 13.6, answer questions 32 and 33.

32. Which of the following vascular structures is identified by arrow *A*?
    a. splenic artery
    b. splenic vein
    c. left renal vein
    d. superior mesenteric vein

33. Which of the following vascular structures is identified by arrow *B*?
    a. celiac axis
    b. splenic artery
    c. gastroduodenal artery
    d. superior mesenteric artery

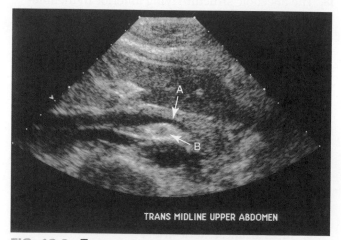

FIG. 13.6 Transverse sonogram of the upper abdomen.

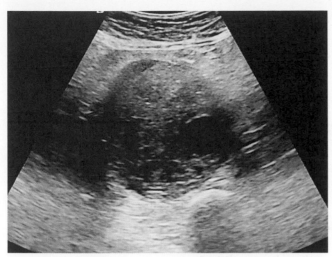

FIG. 13.7 Transverse sonogram of the abdominal aorta.

Using Figure 13.7, answer question 34.

34. The findings in this sonogram are most suspicious for which of the following conditions?
a. pseudoaneurysm
b. dissecting aneurysm
c. ruptured aneurysm
d. aneurysm with chronic thrombus

Using Figure 13.8, answer questions 35 and 36.

35. Arrow *A* is most likely identifying which of the following vascular structures?
a. hepatic vein
b. main portal vein
c. inferior vena cava
d. right renal vein

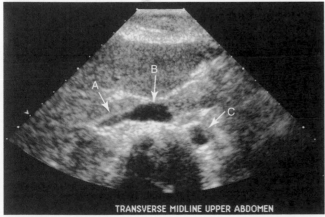

TRANSVERSE MIDLINE UPPER ABDOMEN

FIG. 13.8 Transverse sonogram of the upper abdomen.

36. The anechoic area identified by arrow *B* is most consistent with which of the following vascular structures?
a. splenic vein
b. inferior vena cava
c. abdominal aorta
d. main portal vein

37. Dilatation of an artery caused by damage to one or more layers of the arterial wall describes a(n):
a. berry aneurysm
b. dissecting aneurysm
c. pseudoaneurysm
d. abdominal aortic aneurysm

38. Diffuse enlargement of the abdominal aorta without distal tapering best describes:
a. ectatic aneurysm
b. pseudoaneurysm
c. aortic ectasia
d. true abdominal aortic aneurysm

39. Which of the following vascular structures courses posterior to the inferior vena cava?
a. splenic artery
b. right renal artery
c. left renal vein
d. inferior mesenteric artery

40. Which of the following vessels lies between the duodenum and the anterior portion of the pancreatic head?
a. gastric artery
b. celiac axis
c. common hepatic artery
d. gastroduodenal artery

41. Which of the following statements about the main renal arteries is true?
a. Duplication of the main renal arteries is rare.
b. The left renal artery courses anterior to the splenic vein.
c. The right renal artery courses posterior to the crus of the diaphragm.
d. The left renal artery courses posterior to the tail of the pancreas.

42. Which of the following arteries supplies the left transverse colon, the descending colon, and the sigmoid?
a. gonadal artery
b. superior mesenteric artery
c. external iliac artery
d. inferior mesenteric artery

43. Patients with Marfan syndrome have a predisposing risk factor for developing a(n):
    a. pseudoaneurysm
    b. pulmonary embolism
    c. abdominal aortic aneurysm
    d. stenosis in the common carotid artery

44. The risk of rupture of an abdominal aortic aneurysm measuring 6.0 cm in diameter is approximately:
    a. 5% within 1 year
    b. 15% within 5 years
    c. 50% within 2 years
    d. 75% within 5 years

45. The amount of blood supplied to the liver from the portal venous system is approximately:
    a. 10%
    b. 30%
    c. 50%
    d. 70%

46. Which of the following vessels course anterior to the abdominal aorta and posterior to the superior mesenteric artery?
    a. portal vein
    b. splenic vein
    c. left renal vein
    d. superior mesenteric vein

47. The inferior mesenteric vein usually drains into the:
    a. splenic vein
    b. main portal vein
    c. superior mesenteric vein
    d. inferior vena cava

48. Which of the following vascular structures is most commonly mistaken as a dilated pancreatic duct?
    a. splenic vein
    b. celiac axis
    c. splenic artery
    d. superior mesenteric vein

49. A dilatation of an artery compared with a more proximal segment describes which of the following abnormalities?
    a. pseudoaneurysm
    b. arteriovenous fistula
    c. ectatic aneurysm
    d. saccular aneurysm

50. Which of the following controls will decrease artifactual echoes only within the abdominal aorta?
    a. Overall gain
    b. Dynamic range
    c. Postprocessing
    d. Time-gain compensation

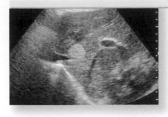

CHAPTER 14

Gastrointestinal Tract

KEY TERMS

cardiac orifice   opening at the upper end of the stomach.

chyme   semiliquid mass composed of food and gastric juices.

Crohn's disease   periods of intestinal inflammation; occurs most frequently in the ileum.

diverticulum   saccular outpouching of the mucous membrane through a tear in the muscular layer of the gastrointestinal tract.

fecalith   a hard-compacted mass of feces in the colon.

gastritis   inflammation of the stomach.

gastroparesis   failure of the stomach to empty; caused by a decrease in gastric motility.

graded compression technique   Gradual increase in pressure on the anterior abdominal wall to displace normal overlying bowel gas. Commonly used when evaluating the appendix.

greater curvature of the stomach   longer, convex, left border of the stomach.

haustra   a recess or sacculation demonstrated in the walls of the colon.

ileus   obstruction of the small intestines.

intussusception   prolapse of one segment of bowel into the lumen of an adjacent segment of bowel.

lesser curvature of the stomach   shorter, concave, right border of the stomach.

ligament of Treitz   muscle fibers within peritoneal folds at the duodenal/jejunum junction.

malrotation   a congenital abnormality of the bowel where the intestine or bowel does not fold or properly rotate in early fetal development. The malrotated intestines are not properly attached to the abdominal wall, which can result in the intestines twisting around one another.

Meckel diverticulum   an anomalous sac protruding from the ileum; caused by an incomplete closure of the yolk stalk.

McBurney sign   extreme pain or tenderness over McBurney point (midway between the umbilicus and the right iliac crest); associated with appendicitis.

mucocele   distention of the appendix or colon with mucus.

peristalsis   rhythmic serial contractions of the smooth muscle of the intestines that forces food through the digestive tract.

pyloric orifice   opening at the lower end of the stomach.

pylorospasm   spasm of the pyloric sphincter; associated with pyloric stenosis.

rugae   ridges or folds in the stomach lining.

target sign   a circular structure demonstrating alternate hyperechoic and hypoechoic wall layers. A target sign may or may not signify pathology in the gastrointestinal tract.

volvulus   abnormal twisting of a portion of the intestines or bowel, which can impair blood flow.

GASTROINTESTINAL (GI) TRACT (Fig. 14.1)

- Extends from the mouth to the anus.
- Divisions include the mouth, pharynx, esophagus, stomach, small intestines, and colon.
- Also called digestive tract, alimentary tract or canal, and intestinal tract.
- Lined with a mucous membrane.
- Largest endocrine organ in the body.

PHYSIOLOGY

Functions of the GI Tract

- Ingest food.
- Digest food.
- Secrete mucus and digestive enzymes.
- Absorb and break down food.

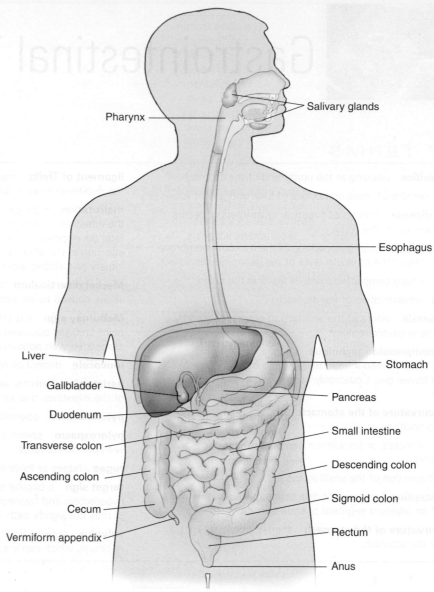

FIG. 14.1   GI anatomy.

- Reabsorb fluid in the intestinal walls to prevent dehydration.
- Form solid feces.
- Release fecal waste.

ANATOMY

Esophagus

- Muscular tube extending from the pharynx to the stomach.
- Courses down the chest through the esophageal hiatus of the diaphragm, terminating at the cardiac orifice of the stomach.
- Wall layers from the outer layer to the lumen include:
  - External or fibrous.
  - Muscularis.
  - Submucosal.
  - Mucosal.

Stomach

- Principal organ of digestion located between the esophagus and small intestines.
- Secretes hydrochloric acid and pepsin.
- Divided into the fundus, body, and pylorus.
- Pylorus divided into the antrum and pyloric canal.
- Wall layers from the outer layer to the lumen include:
  - Serosal.
  - Muscularis propria.
  - Submucosal.
  - Muscular.
  - Mucosal or rugae.

Small Intestines

- Elaborate tube extending from the pyloric opening to the ileocecal valve.
- Secretes mucus and receives digestive enzymes.
- Divided into the duodenum, jejunum, and ileum.
- Majority of food absorption occurs in the small intestines.
- Wall layers from outer layer to lumen include:
  - Serous.
  - Muscular.
  - Submucosal.
  - Mucosal.

Duodenum

- Divided into the superior, descending, transverse, and ascending portions.
- Secretes large quantities of mucus, protecting the small intestines from the strongly acidic chyme.
- Enzymes from the duct of Wirsung and bile from the common bile duct empty into the descending portion.

Jejunum

- Begins at the ligament of Treitz.
- Extends from the duodenum to the ileum.

Ileum

- Extends from the jejunum to the junction with the cecum (ileocecal junction).

Colon

- Extends from the terminal ileum to the anus.
- Secretes large quantities of mucus.
- Divisions include the cecum, appendix, ascending colon, transverse colon, descending colon, sigmoid, rectum, and anus.
- Bacteria in the colon produce vitamin K and some B-complex vitamins.
- Wall layers from the outer layer to the lumen include:
  - Serous.
  - Muscular or haustra.
  - Submucosal.
  - Mucosal.

Cecum

- Blind pouch of the colon located in the right lower quadrant directly posterior to the abdominal wall and lateral to the ileum.
- Largest diameter.

Appendix

- Narrow, blind-end, tubular structure communicating with the cecum.
- Nonperistaltic structure generally located in the right lower quadrant.
- Contains lymphoid tissue.

Ascending Colon

- Extends superiorly from the cecum.
- Curves to the left, forming the hepatic flexure.
- Lodged in a shallow depression on the undersurface of the right lobe of the liver and to the right of the gallbladder.

Transverse Colon

- Courses transversely from the right to the left side of the upper abdomen.
- Curves inferiorly, forming the splenic flexure.

Descending Colon

- Begins inferior to the spleen and terminates at the sigmoid.
- Passes inferiorly along the left flank to the iliac crest.

Sigmoid

- Narrowest portion of the colon, terminating at the rectum.
- Mobile structure in contact with the psoas muscle.

Rectum

- Terminal portion of the colon located between the sigmoid and anus.
- Capable of considerable distention.
- Terminates at the anal sphincter.

Anal Canal

- Lower portion of the rectum.
- Extends upward and forward, then turns backward following the sacral canal.

LOCATION

Esophagus

- Located to the left of midline, posterior to the left lobe of the liver and anterior to the abdominal aorta.
- Gastroesophageal junction is located anterior to the aorta; posterior to the left lobe of the liver; superior to the celiac axis; inferior to diaphragm.
- Right margin is contiguous with the lesser curvature of the stomach.
- Left margin is contiguous with the greater curvature of the stomach.

Stomach

- Located in the left upper quadrant extending transversely and slightly to the right of midline.
- Located inferior to the diaphragm; anteromedial to the spleen, left adrenal gland, and left kidney; anterior to the pancreas; superior to the splenic flexure.
- Pylorus lies in a transverse plane slightly to the right of midline.

Small Intestines

- Located in the central and lower portion of the abdominal cavity.
- Surrounded superiorly and laterally by the colon.

Duodenum

- **Superior portion (1st)** of the duodenum is located anterior to the gastroduodenal artery, head of the pancreas, common bile duct, common hepatic artery and portal vein; posterior to the gallbladder and liver.
- **Descending portion (2nd)** of the duodenum is located anterior to the right kidney and ureter; posterior to the transverse colon and common bile duct; superior to the gallbladder neck.
- **Transverse portion (3rd)** of the duodenum is located anterior to the great vessels; posterior to the superior mesenteric artery and vein.
- **Ascending portion (4th)** of the duodenum is located anterior to the left psoas muscle and inferior to the first lumbar vertebrae.

Jejunum

- Located in the umbilical and left iliac regions.
- Located anterior to the left psoas muscle and left kidney.

Ileum

- Located in the umbilical and right iliac regions.
- Located anterior to the right psoas muscle, right iliac vessels, right kidney and ureter.

Colon

- Forms an upside-down U shape extending from the right lower quadrant to the left lower quadrant.
- **Cecum**—located anterior to the right psoas muscle and inferior to the ascending colon.
- **Appendix**—variable location; typically located anterior to the right iliac vessels and posterior to the ileocecal valve.
- **Ascending colon**—located anterior to the right kidney and lateral to the right quadratus lumborum muscle; inferior to the right lobe of the liver.
- **Transverse colon**—located anterior to the descending duodenum and pancreas; inferior to the right lobe of the liver.
- **Descending colon**—located anterior to the left iliac crest and inferior to the spleen.
- **Sigmoid**—located anterior to the sacrum, external iliac vessels and left ureter; posterior to the bladder; superior to the rectum.
- **Rectum**—located adjacent to the posterior border of the urinary bladder in males and posterior to the vagina and uterus in females.

SIZE

- Stomach wall should not exceed 5 mm in thickness when distended.
- Normal bowel wall should not exceed 4 mm in thickness.
- Normal appendix should not exceed 2 mm in wall thickness or 6 mm in anterior posterior diameter.
- Small intestines decrease in size from the pylorus to the ileocecal valve.
- Colon is largest at the cecum and gradually decreases in size toward the rectum.

SONOGRAPHIC APPEARANCE

- Walls of the gastrointestinal tract demonstrate alternating hyperechoic and hypoechoic circular echo patterns (mucosal layer appears hyperechoic).
- From outer wall layer to lumen:
  - **Serosal layer**—hyperechoic.
  - **Muscular propia layer**—hypoechoic.
  - **Submucosa layer**—hyperechoic.
  - **Intramural layer**—hypoechoic.
  - **Mucosal layer**—hyperechoic.

- Gastroesophageal junction appears as a target structure lying posterior to the liver and slightly to the left of midline.
- Stomach appears as a target structure when empty and an anechoic structure with swirling hyperechoic echoes when distended with fluid.
- Small intestines are usually gas-filled.
- Jejunum and ileum demonstrate small folds in the wall, termed the *keyboard sign.*
- The colon is identified by haustral wall markings (3–5 cm apart).
- Descending colon is seen as a tubular structure with echogenic wall margins.
- Peristalsis should be observed in the stomach and small and large intestines.
- Rectum is best evaluated with an endorectal transducer.
- Vascularity is imperceptible in the normal bowel wall.

EXAMINATION TECHNIQUES, PROTOCOLS, AND IMAGE OPTIMIZATION

Preparation

- Fasting may improve visualization of the gastrointestinal tract.
- Two-hour fasting is recommended for pyloric examinations.
- Ingestion of 16 to 32 oz. of water allows imaging of the stomach wall.
- In cases of emergency, a gastrointestinal tract ultrasound can still be performed successfully without fasting.

Transducer Selection

- Use the highest frequency possible to obtain optimal resolution for penetration depth.
  - Adults—5.0 to 9 MHz linear.
  - Children and small adults—7.5 to 15 MHz.
  - Obese patients or deeper structures may require a lower frequency.
- Linear transducer preferred.
- Curvilinear transducer may be used.
- Sector or vector transducers have a smaller footprint great for imaging the pylorus.

Patient Positioning

Stomach

- Semi-Fowler—places fluid in the body of the stomach.
- Right posterior oblique—places fluid in the pylorus of the stomach.
- Right lateral decubitus—places fluid in the duodenum.
- Supine—places the fluid in the fundus of the stomach.

Bowel

- Supine, posterior obliques, and lateral decubitus.

Examination Protocol

- Systematic approach in the sagittal, coronal, and transverse planes carefully examining and imaging the focused area of interest using the national or institution protocol.
- Evaluate for normal bowel peristalsis.
- Abnormalities of the gastrointestinal tract should be documented and when applicable measured in two imaging planes. Color and/or spectral Doppler evaluation of the abnormality should be included.
- **Pyloric canal:**
  - Measure the thickness of the pyloric muscle in the transverse and sagittal planes. This is the most important measurement when evaluating for pyloric stenosis.
  - Measure length of pyloric canal.
  - Demonstrate stomach contents passing through the pyloric canal into the superior portion of duodenum.

- **Appendix:**
  - Starting from the hepatic flexure or terminal ileum, using graded compression slowly move inferior following the cecum to the area of the appendix.
  - Measure anterior posterior diameter and if needed wall thickness of the appendix.
  - Increase transducer pressure over the appendix to determine compressibility. The abnormal appendix is usually noncompressible.
  - Color and/or spectral Doppler evaluation of the abnormality should be included.
  - Following compression, quickly release transducer pressure to determine whether the patient demonstrates a positive or negative McBurney sign.
- **Intussusception:**
  - Systematic survey and imaging of the entire abdomen, beginning in the right lower quadrant in the transverse plane.
  - Sagittal images should also be included.
  - Color and/or spectral Doppler evaluation of the abnormality should be included.

Image Optimization

- Place gains settings to display the to the normal liver parenchyma a medium shade of gray with adjustments to reduce artifactually produced echoes within normally anechoic structures.
- Focal zone(s) should be placed at or below the area of interest. The use of multiple focal zones increases detail resolution and decreases temporal resolution.
- Sufficient imaging depth to visualize structures immediately posterior to the area of interest.
- Harmonic imaging and decreasing system compression (dynamic range) can be used to reduce artifactual echoes in obese and gassy patients.
- Spatial compounding can be used to improve visualization of structures posterior to highly attenuating bowel gas.
- Doppler settings should be adjusted to minimize flash artifact.
- The use of multiple patient positions may redistribute overlying bowel gas.

Examination Limitations

- Gastrointestinal gas.
- Obesity.
- Patient cooperation (e.g., pain).

Helpful Hints

- The appendix is generally found midway between the right side of the umbilicus and the right anterior superior iliac spine.
- Remember to use a graded compression technique when evaluating the appendix.
- The normal appendix is not visualized in many cases.
- Having the infant drink water is the best when imaging the pylorus. Infants prefer glucose water.

Indications for Examination

- Abdominal or right lower quadrant pain.
- Leukocytosis.
- Vomiting.
- Weight loss.
- Fever.
- Abdominal mass.
- Diarrhea.
- Absence of bowel sounds.

GASTROINTESTINAL HORMONES

Cholecystokinin

- Hormone produced in the walls of the small intestines in response to high level proteins and fat in the chyme.

Gastrin

- Hormone released by the stomach that stimulates secretion of gastric acids.

Pepsin

- Protein-digesting enzyme produced by the stomach.

Secretin

- Hormone produced in the small intestines that stimulates secretion of bicarbonate to decrease the acid content of the intestines.

Pathology of the Stomach

PATHOLOGY	ETIOLOGY	CLINICAL FINDINGS	SONOGRAPHIC FINDINGS	DIFFERENTIAL CONSIDERATIONS
Carcinoma	Adenocarcinoma in 80% of cases Male prevalence	Upper abdominal discomfort Nausea/vomiting Decrease in appetite Fatigue Weight loss Abdominal mass	Target tumor of the stomach Hypervascular mass Gastric wall thickening Left upper quadrant mass	Polyp Ulcer Lymphoma Metastases
Gastric dilatation	Gastric obstruction Gastroparesis Duodenal ulcer Inflammation Pylorospasm Neurological disease Neoplasm Medication	Abdominal pain Nausea/vomiting Bloating	Distended stomach Swirling hyperechoic internal echoes Decrease or lack of forward peristalsis of stomach contents Thin gastric wall margins	Omental cyst Renal cyst Liver cyst Pancreatic pseudocyst
Gastric ulcer	Bacterial infection (75%) Stress Malignant neoplasm	Epigastric pain Postprandial pain Bloating Nausea Heartburn	Thick gastric wall margins Hypervascular gastric wall Most commonly located in the lesser curvature of the stomach	Gastritis Neoplasm
Gastritis	Bacterial infection Bile reflux Smoking Excessive alcohol consumption Radiation	Upper abdominal discomfort Decrease in appetite Belching Nausea/vomiting Fatigue Fever	Diffuse or localized thickening in the gastric wall Enlarged and prominent rugae	Gastric ulcer Neoplasm
Hypertrophied pyloric stenosis	Marked thickening of the circular muscle fibers of the pylorus Male prevalence (4:1) Between 2–10 weeks of age (most common)	Projectile vomiting Weight loss or poor weight gain Decreased urination Palpable upper abdominal mass (olive sign) Lethargy Change in stools (decrease in number and size)	Target pattern medial to the porta hepatis and gallbladder Pyloric muscle thickness above 3–4 mm (most important measurement) Length of the pyloric canal exceeding 17 mm Stomach contents does not flow through the pyloric canal	Normal pyloric canal

Pathology of the Stomach—(cont'd)

PATHOLOGY	ETIOLOGY	CLINICAL FINDINGS	SONOGRAPHIC FINDINGS	DIFFERENTIAL CONSIDERATIONS
Leiomyoma	Benign neoplasm of the smooth muscle Found in small intestines and stomach	Asymptomatic Weight loss	Intraluminal solid gastric mass Well-defined wall margins	Polyp Carcinoma Leiomyosarcoma Gastritis
Leiomyosarcoma	Malignant neoplasm of the smooth muscle	Asymptomatic Epigastric pain GI obstruction Weight loss	Intraluminal mass of variable echogenicity	Leiomyoma Polyp
Polyp	Abnormal growth of the mucous membrane tissue Most common tumor of the stomach	Asymptomatic	Hypoechoic lesion protruding from the gastric wall Smooth wall margins	Carcinoma Leiomyoma Gastritis

Pathology of the Small Intestines

PATHOLOGY	ETIOLOGY	CLINICAL FINDINGS	SONOGRAPHIC FINDINGS	DIFFERENTIAL CONSIDERATIONS
Crohn disease **Complications** Fistula formation Abscess Perianal ulcerations Luminal narrowing	Chronic inflammation of the intestines	Abdominal cramping Blood in stool Diarrhea Fever Decrease in appetite Weight loss	Noncompressible thick walled loops of bowel Loss of wall differentiation Hyperemic bowel Hypoactive or absence of peristalsis Increase in echogenicity of the surrounding mesentery (creeping fat)	Ileus Diverticular abscess
Ileus	Bowel obstruction Peritonitis Renal colic Acute pancreatitis Bowel ischemia Neoplasm	Abdominal pain Constipation Fever Nausea/vomiting Absence of bowel sounds	Distention of the small bowel with air or fluid Hypoactive or absent peristalsis	Intussusception Crohn disease
Intussusception	Telescoping of one part of the intestines into the lumen of an adjacent part	Acute abdominal pain Palpable mass Bilious vomiting Mucous and blood in stool (currant jelly) Lethargy	Edematous bowel Multiple circular rings "Donut sign" Hypovascular intestinal wall Hypervascular mesentery	Ileus Crohn disease Appendicitis Cecal volvulus
Lymphoma	Hodgkin's or non-Hodgkin's	Lymphadenopathy Left upper quadrant pain Fever Blood loss Leukopenia Weight loss Anorexia Abdominal mass	Circumferential wall thickening (most common) Hypoechoic or anechoic but can be variable Aneurysmal distention of the bowel.	Lymphadenopathy Retroperitoneal pathology
Meckel diverticulum	Incomplete closure of the yolk stalk	Asymptomatic Abdominal or pelvic pain Rectal bleeding	Anechoic or complex mass located slightly to the right of the umbilicus Thick wall margins Round or oval in shape	Diverticular abscess Appendicitis Ovarian pathology

Pathology of the Colon

PATHOLOGY	ETIOLOGY	CLINICAL FINDINGS	SONOGRAPHIC FINDINGS	DIFFERENTIAL CONSIDERATIONS
Acute appendicitis	Obstructed appendix	Periumbilical or right lower quadrant (RLQ) pain Fever Nausea/vomiting Leukocytosis McBurney sign	Noncompressible tubular structure generally located in the RLQ Anterior-posterior diameter of the appendix exceeding 6 mm Wall thickness exceeding 2 mm Hypervascular structure Rebound pain at McBurney point Fecalith or calculus formation	Bowel obstruction Diverticulum Normal cecum Ovarian pathology Ectopic pregnancy
Appendiceal abscess	Infection	Tender palpable RLQ mass Spiking fever Marked leukocytosis McBurney sign	Poorly defined hypoechoic mass Posterior acoustic enhancement Noncompressible	Diverticular abscess Tuboovarian abscess Ovarian torsion Ectopic pregnancy
Carcinoma	50% are located in the rectum 25% are located in the sigmoid	Asymptomatic Rectal bleeding Change in bowel patterns GI obstruction	Hypoechoic thickening of the bowel wall Hyperechoic mass Compressed wall layers Target appearance	Polyp Diverticulum Abscess Crohn disease
Diverticular abscess	Infection	Asymptomatic Lower abdominal pain Fever Leukocytosis Rectal bleeding	Hypoechoic circular or oval mass adjacent to the colon Thickening of the colon wall Hypervascular periphery	Neoplasm Appendicitis Lymphadenopathy
Mucocele	Inflammatory scarring—most common Neoplasm Fecalith Polyp	Palpable abdominal mass Abdominal pain	Cystic to hypoechoic intraluminal bowel mass Posterior acoustic enhancement Irregular inner wall margin May demonstrate calcification(s)	Cystadenoma Ovarian cyst Appendiceal abscess Diverticulum
Polyp	Abnormal growth of mucous membrane tissue	Asymptomatic Rectal bleeding Abdominal pain Diarrhea or constipation	Hypoechoic mass of the bowel wall protruding into the lumen	Carcinoma Diverticulum Fecal material
Volvulus	Torsion of a segment of bowel (emergent surgery) Malrotation Colonic most common	Acute abdominal pain Bilious vomiting	Dilated loops of bowel Superior mesenteric vein (SMV) wraps around the superior mesenteric artery (SMA) Whirlpool sign on color Doppler at the level of the superior mesenteric vein and artery	Ileus Intussusception

GASTROINTESTINAL TRACT REVIEW

1. The esophagus begins at the pharynx and terminates at the:
   a. cardiac orifice of the stomach
   b. pyloric orifice of the stomach
   c. gastric orifice of the stomach
   d. esophageal hiatus of the stomach

2. Male infants have a predisposing factor for developing which of the following gastrointestinal conditions?
   a. ileus
   b. gastritis
   c. intussusception
   d. hypertrophied pyloric stenosis

3. Which of the following is a clinical symptom of acute appendicitis?
   a. heartburn
   b. leukopenia
   c. periumbilical pain
   d. positive Murphy sign

4. Which portion of the gastrointestinal tract is most likely to demonstrate rugae?
   a. esophagus
   b. stomach
   c. duodenum
   d. transverse colon

5. Bilious vomiting is a symptom of:
   a. appendicitis
   b. Crohn's disease
   c. intussusception
   d. hypertrophied pyloric stenosis

6. Which of the following is considered a function of the duodenum?
   a. secrete pepsin
   b. produce lipase
   c. secrete large quantities of mucus
   d. produce vitamin K and B complex

7. Crohn disease most commonly occurs in which of the following regions?
   a. duodenum
   b. ileum
   c. cecum
   d. sigmoid

8. Prolapse of one section of bowel into the lumen of another bowel segment describes which of the following conditions?
   a. ileus
   b. diverticulitis
   c. intussusception
   d. volvulus

9. The gastroesophageal junction is located:
   a. anterior to the aorta
   b. superior to the diaphragm
   c. inferior to the celiac axis
   d. anterior to the left lobe of the liver

10. Twisting of a portion of the bowel describes:
    a. volvulus
    b. malrotation
    c. pylorospasm
    d. intussusception

11. The right margin of the esophagus is contiguous with the:
    a. pyloric canal
    b. tail of the pancreas
    c. lesser curvature of the stomach
    d. greater curvature of the stomach

12. Which of the following structures demonstrate haustral wall markings?
    a. ileum
    b. appendix
    c. stomach
    d. colon

13. The small intestine is a region of the gastrointestinal tract extending from the:
    a. duodenum to the ileum
    b. pyloric opening to the appendix
    c. duodenum to the cecum
    d. pyloric opening to the ileocecal valve

14. Which of the following is the most accurate measurement when evaluating for hypertrophied pyloric stenosis?
    a. length of the pyloric canal
    b. transverse diameter of pyloric canal
    c. wall thickness of pyloric muscle
    d. anterior posterior diameter of the pyloric canal

15. The anterior-posterior diameter of the normal adult appendix should not exceed:
    a. 2 mm
    b. 4 mm
    c. 6 mm
    d. 10 mm

16. Extreme pain over McBurney point is most commonly associated with:
    a. cholecystitis
    b. intussusception
    c. appendicitis
    d. diverticulitis

17. Malignant neoplasms involving the large intestines are most frequently located in which of the following regions?
    a. ileum
    b. rectum
    c. sigmoid
    d. descending colon

18. The common bile duct enters which of the following sections of the duodenum?
    a. superior
    b. descending
    c. ascending
    d. transverse

19. An episode of excessive alcohol consumption is most commonly associated with which of the following conditions?
    a. ileus
    b. colitis
    c. gastritis
    d. appendicitis

20. Which of the following organs is considered the principal organ of digestion?
    a. mouth
    b. esophagus
    c. stomach
    d. small intestines

21. Which of the following gastrointestinal regions is composed of five individual wall layers?
    a. esophagus
    b. stomach
    c. duodenum
    d. rectum

22. McBurney point is best described as a point between the:
    a. umbilicus and inguinal canal
    b. symphysis pubis and right iliac crest
    c. umbilicus and right iliac crest
    d. right costal margin and right iliac crest

23. The duodenum is divided into ascending, descending,
    a. inferior, and horizontal portions
    b. superior, and transverse portions
    c. transverse, and vertical portions
    d. superior, and inferior portions

24. Which portion of the duodenum is located posterior to the transverse colon?
    a. superior
    b. descending
    c. inferior
    d. transverse

Using Figure 14.2, answer question 25.

25. The finding *(arrow)* in the sonogram is most suspicious for a(n):
    a. polyp
    b. abscess
    c. diverticulum
    d. carcinoma

Using Figure 14.3, answer question 26.

26. The finding in this sonogram is most suspicious for:
    a. gastritis
    b. pancreatitis
    c. pyloric stenosis
    d. intussusception

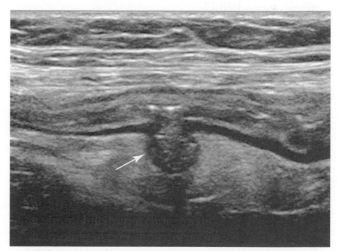

FIG. 14.2   Sonogram of the descending colon.

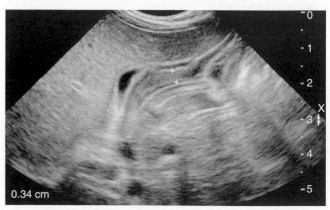

FIG. 14.3   Sonogram of the upper abdomen.

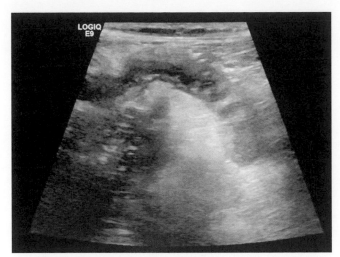

FIG. 14.4   Sonogram of the right lower quadrant.

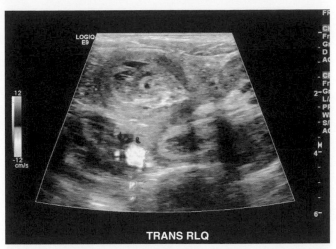

FIG. 14.5   Transverse sonogram of the right lower quadrant.

Using Figure 14.4, answer question 27.

27. A sagittal oblique image lateral to the right ovary is most likely demonstrating which of the following?
  a. volvulus
  b. appendicitis
  c. paraovarian cyst
  d. Meckel diverticulum

Using Figure 14.5, answer question 28.

28. Which of the following abnormalities is demonstrated in this sonogram of the right lower quadrant?
  a. an ileus
  b. Crohn's disease
  c. an appendicitis
  d. intussusception

Using Figure 14.6, answer question 29.

29. Which of the following normal gastrointestinal structures is demonstrated in this midline sonogram of the upper abdomen?
  a. duodenum
  b. pyloric canal
  c. pyloric antrum
  d. gastroesophageal junction

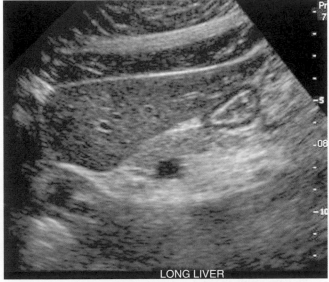

FIG. 14.6   Longitudinal midline sonogram of the upper abdomen.

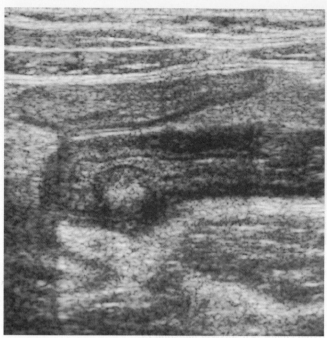

FIG. 14.7 Sonogram of the small intestines.

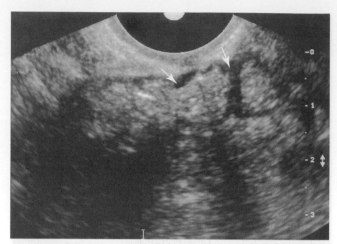

FIG. 14.8 Sonogram of the ascending colon.

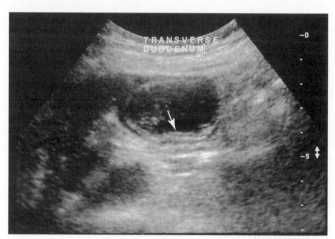

FIG. 14.9 Transverse sonogram of the duodenum.

Using Figure 14.7, answer question 30.

30. A 30-year-old woman presents with a history of chronic abdominal cramping. On the basis of this clinical history, the finding in this sonogram is most consistent with:
   a. intussusception
   b. diverticulitis
   c. Crohn disease
   d. acute appendicitis

Using Figure 14.8, answer question 31.

31. Which of the following are identified by the arrows?
   a. polyps
   b. wall thickening
   c. diverticulums
   d. haustral wall markings

Using Figure 14.9, answer question 32.

32. The intestinal wall layer identified by the arrow is most likely the:
   a. submucosal layer
   b. muscular layer
   c. mucosal layer
   d. serosal layer

33. A Meckel diverticulum is generally located:
   a. adjacent to the appendix
   b. slightly to the right of the umbilicus
   c. adjacent to the cecum
   d. in the left lower quadrant

34. To be considered within normal limits, the wall thickness of the pyloric canal should not exceed:
   a. 2 mm to 3 mm
   b. 3 mm to 4 mm
   c. 4 mm to 5 mm
   d. 5 mm to 6 mm

35. Hypertrophied pyloric stenosis most commonly develops in infants between:
    a. 1 to 2 months of age
    b. 1 to 6 weeks of age
    c. 2 to 3 months of age
    d. 2 to 10 weeks of age

36. Ulcers are more commonly located in which of the following regions of the stomach?
    a. body
    b. pylorus
    c. lesser curvature
    d. greater curvature

37. A patient presents with a history of abdominal distention and pain. A sonogram of the periumbilical area demonstrates distended fluid-filled loops of small bowel with minimal peristalsis. On the basis of the clinical history, the sonographic findings are most suspicious for which of the following conditions?
    a. ileus
    b. intussusception
    c. diverticulitis
    d. Crohn's disease

38. Graded compression technique is most commonly used when evaluating for:
    a. ileus
    b. an appendicitis
    c. diverticulitis
    d. intussusception

39. The duodenum protects the small intestines from chyme by secreting:
    a. pepsin
    b. mucous
    c. sodium bicarbonate
    d. cholecystokinin

40. The ileum is a section of the gastrointestinal tract extending from the:
    a. duodenum to the cecum
    b. jejunum to the appendix
    c. cecum to the ascending colon
    d. jejunum to the ileocecal junction

41. The majority of food absorption occurs in which portion of the gastrointestinal tract?
    a. stomach
    b. cecum
    c. small intestines
    d. ascending colon

42. Which of the following is a protein-enzyme produced by the stomach?
    a. gastrin
    b. pepsin
    c. secretin
    d. cholecystokinin

43. Forward movement of intestinal contents caused by rhythmic contractions of the intestines is termed:
    a. rugae
    b. pylorospasm
    c. cramping
    d. peristalsis

44. A febrile female patient complaining of periumbilical pain and vomiting presents to the emergency department. Her last menstrual period was 2 weeks earlier. Based on this clinical presentation, the referring physician should order a(n):
    a. pelvic ultrasound to rule out ovarian cyst
    b. pelvic ultrasound to rule out ectopic pregnancy
    c. abdominal ultrasound to rule out appendicitis
    d. abdominal ultrasound to rule out gallstones

45. Which portion of the colon follows the sacral canal?
    a. rectum
    b. sigmoid
    c. anal canal
    d. descending

46. Which of the following patient positions is the best for viewing fluid in the pylorus?
    a. supine
    b. semi-Fowler
    c. right lateral decubitus
    d. right posterior oblique

47. The superior portion of the duodenum is located anterior to the:
    a. liver
    b. gallbladder
    c. common bile duct
    d. transverse colon

48. Which of the following abnormalities is *not* associated with a mucocele?
    a. polyp
    b. fecalith
    c. gastritis
    d. scarring

49. Which portion of the large intestines demonstrates the narrowest lumen?
    a. cecum
    b. sigmoid
    c. ascending
    d. descending

50. An asymptomatic patient demonstrates a small, intraluminal hypoechoic mass on ultrasound. The mass appears to protrude from a gastric wall. This is most suspicious for which of the following gastric pathologies?
    a. polyp
    b. ulcer
    c. adenoma
    d. leiomyoma

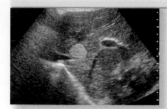

CHAPTER 15

Abdominal Wall, Musculoskeletal Sonography, and Pediatric Hip

KEY TERMS

abdominal wall hernia   protrusion of peritoneal contents through a defect in the abdominal wall muscle.

Achilles tendon   attaches the gastrocnemius and soleus muscles.

anisotropy artifact   hypoechoic sonographic artifact caused when the ultrasound beam is not perpendicular to the fibrillar structure of a tendon.

aponeurosis   a broad, flat sheet of fibrous connective tissue that serves as a tendon to attach muscle to bone, or as fascia to bind muscles together, or other tissues at their origin or insertion.

Baker cyst   a synovial cyst adjacent and posterior to the knee joint.

Barlow maneuver   determines whether hip can be dislocated. Hip is flexed and the thigh adducted while gently placing posterior pressure on the femoral head.

biceps tendon   connects the biceps muscle to the shoulder joint in two places are called the proximal biceps tendons. The tendon that attaches the biceps muscle to the bones of the forearm (radius and ulna) is called the distal biceps tendon.

Development displacement of the hip (DDH)   preferred term to describe the abnormal relationship of the femoral head to the acetabulum; a congenital or acquired deformation or misalignment of the hip joint.

direct inguinal hernia   protrudes into the inguinal canal "directly" from posteriorly

dorsal   pertaining to the back or posterior.

femoral hernia   herniation within the femoral canal, inferior to the inguinal ligament and superior to the saphenofemoral junction.

fibril   a small filamentous fiber that is often a component of a cell.

ganglion cyst   small tumor or fluid collection that can occur at the connection of any tendon

indirect inguinal hernia   protrudes into the inguinal canal "indirectly" from a superolateral direction after passing through the internal inguinal ring.

linea alba   a thick layer of aponeurosis that separates the rectus abdominis muscles.

linea semilunaris   lateral borders of the rectus abdominis muscles

Morton's neuroma   a nonneoplastic fusiform enlargement of a digital branch of the medial or lateral plantar nerves.

musculoskeletal system   consists of all the muscles, bones, joints, ligaments, and tendons that function in the movement of the body and organs.

Ortolani maneuver   relocates the femoral head within the acetabulum. Hip is flexed and abducted while gently pulling anteriorly. Demonstrates whether the dislocated hip is reducible.

rectus abdominis muscle   one of a pair of anterolateral abdominal wall muscles located lateral to the linea alba.

rheumatoid arthritis   autoimmune disorder affecting the lining of joints.

rotator cuff   a musculotendinous structure about the capsule of the shoulder joint, formed by the inserting fibers of the supraspinatus, infraspinatus, teres minor, and subscapularis muscles, which blend with the capsule and provide mobility and strength to the shoulder joint.

spigelian hernia   is usually considered an anterior abdominal wall hernia that occurs inferior to the umbilicus at the linea semilunaris border (lateral) of the rectus abdominis muscle.

sprain   a painful wrenching or laceration of the ligaments of a joint.

strain   to injure or impair by overuse or overexertion; wrench.

tendinosis   term used to describe degenerative changes in a tendon without signs of tendon inflammation; associated with overuse injuries.

Thompson test   a test used to evaluate the integrity of the Achilles tendon where the toes are pointing down while squeezing the calf.

volar   relating to the palm of the hand or sole of the foot.

PHYSIOLOGY

Function of the Anterior Abdominal Wall

- Movement of the torso.

Function of the Musculoskeletal System

- Movement of body parts and organs.

ANTERIOR ABDOMINAL WALL ANATOMY (Fig. 15.1)

- Consists of several layers of fat, fascia, and muscle.
- Subcutaneous tissue located anterior to the muscle groups.
- Fascial interface located anterior to the peritoneum.

Linea Alba

- Midline tendon extending from the xiphoid process to the symphysis pubis separating the rectus abdominis muscles.
- Located posterior to the subcutaneous fat.

Rectus Abdominis Muscles

- Located on either side of the linea alba.
- Extend the entire length of the anterior abdominal wall.
- Each rectus muscle is contained within a rectus sheath.

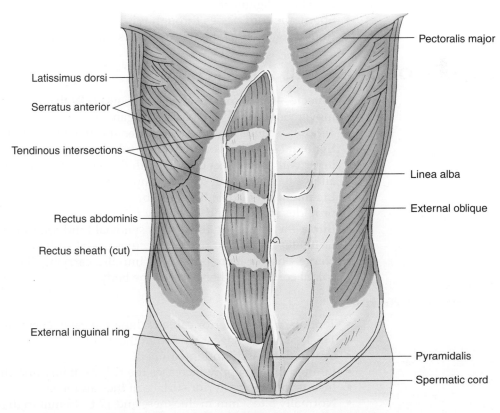

FIG. 15.1 Anterior abdominal wall anatomy.

Rectus Sheath

- Tendinous sheet that covers the anterior and posterior rectus abdominis muscle.
- Formed by the aponeuroses of the external, internal, and transverse abdominis muscles laterally.
- Fuses at the midline to form the linea alba.

External Oblique Muscles

- Most external of the anterolateral abdominal wall muscles.
- Located anterior to the internal oblique and transverse abdominis muscles.

Internal Oblique Muscles

- Middle muscle of the anterolateral abdominal wall muscles.
- Located posterior to the external oblique muscle and anterior to the transverse abdominis muscle.
- Acts with the contralateral external oblique muscle to achieve side bends of the trunk.

Transversus Abdominis Muscle

- Most internal of the anterolateral abdominal wall muscles.
- Located immediately posterior to the internal and external oblique muscles.

Inguinal Ligament

- Runs between the pubic tubercle and the anterior superior iliac spine (ASIS).
- Landmark for the separation of the body wall and thigh.

Inguinal Canal

- Opening in the medial inferior aspect of the inguinal ligament between the muscle fascia and ligament.
- Spermatic cord passes through this point into scrotum in males.
- Round ligament of the uterus passes through this point to the labia majora.

MUSCULOSKELETAL ANATOMY

- **Muscle**—tissue composed of fibers and cells that are able to contract, causing movement of the body parts or organs.
- **Tendon**—bands of dense, fibrous connective tissue that attach muscle to bone.
- **Synovial sheath**—double-walled tubular structures surrounding some tendons; inner wall is in direct contact with the tendon; small amount of synovial fluid allows the inner wall to glide smoothly within the outer wall.
- **Ligament**—a flexible band of fibrous tissue binding joints together (bone to bone); provides strength and flexibility to a joint.
- **Bursa**—a fibrous sac filled with synovial fluid found between the tendon and bone; facilitates movement of the musculoskeletal system.
- **Nerve**—one or more bundles of impulse-carrying fibers that connect the brain and spinal cord with other parts of the body.

Achilles Tendon

- Tendon of the posterior calf attaching the gastrocnemius and soleus muscles.
- Thickest and strongest tendon in the body.
- Covered by fascia and integument.
- Limited blood supply increases the risk for injury and difficulty in healing.
- Inserts into the posterior surface of the calcaneus.
- Normally 5 to 7 mm in thickness and 12 to 15 mm in diameter.
- Increase in the normal size has been documented in athletes.

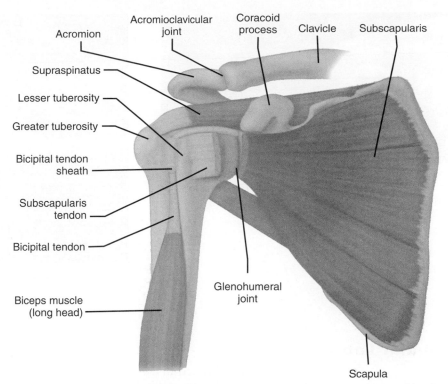

FIG. 15.2 Illustration of the long head biceps tendon in the rotator interval in the bicipital groove.

Knee Joint

- A complex hinge joint.
- Condyloid joint connecting the femur and the tibia.
- Arthrodial joint connecting the patella and the femur.

Shoulder Joint (Fig. 15.2)

- Most mobile joint of the body.
- Bicep tendon found in the bicipital groove extending down the anterior surface of the humerus.
- Subscapularis tendon is located anterior medially on the rotator cuff.
- Infraspinatus tendon is located lateral and posterior to the shoulder.
- Supraspinatus tendon is located superior to the humeral head under the acromion.

Wrist Joint

- Flexus retinaculum space—carpal tunnel.
- Flexus pollicis—most radial tendon in the carpal tunnel.

PEDIATRIC HIP ANATOMY

Pelvic Girdle

- Ilium—broad portion of the hip bone.
- Ischium—lower posterior portion of the hip bone.
- Pubis—lower anterior portion of the hip bone.

Acetabulum

- Located on the lateral surface of the hip bone.
- Receives the head of the femur.

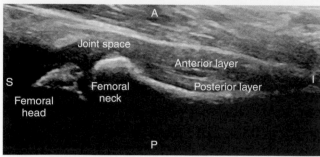

FIG. 15.3 Sagittal oblique image of the normal anterior hip joint. *A,* Anterior; *I,* inferior; *P,* posterior; *S,* superior.

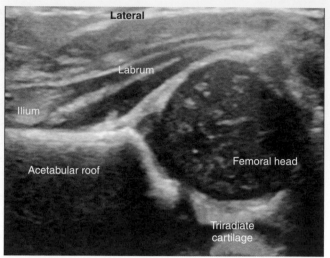

FIG. 15.4 Coronal sonogram of a normal pediatric hip.

Acetabular Labrum

- Fibrocartilage located in the acetabular rim.
- Extends over the superolateral aspect of the hip joint.
- Increases surface strength of the hip joint.

Iliofemoral Ligament

- Triangular ligament attached inferiorly to the intertrochanteric line of the femur.
- Attached by its apex to the anterior spine of the ilium and rim of the acetabulum.
- Limits extension of the hip joint.

Triradiate Cartilage

- Separates bony ossification centers in the ilium, ischium, and pubis to form the acetabulum.
- "Y" configuration.

Femur

- Femoral head—most superior rounded portion of the femur that fits in the acetabulum of the hip bone.

Joint Capsule

- Contains an outer fibrous membrane and inner synovial membrane.
- Consists of an anterior and posterior layer (area fluid collections occur).

SONOGRAPHIC APPEARANCE OF THE ANTERIOR ABDOMINAL WALL

- Superficial fat demonstrates a medium shade of gray echogenicity.
- Muscles demonstrate a low to medium shade of gray echo pattern with hyperechoic striations.
- The peritoneal line appears as a hyperechoic linear structure anterior to the peritoneal cavity in the deepest layer of the abdominal wall.

SONOGRAPHIC APPEARANCE OF THE MUSCULOSKELETAL SYSTEM

- Muscles demonstrate a low to medium shade of gray echo pattern with hyperechoic striations in the sagittal plane and punctate echogenic areas within the hypoechoic muscle in the transverse plane.
- Tendons appear homogeneous with hyperechoic linear bands throughout when viewed in the longitudinal plane.
- Ligaments appear homogeneous with compacted hyperechoic linear bands throughout when viewed in the longitudinal plane. In transverse plane, ligaments have a spotted appearance.
- Bursae appear as a thin linear hypoechoic structure that merges with the surrounding fat in the sagittal plane. Difficult to visualize in the transverse plane.
- Synovial sheaths appear as thin hypoechoic line beneath the tendon.
- Peripheral nerves appear as echogenic structures and tend to be slightly hypoechoic compared with the tendons and ligaments.

SONOGRAPHIC APPEARANCE OF THE PEDIATRIC HIP

- The bony structures of the pediatric hip joint appear hyperechoic.
- Femoral head appears hypoechoic compared with the adjacent bone.
- A hyperechoic ossification center may be demonstrated in the femoral head around 2 months of age.
- Joint capsule appears hypoechoic compared with the femur and hyperechoic to the adjacent muscle.

EXAMINATION TECHNIQUES, PROTOCOLS, AND IMAGE OPTIMIZATION

Preparation

- No preparation is necessary for a sonogram of the anterior abdominal wall, pediatric hip, or musculoskeletal system.

Transducer Selection

Anterior Abdominal Wall

- Use the highest frequency possible to obtain optimal resolution for penetration depth.
- Adults—7.5 to 12 MHz linear.
- 3.5 MHz curvilinear transducer may be necessary in obese patients.

Musculoskeletal System

- Use the highest frequency possible to obtain optimal resolution for penetration depth.
- Adults—10 to 17 MHz linear.

Pediatric Hip

- Use the highest frequency possible to obtain optimal resolution for penetration depth.
- 9 to 15 MHz linear.

Patient Positioning

Anterior Abdominal Wall

- Abdominal wall fluid collection—supine.
- Abdominal wall and inguinal hernia—supine and upright.

Musculoskeletal System

- Dependent on which area of the body evaluated.
- **Ankle:**
  - *Achille's tendon*—prone or kneeling on a chair with foot overhanging end of stretcher or chair.
- **Knee:**
  - *Popliteal fossa*—prone or supine with leg bent into a frog position.
  - *Suprapatellar recess*—supine.
  - *Medial and lateral meniscus*—right or left lateral decubitus.
- **Shoulder:**
  - *Biceps tendon*—sitting with arm resting close to the body and palm facing up.
  - *Subscapsularis tendon*—sitting with arm held closely to body and elbow bent 90 degrees.
  - *Supraspinatus tendon*—sitting with arm behind the back, as if placing their hand in the opposite back pocket.
  - *Infraspinatus tendon*—sitting placing their hand on the contralateral shoulder.
- **Wrist:**
  - Median nerve, flexor tendons, volar joint recess, volar ganglion cyst, ulnar nerve and artery—volar position (palm up).
  - Extensor tendons, dorsal joint space, dorsal ganglion cyst, triangular fibrocartilage complex—dorsal position (palm down).

Pediatric Hip

- **Hip effusion**—supine with leg in the neutral position.
- **Developmental dysplasia of the hip**—supine or right lateral and left lateral decubitus with leg in neutral and flexion positions.

Examination Protocol

- **Anterior abdominal wall fluid collection.**
  - Evaluate, annotate, and document the area of concern in two orthogonal planes.
  - Abnormalities should be documented and when applicable measured in two imaging planes. Color and/or spectral Doppler evaluation of the abnormality should be included.
- **Anterior abdominal wall hernia.**
  - Measure the fascial defect in the short axis.
  - Determine the type of herniated abdominal contents (e.g., fat, bowel).
  - Measure the length, height, and width of herniated contents.
  - Cine clip in the short axis and/or long axis during Valsalva maneuver to demonstrate movement of abdominal contents through the defect.
  - Cine clip in the short and/or long axis using transducer compression to evaluate and document reducibility of herniated contents.
  - Color Doppler evaluation of the hernia should be included.
- **Inguinal hernia.**
  - Document the inferior epigastric arteries with color Doppler in the transverse plane.
  - Document spermatic cord from the inguinal ring to the scrotal sac in males or the round ligament in females.
  - Measure the fascial defect in the short axis.
  - Determine the type of herniated abdominal contents (e.g., fat, bowel).
  - Cine clip in the short axis and/or long axis during Valsalva maneuver to demonstrate and document movement of abdominal contents through the defect.
  - Cine clip in the short and/or long axis using transducer compression to evaluate and document reducibility of herniated contents.
  - Color Doppler evaluation of the hernia should be included.

- **Musculoskeletal system.**
  - Evaluate and document the area of interest in the sagittal, coronal, and transverse planes.
  - Cine clip of joint or hand movement.
  - Comparison of images and cine clip of contralateral side when indicated.
  - Abnormalities should be documented and when applicable measured in two imaging planes. Color and/or spectral Doppler evaluation of the abnormality should be included.
- **Pediatric hip for effusion.**
  - In the sagittal plane, evaluate and document the anterior posterior measurement of both hip joint capsules.
  - Color Doppler image of both joint capsules.
- **Pediatric hip for development dysplasia of the hip.**
  - Coronal image with and without Graf angles with the leg in the neutral and/or flexed position bilaterally.
  - Graf angles should demonstrate an alpha angle of 60 degrees or greater and beta angle less than 55 degrees. The femoral head should be in contact with the acetabulum to be considered normal.
  - In the coronal plane, using the Barlow maneuver evaluate and document lateral movement of the femoral head bilaterally.
  - Transverse image with the leg in a flexed position bilaterally.

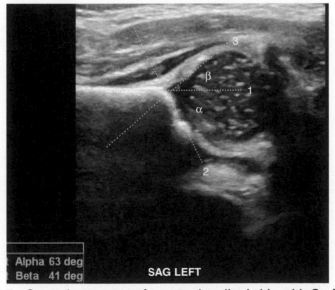

FIG. 15.5   Coronal sonogram of a normal pediatric hip with Graf angles.

Image Optimization

- Place gains settings to display muscle a low to medium shade of gray with hyperechoic striations.
- Focal zone(s) should be placed at or below the area of interest. The use of multiple focal zones increases detail resolution and decreases temporal resolution.
- Sufficient imaging depth to visualize structures immediately posterior to the area of interest.
- Harmonic imaging and decreasing system compression (dynamic range) can be used to reduce artifactual echoes.

- Spatial compounding can be used to improve visualization of structures posterior to highly attenuating structures.
- Doppler settings should be adjusted for a slow flow rate.

Examination Limitations

- Patient cooperation.
- Patient limitations.
- Near field reverberation.

Helpful Hints

- Power Doppler may aid in detecting low flow velocities.
- **Anterior abdominal wall**
  - Hernias may only be visible when the patient is standing.
  - In the supine position raising chest and head keeping abdomen tense can be used if patient is unable to perform a Valsalva maneuver.

Musculoskeletal System

- Small hockey-stick linear transducer when evaluating small structures.
- Achilles tendon measurements should be made in the transverse plane.

Pediatric Hip

- A happy baby makes for a better examination.
  - Feed the baby if hungry.
  - Place the baby on top of a warm blanket.
  - Entertain the baby with toys or a video on the parent's cell phone.

Indications for an Anterior Abdominal Wall Examination

- Trauma.
- Hernia.
- Palpable mass.
- Postsurgery.
- Evaluate mass from previous medical imaging study (e.g., CT)

Indications for a Musculoskeletal Examination

- Trauma.
- Pain.
- Palpable mass.
- Decrease in motion.
- Evaluate mass from previous medical imaging study (e.g., CT).

Indications for a Pediatric Hip Examination

- Breech presentation.
- Hip click.
- Asymmetry of thigh folds.
- Hip pain.

Anterior Abdominal Wall Pathology

PATHOLOGY	ETIOLOGY	CLINICAL FINDINGS	SONOGRAPHIC FINDINGS	DIFFERENTIAL CONSIDERATIONS
Abdominal wall abscess	Infection	Palpable abdominal wall mass Fever Leukocytosis	Hypoechoic or anechoic mass anterior to the peritoneal fascial plane Thick irregular borders May demonstrate posterior acoustic enhancement or shadowing	Hematoma Hernia Seroma
Diastasis recti abdominis	Prolonged increased abdominal pressure weakens the linea alba May include: Pregnancy Morbid obesity Ascites	Bulging of the anterior abdominal wall	Increase in distance between the rectus abdominis muscles Anterior bulging of the epigastric segment of the linea alba	Epigastric linea alba hernia Ventral hernia
Femoral hernia	Weakness of the femoral canal	Asymptomatic Palpable mass Groin pain	Fascial defect Herniation of fat, bowel or both through the femoral canal Located superior to the saphenofemoral junction, inferior to the inguinal canal, medial to the common femoral vein	Inguinal hernia Lipoma Lymph node
Inguinal hernia Subdivided into direct and indirect using the inferior epigastric artery as a vascular landmark	Weakness of the internal inguinal ring Patent processus vaginalis	Asymptomatic Palpable mass Groin pain	Fascial defect Herniation of fat, bowel or both into the inguinal canal **Direct**—arises inferior and medial to the inferior epigastric artery (IEA) **Indirect**—arises superior and lateral to the IEA	Technical error Undescended testis
Lipoma	Growth of fat cells in a thin, fibrous capsule	Palpable superficial mass	Isoechoic to hypoechoic superficial mass Smooth wall margins	Lymph node Leiomyoma
Rectus sheath hematoma	Trauma Pregnancy Long-term steroid use Coughing Sneezing Heavy exercise Anticoagulant therapy	Abdominal pain Abdominal mass Decreased hematocrit	Mass located in the rectus muscle or between the sheath and muscle **Acute hematoma** Hypoechoic mass **Subacute hematoma** Complex mass **Chronic hematoma** Anechoic	Abscess Hernia
Ventral and umbilical hernia	Defect in the abdominal muscles	Visual or palpable ventral or umbilical mass Abdominal pain	Extension of the intestines and/or omentum through a defect in the abdominal wall	Hematoma Abscess Diastasis recti abdominis Technical error

Musculoskeletal Pathology

PATHOLOGY	ETIOLOGY	CLINICAL FINDINGS	SONOGRAPHIC FINDINGS	DIFFERENTIAL CONSIDERATIONS
Achilles tendonitis	Inflammation Trauma	Pain or tenderness at the site of insertion Palpable mass Decreased range of motion in the foot or ankle joint	Thickening of the tendon Tendon thickness exceeding 7 mm Prominent hypoechoic areas interspersed between the fibrous tissues Irregular wall margins Hypervascularity Calcifications in chronic cases	Partial tear Anisotropy artifact Tendinosis
Achilles tendon tear	Trauma	Painful tendon Positive Thompson test Focal cleft at tendon insertion	**Complete Tear** Irregular tendon contour Hematoma surrounding the defect Most commonly located in the distal portion 2-6 cm from the calcaneus **Partial Tear** Focal disruption in the tendon Fluid collection within the tendon Most commonly located in the distal portion	Anisotropy artifact Tendonitis Tendinosis
Baker cyst	Knee trauma Rheumatoid arthritis Osteoarthritis Chronic knee dysfunction	Pain in knee or proximal calf Knee swelling Palpable mass	Anechoic mass in the medial and posterior aspect of the knee May contain internal echoes May extend into the calf Rarely extends into the thigh Fluid collections dissect inferiorly into the muscular fascial planes when ruptured	Joint effusion Abscess Hematoma
Carpal tunnel syndrome	Repetitive motion	Positive Phalen's and Tinel's signs Nocturnal paresthesia Atrophy in the palm muscle	Flattening of the medial nerve at the level of the hamate bone Bulging of the flexor retinaculum Fat layer or large fluid collection around the tendons Decreased movement of the nerve through tunnel when fingers are flexed	
Cellulitis	Inflammation of the cellular or connective tissue Infection in or close to the skin Rapid spread of infection may become life threatening	Swollen, red skin that is hot and tender to the touch	**Early Stage** Skin and subcutaneous tissue are thickened and hyperechoic **Later Stage** Anechoic fluid within the echogenic cellular tissue Increased blood flow	Abscess Superficial thrombophlebitis

Musculoskeletal Pathology—(cont'd)

PATHOLOGY	ETIOLOGY	CLINICAL FINDINGS	SONOGRAPHIC FINDINGS	DIFFERENTIAL CONSIDERATIONS
Ganglion cyst	Idiopathic Repetitive motion	Small bulge found on the wrist, but can occur with any tendon Pain	Anechoic fluid collection at tendon connection to bone Single or multiple Variable size	Tenosynovitis Synovial sarcoma
Morton's neuroma	Benign growth of the plantar nerve tissue	Sharp burning pain radiating from the foot to the toes Numbness of the ball of the foot	Hypoechoic intermetatarsal mass	Ganglion cyst Giant cell tumor
Muscle tear	Sprain or strain **Risk Factors** Increase in age Lifting above the head Sports strains Cigarette smoking Corticosteroid medications	Pain Swelling Decrease in range of motion	Heterogeneous mass Focal disruption of the normal muscle Perifascial fluid	Giant cell tumor Neuroma
Tendon tear	Trauma Chronic inflammation	Pain with movement Limited movement	**Partial Tear** Disruption of tendon Anechoic or hypoechoic clefts within the tendon **Complete** Nonvisualization of tendon in expected location Surrounding muscle atrophy	Technical error
Tenosynovitis	Inflammation of the tendon sheath caused by trauma or infection	Pain Swelling Difficulty moving joint	**Acute** Anechoic fluid within a tendon sheath **Chronic** Hypoechoic thickening of the synovial sheath Little or no fluid May demonstrate hyperemia	Partial tendon tear

RHEUMATOID ARTHRITIS	SONOGRAPHIC FINDINGS

Autoimmune disorder causing chronic inflammation eventually resulting in bone erosion and joint deformity
Sonography is used for monitoring therapy, guiding intervention and early detection
	Hyperemia (early stage)
	Synovial proliferation
	Joint effusion
	Cortical irregularity adjacent to synovitis (erosion)
	Bursitis
	Tendon disease (late stage)
	   Tenosynovitis
	   Tendinosis
	   Tear

Pathology of the Pediatric Hip

PATHOLOGY	ETIOLOGY	CLINICAL FINDINGS	SONOGRAPHIC FINDINGS	DIFFERENTIAL CONSIDERATIONS
Development displacement of the hip	Loose, elastic joint capsule Genetic Mechanical Physiological **Risk Factors** Family history of congenital dislocation of the hip Female infant Breech presentation Pregnancies with oligohydramnios Foot deformity that requires further treatment Neonatal torticollis	Hip click on the Barlow or Ortolani maneuvers Limited abduction Asymmetry of thigh folds Limb shortening Abnormal leg posture	Alpha angle less than 60 degrees Beta angle 55 degrees or greater Shallow acetabulum Femoral head not in contact with acetabular floor	Immature hip Technical error
Joint effusion Aka: synovitis Most common cause of hip pain in children	Transient in 90% of cases Infection	Hip pain Limping or change in gait Recent illness	Increase thickness of the joint capsule Bulging of joint capsule Anechoic or hypoechoic fluid between the anterior and posterior layers of the joint capsule Asymmetry in the anterior hip recess exceeding 2 mm compared with the contralateral hip	Technical error Septic hip

ABDOMINAL WALL, MUSCULOSKELETAL SONOGRAPHY, AND PEDIATRIC HIP REVIEW

1. A direct inguinal hernia arises:
   a. inferior and medial to the inferior epigastric artery
   b. superior and medial to the superior epigastric artery
   c. inferior and medial to the superior epigastric artery
   d. superior and lateral to the inferior epigastric artery

2. Which of the following joints has the largest range of motion?
   a. hip
   b. wrist
   c. knee
   d. shoulder

3. Which of the following is NOT a risk factor for developmental dysplasia of the hip?
   a. club foot
   b. male infant
   c. neonatal torticollis
   d. breech presentation

4. Which of the following joints is associated with a positive Tinel's sign?
   a. knee
   b. wrist
   c. ankle
   d. shoulder

5. Which of the following most accurately describes the location of the transversus abdominis muscle?
   a. medial to the external oblique muscle
   b. posterior to the internal oblique muscle
   c. lateral to the internal oblique muscle
   d. anterior to the external oblique muscle

6. When evaluating the Achilles tendon, the patient should be placed in which of the following positions?
   a. prone with leg abducted
   b. supine with leg in frog position
   c. lateral with foot supported on a pillow
   d. prone with foot overhanging the stretcher

7. Which of the following artifacts is likely to occur when the ultrasound beam is not perpendicular with a fibrillar tendon?
   a. duplication
   b. refraction
   c. anisotropy
   d. shadowing

8. Which of the following patient positions is used when evaluating the supraspinatus tendon?
   a. sitting with hand on opposite shoulder
   b. sitting with arm behind back
   c. sitting with arm close to the body and palm up
   d. sitting with arm close to the body and elbow bent at 90 degrees

9. Which of the following is an early stage of rheumatoid arthritis?
   a. tendon tear
   b. tendinosis
   c. hyperemia
   d. tenosynovitis

10. The triradiate cartilage is located:
    a. superior to the labrum
    b. lateral to the ilium
    c. posterior to the femoral head
    d. medial to the femoral head.

11. An indirect inguinal hernia arises:
    a. inferior and medial to the inferior epigastric artery
    b. inferior and medial to the superior epigastric artery
    c. superior and lateral to the inferior epigastric artery
    d. superior and lateral to the superior epigastric artery

12. What is the *normal* alpha angle when evaluating for developmental displacement of the hip in a 2-month old infant?
    a. less than 50 degrees
    b. 50 degrees or greater
    c. less than 60 degrees
    d. 60 degrees or greater

13. Bursae appear on ultrasound as:
    a. thin, linear hypoechoic structures
    b. thick, convex hypoechoic structures
    c. thin, linear hyperechoic structures
    d. thick, concave hyperechoic structures

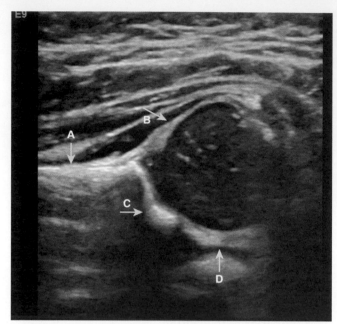

FIG. 15.6 Coronal sonogram of pediatric hip.

Using Figure 15.6, answer questions 14 to 17.

14. Which of the following structures is identified by the letter A?
- **a.** ilium
- **b.** ischium
- **c.** femur
- **d.** symphysis pubis

15. Which of the following structures is identified by the letter B?
- **a.** ischium
- **b.** labrum
- **c.** acetabular roof
- **d.** triradiate cartilage

16. Which of the following structures is identified by the letter C?
- **a.** ilium
- **b.** ischium
- **c.** labrum
- **d.** acetabular roof

17. Which of the following structures is identified by the letter D?
- **a.** labrum
- **b.** ischium
- **c.** triradiate cartilage
- **d.** acetabular roof

18. An increase in distance between the rectus abdominis muscles is a sonographic finding associated with:
- **a.** a ventral hernia
- **b.** an umbilical hernia
- **c.** an epigastric hernia
- **d.** diastasis recti abdominis

19. Flattening of the medial nerve is a sonographic finding associated with:
- **a.** rotator cuff tear
- **b.** ganglion cyst
- **c.** carpal tunnel syndrome
- **d.** Morton's neuroma

20. A defect in the muscles of the abdominal wall is most likely related to a:
- **a.** cyst
- **b.** polyp
- **c.** hernia
- **d.** diverticulum

21. The Thompson test is used to check the integrity of the:
- **a.** calf muscles
- **b.** rotator cuff
- **c.** Achilles tendon
- **d.** anterior abdominal wall

22. Which of the following patient positions is used when evaluating the biceps tendon?
- **a.** sitting with arm resting close to the body and palm facing down
- **b.** sitting with arm held closely to body and elbow bent at 90 degrees
- **c.** sitting with hand resting on contralateral shoulder
- **d.** sitting with arm resting close to body and palm facing up

23. Anechoic fluid within a tendon sheath is most suspicious for:
- **a.** a tendon tear
- **b.** tendinosis
- **c.** tenosynovitis
- **d.** a Baker's cyst

24. Muscle attaches to bone by which of the following structures?
- **a.** tendon
- **b.** fibril
- **c.** ligament
- **d.** synovial membrane

25. Which of the following is an autoimmune disorder affecting the lining of joints?
- **a.** tendinosis
- **b.** osteoarthritis
- **c.** tendonitis
- **d.** rheumatoid arthritis

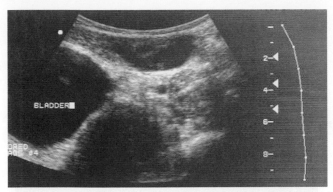

FIG. 15.7 Transverse sonogram of the left anterior abdominal wall.

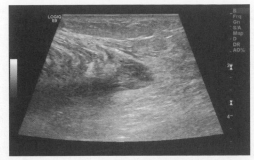

FIG. 15.9 Sagittal image of the posterior calf.

Using Figure 15.7, answer question 26.

26. A patient hospitalized with pneumonia presents with a palpable abdominal wall mass. This finding is most suspicious for a(n):
   a. urachal sinus
   b. umbilical hernia
   c. rectus sheath hematoma
   d. ovarian cyst

Using Figure 15.8, answer question 27.

27. The anechoic structure is most suspicious for a:
   a. torn ligament
   b. synovial cyst
   c. joint effusion
   d. thrombosed superficial vein

Using Figure 15.9, answer question 28.

28. A patient complains of severe calf pain following hyperextension of the knee while playing soccer. The sonographic finding is most suspicious for:
   a. a muscle tear
   b. a synovial cyst
   c. tenosynovitis
   d. a lipoma

Using Figure 15.10, answer question 29.

29. A patient presents to the ultrasound department with a palpable umbilical mass. The finding in this sonogram is most consistent for a(n):
   a. abscess
   b. hematoma
   c. hernia
   d. urachal sinus

30. Degenerative changes in a tendon without signs of inflammation is termed:
   a. strain
   b. sprain
   c. tendinosis
   d. anistrophy

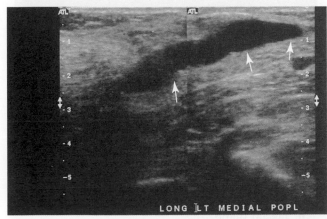

FIG. 15.8 Sagittal sonogram of the medial popliteal fossa.

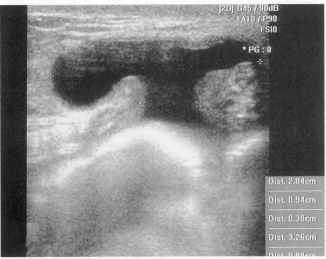

FIG. 15.10 Transverse sonogram of the anterior abdominal wall.

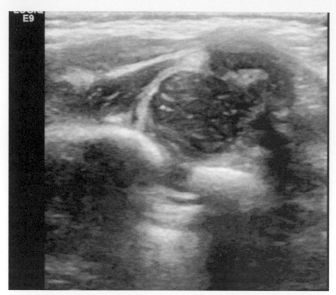

FIG. 15.11 Coronal image of a pediatric hip.

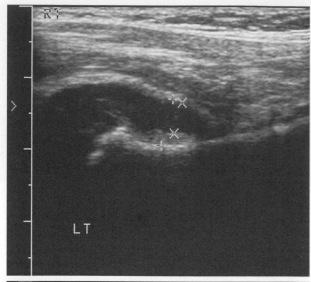

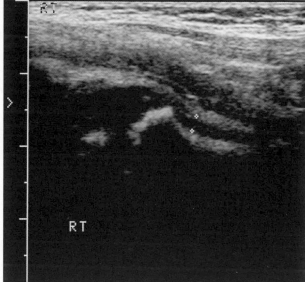

FIG. 15.12 Sagittal sonograms of the left and right hip.

Using Figure 15.11, answer question 31.

31. The sonogram is most likely demonstrating a(n):
   a. normal hip
   b. immature hip
   c. subluxed hip
   d. dislocated hip

32. Which of the following tendons is located under the acromion?
   a. biceps
   b. subcapsularis
   c. infraspinatus
   d. supraspinatus

Using Figure 15.12, answer question 33.

33. A toddler presents with a history of limping. On the basis of the clinical history, the sonographic finding is most suspicious for which of the following conditions?
   a. joint effusion
   b. hip dislocation
   c. hip subluxation
   d. synovial cyst formation

Using Figure 15.13, answer question 34.

34. A soft tissue image over the area of discomfort demonstrates a hyperechoic linear structure outlined by the calibers. This is most suspicious for a:
   a. lipoma
   b. ligament
   c. foreign body
   d. fascial plane

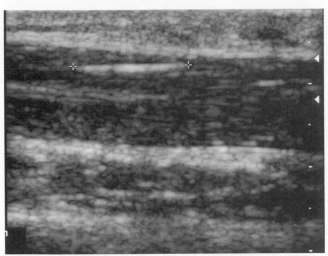

FIG. 15.13   Sonogram of the forearm.

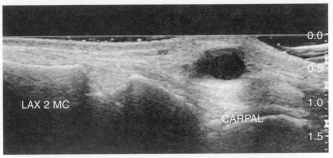

FIG. 15.15   Axial sonogram of the left wrist.

Using Figure 15.14, answer question 35.

35. A sagittal image of the Achilles tendon shows which of the following findings?
    a. normal tendon
    b. tendonitis
    c. complete tear
    d. incomplete tear

36. A femoral hernia is located:
    a. superior to the inguinal ligament
    b. inferior to the great saphenous vein
    c. lateral to the common femoral vein
    d. superior to the saphenofemoral junction

37. The thickness of a normal Achilles tendon should not exceed:
    a. 3 mm
    b. 5 mm
    c. 7 mm
    d. 10 mm

Using Figure 15.15, answer question 38.

38. The pathology demonstrated in this sonogram is most suspicious for a:
    a. Baker's cyst
    b. joint effusion
    c. ganglion cyst
    d. radial artery aneurysm

39. The location of the rectus abdominis muscles is described as lateral to the:
    a. iliac crests
    b. linea alba
    c. external oblique muscles
    d. internal oblique muscles

40. The fascial interface of the anterior abdominal wall is located directly anterior to the:
    a. linea alba
    b. peritoneum
    c. subcutaneous fat
    d. rectus abdominis muscles

41. The Valsalva maneuver is a common technique used when evaluating the:
    a. pediatric hip
    b. Achilles tendon
    c. anterior abdominal wall
    d. gastrointestinal tract

42. A teenager arrives at the emergency department following a skiing injury. A nonvascular hypoechoic mass is identified in the posterior popliteal fossa. This mass most likely represents a(n):
    a. Baker cyst
    b. lymph node
    c. hematoma
    d. pseudoaneurysm

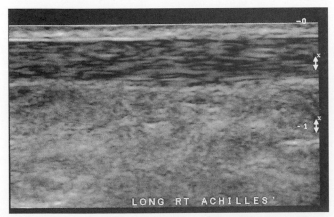

FIG. 15.14   Sagittal sonogram of the Achilles tendon.

43. Which approach is used to evaluate for hip effusion?
    a. medial
    b. lateral
    c. anterior
    d. posterior

44. The Graf technique is used to evaluate which of the following joints?
    a. hip
    b. knee
    c. wrist
    d. shoulder

Using Figure 15.16, answer question 45.

45. A patient presents with a history of sharp burning foot pain radiating to the third and fourth toes. Based on this clinical history, the calipers are most likely measuring a:
    a. lipoma
    b. muscle tear
    c. synovial cyst
    d. Morton neuroma

46. Measurement of the Achilles tendon should be made in the:
    a. sagittal plane
    b. transverse plane
    c. coronal plane
    d. supine position

47. A complete tear of the Achilles tendon is most commonly located:
    a. at the superior insertion
    b. in the medial portion of the tendon near the medial malleolus
    c. approximately 2 to 6 cm from the superior tendon insertion
    d. in the distal portion of the tendon near the calcaneus

48. Which of the following muscles extends the entire length of the anterior abdominal wall?
    a. linea alba
    b. external oblique
    c. rectus abdominis
    d. internal oblique

49. Which of the following vascular structures is a key sonographic landmark used when evaluating for an inguinal hernia
    a. internal iliac artery
    b. common femoral artery
    c. inferior epigastric artery
    d. superior epigastric artery

50. A lipoma located in the anterior abdominal wall most commonly appears on ultrasound as a:
    a. anechoic mass
    b. complex mass
    c. hyperechoic mass
    d. hypoechoic mass

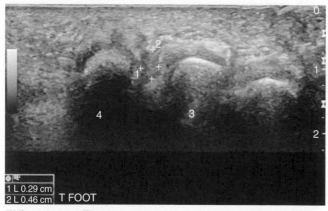

FIG. 15.16 Transverse sonogram of the left metatarsal bones.

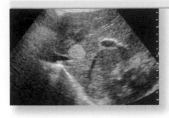

CHAPTER 16

Male Pelvis

KEY TERMS

appendix testis   a small solid structure located posterior to the epididymal head.

central zone (CZ)   cone-shaped area of the prostate gland located deep in the peripheral zone.

corpus cavernosa   the two columns of erectile tissue forming the body of the penis.

corpus spongiosum   the mass of spongy tissue surrounding the urethra.

cryptorchidism   undescended testis.

Denonvilliers' fascia   separates the prostate and rectum; important landmark for radical prostatectomy.

epididymis   long, tightly coiled ducts that carry sperm from the testis to the vas deferens.

epididymitis   inflammation of the epididymis; commonly caused by a urinary tract infection; most common cause of acute scrotal pain.

hydrocele   abnormal accumulation of serous fluid between the two layers of tunica vaginalis.

hypospadias   urethra opening is located somewhere along the undersurface of the penis.

mediastinum testis   thick portion of the tunica albuginea.

peripheral zone (PZ)   the largest area of the prostate gland located just beneath the capsule.

periurethral glands   glandular tissue lining the proximal prostatic urethra.

Peyronie's disease   Fibrous scar tissue most commonly along the dorsal portion of the penis within tunica albuginea that may progress to calcification(s).

polyorchidism   more than two testes.

prostate specific antigen (PSA)   a protein produced by the prostate; elevation is associated with carcinoma of the prostate gland.

orchitis   inflammation of the testis; commonly caused by chlamydia.

rete testis   network of ducts formed in the mediastinum testis connecting the epididymis with the superior portion of the testis.

space of Retzius   retropubic space between the symphysis pubis and urinary bladder.

spermatic cord   supporting structure on the posterior border of the testes that courses through the inguinal canal.

spermatocele   a cyst arising from the rete testis.

surgical capsule   hypoechoic connective tissue dividing the peripheral and central zones.

testicular torsion   twisting of the spermatic cord upon itself, obstructing the blood vessels supplying the epididymis and testis; also known as bell clapper.

transitional zone (TZ)   two small areas of the prostate gland adjacent to the proximal urethral space.

transurethral resection prostatectomy (TURP)   a surgical procedure to relieve symptoms of benign prostatic hypertrophy; demonstrates as an anechoic space in the center of the prostate.

varicocele   dilatation of the spermatic veins; most common cause of male infertility.

vas deferens   a small tube that transports the sperm from each testis to the prostatic urethra.

verumontanum   divides the urethra into proximal and distal segments.

PHYSIOLOGY

Function of the Scrotum

- Allows maintenance of a lower body temperature necessary for sperm survival.

Functions of the Epididymis

- Store and transport sperm produced by the testes.
- Mature the sperm.

Functions of the Testis

- Produce testosterone.
- Germinate sperm.

Functions of the Prostate Gland

- Secretes alkaline fluid to transport sperm.
- Secretions contain alkaline phosphatase, citric acid, and prostate specific antigen (PSA).
- Produces 80% to 85% of the ejaculation fluid.
- Produces PSA.
- Testosterone and dihydrotestosterone regulate prostate growth and function.

Functions of the Penis

- Transport urine out of the body.
- Male sex organ.

ANATOMY

Scrotum (Fig. 16.1)

- A two-compartment pouch that contains and supports each testis.
- Divided by a medium raphe or septum.
- Contains a number of tissue layers and vascular structures.

Epididymis

- Empties into the ductus deferens (vas deferens).
- Located lateral and posterior to the testis.
- Extends from the superior to the inferior pole of each testis.
- Divided into:
  - Head—located posterior and superior to the testis.
  - Body—located directly posterior to the testis.
  - Tail—located posterior and inferior to the testis.

Testes

- Paired male reproductive organs located in the scrotum.
- Endocrine and exocrine glands.
- Composed of multiple lobules.

Tunica Albuginea

- Fibrous sheath enclosing each testis.

Tunica Vaginalis

- Two layers of serous membrane (visceral and parietal) covering the anterior and lateral portions of the testis and epididymis.

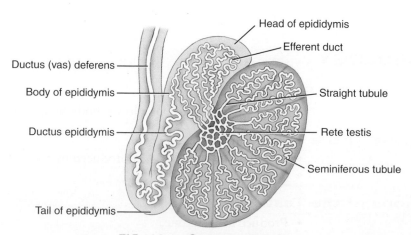

FIG. 16.1 Scrotum anatomy.

- Visceral layer surrounds the tunica albuginea and parietal layer lines the scrotal sac.
- Small amount of fluid is normal within these layers to prevent friction.
- Potential space for fluid collections (e.g., hydrocele).

Mediastinum Testis

- Thick portion of the tunica albuginea.
- Located in the posterior medial border of the testis.

Rete Testis

- Network of ducts formed in the mediastinum testis.
- Transports seminal fluid from the testis to the epididymis.
- Connects the epididymis to the superior testis.

Spermatic Cord

- Support structure located on the posterior border of the testes.
- Courses between the abdominal cavity and scrotum
- Located in the inguinal canal superior to the testicles.
- Made up of arteries, veins, nerves, lymphatics, seminal duct, fatty and connective tissues.

Vas Deferens

- A small tube that transports sperm from each testis to the prostatic urethra.
- Also called ductus deferens.

Prostate Gland (Fig. 16.2)

- A cone-shaped retroperitoneal structure.
- Inferior border (apex) provides an exit for the urethra.
- Superior border (base) is in contact with the urinary bladder.
- Consists of five lobes: anterior, middle, posterior, and two lateral lobes.
- Divided into three zones: central, peripheral, and transitional zones.
- Lies inferior to the seminal vesicles and urinary bladder.
- Lies posterior to the symphysis pubis and anterior to the rectal ampulla (space of Retzius).
- Lies anterior to Denonvilliers' fascia, which separates the prostate and rectum.
- Attached to the symphysis pubis by prostatic ligaments.
- The urethra is the anatomical landmark dividing the prostate into anterior (fibromuscular) and posterior (glandular) sections.

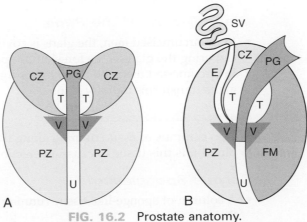

FIG. 16.2   Prostate anatomy.

Central Zone (CZ)

- Comprises approximately 25% of the glandular tissue.
- Resistant to disease.
- Midline wedge at the base of the prostate between the peripheral and transitional zones.

Peripheral Zone (PZ)

- Comprises approximately 70% of the glandular tissue.
- Surrounds the distal urethral segment.
- Separated from the central zone by the surgical capsule.
- Occupies the posterior, lateral, and apical regions of the prostate.
- Site for most prostate cancer.

Transitional Zone (TZ)

- Comprises 5% of the glandular tissue and periurethral glands.
- Two small glandular areas adjacent to the proximal urethral sphincter.
- Bound caudally by the verumontanum.
- Separated laterally and posteriorly from the outer glands by the surgical capsule.
- Area where benign prostatic hypertrophy (BPH) originates.

Periurethral Glands

- Comprise 1% of glandular tissue.
- Tissue lines the prostatic urethra.

Seminal Vesicles

- Paired structures lying superior to the prostate, posterior to the bladder, and lateral to the vas deferens.
- Ducts of the seminal vesicles enter the central zone.
- Joins the vas deferens to form the ejaculatory ducts.
- Stores sperm.

Surgical Capsule

- Connective tissue separating the peripheral and central zones.
- Surgical boundary line used in transurethral resection procedures.
- Not a true capsule.

Verumontanum

- Divides the urethra into proximal and distal segments.
- Region where the ejaculatory ducts enter the urethra.

Penis (Fig. 16.3)

- The penis is made of several parts:

Glans (Head) of the Penis

- In uncircumcised men, the glans is covered with pink, moist tissue called mucosa.
- Covering the glans is the foreskin (prepuce).
- In circumcised men, the foreskin is surgically removed and the mucosa on the glans transforms into dry skin.

Corpus Cavernosum

- Two columns of tissue running along the sides of the penis.
- Blood fills this tissue to cause an erection.

Corpus Spongiosum

- A column of sponge-like tissue running along the front of the penis and ending at the glans penis.
- The urethra runs through the corpus spongiosum.

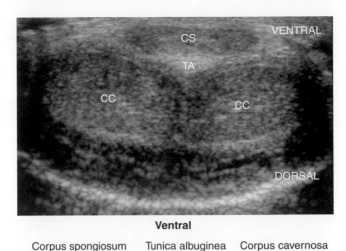

Ventral

Corpus spongiosum   Tunica albuginea   Corpus cavernosa

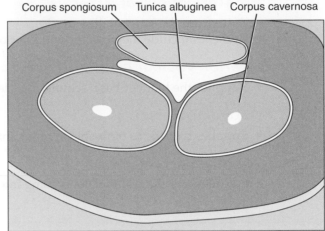

Dorsal

FIG. 16.3 Transverse scanning plane image of an axial section of the penis.

- It fills with blood during an erection, keeping the urethra open.
- The three corpora are separated by the tunica albuginea.
- Thick, fibrous, loose skin covers the penis, termed Buck's fascia.

VASCULAR ANATOMY

Scrotum

Testicular Arteries

- Arise from the anterior aspect of the abdominal aorta.
- Branch in the posterior portion of the superior testis.
- Course along the periphery toward the mediastinum testis.
- Low-resistance flow, demonstrating low-flow velocity (15 cm/s).

Centripetal Arteries

- Arise from the capsular arteries coursing from the testicular surface toward the mediastinum and branch into multiple rami arteries.
- Low-resistance blood flow, demonstrating low-flow velocity (5 to 20 cm/s).

Cremasteric and Deferential Arteries

- Contained in the spermatic cord.
- Supply the extratesticular structures.
- Cremasteric arteries supply peritesticular tissues.

- Deferential arteries supply the epididymis and vas deferens.
- Anastamose with the testicular artery provide flow to the testis.
- High-resistance blood flow.

Testicular Veins

- Left testicular vein empties into the left renal vein.
- Right testicular vein empties directly into the inferior vena cava.

Spermatic Vein

- Normal size 1 to 2 mm.
- Dilated when diameter exceeds 2 mm.

Prostate

Prostaticovesical Arteries

- Arise from the internal iliac arteries.
- Branches include the prostatic and inferior vesical arteries.

Inferior Vesical Artery

- Supplies the bladder base, seminal vesicles, and the ureter.

Capsular Arteries

- Supplies two-thirds of the blood going into the prostate.

Urethral Artery

- Supplies one-third of the blood going into the prostate.

Penis

Arterial Supply

- Blood supply to the penis and urethra is through the paired internal pudendal arteries (branches of the internal iliac arteries).
- The internal pudendal arteries subdivided into a deep cavernosal artery of the penis and bulbouretheral artery.
- Deep cavernosal artery supplies the corpus cavernosum.
- Branches of the dorsal artery and bulbouretheral artery supply the corpus spongiosum, glans penis, and urethra.

Venous Drainage

- Superficial dorsal and the deep dorsal veins are the main source of venous drainage.
- Superficial dorsal vein lies outside of Buck's fascia while the deep dorsal vein lies beneath Buck's fascia.
- Superficial and deep dorsal veins connect with the pudendal venous plexus that ultimately drains into the internal pudendal vein and then the internal iliac veins.

Congenital Anomalies—Male Pelvis

ANOMALY	DESCRIPTION	CLINICAL FINDINGS	SONOGRAPHIC FINDINGS	DIFFERENTIAL CONSIDERATIONS
Cryptorchidism	Undescended testis 80% are located in the inguinal canal Associated with a herniated scrotal sac and an increased risk of infertility, torsion, and malignancy Normal testes will descend by 6 months of age	Absence of testis in the scrotum Palpable inguinal mass	Absence of testis in the scrotum Oval-shaped homogeneous, hypoechoic mass in the inguinal canal, pelvis, or retroperitoneum May measure smaller than a normal testis Generally mobile within inguinal canal	Lymph node Hematoma Bowel
Polyorchidism	Presence of more than two testes Associated with inguinal hernia, testicular torsion, and malignancy	Asymptomatic Enlarged scrotum Palpable scrotal mass	Small echogenic extratesticular mass similar to the testis Usually located in the superior medial aspect of the scrotum	Epididymal neoplasm Testicular neoplasm Epididymitis
Agenesis of the seminal vesicles	Absence of seminal vesicles Associated with ipsilateral renal agenesis	Asymptomatic Urinary retention Perirenal pain	Absence of the hypoechoic seminal vesicles	Technical error Epididymal neoplasm
Megalourethra	Agenesis of the corpus cavernosa and/ or corpus spongiosum **Classifications** Fusiform Complete agenesis of all corpora Scaphoid (most common and least severe) Associated with Prune belly syndrome	Grossly enlarged penis Dilation of the penile shaft with voiding Associated with hydronephrosis and hydroureters	Anechoic area in anterior penis Distended bladder Thick bladder wall Associated with bilateral hydronephrosis and hydroureters Posterior urethra may be dilated	Urethral diverticulum Posterior urethral valve Urethral agenesis

SIZE

Adult

- Testis: 3 to 5 cm in length, 3 cm in height, and 2 to 4 cm in width.
- Epididymis: 10 to 12 mm in the superior portion (head), 2 to 4 mm in the posterior portion (body), and 2.5 mm in the inferior portion (tail).
- Prostate: 2 cm in length, 3 cm in height, and 4 cm in width.

Prepuberty

- Testis: 2.0 to 2.5 cm in length.

Infant

- Testis: 1.0 to 1.5 cm in length.

SONOGRAPHIC APPEARANCE

Scrotum

- Thin hyperechoic wall measuring 2 to 8 mm in thickness.
- Small amount of anechoic fluid surrounds each testis.
- Vascular structures are prominent inferiorly.

Testes

- Homogeneous parenchyma demonstrating a medium-level to low-level echo pattern.
- Ovoid in shape.
- The mediastinum testis appears as a hyperechoic linear structure located in the medial and posterior aspect of each testis.
- Low-resistance, low-velocity intratesticular blood flow demonstrating continuous flow throughout diastole.
- Hypoechoic parenchyma is demonstrated in infants and children.
- The echogenicity of the testes should be symmetrical.
- Intratesticular Doppler blood flow should be symmetrical.

Epididymis

- Homogeneous structure demonstrating a medium-level to low-level echo pattern.
- Isoechoic to hypoechoic compared with the normal testis.
- Coarser echo pattern compared with the normal testis.
- Minimal or no discernible internal blood flow.

Spermatic Cord

- Hypoechoic to isoechoic structure superior to the testicles.
- Multiple linear strands in sagittal orientation.
- Round or oval in shape in transverse orientation.

Prostate

- Homogeneous structure demonstrating a medium-level echo pattern.
- Peripheral zone appears uniform in texture and slightly more echogenic than the central zone.
- Hyperechoic band (surgical capsule) separates the peripheral and central zones.
- Seminal vesicles appear as hypoechoic structures superior to the prostate gland.
- Verumontanum appears hyperechoic compared with the parenchyma.

Penis

- Corpus spongiosum is located in the midline with a homogeneous medium-level echo pattern.
- Corpus cavernosa are symmetrical, display a medium-level echo pattern and are located posterior to the corpus spongiosum.
- Corpus cavernosa are covered by a highly echogenic tunica albuginea.
- Centrally located within the corpus cavernosa are the cavernous arteries.

EXAMINATION TECHNIQUES, PROTOCOLS, AND IMAGE OPTIMIZATION

Preparation

- No preparation is necessary for a sonogram of the scrotum and penis.
- Prostate—transrectal approach is the preferred technique.
  - Transabdominal—full urinary bladder.
  - Transrectal—empty urinary bladder.

Transducer Selection

Scrotum

- Use the highest frequency possible to obtain optimal resolution for penetration depth.
  - Adults—7.5 MHz to 12 MHz linear.
  - Children and small adults—10 MHz to 15 MHz linear.
- Lower frequency and/or curvilinear transducer may be used with an extremely swollen scrotum.

Prostate

- Use the highest frequency possible to obtain optimal resolution for penetration depth.
  - Transabdominal—3 MHz to 5 MHz curvilinear.
  - Transrectal—5 MHz to 8 MHz transrectal.

Penis

- Use the highest frequency possible to obtain optimal resolution for penetration depth.
  - 12 MHz to 15 MHz linear.
  - 10 MHz to 15 MHz linear for deeper structures.

Patient Positioning

Scrotum

- Supine with the legs slightly apart and a rolled towel place under scrotum for support.
- Cover the patient's pelvis with a towel and ask patient to place his penis on his abdomen.

Prostate

- Transabdominal.
  - Supine.
- Transrectal.
  - Left lateral decubitus with knees flexed toward the chest.

Penis

- Supine with dorsum of the penis lying against the abdomen.

Examination Protocol

Scrotum

- Systematic evaluation and bilateral imaging of the head, body, and tail of the epididymis and upper, mid, and lower portions of the testes in the sagittal and transverse planes.
- Measure length, height, and width of each testis.
- Measure the head, body, and/or tail of each epididymis.
- Duplex imaging of testes to evaluate vascular flow.
- Evaluate each testicle and epididymis using the same gray-scale and Doppler settings to compare symmetry of parenchymal echogenicity and vascularity.
- Abnormalities of the scrotum and/or scrotal contents should be documented and when applicable measured in two imaging planes. Color and/or spectral Doppler evaluation of the abnormality should be included.
- Varicocele—measure the size of the vein(s) with and without Valsalva.

Prostate

- Transabdominal.
  - Angle caudally through the urinary bladder to visualize the prostate.

- Measure length, height, and width of the prostate.
- Color Doppler to evaluate for normal vascular flow.
- Abnormalities of the prostate should be documented and when applicable measured in two imaging planes. Color and/or spectral Doppler evaluation of the abnormality should be included.

Transrectal

- Invert the ultrasound image so the near field is at the bottom of the screen.
- Sagittal—the base of the prostate will be on the left of the screen; rectal wall can be seen in the near field; bladder in the far field.
- Transverse imaging plane starting at the level of the seminal vesicles then angle caudally, to evaluate and image the entire prostate from the base to the apex.
- Sagittal imaging plane angling both left and right evaluating and imaging the prostate gland, urethra, and the verumontanum.
- Measure length, height, and width of prostate.
- Color Doppler imaging to evaluate for normal vascular flow.
- Abnormalities of the prostate should be documented and when applicable measured in two imaging planes. Color and/or spectral Doppler evaluation of the abnormality should be included.

Penis

- Systematic dorsal, lateral, or ventral approach in the sagittal, coronal, and transverse planes carefully examining and imaging the focused area of interest using the national or institution protocol.
- Visualization of all three cylindrical portions of the penis in the area of interest.
- Evaluate both corpus cavernosa for symmetry in echogenicity, shape and size.
- Palpable areas and areas of interest should be annotated on image.
- Abnormalities of the penis should be documented and when applicable measured in two imaging planes. Color and/or spectral Doppler evaluation of the abnormality should be included.

Image Optimization

- Place gains settings to display the to the normal testicle, prostate or corpus cavernosa parenchyma a medium shade of gray with adjustments to reduce artifactually produced echoes within normally anechoic structures.
- Focal zone(s) should be placed at or below the area of interest. The use of multiple focal zones increases detail resolution and decreases temporal resolution.
- Sufficient imaging depth to visualize structures immediately posterior to the area of interest.
- Harmonic imaging and decreasing system compression (dynamic range) can be used to reduce artifactual echoes.
- Spatial compounding can be used to improve visualization of structures posterior to highly attenuating structures (e.g., calcification).
- Doppler settings should be adjusted for a slow flow rate.

Examination Limitations

- Patient cooperation (e.g., pain, modesty).
- Near-field reverberation.

Helpful Hints

- Power Doppler may aid in detecting low flow velocities.

Scrotum

- Pressing down on the ipsilateral medial superior thigh can aid in transducer/skin contact.

Prostate

- Central zone comprises the majority of the base of the prostate.
- Vas deferens can be seen between the seminal vesicles.

Penis

- Use of a stand-off pad can improve visualization of superficial pathology.
- Visualization of the cavernosal arteries may be difficult to identify in a flaccid penis.
- Warm compresses along penis will help accentuate small arteries.

Indications for Scrotal Examination

- Scrotal pain.
- Scrotal trauma.
- Enlarged scrotum.
- Palpable scrotal mass.
- Infertility.
- Undescended testis.
- Evaluate mass from previous medical imaging study (e.g., computed tomography).

Indications for Prostate Examination

- Enlarged prostate.
- Changes in urination.
- Elevated PSA level.
- Infertility.
- Routine screening starting at age 50.
- Evaluate mass from previous medical imaging study (e.g., computed tomography).

Indications for Penis Examination

- Vasculogenic impotence.
- Painful erection.
- Palpable mass.
- Trauma.
- Evaluate mass from previous medical imaging study (e.g., computed tomography).

LABORATORY VALUES

Prostate Specific Antigen

- Normal monoclonal PSA 4.0 ng/mL.
- Protein produced by the prostate.
- Level greater than 20 ng/mL indicates a strong likelihood for carcinoma.
- Elevation of 20% in 1 year is considered abnormal.

Scrotal Pathology

PATHOLOGY	ETIOLOGY	CLINICAL FINDINGS	SONOGRAPHIC FINDINGS	DIFFERENTIAL CONSIDERATIONS
Calculus Aka: scrotal pearl	Inflammation of the tunica vaginalis Torsion of the appendix testis or epididymis	Asymptomatic Palpable scrotal mass	Hyperechoic focus Mobile Posterior acoustic shadowing Round in shape	Arterial calcification
Edema	Idiopathic Peritoneal dialysis Heart or liver failure Lymphatic or venous obstruction	Swollen scrotum Erythema	Hypoechoic or complex scrotal wall thickening Scrotal wall may demonstrate striations Scrotal wall may demonstrate hypervascularity May demonstrate reactive hydrocele Normal testes	Technical error
Hematocele	Trauma Ruptured varicocele	Scrotal pain Scrotal mass	Anechoic fluid collection with swirling debris. Thickened scrotal wall with septations when chronic	Chronic hydrocele Loculated hydrocele Testicular torsion
Hernia	Weak abdominal wall muscles Inguinal hernia may extend into the scrotum	Scrotal mass Abdominal pain	Complex extratesticular mass Mass can be traced to the inguinal canal May contain bowel and/or omentum	Testicular torsion Hematocele
Hydrocele	Inflammation Idiopathic Congenital Associated with torsion, trauma, or malignancy	Enlarged scrotum Asymptomatic Scrotal mass Scrotal pain	Anechoic fluid collection lateral and anterior to the testis Strong posterior acoustic enhancement Thin scrotal wall when acute Diffuse scrotal wall thickening when chronic May demonstrate internal echoes or septations	Epididymal cyst Spermatocele Hematocele Hernia
Varicocele	Idiopathic Incompetent valves in the spermatic vein	Asymptomatic Infertility Tender scrotal mass Scrotal ache	Tortuous venous structures exceeding 2 mm in diameter Most commonly located on the left and in the inferior portion of the scrotum Veins increase in size with Valsalva maneuver or while patient is standing	Loculated hydrocele Epididymal cyst

Epididymal Pathology

PATHOLOGY	ETIOLOGY	CLINICAL FINDINGS	SONOGRAPHIC FINDINGS	DIFFERENTIAL CONSIDERATIONS
Adenomatoid tumor	Most common benign tumor Found commonly in the epididymis	Asymptomatic	Variable echogenicity from hypo- to hyperechoic Small in size (less than 2 cm)	Focal epididymitis
Cyst	Cystic dilatation of epididymal tubules Vasectomy	Asymptomatic Palpable scrotal mass	Anechoic mass in the epididymis Compression of the testis Absence of internal blood flow	Spermatocele Loculated hydrocele Varicocele

Epididymal Pathology—(cont'd)

PATHOLOGY	ETIOLOGY	CLINICAL FINDINGS	SONOGRAPHIC FINDINGS	DIFFERENTIAL CONSIDERATIONS

Epididymitis	Lower urinary infection
	Idiopathic
	Trauma
		Acute scrotal pain
		Palpable posterior
		  mass
		Leukocytosis
		Fever
		Dysuria
			Enlarged hypoechoic
			  epididymis
			Hypervascular epididymis
			Hyperechoic with calcifica-
			  tions when chronic
			Small cysts may be
			  visualized
				Testicular torsion
				Varicocele

Spermatocele	Retention cyst arising
	  from the rete testis
	Idiopathic
	Infection
	Trauma
		Asymptomatic
		Palpable scrotal
		  mass
			Anechoic mass lying
			  superior to the testis
			Round or oval in shape
			Does not compress testis
			Absence of internal
			  vascular flow
				Loculated hydrocele
				Epididymal cyst

Testicular Pathology

PATHOLOGY	ETIOLOGY	CLINICAL FINDINGS	SONOGRAPHIC FINDINGS	DIFFERENTIAL CONSIDERATIONS

Abscess	Complication of
	  untreated
	  epididymo-orchitis
		Fever
		Scrotal pain
		Scrotal swelling
			Complex testicular or
			  epididymal mass
			Hypervascular peripheral
			  flow
			Lack of blood flow within
			  mass
				Neoplasm

Cyst	Incidence increases
	  with age
		Asymptomatic	Anechoic mass within the
			  testis
			Smooth wall margins
			Posterior acoustic
			  enhancement
			Absence of internal
			  vascular flow
				Resolving hematoma
				Vascular structure
				Neoplasm

Malignant
neoplasm
	Germ cell neoplasm—
	  most common
	  seminoma
	Teratoma
	Stromal neoplasm
	Metastases
		Asymptomatic
		Palpable scrotal
		  mass
		Scrotal swelling
			Solid hypoechoic
			  intratesticular mass
			May appear complex
			Hypervascular mass
			  periphery
			Reactive hydrocele
				Abscess
				Hematoma
				Focal orchitis

Microcalcifications	Idiopathic
	Calcified vessels
	Granulomatosis
		Asymptomatic	Multiple small hyperechoic
			  foci dispersed in the
			  testis parenchyma
			Usually bilateral
			Associated with a neoplasm
			  in 40% of cases
				Neoplasm
				Chronic orchitis
				Resolving hematoma

Orchitis	Chlamydia—most
	  common
	Secondary to
	  epididymitis
		Scrotal pain
		Scrotal swelling
		Fever
		Nausea/vomiting
		Elevated WBC
			Enlarged hypoechoic testis
			  parenchyma
			Increase in intratesticular
			  vascular flow
			Hydrocele
			Complex areas of necrosis
			Atrophy and intratesticular
			  calcifications are
			  demonstrated in
			  chronic cases
				Testicular torsion
				Neoplasm

Continued

Testicular Pathology—(cont'd)

PATHOLOGY	ETIOLOGY	CLINICAL FINDINGS	SONOGRAPHIC FINDINGS	DIFFERENTIAL CONSIDERATIONS
Tubular ectasia of the rete testis	Usually associated with epididymal obstruction resulting from trauma or inflammation	Asymptomatic	Cystic lesion demonstrated in the region of the mediastinum testis Variable in size Usually bilateral and asymmetrical	Carcinoma
Testicular rupture	Trauma	Scrotal pain Scrotal swelling Palpable scrotal mass	Irregular fibrous testicular capsule Extrusion of the testis into the scrotal sac Hematocele	Neoplasm Hematoma
Testicular torsion **Salvage rate** 80%–100% within 6 hours 70% within 6–12 hours Greater than 12 hours can result in complete infarction	Twisting of the spermatic cord on itself, obstructing the blood vessels supplying the epididymis and testis Epididymis and testis are not properly anchored "bell clapper"	Sudden onset of groin or scrotal pain Lower abdominal pain Nausea/vomiting Scrotal swelling	Hypoechoic parenchyma (acute) Hetergeneous parenchyma (chronic) May appear enlarged Markedly absent or decreased intratesticular blood flow Hydrocele	Neoplasm Hematoma Improper Doppler settings and angle

Prostate Pathology

PATHOLOGY	ETIOLOGY	CLINICAL FINDINGS	SONOGRAPHIC FINDINGS	DIFFERENTIAL CONSIDERATIONS
Benign prostatic hypertrophy	Noninflammatory enlargement of the prostate gland Usually occurs in the transitional zone	Urinary frequency Dysuria Decreased urinary output Urinary tract infection	Symmetrical prostate enlargement Hypoechoic parenchyma May demonstrate nodules, cysts, or calcifications Associated hydronephrosis	Carcinoma
Carcinoma	Idiopathic Associated with hormone production	Asymptomatic Hematuria Bladder obstruction Elevated PSA	Small hypoechoic nodules Smooth or irregular wall margins Asymmetrical prostate enlargement Thickening of the bladder wall Majority located in the peripheral zone	Seminal vesicle Benign prostatic hypertrophy
Cyst	Congenital or acquired Occurs laterally in any of the three zones	Asymptomatic Benign prostatic hypertrophy	Anechoic prostate mass Smooth wall margins Posterior acoustic enhancement Lack of internal vascular flow	Resolving hematoma Vascular structure Post-TURP scar
Prostatitis	Infection Acute or chronic inflammation of the prostate gland	**Acute** Rectal and prostate tenderness Fever **Chronic** Urinary frequency and urgency Dysuria	**Acute** Normal prostate Diffuse hyperechoic parenchyma Hypervascularity **Chronic** Heterogenous parenchyma Calcification(s) Capsular thickening Prostate atrophy	Calcifications

Penile Pathology

PATHOLOGY	ETIOLOGY	CLINICAL FINDINGS	SONOGRAPHIC FINDINGS	DIFFERENTIAL CONSIDERATIONS
Peyronie's disease	Idiopathic Trauma Medication side effect	Pain with marked curvature of the penis Erectile dysfunction Palpable mass(es)	Focal hyperechoic thickening, echogenic plaque or calcifications located in the tunica albuginea May demonstrate posterior acoustic shadowing	Congenital curvature of the penis Arterial calcification(s)
Trauma	Penile injury during erection	Popping sound with sharp pain followed by rapid decrease in erection Penile discoloration Penile deformity	Irregular hypo- or hyperechoic area that courses transversely Adjacent hypoechoic to complex mass (hematoma) Most commonly located on the ventral surface Evaluate tunica albuginea for interruption	Thrombosis of deep or superficial dorsal veins

SCROTUM AND PROSTATE REVIEW

1. A hydrocele is defined as an abnormal fluid collection between the:
   a. tunica albuginea and the tunica vaginalis
   b. two layers of the tunica vaginalis
   c. spermatic cord and the tunica vaginalis
   d. two layers of the tunica albuginea

2. "Bell clapper" is another term used to describe which of the following abnormalities?
   a. hydrocele
   b. microcalcifications
   c. testicular torsion
   d. cryptorchidism

3. Normal testes will descend into the scrotal sac by:
   a. 6 months of age
   b. 12 months of age
   c. 2 years of age
   d. 3 years of age

4. Carcinoma of the prostate gland most commonly develops in the:
   a. central zone
   b. peripheral zone
   c. seminal vesicles
   d. transitional zone

5. Which of the following is a common sonographic finding in Peyronie's disease?
   a. Hyperechoic focus within the scrotal sac
   b. Aneurysm of the internal pudendal arteries
   c. Calcifications located in the tunica albuginea
   d. Thrombosis of the superficial dorsal vein

6. A fibrous sheath enclosing the testis describes which of the following structures?
   a. rete testis
   b. vas deferens
   c. tunica albuginea
   d. tunica vaginalis

7. Which of the following functions is considered a responsibility of the prostate gland?
   a. stores sperm
   b. matures sperm
   c. germinates sperm
   d. produces ejaculation fluid

8. The thickened portion of the tunica albuginea is termed the:
   a. rete testis
   b. vas deferens
   c. seminal vesicles
   d. mediastinum testis

9. Which of the following structures supports the posterior border of the testes?
   a. epididymis
   b. rete testes
   c. spermatic cord
   d. mediastinum testis

10. Which of the following structures divides the male urethra into proximal and distal segments?
    a. seminal vesicles
    b. surgical capsule
    c. vas deferens
    d. verumontanum

11. An anechoic structure arising from the rete testes describes which of the following structures?
    a. epididymal cyst
    b. testicular cyst
    c. spermatocele
    d. prostate cyst

12. A scrotal pearl demonstrates on ultrasound as a(n):
    a. immobile hypoechoic focus
    b. mobile hyperechoic focus
    c. mobile hypoechoic focus
    d. immobile hyperechoic focus

13. A spermatic vein is considered dilated after the diameter exceeds:
    a. 2 mm
    b. 4 mm
    c. 6 mm
    d. 8 mm

14. The scrotum is divided into two separate compartments by the:
    a. medium raphe
    b. tunica vaginalis
    c. mediastinum testis
    d. spermatic cord

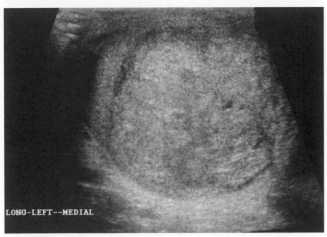

FIG. 16.4 Sagittal sonogram of the left testis.

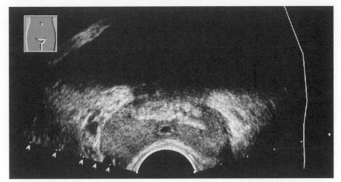

FIG. 16.6 Sonogram of the prostate gland.

Using Figure 16.4, answer question 15.

15. A 35-year-old patient presents with a palpable scrotal mass. The sonographic finding is most suspicious for which of the following abnormalities?
    a. acute orchitis
    b. testicular carcinoma
    c. epididymitis
    d. scrotal herniation

Using Figure 16.5, answer question 16.

16. The sonographic finding is most suspicious for:
    a. testicular rupture
    b. testicular carcinoma
    c. epididymitis
    d. scrotal hernia

Using Figure 16.6, answer question 17.

17. Hyperechoic foci are identified in which of the following regions of the prostate gland?
    a. peripheral zone
    b. surgical capsule
    c. central zone
    d. seminal vesicles

Using Figure 16.7, answer questions 18 and 19.

18. A 30-year-old patient presents with a tender scrotal mass. The sonographic finding is most suspicious for which of the following abnormalities?
    a. orchitis
    b. a scrotal hernia
    c. a varicocele
    d. epididymitis

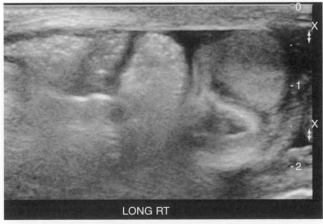

FIG. 16.5 Sagittal image of the right scrotum.

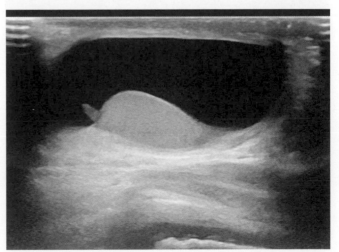

FIG. 16.7 Transverse sonogram of the inferior border of the left scrotum.

19. Which of the following complications is associated with this diagnosis?
    a. infertility
    b. reactive hydrocele
    c. testicular torsion
    d. deep vein thrombosis

Using Figure 16.8, answer questions 20 and 21.

20. The sonographic finding in this image is most consistent with a:
    a. hydrocele
    b. urinoma
    c. spermatocele
    d. scrotal edema

21. The echogenic structure superior to the testis most likely represents the:
    a. spermatic cord
    b. scrotal pearl
    c. polyorchidism
    d. appendix testis

22. Which of the following conditions most commonly causes epididymitis?
    a. hydrocele
    b. varicocele
    c. bladder infection
    d. inguinal hernia

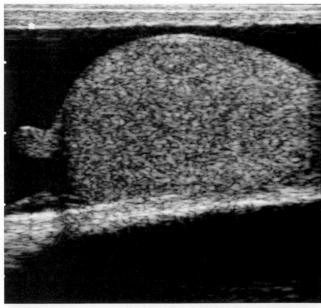

FIG. 16.8   Sagittal sonogram of the right scrotum.

23. Which of the following regions in the prostate most commonly develops benign prostatic hypertrophy (BPH)?
    a. central zone
    b. peripheral zone
    c. transitional zone
    d. periurethral glands

24. Twisting of the spermatic cord on itself is a predisposing factor of which of the following abnormalities?
    a. orchitis
    b. epididymitis
    c. spermatocele
    d. testicular torsion

25. Which of the following conditions is the most common cause of orchitis?
    a. epididymitis
    b. microlithiasis
    c. malignant neoplasm
    d. sexually transmitted infection

26. Sudden onset of severe scrotal pain in an adolescent patient is most suspicious for:
    a. orchitis
    b. varicocele
    c. epididymitis
    d. testicular torsion

27. The epididymis connects to the testis by which of the following structures?
    a. medium raphe
    b. vas deferens
    c. rete testis
    d. spermatic cord

28. The corpus spongiosum is located:
    a. anterior to the corpus cavernosa
    b. posterior to the corpus cavernosa
    c. lateral to the corpus cavernosa
    d. medial to the cavernous artery.

29. The majority of blood supplied to the prostate gland is through the:
    a. urethral artery
    b. capsular artery
    c. inferior vesical artery
    d. prostaticovesical arteries

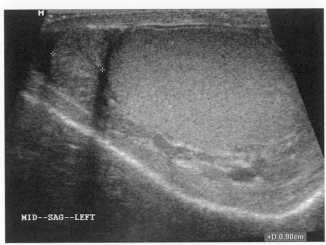

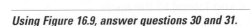

FIG. 16.9 Sonogram of the left scrotum.

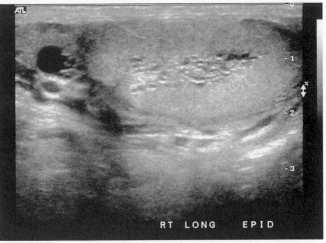

FIG. 16.10 Sagittal sonogram of the right scrotum.

Using Figure 16.9, answer questions 30 and 31.

30. The finding in the sonogram of the left scrotum is most suspicious for which of the following abnormalities?
a. hematocele
b. varicocele
c. epididymitis
d. scrotal hernia

31. An echogenic mass is identified superior to the testis and outlined by the calibers. This most likely represents which of the following structures?
a. inguinal hernia
b. adenomatoid tumor
c. head of the epididymis
d. appendix testis

Using Figure 16.10, answer questions 32 and 33.

32. The right testicle is demonstrating which of the following conditions?
a. acute orchitis
b. microcalcifications
c. malignant neoplasm
d. tubular ectasia of the rete testis

33. The contralateral testis in this patient will most likely demonstrate a:
a. spermatocele
b. cryptorchidism
c. normal appearance
d. tubular ectasia of the rete testis

Using Figure 16.11, answer question 34.

34. A palpable right scrotal mass is discovered during a recent physical examination. The sonographic finding is most consistent with which of the following abnormalities?
a. varicocele
b. hydrocele
c. testicular cyst
d. spermatocele

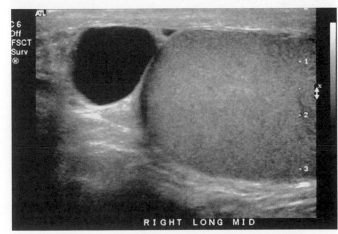

FIG. 16.11 Sagittal image of the right testis.

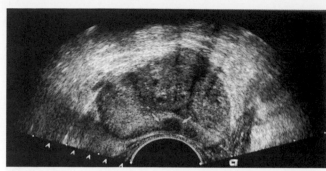

FIG. 16.12 Transrectal image of the prostate gland.

Using Figure 16.12, answer question 35.

35. The neoplasm identified by the arrows is located in which region of the prostate gland?
a. central zone
b. seminal vesical
c. transitional zone
d. peripheral zone

Using Figure 16.13, answer question 36.

36. This sagittal image of the left inguinal canal in an 8-month-old male infant is most likely demonstrating a(n):
a. lipoma
b. inguinal hernia
c. undescended testicle
d. enlarged lymph node

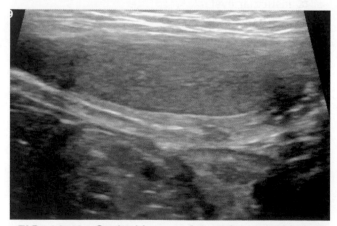

FIG. 16.13 Sagittal image of the left inguinal canal.

37. The normal monoclonal level of prostate specific antigen (PSA) should not exceed:
a. 2 ng/mL
b. 4 ng/mL
c. 6 ng/mL
d. 8 ng/mL

38. Decreased urine output is most commonly linked with an abnormality in which of the following structures?
a. testis
b. scrotum
c. epididymis
d. prostate gland

39. The location of the epididymis is most accurately described as:
a. posterior to the testis
b. posterior and medial to the testis
c. posterior and lateral to the testis
d. anterior and medial to the testis

40. Blood is supplied directly to the epididymis through which of the following arteries?
a. capsular
b. testicular
c. cremasteric
d. centripetal

41. Which of the following veins receives the left testicular vein?
a. left renal vein
b. inferior vena cava
c. left suprarenal vein
d. left internal iliac vein

42. Which of the following pathologies is the most common cause of acute scrotal pain in the adult patient?
a. orchitis
b. varicocele
c. epididymitis
d. testicular torsion

43. Which of the following most accurately describes the echogenicity and location of the seminal vesicles?
a. heterogeneous structures located anterior to the urinary bladder
b. homogeneous structures located inferior to the prostate gland
c. hypoechoic structures located superior to the prostate gland
d. homogeneous structures located medial to the vas deferens

44. Which of the following arteries is contained in the spermatic cord?
a. cremasteric
b. inferior vesical
c. centripetal
d. capsular

45. A 60-year-old patient presents with a history of urinary frequency and a decrease in urinary output. These clinical symptoms are most commonly associated with:
a. prostatitis
b. orchitis
c. prostate carcinoma
d. benign prostatic hypertrophy (BPH)

46. Cryptorchdism is associated with an increased risk in developing:
a. orchitis
b. epididymitis
c. testicular torsion
d. microcalcifications

47. Which region of the prostate gland comprises only 5% of the glandular tissue?
a. central zone
b. peripheral zone
c. transitional zone
d. periurethral glands

48. Which of the following structures lines the prostatic urethra?
a. vas deferens
b. verumontanum
c. periurethral glands
d. seminal vesicles

49. The lobes of the prostate gland are termed the:
a. anterior, posterior, and two lateral lobes
b. central, peripheral, and transitional lobes
c. superior, inferior, anterior, and posterior lobes
d. anterior, middle, posterior, and two lateral lobes

50. The sonographic appearance of the mediastinum testis is best described as a(n):
a. hyperechoic linear structure located in the posterior medial aspect of the testis
b. hypoechoic ovoid-shaped structure located in the posterior lateral aspect of the testis
c. hypoechoic linear structure located in the anterior medial aspect of the testis
d. hyperechoic tortuous structure located in the anterior medial aspect of the testis

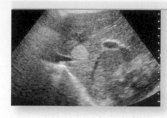

CHAPTER 17

Neck and Salivary Glands

KEY TERMS

brachial cleft cyst a congenital diverticulum of the brachial cleft located directly below the angle of the mandible.

exophthalmos bulging of the eyeballs; associated with hyperthyroidism.

de Quervain syndrome subacute thyroiditis secondary to a viral infection.

goiter a pronounced swelling of the neck caused by an enlarged thyroid gland.

Graves disease a multisystemic autoimmune disorder characterized by pronounced hyperthyroidism; usually associated with an enlarged thyroid and exophthalmos.

Hashimoto disease a progressive autoimmune inflammatory disorder of the thyroid gland; most common cause of hypothyroidism; associated with an increased risk of developing a thyroid malignancy. Most common cause of thyroid enlargement in children and hypothyroidism in adults.

hypercalcemia an excessive amount of calcium in the blood; associated with hyperparathyroidism.

hyperparathyroidism excessive function of the parathyroid glands; may lead to osteoporosis and nephrolithiasis.

hyperthyroidism hyperactivity of the thyroid gland; associated with Graves disease.

hypocalcemia a deficiency of calcium in the blood; associated with hypoparathyroidism.

hypoparathyroidism a condition of insufficient secretion of the parathyroid glands; associated with hypocalcemia and primary parathyroid dysfunction.

hypothyroidism decreased activity of the thyroid gland; associated with Hashimoto disease.

longus colli muscles neck muscles located on the anterior surface of the vertebral column, between the atlas and the third thoracic vertebra; commonly associated with whiplash injuries.

myxoedema the most severe form of hypothyroidism; characterized by swelling of the hands, face, and feet; may lead to coma and death.

postpartum thyroiditis a transient thyroiditis seen following pregnancy.

sternocleidomastoid muscles lateral and superficial neck muscles that attach to the sternum, clavicle, and the mastoid process of the temporal bone; act to flex and rotate the head.

strap muscles a group of long and flat muscles located anterior and lateral to each thyroid lobe; includes the sternohyoid, sternothyroid, and omohyoid muscles.

thyroglossal cyst an embryonic remnant cyst located between the isthmus of the thyroid and the tongue.

PHYSIOLOGY

Function of the Thyroid Glands

- Maintain body metabolism, growth, and development.
- Iodine is processed to manufacture, store, and secrete hormones: thyroxine, triiodothyronine, and calcitonin.
- Secretion of thyroid hormones is primarily controlled by the thyroid-stimulating hormone produced by the pituitary gland.
- Functions to control the basil metabolic rate (BMR).

Function of the Parathyroid Glands

- Maintain homeostasis of blood calcium concentrations.
- Secretes parathormone.

Function of the Salivary Glands

- Exocrine glands that secrete enzymes as saliva to aid in mouth lubrication, digestion, maintain tooth integrity, and antibacterial activity.

Function of the Carotid Arteries

- Supply blood to the head and neck.

Function of the Jugular Veins

- Drain blood from the head and neck.

ANATOMY (Fig. 17.1)

Muscles of the Neck

- Paired muscles located around the thyroid gland.

Longus Colli Muscles

- Located on the anterior surface of the vertebral column.
- Lie adjacent to the trachea and posterior to the thyroid lobe and common carotid artery.
- May be mistaken for an enlarged parathyroid gland.

Platysma Muscles

- Superficial muscles located in the lateral neck.
- Located posterior to the subcutaneous tissues.

Sternocleidomastoid Muscles

- Lateral and superficial neck muscles.
- Located lateral to the thyroid lobes, sternohyoid muscle and sternothyroid muscle.

Strap Muscles

- A collective group of long flat neck muscles.
- Located anterior and lateral to the thyroid gland.
- Include the:
  - **sternothyroid** – located directly superficial to the thyroid gland.
  - **omohyoid** – located lateral to the sternothyroid muscles.
  - **sternohyoid** – located anterior to the sternothyroid muscles.

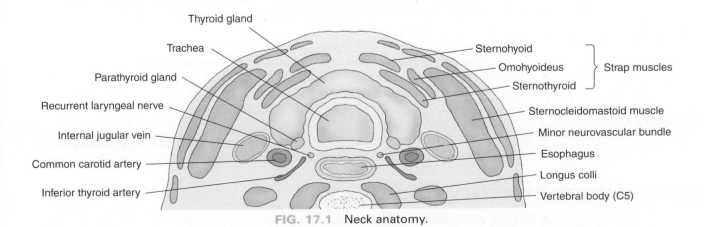

FIG. 17.1 Neck anatomy.

VASCULATURE OF THE NECK

Common Carotid Arteries

- Left originates from the aortic arch.
- Right arises from the innominate (brachiocephalic) artery.
- Ascend the anterolateral aspect of the neck.
- Lie medial to the internal jugular vein and lateral to the thyroid lobe.
- Course deep to the sternocleidomastoid muscles.
- Typically, no branches.
- Bifurcate into the external and internal carotid arteries.

External Carotid Arteries

- Supplies the neck, scalp, and face with blood.
- Lies anterior and medial to the internal carotid artery.
- Multiple extracranial branches.
- Superior thyroid artery is the first branch of the external carotid arteries.

Internal Carotid Arteries

- Main blood supply to the eyes and brain.
- Lie posterior and lateral to the external carotid artery.
- Terminate at the circle of Willis.
- No extracranial branches.
- Ophthalmic artery is the first branch of the internal carotid artery.

Vertebral Arteries

- Arise from the first segment of the subclavian artery.
- Provide blood to the posterior brain.
- Lie in the posterior neck, ascending through the transverse processes of the spine.
- Left and right vertebral arteries join to form the basilar artery at the base of the skull.
- Basilar artery terminates in the posterior aspect of the circle of Willis.
- Multiple extracranial branches.

Internal Jugular Veins

- Receive the major portion of blood from the brain, neck, and superficial parts of the face.
- Course lateral to the carotid artery.
- Unite with the subclavian vein, forming the innominate (brachiocephalic) vein.
- Right and left innominate veins join, forming the superior vena cava.

External Jugular Veins

- Receive blood from the exterior cranium and deep parts of the face.
- Located in the superficial fascia of the lateral neck.
- Empty into the subclavian vein.

Vertebral Veins

- Receive blood from the posterior brain and empty into the brachiocephalic vein.
- Located anterior to the corresponding vertebral artery.

ANATOMY OF THE THYROID GLANDS

- Largest endocrine gland in the human body.
- Divided into the right and left lobes with a connecting isthmus.
- Right lobe is usually larger than the left.
- Isthmus connects the lower third of the thyroid lobes.
- Consists of follicles, connective tissue, nerves, lymphatics, and stroma.
- Covered by two layers of connective tissue.

VASCULATURE OF THE THYROID GLANDS

- Superior thyroid arteries supply blood flow to the superior portion of the thyroid gland.
- Inferior thyroid arteries supply blood flow to the inferior portion of the thyroid gland.
- Superior thyroid artery arises from the external carotid artery.
- Inferior thyroid artery arises from the thyrocervical artery.
- Superior, middle thyroid veins drain into the internal jugular vein; inferior thyroid vein drains into the innominate vein.

ANATOMY OF THE PARATHYROID GLANDS

- Two paired, bean-shaped glands located posterior to the thyroid gland.

ANATOMY OF THE SALIVARY GLANDS

- Exocrine glands divided into lobules with a hilum where branching blood vessels, ducts and nerves are present.
- **Parotid gland.**
  - Largest of the salivary glands.
  - Shaped like an inverted pyramid.
  - Contains Stenson's duct (excretory duct).
  - Only salivary gland that has intraparenchymal lymph nodes.
- **Submandibular gland.**
  - Produce 70% of saliva.
  - Triangular in shape.
  - Contains Wharton's duct.
  - Glandular processes may connect the submandibular gland with the parotid and sublingual glands.
- **Sublingual gland.**
  - Small and oval in shape.
  - Contains 8 to 20 excretory glands.

LOCATION

Esophagus

- Located medial to the left thyroid lobe and posterior to the trachea.

Trachea

- Forms the medial border of the thyroid glands.

Thyroid Lobes

- Medial and anterior to the corresponding common carotid artery and internal jugular vein.
- Posterior and medial to the sternocleidomastoid and strap muscles.
- Anterior to the longus colli muscle.
- Anterolateral to the trachea and esophagus.
- Inferior to the thyroid cartilage of the larynx.

Thyroid Isthmus

- Anterior to the trachea.
- Medial and anterior to the common carotid arteries and internal jugular veins.

Parathyroid Glands

- Posterior to the thyroid glands.
- Anterior to the longus colli muscles.

Salivary Glands

Parotid Gland

- Anterior to the ear near the ramus of the mandible.
- Retromandibular vein separates the superior and deep lobes of the gland.

Submandibular Gland

- Located beneath the anterior mandible, inferior and lateral to the mylohoid muscle.

Sublingual Gland

- Located beneath the muscles of the tongue, medial to the mylohoid muscle and lateral to the hypoglossal muscle.

CONGENITAL ANOMALIES

Pyramidal Lobe

- Third lobe arising from the superior portion of the isthmus.
- Ascends to the level of the hyoid bone.
- Appears in 10% to 40% of patients.
- Begins to atrophy in adulthood.
- Appears isoechoic to the normal thyroid gland.

Absent Isthmus

- Thyroid consists of two distinct lobes.

Ectopic Parathyroid Gland Location

- May be found near the carotid bifurcation or posterior to the carotid artery.
- May also be located retroesophageal, substernal, submandibular, or intrathyroid.

SIZE

- Isthmus—0.2 to 0.6 cm in height.
- Thyroid glands (adult)—4.0 to 6.0 cm in length, 1.3 to 1.8 cm in height, and 1.5 to 2.0 cm in width.
- Thyroid glands (pediatric)—2.0 to 3.0 cm in length, 0.2 to 1.2 cm in height, and 1 to 1.5 cm in width.
- Parathyroid glands—up to 6 mm in length, 2 mm in height, and 4 mm in width.
- Parotid glands – up to 7 cm in length, and 3.5 cm in both height and width.
- Submandibular glands – averages 3.5 cm in length.
- Sublingual gland – up to 2.5 cm in length.

SONOGRAPHIC APPEARANCE

- **Thyroid lobes and isthmus** appear as homogeneous solid structures demonstrating a medium-gray echo pattern with a surrounding thin hyperechoic line.
- **Sternocleidomastoid muscle** are large and oval in shape appearing hypoechoic compared with the normal thyroid gland.
- **Strap muscles** are thin and hypoechoic compared with the normal thyroid gland.

- **Longus colli muscles** appear hypoechoic compared with the normal thyroid gland.
- **Parathyroid glands** are flat, bean-shaped hypoechoic structures located posterior and medial to the thyroid lobes.
- **Salivary glands** – homogeneous and hyperechoic compared with the normal surrounding muscle. Degree of echogenicity depends on the amount intraglandular fatty tissue.
- **Carotid arteries and jugular veins** appear as anechoic tubular structures demonstrating internal vascular flow.

EXAMINATION TECHNIQUES, PROTOCOLS, AND IMAGE OPTIMIZATION

Preparation

- No preparation is necessary for a sonogram of the neck or salivary glands.

Transducer Selection – Thyroid, Parathyroid, and Salivary Glands

- Use the highest frequency possible to obtain optimal resolution for penetration depth.
  - Adults – 5 MHz to 12 MHz linear.
  - Adults – 3.5 MHz curvilinear transducer may be necessary for measuring the length of an enlarged thyroid gland.
  - Children and small adults - 10 MHz to 15 MHz linear.

Patient Positioning

- Supine with chin up and neck extended to view thyroid gland, submandibular and sublingual glands.
- Slight turn of head toward the left to view the right thyroid lobe and/or parotid gland.
- Slight turn of the head toward the right to view the left thyroid lobe and/or parotid gland.
- Pillows may be placed behind the patient's upper back to aid in neck extension.

Examination Protocol

- **Thyroid and Parathyroid Glands.**
  - Beginning superior to the thyroid gland, systematic evaluation and bilateral imaging of the upper, mid, and lower thyroid lobes and isthmus in the sagittal and transverse planes.
  - Measure length, height, and width of each thyroid lobe.
  - Measure height of thyroid isthmus.
  - Duplex imaging of the thyroid gland to evaluate vascular flow.
  - Abnormalities of the thyroid or parathyroid glands should be documented and when applicable measured in two imaging planes. Color and/or spectral Doppler evaluation of the abnormality should be included.
  - In serial imaging of a multinodular goiter measure length, height and width of thyroid lobe(s) along with length, height, and width of the largest nodule(s).
  - Evaluation and imaging of the anterior neck and submandibular region for lymphadenopathy.
- **Salivary Glands.**
  - Evaluate and image entire specified salivary gland(s) in the sagittal and transverse planes, including imaging of the contralateral salivary gland for comparison.

- Measure length, height, and width of the salivary gland.
- Color Doppler to evaluate for normal vascular flow.
- Abnormalities of the salivary glands should be documented and when applicable measured in two imaging planes. Color and/or spectral Doppler evaluation of the abnormality should be included.

Image Optimization

- Place gains settings to display the normal thyroid and salivary glands a medium shade of gray with adjustments to reduce artifactually produced echoes within normally adjacent anechoic structures.
- Focal zone(s) should be placed at or below the area of interest. The use of multiple focal zones increases detail resolution and decreases temporal resolution.
- Sufficient imaging depth to visualize structures immediately posterior to the area of interest.
- Harmonic imaging and decreasing system compression (dynamic range) can be used to reduce artifactual echoes.
- Spatial compounding can be used to improve visualization of structures posterior to highly attenuating structures (e.g., calcification).
- Doppler settings should be adjusted for a slow flow rate.
- Standoff pads may be necessary in patients with thin necks or extremely superficial structures.

Examination Limitations

- Enlargement of the thyroid gland and attenuation of nodules may limit imaging detail and measurement accuracy.
- Patient inability to extend neck or raise chin.
- Shadowing from the mandible may make it difficult to visualize the parotid gland in its entirety.
- Sublingual gland may be difficult to image behind the tongue.

Helpful Hints

- Musculature of the neck is best identified in the transverse plane.
- Using the trapezoid imaging feature of some linear transducers increases the field of view allowing visualization of both thyroid lobes in the transverse plane and increases the ability to image the entire length of the thyroid gland in the sagittal plane.

Indications for Examination

Thyroid and Parathyroid Glands

- Palpable neck mass.
- Abnormal thyroid function tests.
- Increase in calcium levels.
- Dysphagia.
- Serial evaluation of thyroid or parathyroid nodule(s).
- Evaluate mass from a previous medical imaging study (e.g., CT).

Salivary Glands

- Palpable mass in the area of the salivary glands.
- Fever with mouth or dental infections.
- Mouth dryness (xerostomia).

LABORATORY VALUES

Thyroid

Thyrotropin (TSH)

- Normal range 3 to 42 ng/mL.
- Thyroid-stimulating hormone (TSH).
- Regulates thyroid hormone secretion and production.
- Secretion controlled by the anterior pituitary gland.
- Prolonged elevation is associated with hyperplasia and thyroid enlargement.
- Decrease in levels is the first indication of thyroid gland failure.

Thyroxine (T$_4$)

- Normal range 4.5 to 12.0 µg/dL.
- Stimulates consumption of oxygen.
- Secreted by the follicular cells of the thyroid.
- Controlled by thyrotropin (TSH).
- 100 to 200 mg of iodide must be ingested per week for normal thyroxine production.
- Decreases associated with thyroid disease and nonfunctioning pituitary gland.

Triiodothyronine (T$_3$)

- Normal range 70 to 190 ng/dL.
- Regulates tissue metabolism.
- Decreases associated with Hashimoto thyroiditis.

Calcitonin

- Normal range <100 pg/mL.
- Lowers calcium and phosphorus concentration in the blood.
- Inhibits bone resorption.
- Secreted by the parafollicular cells (C-cells) of the thyroid gland.
- Elevation associated with medullary thyroid carcinoma.
- Decreases are associated with surgical removal or nonfunctioning thyroid glands.

Parathyroid

Parathormone (PTH)

- Normal range 12 to 68 pg/mL.
- Regulates calcium metabolism in conjunction with calcitonin.
- Released in response to low extracellular concentration of free calcium.
- Elevation associated with hyperparathyroidism.

Calcium

- Normal range 8.5 to 10.5 mg/dL.
- Aids in the transportation of nutrients through the cell membranes.
- Elevation associated with hyperparathyroidism, hyperthyroidism, and malignancy.
- Levels exceeding 14.5 mg/dL can be life-threatening.
- Decreases are associated with nonfunctioning or surgical removal of the parathyroid glands.

THYROID PATHOLOGY

Hyperthyroidism

- Hyperactivity of the thyroid gland.
- Symptoms include nervousness, exophthalmos, tremors, constant hunger, weight loss, heat intolerance, palpitations, increased heart rate, and diarrhea.

- Causes include toxic adenoma, Graves disease, and trophoblastic tumors.
- If untreated, may lead to cardiac failure.
- Sonographic appearance – normal or enlarged heterogeneous hypervascular thyroid gland.

Hypothyroidism

- Inadequate production of triiodothyronine (T3) and thyroxine (T4).
- Symptoms include weight gain, hair loss, mental and physical lethargy, skin dryness, feeling cold, muscle cramps, constipation, arthritis, slow metabolic rate, and decreased heart rate.
- Caused by iodine deficiency, chronic autoimmune thyroiditis, thyroid hormone failure, and disease of the pituitary gland or hypothalamus.
- If untreated, may lead to myxedema, coma, or death.
- Sonographic appearance – enlarged, heterogeneous irregular thyroid gland with possible calcifications.

Thyroid Nodules

- 60% are benign.
- 20% are cysts.
- 20% are malignant.

Benign Thyroid Neoplasms

BENIGN MASS	ETIOLOGY	CLINICAL FINDINGS	SONOGRAPHIC FINDINGS	DIFFERENTIAL CONSIDERATIONS
Adenoma	Composed of epithelial tissue Most common thyroid neoplasm	Asymptomatic Hyperthyroidism Female prevalence (7:1)	Homogeneous echogenic mass Prominent hypoechoic peripheral halo Peripheral blood flow May degenerate and appear complex "Cold" nodule on nuclear medicine scan	Carcinoma Cyst Goiter
Cyst 10%-15% of solitary thyroid nodules	Simple cyst	Asymptomatic Palpable neck mass	Anechoic mass Smooth wall margins Posterior acoustic enhancement May demonstrate internal debris	Cystic degeneration of a solid nodule
Goiter	Thyroid hormone deficiency Iodine deficiency Graves' disease Thyroiditis	Palpable neck mass Dysphagia Dyspnea Hyperthyroidism or hypothyroidism	Enlarged thyroid lobe(s) Diffusely heterogeneous Areas of cystic degeneration May demonstrate calcification(s)	Thyroiditis
Hashimoto disease	Chronic lymphatic inflammatory disease	Often painless Hypothyroidism Leukocytosis Sore throat Fever	Enlarged hypoechoic thyroid glands Hypervascular parenchyma	Graves disease deQuervain syndrome
Thyroiditis	Hashimoto disease de Quervain syndrome Viral infection	Hyperthyroidism followed by hypothyroidism Fatigue Fever Leukocytosis Neck pain Dysphagia	Enlarged hypoechoic gland Hypervascular parenchyma Discrete nodules	Graves disease

Cysts of the Neck

CYST	ETIOLOGY	CLINICAL FINDINGS	SONOGRAPHIC FINDINGS	DIFFERENTIAL CONSIDERATIONS
Brachial cleft cyst	Congenital diverticulum of the brachial cleft	Asymptomatic Palpable lateral neck mass	Anechoic superficial neck mass Located directly below the angle of the mandible Located anterior to the sternocleidomastoid muscle May demonstrate internal debris	Thyroglossal cyst Thyroid cyst
Cystic hygroma	Inadequate drainage of lymph fluid into the jugular vein Increased secretion from the epithelial lining Associated with Turners syndrome	Asymptomatic Posterior neck mass	Thin-walled, multilocular cystic structure	
Thyroglossal cyst	Embryonic remnant	Asymptomatic Palpable superficial anterior neck mass	Anechoic superficial neck mass Located between the tongue and the thyroid isthmus May demonstrate internal debris Document relationship to hyoid bone (e.g. inferior)	Thyroid cyst Brachial cleft cyst

Malignant Thyroid Neoplasms

MALIGNANT THYROID NEOPLASMS	ETIOLOGY	CLINICAL FINDINGS	SONOGRAPHIC FINDINGS	DIFFERENTIAL CONSIDERATIONS
Carcinoma	Papillary (80%) Follicular (5%-15%) Medullary (5%) Anaplastic (2%)	Palpable neck mass Dysphagia Dyspnea Hoarseness Neck pain Lymphadenopathy	Hypoechoic mass Irregular borders Thick incomplete peripheral halo Microcalcification(s) May degenerate Increase in size from previous examination Metastases to cervical lymph nodes, lung, bone, and larynx	Cystic degeneration of a benign nodule Nodular goiter Abscess

PARATHYROID PATHOLOGY

Hypercalcemia

- Elevated calcium in the blood.
- Symptoms include confusion, anorexia, abdominal pain, muscle pain and weakness, stone formation, gout, arthritis, weight loss, and bone demineralization.
- Associated with hyperparathyroidism, metastatic bone tumor, Paget disease, and osteoporosis.
- Extremely high levels may result in coma, shock, kidney failure, or death.

Hyperparathyroidism

- Excessive function of the parathyroid glands.
- Most commonly caused by a parathyroid adenoma (80%).
- May lead to osteoporosis and nephrolithiasis.
- Elevated levels of parathormone.

Hypocalcemia

- Deficiency of calcium in the blood.
- Symptoms may include cardiac arrhythmia, hyperparesthesia of the hands, feet, lips, and tongue; muscle cramps; anxiety; and fatigue.
- Associated with hypoparathyroidism, kidney failure, acute pancreatitis, and inadequate amount of magnesium and protein.

Hypoparathyroidism

- Insufficient function of the parathyroid glands.
- Associated with hypercalcemia and primary parathyroid dysfunction.

Parathyroid Pathology

PATHOLOGY	ETIOLOGY	CLINICAL FINDINGS	SONOGRAPHIC FINDINGS	DIFFERENTIAL CONSIDERATIONS
Adenoma	Exposure to ionizing radiation	Hypercalcemia Decrease in serum phosphorus Increase in parathormone Hypertension Nephrolithiasis Cholelithiasis Pancreatitis	Hypoechoic mass located posterior and medial to the thyroid gland Oval in shape Internal vascular flow within larger lesions	Lymph node Thyroid nodule
Carcinoma	Epithelial neoplasm Slow-growing Tend to infiltrate surrounding tissues	Hypercalcemia Elevated parathormone level Firm palpable neck mass	Hypoechoic lobulated mass Round or oval in shape Attenuation of sound (dense) Hypervascular	Parathyroid adenoma Lymph node Thyroid neoplasm Graves disease
Cyst	Uncommon	Asymptomatic Female prevalence 60-70 years of age	Anechoic mass located posterior and medial to the thyroid gland Smooth wall margins Posterior acoustic enhancement	Thyroid cyst Thyroglossal cyst

Salivary Gland Pathology

PATHOLOGY	ETIOLOGY	CLINICAL FINDINGS	SONOGRAPHIC FINDINGS	DIFFERENTIAL CONSIDERATION
Hemangioma	Most common vascular mass in infants Usually located in the parotid gland (80%)	Painless Compressible, slow growing mass May have red or blue skin coloring	Heterogeneous, hypoechoic enlargement or mass Hypervascular Well circumscribed Usually located in the parotid gland (80%)	Sialadenitis Arteriovenous (AV) fistula
Parotitis	Chronic sialadenitis Present 3 years to 6 years of age More common in males	Pain and swelling especially postprandial	Enlarged heterogeneous gland(s) Excretory duct(s) may be dilated. Sialolithiasis Normal vascular flow	Normal parotid gland Hemangioma

Salivary Gland Pathology—(cont'd)

PATHOLOGY	ETIOLOGY	CLINICAL FINDINGS	SONOGRAPHIC FINDINGS	DIFFERENTIAL CONSIDERATION
Sialadenitis	Acute viral or bacterial infection	Painful swelling bilaterally Swelling during eating Postprandial pain Reddening of skin	Enlarged, diffusely hypoechoic gland Complex appearance Hypervascular Cervical lymphadenopathy	Parotitis
Sialolithiasis Submandibular in 60%-90% of cases Parotid in 10%-20% of cases	Infection in 50% of cases	Pain and swelling during eating Palpable mass	Intraductal or intraglandular echogenic focus(i) Posterior acoustic shadowing	Calcified vessel
Sialosis	Associated with: Endocrine diseases Hepatic cirrhosis Chronic alcoholism Malnutrition	Recurrent, painless gland swelling	Enlarged, hyperechoic gland with increased attenuation No increase in vascularity	
Sjogren's syndrome	Chronic autoimmune disease	Eye and mouth dryness Severe dental caries Frothy saliva	Inhomogeneous gland with small, oval hypoechoic or anechoic areas. May demonstrate hypervascularity	

NECK AND SALIVARY GLANDS REVIEW

1. Which of the following veins empties directly into the internal jugular vein?
   a. subclavian
   b. brachiocephalic
   c. superior thyroid
   d. external jugular

2. Which of the following structures produces thyroid stimulating hormone?
   a. thyroid glands
   b. pituitary gland
   c. parathyroid glands
   d. hypothalamus

3. Which of the following symptoms is commonly associated with hyperthyroidism?
   a. constipation
   b. weight gain
   c. exophthalmos
   d. skin dryness

4. Which of the following conditions is most commonly associated with hypothyroidism?
   a. Graves disease
   b. Addison disease
   c. Hashimoto disease
   d. de Quervain syndrome

5. Which of the following is considered a function of the parathyroid gland?
   a. producing hormones
   b. secreting calcitonin
   c. regulating serum electrolytes
   d. maintaining homeostasis of blood calcium concentrations

6. The vertebral arteries join at the base of the skull to form the:
   a. circle of Willis
   b. basilar artery
   c. carotid sinus
   d. brachiocephalic artery

7. A superficial cystic structure lying directly below the angle of the mandible is most suspicious for which of the following?
   a. cystic hygroma
   b. thyroglossal cyst
   c. brachial cleft cyst
   d. parotid cyst

8. A congenital anomaly associated with an additional thyroid lobe is termed a(n):
   a. accessory lobe
   b. pyramidal lobe
   c. ectopic lobe
   d. duplicated isthmus

9. Which of the following transducers may aid in measuring the length of an enlarged thyroid gland?
   a. 3.5 MHz curvilinear
   b. 9.0 MHz linear
   c. 15 MHz linear
   d. 10 MHz sector

10. The first indication of thyroid gland failure is linked with a decrease in:
    a. thyroxine
    b. calcitonin
    c. thyrotropin
    d. triiodothyronine

11. A prominent hypoechoic ring surrounds a thyroid nodule. This sonographic finding is most consistent with which of the following neoplasms?
    a. lipoma
    b. adenoma
    c. lymph node
    d. complex cyst

12. Which of the following salivary glands demonstrates an intraparenchymal lymph node?
    a. parotid gland
    b. sublingual gland
    c. submandibular gland
    d. parotid and submandibular glands

13. Hyperthyroidism followed by hypothyroidism is a clinical finding for which of the following conditions?
    a. goiter
    b. thyroiditis
    c. hyperplasia
    d. metastatic disease

14. A thyroglossal cyst is located between which of the following structures?
   a. hyoid bone and thyroid gland
   b. left thyroid lobe and tongue
   c. thyroid isthmus and tongue
   d. trachea and thyroid gland

15. The majority of blood supplied to the brain is through the:
   a. vertebral arteries
   b. external carotid arteries
   c. internal carotid arteries
   d. common carotid arteries

Using Figure 17.2, answer questions 16 to 18.

16. The anechoic structures identified by arrow *A* most likely represent which of the following structures?
   a. thyroid cyst
   b. carotid artery
   c. strap muscles
   d. parathyroid cyst

17. The echogenic structure identified by arrow *B* most likely represents which of the following structures?
   a. esophagus
   b. strap muscles
   c. thyroid isthmus
   d. longus colli muscle

18. The hypoechoic structure identified by arrow *C* most likely represents which of the following structures?
   a. trachea
   b. strap muscles
   c. longus colli muscle
   d. sternocleidomastoid muscle

Using Figure 17.3, answer questions 19 and 20.

19. A 32-year-old woman presents with a 2-month history of fatigue, sore throat, and dysphagia following an episode of cellulitis. The results of laboratory tests are pending. On the basis of this clinical history, the sonographic findings are most consistent with:
   a. Graves disease
   b. metastatic disease
   c. Hashimoto disease
   d. carotid body tumor

20. On the basis of the clinical symptoms and sonographic findings, the laboratory results will most likely demonstrate:
   a. hypercalcemia
   b. hypothyroidism
   c. hyperthyroidism
   d. hypoparathyroidism

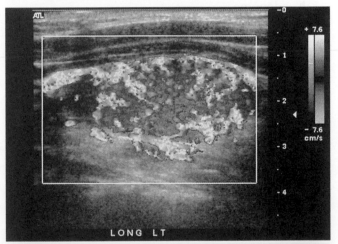

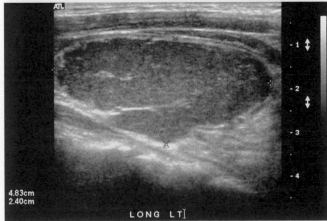

FIG. 17.3 Longitudinal sonograms of the thyroid gland.

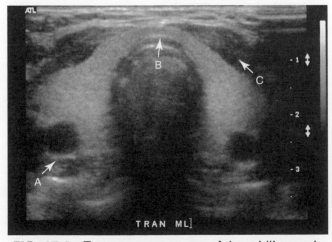

FIG. 17.2 Transverse sonogram of the midline neck.

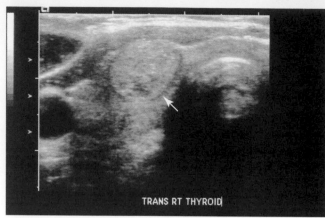

TRANS RT THYROID

FIG. 17.4 Transverse sonogram of the thyroid gland.

Using Figure 17.4, answer question 21.

21. Which of the following abnormalities is identified in this sonogram of the thyroid gland?
    a. goiter
    b. adenoma
    c. carcinoma
    d. hemangioma

Using Figure 17.5, answer question 22.

22. A patient presents with a palpable anterior neck mass. On the basis of this clinical history, the sonographic finding is most suspicious for a:
    a. cystic hygroma
    b. brachial cleft cyst
    c. thyroglossal cyst
    d. submandibular salivary gland cyst

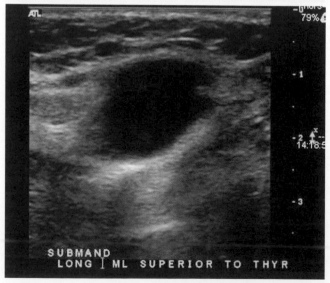

SUBMAND
LONG ML SUPERIOR TO THYR

FIG. 17.5 Sagittal sonogram of the midline neck.

23. How many parathyroid glands are found in the majority of the population?
    a. 2
    b. 3
    c. 4
    d. 6

24. Which of the following arteries arises first from the internal carotid artery?
    a. basilar artery
    b. ophthalmic artery
    c. superior thyroid artery
    d. middle cerebral artery

25. Which of the following symptoms is most likely related to hypercalcemia?
    a. fatigue
    b. palpitations
    c. tingling feet
    d. abdominal pain

26. Pancreatitis, hypertension, and hypercalcemia are clinical findings associated with which of the following neoplasms?
    a. multinodular goiter
    b. parathyroid adenoma
    c. thyroid carcinoma
    d. parathyroid carcinoma

27. The parathyroid glands are located:
    a. anterior to the thyroid lobe and longus colli muscle
    b. posterior to the thyroid lobe and longus colli muscle
    c. anterior to the thyroid gland and posterior to the longus colli muscle
    d. posterior to the thyroid gland and anterior to the longus colli muscle

28. A cystic hygroma is most likely related to which of the following abnormalities?
    a. thyroglossal cyst
    b. arteriovenous fistula
    c. inadequate drainage of lymph fluid
    d. impaired synthesis of thyroid hormones

29. Which of the following statements about the carotid artery is *true*?
    a. The right common carotid artery arises from the aortic arch.
    b. The external carotid artery courses lateral to the internal carotid artery.
    c. The internal carotid artery terminates at the circle of Willis.
    d. The internal carotid artery lies anterior to the external carotid artery.

30. Inflammation of the thyroid gland secondary to a viral infection is most commonly associated with which of the following conditions?
    a. Graves disease
    b. Caroli disease
    c. Mirizzi syndrome
    d. de Quervain syndrome

31. Which of the following muscles is located posterior to the thyroid lobes?
    a. sternohyoid
    b. omohyoid
    c. longus colli
    d. sternocleidomastoid

32. The most common thyroid neoplasm is a(n):
    a. cyst
    b. goiter
    c. adenoma
    d. carcinoma

33. Exposure to ionizing radiation is a predisposing factor for development of which of the following neoplasms?
    a. thyroglossal cyst
    b. thyroid adenoma
    c. parathyroid cyst
    d. parathyroid adenoma

34. Primary carcinoma of the thyroid gland is known to extend to which of the following structures?
    a. bone
    b. liver
    c. brain
    d. pancreas

35. Which of the following conditions is considered a predisposing factor for developing a thyroid malignancy?
    a. Graves disease
    b. Hashimoto disease
    c. de Quervain syndrome
    d. Marfan syndrome

36. The normal length of an adult thyroid lobe is approximately:
    a. 1.0 to 2.0 cm
    b. 2.0 to 4.0 cm
    c. 4.0 to 6.0 cm
    d. 5.0 to 7.0 cm

37. Including iodide in your diet is required for the normal production of:
    a. calcium
    b. thyroxine
    c. calcitonin
    d. thyrotropin

38. Chronic sialadenitis is associated with which of the following conditions?
    a. sialolithiasis
    b. Sjogren's syndrome
    c. parotitis
    d. thyroglossal cyst

39. Which of the following symptoms is associated with hypothyroidism?
    a. tremors
    b. weight loss
    c. muscle cramps
    d. exophthalmos

40. Which of the following arteries is the first branch of the external carotid artery?
    a. lingual artery
    b. fascial artery
    c. superior thyroid artery
    d. ascending pharyngeal artery

41. Serial evaluation of a multinodular goiter should include measurements of the overall length, height, and width of a thyroid lobe along with measurements of the length, height, and width of:
    a. each individual nodule
    b. the largest nodule(s)
    c. the complex nodule(s)
    d. the hypervascular nodule(s)

42. The majority of the thyroid nodules identified on ultrasound are:
    a. benign
    b. fluid filled
    c. hypervascular
    d. multilocular

43. Multilocular nodules are demonstrated on a sonogram of a thyroid gland. This is most consistent with which of the following conditions?
    a. Graves disease
    b. de Quervain syndrome
    c. Hashimoto disease
    d. Addison syndrome

44. Development of which of the following conditions is linked to hyperparathyroidism?
    a. kidney failure
    b. acute pancreatitis
    c. osteoporosis
    d. hepatomegaly

45. A solitary hypoechoic thyroid nodule demonstrating irregular borders and microcalcifications is most suspicious for:
    a. carcinoma
    b. an adenoma
    c. diffuse hyperplasia
    d. a hemangioma

46. A parathyroid mass may be suspected when an abnormality is located:
    a. superior to the thyroid isthmus
    b. lateral to a thyroid lobe
    c. posterior to a thyroid lobe
    d. anterior to the thyroid isthmus

47. Which of the following muscles is located lateral to the thyroid lobes just beneath the subcutaneous tissues in the neck?
    a. sternohyoid
    b. platysma
    c. omohyoid
    d. sternocleidomastoid

48. Which of the following muscles is most often affected by a whiplash injury?
    a. scalene
    b. sternohyoid
    c. longus colli
    d. sternocleidomastoid

49. Pronounced swelling of the neck is most often caused by a(n):
    a. thyroglossal cyst
    b. carotid body tumor
    c. enlarging thyroid gland
    d. aneurysm of the carotid artery

50. Which of the following is the most common etiology of hyperparathyroidism?
    a. carotid body tumor
    b. adenoma of a parathyroid gland
    c. hyperplasia of a parathyroid gland
    d. multinodular goiter of a thyroid gland

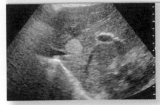

CHAPTER 18

Peritoneum, Noncardiac Chest, Invasive Procedures, and Patient Care

KEY TERMS

ascites abnormal collection of serous fluid in the peritoneal cavity.

bare area a large triangular area devoid of peritoneal covering located between the two layers of the coronary ligament.

biopsy the removal of a small piece of living tissue for microscopic analysis.

coronary ligaments left coronary ligament suspends the left lobe of the liver from the diaphragm; right coronary ligament serves as a barrier between the subphrenic space and Morison pouch.

chylous ascites an accumulation of chyle and emulsified fats in the peritoneal cavity; most commonly associated with an abdominal neoplasm.

exudative ascites an accumulation of fluid, pus, or serum in the peritoneal cavity; most commonly associated with malignant or infectious processes.

fine-needle aspiration a thin needle and gentle suction is used to obtain tissue samples for pathological testing.

greater omentum a double-fold of peritoneum attached at the greater curvature of the stomach and superior portion of the duodenum; covers the transverse colon and small intestines.

hemoperitoneum the presence of extravasated blood in the peritoneal cavity.

hemothorax an accumulation of blood and fluid in the pleural cavity.

lesser omentum a portion of peritoneum extending from the portal fissure of the liver to the diaphragm; encloses the lower end of the esophagus.

loculated ascites the presence of numerous small fluid spaces in the peritoneal cavity.

lymphocele a collection of lymph from injured lymph vessels.

mesenteric a double layer of peritoneum suspending the intestine from the posterior abdominal wall.

mesenteric cyst a congenital thin-walled cyst located between the leaves of the mesentery; most commonly located in the small-bowel mesentery.

paracentesis a cannula or catheter is passed into the abdominal cavity to allow outflow of fluid into a collecting device for diagnostic or therapeutic purposes.

peritoneum a serous membrane containing lymphatics, vessels, fat, and nerves.

pleural cavity a thin space located between the two layers of pleura.

pleural effusion an accumulation of fluid within the pleural cavity between the parietal and visceral pleural membranes.

pouch of Douglas a pouch formed by the inferior portion of the parietal peritoneum.

omentum an extension of the peritoneum surrounding one or more organs adjacent to the stomach.

seroma benign pocket of serous fluid that may develop after surgery, trauma, or inflammation.

thoracentesis a needle is inserted through the chest wall and pleural cavity to aspirate fluid for diagnostic or therapeutic purposes.

transudative ascites an accumulation of a fluid in the peritoneal cavity containing small protein cells; most commonly associated with cirrhosis or congestive heart failure.

PHYSIOLOGY

Functions of the Peritoneum

- Secretes serous fluid to reduce friction between structures.
- Suspends and enfolds organs.

PERITONEUM ANATOMY (Fig. 18.1)

- An extensive serous membrane lining the entire abdominal wall.
- Composed of two layers: parietal (lines the cavity) and visceral (covers the organs).
- Folds of peritoneum form several potential spaces.
- Suspensory ligaments extend between organs.

Greater Omentum

- A transparent double fold of peritoneum that spreads like an apron inferiorly to cover most of the abdominopelvic cavity.
- In cases of trauma, will often seal hernias and wall off infections.
- Keeps the small intestines warm.

Lesser Omentum (Gastrohepatic Omentum)

- Membranous extension from the portal fissure to the lesser curvature of the stomach and first portion of the duodenum.
- Provides support for the hepatic vessels.

Intraperitoneal Organs Include:

- Appendix.
- Cecum.
- Duodenal bulb.
- Gallbladder.
- Ileum.
- Jejunum.
- Liver.

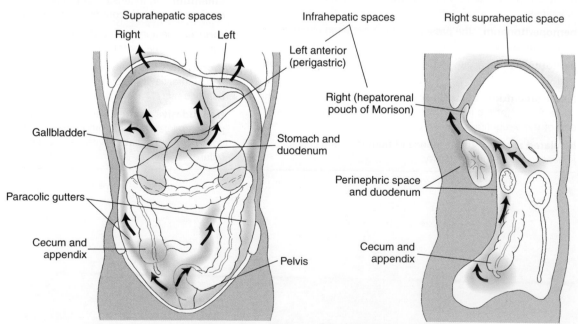

FIG. 18.1   Peritoneal anatomy.

- Ovaries.
- Sigmoid colon.
- Spleen.
- Stomach.
- Transverse colon.
- Upper one-third of the rectum.
- Uterine body.

Intraperitoneal Ligaments/Mesentery Include:

- Falciform.
- Coronary.
- Triangular.
- Hepatoduodenal.
- Hepatogastric.
- Gastrocolic.
- Gastrosplenic.
- Transverse mesocolon.
- Sigmoid mesocolon.
- Small bowel mesentery.

Extraperitoneal Organs Include:

- Urinary bladder.
- Distal ureters.
- Uterus/fallopian tubes.
- Prostate/seminal vesicles.
- Distal one-third of the rectum.

PERITONEAL SPACES

Lesser Sac (Omental Bursa)

- Located anterior to the pancreas and posterior to the stomach.
- Located between the diaphragm and transverse colon.
- Communicates with the subhepatic space through the foramen of Winslow (epiploic foramen).

Morison Pouch (Hepatorenal Pouch)

- Located superior and anterior to the right kidney and posterior to the lateral portion of the right lobe of the liver.
- Unable to communicate with the subphrenic space because of the right coronary ligament (bare area).
- Communicates with the right paracolic gutter.
- Frequent site for fluid to collect.

Paracolic Gutters

- Located lateral to the colon.
- Serve as conduits for fluid between the deep pelvis and upper abdomen.
- Left paracolic gutter is shallow.
- Right paracolic gutter demonstrates less resistance and is the more common route of fluid extension.

Pelvic Spaces

- Retrovesical pouch is located posterior to the urinary bladder and anterior to the rectum.
- Retrouterine pouch is located posterior to the uterus and anterior to the rectum. Also called posterior cul de sac or pouch of Douglas.

- Vesicouterine pouch is located anterior to the uterus and posterior to the urinary bladder. Also called anterior cul de sac.
- Prevesical or retropubic space is located anterior to the urinary bladder and posterior to the symphysis pubis. Also known as space of Retzius.

Subhepatic Space

- Extends from the inferior border of the liver to a deep recess anterior to the right kidney.
- Most common site for fluid to collect.

Subphrenic Spaces

- Divided into the left and right subphrenic spaces by the falciform ligament.
- Left subphrenic space is located inferior to the diaphragm and superior to the spleen.
- Left subphrenic space includes spaces between the left diaphragm, left lobe of the liver, stomach, and spleen.
- Right subphrenic space is located inferior to the diaphragm and superior to the liver.
- Right subphrenic space extends over several rib spaces to the right coronary ligament (bare area).

LOCATION OF THE PERITONEUM

- Extends from the anterior abdominal wall to the retroperitoneum and paraspinal tissues.
- Extends from the diaphragm to the deep pelvic spaces around the bladder.

ANATOMY OF THE PLEURA

- A delicate serous membrane composed of a visceral and parietal layer.
- Visceral pleura is the outmost coat of the lung and has a low sensitivity to pain.
- Parietal pleura lines the thoracic cavity (chest wall) and has a high sensitivity to pain.
- Pleural cavity is a thin space between the two layers of the pleura.
- Pleural fluid lubricates the pleural surfaces.
- Pleural membrane separates the two lungs.

SONOGRAPHIC APPEARANCE

- Fluid collections are not generally demonstrated in the chest or abdominal cavity.
- A small amount of pelvic fluid may be identified in ovulatory patients.
- Parietal peritoneum appears as a thin continuous hyperechoic line deep to the anterior abdominal musculature, separating the abdominal wall from the peritoneal cavity.
- Lung-Air/Visceral pleura interface appears hyperechoic.

EXAMINATION TECHNIQUES, PROTOCOLS, AND IMAGE OPTIMIZATION

Preparation

- No preparation is necessary for a sonogram of the peritoneal or thoracic cavity.
- Preparation will vary with the type of invasive procedure.

Transducer Selection

- Use the highest frequency possible to obtain optimal resolution for penetration depth.
  - 2.5 MHz to 4.0 MHz curvilinear or vector transducer for the peritoneum and thoracic cavity.
  - 9.0 MHz to 15 MHz linear transducer for superficial structures.

Patient Positioning

- **Peritoneal Cavity and Paracentesis.**
  - Supine.
- **Non-Cardiac Chest.**
  - Supine or sitting.
- **Thoracentesis.**
  - Sitting leaning slightly forward, with arms resting on a table for stability.
- **Fine Needle Aspiration and Biopsy.**
  - Position will vary.

Examination Protocol

- **Peritoneal Ascites.**
  - Systematic approach in the sagittal, coronal, and transverse planes carefully examining and imaging the abdomen and pelvic cavities in two orthogonal planes.
  - Abnormalities should be documented and when applicable measured in two imaging planes. Color and/or spectral Doppler evaluation of the abnormality should be included.
- **Peritoneal Mass.**
  - Systematic approach in the sagittal, coronal, and transverse planes carefully examining and imaging the area of concern in two orthogonal planes.
  - Abnormalities should be documented and when applicable measured in two imaging planes. Color and/or spectral Doppler evaluation of the abnormality should be included.
- **Invasive Procedures.**
  - Explain procedure to patient.
  - Have patient sign consent form.
  - Localize the area of interest in two orthogonal planes remaining perpendicular to the table or floor.
  - Document and annotate the area of interest including depth from skin to fluid collection or mass.
  - Perform a "time out" before beginning an invasive procedure.
    - Verify site of procedure.
    - Verify the correct invasive procedure is being performed.
    - Verify the patient's name and birthdate with patient.
  - Assist physician performing invasive procedure. (e.g., sterile tray, ultrasound system controls, etc.).
  - Visualization of the needle is obtained at a plane parallel with the needle path.
  - Postprocedure – evaluate and document area of needle path for any evidence of postprocedural bleeding.

Sterile Procedure Technique

- A sterile field should be prepared **just before** the invasive procedure.
- Wash hands thoroughly.
- Place sterile wrapped package on a clean and stable work surface.
- Open the sterile wrapped pack starting with the outermost flap of the drape placing it on the work surface. Repeat with adjacent flap of the drape placing it on the work surface.

- Additional sterile items should be "dropped" directly onto the sterile portion of the package.
- Sterile gloves must be used when touching any item in the sterile field.
- A sterile transducer sheath may be necessary to cover the transducer and cord.
- Sterile ultrasound gel should be used on patient's skin.

Image Optimization

- Place gains settings to display normal liver parenchyma as a medium shade of gray with adjustments to reduce artifactually produced echoes within the hepatic vessels and gallbladder.
- Focal zone(s) should be placed at or below the area of interest. The use of multiple focal zones increases detail resolution and decreases temporal resolution.
- Sufficient imaging depth to visualize structures immediately posterior to the area of interest.
- Harmonic imaging and decreasing system compression (dynamic range) can be used to reduce artifactual echoes.
- Spatial compounding can be used to improve visualization of structures posterior to highly attenuating structures.
- Doppler settings should be adjusted for a slow flow rate.

Examination Limitations

- Patient cooperation.
- Patient limitations.

Helpful Hints

- Limit the amount of transducer pressure used when making a depth measurement for an invasive procedure.

Indications for Peritoneal Cavity Examination

- Increase in abdominal girth.
- Chronic liver disease.
- Congestive heart failure.
- Ultrasound-guided paracentesis or biopsy.
- Evaluate pathology demonstrated on a previous medical imaging study (e.g., CT).

Indications for Pleural Cavity Examination

- Shortness of breath.
- Ultrasound-guided thoracentesis.
- Evaluate fluid collection demonstrated on previous medical imaging study (e.g., chest x-ray examination).

LABORATORY VALUES

- Laboratory values will vary with individual cases.
- Decreased hematocrit is suspicious for internal bleeding.
- Leukocytosis is suspicious for infection.

Peritoneal Fluid Collections

FLUID COLLECTION	ETIOLOGY	CLINICAL FINDINGS	SONOGRAPHIC FINDINGS	DIFFERENTIAL CONSIDERATIONS
Abscess	Infection	Abdominal pain Fever Leukocytosis Fatigue Nausea/vomiting	Complex mass is most common Thick, irregular wall margins Displacement of adjacent structures Nonvascular mass May demonstrate septations, shadowing (air), or mild acoustic enhancement	Hematoma Complex ascites Lymphadenopathy
Benign ascites	Congestive heart failure Cirrhosis Hypoalbuminemia Infection Inflammation Portal venous obstruction Postoperative complication	Dependent on etiology Abdominal distention Abdominal pain Shortness of breath with large collections	Anechoic fluid accumulation in the peritoneal cavity Fluid conforms to surrounding structures Mobility of fluid with patient position change Bowel may appear "floating" within the fluid Most commonly located in the subhepatic space followed by the paracolic gutters, and posterior pelvic cul de sac Thick-appearing gallbladder wall with adjacent ascites	Fluid-filled loops of bowel Abscess Hemoperitoneum Lymphocele Cystic neoplasm
Hemoperitoneum	Surgery Ruptured blood vessel Trauma Fistulas Necrotic neoplasm	Abdominal pain Decrease in hematocrit Shock	Hypoechoic fluid collection(s) Swirling low-level echoes Hyperechoic mass(es) within the fluid representing clot formation	Ascites Pseudomyxoma peritonei
Lymphocele	Disruption of the lymphatic system Complication of a renal transplant or vascular, urological, or gynecological surgery	Asymptomatic Abdominal pain or discomfort	Anechoic cystic mass frequently containing septations Round or oval in shape Well-defined wall margins Posterior acoustic enhancement Usually found medial to a renal transplant	Seroma Resolving hematoma Urinoma Loculated ascites
Malignant ascites	Metastasis	Abdominal distention Abdominal pain or discomfort	Anechoic or complex fluid accumulation in the peritoneal cavity Septations Does not change with patient position Does not conform to surrounding structures Matted bowel Gallbladder wall measuring 3 mm or less with adjacent ascites	Benign ascites Pseudomyxoma peritonei

Continued

Peritoneal Fluid Collections—(cont'd)

FLUID COLLECTION	ETIOLOGY	CLINICAL FINDINGS	SONOGRAPHIC FINDINGS	DIFFERENTIAL CONSIDERATIONS
Pseudomyxoma peritonei	Metastasis Ruptured mucinous cystadenoma Ruptured appendix	Abdominal pain Abdominal distention Constipation	Multiseptated cystic areas in the peritoneal cavity Internal echoes or echogenic linear strands Matted bowel loops compressed posteriorly	Loculated ascites Hemoperitoneum
Seroma	Trauma Surgery Inflammation	Asymptomatic Abdominal pain or discomfort	Anechoic mass Smooth wall margins May conform to the surrounding structures	Biloma Urinoma Lymphocele Resolving hematoma

Peritoneal Masses

MASS	ETIOLOGY	CLINICAL FINDINGS	SONOGRAPHIC FINDINGS	DIFFERENTIAL CONSIDERATIONS
Mesenteric cyst	Wolffian or lymphatic duct in origin	Colicky abdominal pain Intestinal obstruction	Cystic structure located in the mesentery Smooth wall margins Is not associated with any adjacent structure Most commonly located in the small-bowel mesentery	Renal cyst Ascites Hematoma Abscess Neoplasm
Mesenteric lymphomatous	Lymphoma	Found more frequently with non-Hodgkin's lymphoma	Anechoic mass containing a central echogenic target ("sandwich sign")	Lymphadenopathy Bowel
Omental cyst	Congenital failure of the mesentery to fuse Trauma	Asymptomatic	Small cystic structure located adjacent to the stomach or lesser sac Mass will contour to the bowel margins Smooth wall margins Honeycomb appearance	Renal cyst Pancreatic pseudocyst Hematoma Abscess Ascites Neoplasm
Peritoneal carcinomatosis	Metastasis	Abdominal distention Abdominal pain	Ascites Irregular masses Echo poor nodules Thickening of peritoneum and omentum	Lymphadenopathy

Noncardiac Chest Abnormality

ABNORMALITY	ETIOLOGY	CLINICAL FINDINGS	SONOGRAPHIC FINDINGS	DIFFERENTIAL CONSIDERATIONS
Diaphragmatic paralysis	Peripheral neuropathy Phrenic nerve palsy Shingles	Shortness of breath Syncope Dyspnea Chest pain	Unusual or absent movement of the diaphragm with normal respiration Absent or paradoxical movement of the diaphragm when sniffing	Technical error
Pleural effusion	Infection Cardiovascular disease Trauma	Shortness of breath Chest pain Nonproductive cough	Anechoic fluid collection in the dependent portion of the thorax Complex fluid typically infectious or malignant response	Subphrenic ascites Hemothorax Artifact

INVASIVE PROCEDURES

- A diagnostic or therapeutic technique that requires entry of a body cavity or interruption of normal body function.

Contraindications for Invasive Procedures

- Bleeding disorder.
- Patient inability to give consent.
- Patient inability to cooperate.

Risk Factors of Procedures

- Bleeding.
- Infection.
- Seeding.
- Inadequate sample.
- Inconclusive results.

Types of Invasive Procedures

Biopsy

- A larger core needle is used to remove a small piece of living tissue.
- The excised tissue is examined by a pathologist.

Fine-Needle Aspiration

- A very slender needle along with gentle suction is used to obtain tissue samples.
- Aspirated material is examined by a pathologist.

Paracentesis

- A cannula or catheter is passed into the abdominal cavity to allow outflow of fluid into a collecting device.
- May be for diagnostic or therapeutic purposes.

Thoracentesis

- Perforating the chest wall and pleural cavity with a needle to aspirate fluid.
- May be for diagnostic or therapeutic purposes.

PATIENT CARE

Vital Signs

- Refers to the temperature, pulse, respiration, and blood pressure.
  - **Temperature.**
    - Normal temperature is 98.6 degrees Fahrenheit.
  - **Pulse.**
    - Radial artery most convenient site.
    - 60 to 65 beats per minute (bpm) – Adults.
    - 120 to 140 bpm – Newborn infants.
  - **Respiration.**
    - Quiet, effortless and regular rhythm.
    - 16 to 20 breaths per minute – Adult.
  - **Blood pressure.**
    - Patient should sit or lie down on his/her back with arm and cuff level with the heart.
    - Center cuff over brachial artery.
    - Inflate high enough to cut off blood flow.

- Release at a rate of 2 to 3 mm/Hg until flow returns (systolic) continuing until the artery can no longer be heard (diastolic).
- Normal systolic pressure in adults ranges from 100 to 120 mm/Hg.
- Normal diastolic pressure in adults ranges from 60 to 80 mm/Hg.

Infection Control – Protective Measures

- Prevent the spread of communicable diseases and microorganisms among patients, personnel, and visitors.
  - **Hand Washing.**
    - Best protection to stop the spread of pathogens.
    - Scrub your hands for a minimum of 20 seconds.
  - **Gloves.**
    - Should cover the wrist.
    - Should only be used once and then discarded.
    - When removing gloves, ensure the inside part is on the outside.
    - Wash hands immediately after removing gloves.
  - **Gowns.**
    - Most protective clothing.
    - Should be long and large enough to cover your clothing.
    - Put gloves on after you have gowned.
  - **Masks.**
    - Used for airborne particle and droplet protection.
  - Eye and Face Shields.
    - Protect the mucous membranes of the face from pathogens.

Patient Safety

- Inspect transducer and cable for fraying or defects.
- Double-check the patient's identity before beginning any ultrasound examination.
- When working with patients in wheelchairs make sure the brakes are locked and the foot rests are lifted before transferring patient.
- Use proper body mechanics when transferring patients from ultrasound stretcher to and from the wheelchair or gurney.
- Know the location of the fire alarm, crash cart and other emergency equipment.
- Perform a "time out" before beginning any invasive procedure.
  - Verify site of procedure.
  - Verify the correct invasive procedure is being performed.
  - Verify the patient's name and birthdate with patient.

PERITONEUM, NONCARDIAC CHEST, INVASIVE PROCEDURES, AND PATIENT CARE REVIEW

1. A patient arrives by ambulance to the emergency department following a motor vehicle accident. On ultrasound, a large hypoechoic fluid collection is identified in the left subphrenic space. On the basis of the clinical history, this fluid collection most likely represents:
   a. ascites
   b. a lymphocele
   c. pleural effusion
   d. hemoperitoneum

2. Which of the following is a predisposing condition associated with the development of a pleural effusion?
   a. hepatitis
   b. pancreatitis
   c. portal hypertension
   d. congestive heart failure

3. Free fluid most commonly accumulates in which of the following peritoneal spaces?
   a. subphrenic space
   b. paracolic gutter
   c. space of Retzius
   d. subhepatic space

4. Which of the following structures lines the abdominal cavity?
   a. mesentery
   b. peritoneum
   c. lesser omentum
   d. greater omentum

5. A patient is most commonly placed in which of the following positions during a thoracentesis procedure?
   a. prone
   b. sitting
   c. decubitus
   d. reverse Trendelenburg

6. The lesser sac communicates with the subhepatic space through the foramen of:
   a. Monro
   b. Ovale
   c. Vater
   d. Winslow

7. Which of the following organs lie within the peritoneum?
   a. spleen
   b. kidneys
   c. pancreas
   d. adrenal glands

8. Chylous ascites is most commonly associated with which of the following abnormalities?
   a. cirrhosis
   b. acute cholecystitis
   c. abdominal neoplasm
   d. congestive heart failure

9. Which of the following peritoneal spaces is located lateral to the intestines?
   a. retrovesical pouch
   b. subhepatic space
   c. paracolic gutter
   d. subphrenic space

10. Which of the following fluid collections is typically located medial to a renal transplant?
    a. seroma
    b. urinoma
    c. lymphocele
    d. hematoma

11. Which of the following invasive procedures accomplishes withdrawal of fluid from the abdominal cavity?
    a. fine-needle aspiration
    b. peritoneal biopsy
    c. thoracentesis
    d. paracentesis

12. Peritoneal ascites is a common complication in which of the following conditions?
    a. malignancy
    b. pneumonia
    c. polycystic liver disease
    d. renal artery stenosis

13. A decrease in hematocrit is most consistent with which of the following conditions?
    a. infection
    b. malignancy
    c. hemorrhage
    d. thrombosis

14. An apron of peritoneum covering the small intestines describes the:
    a. linea alba
    b. perineum
    c. mesentery
    d. greater omentum

15. The peritoneum is described as extending from the:
    a. posterior abdominal wall to the retroperitoneum
    b. diaphragm to the umbilicus
    c. diaphragm to the deep pelvic recesses
    d. posterior abdominal wall to the paraspinal tissues

16. Which of the following peritoneal spaces is located anterior to the uterus and posterior to the urinary bladder?
    a. prevesical
    b. vesicouterine
    c. retropubic
    d. retrovesical

17. A delicate serous membrane composed of a visceral and a parietal layer *best* describes the:
    a. pleura
    b. mesentery
    c. omentum
    d. peritoneum

18. On ultrasound, visualization of a biopsy needle is obtained in a plane:
    a. perpendicular to the examination table
    b. parallel with the needle path
    c. perpendicular to the needle path
    d. parallel to the examination table

19. Which of the following structures is located within the right coronary ligament?
    a. pleura
    b. bare area
    c. diaphragmatic crura
    d. inferior vena cava

20. A thin needle is used to obtain tissue samples in which of the following invasive procedures?
    a. thoracentesis
    b. paracentesis
    c. amniocentesis
    d. fine-needle aspiration

Using Figure 18.2, answer question 21.

21. Which of the following peritoneal spaces is most likely identified by the arrow?
    a. pleural space
    b. subphrenic space
    c. Morison pouch
    d. pouch of Douglas

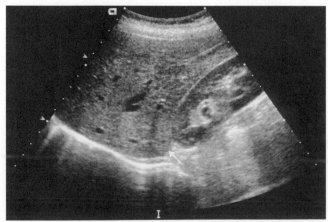

FIG. 18.2 Sagittal sonogram of the right upper quadrant.

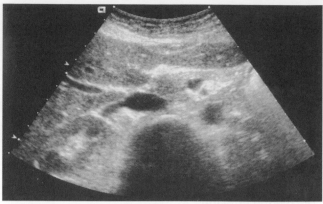

FIG. 18.3 Transverse sonogram of the upper abdomen.

Using Figure 18.3, answer question 22.

22. Which of the following structures is located within the peritoneal cavity?
    a. aorta
    b. liver
    c. pancreas
    d. inferior vena cava

Using Figure 18.4, answer questions 23 to 25.

23. Arrow *A* is most likely identifying which of the following structures?
    a. pleura
    b. diaphragm
    c. coronary ligament
    d. hepatic flexure

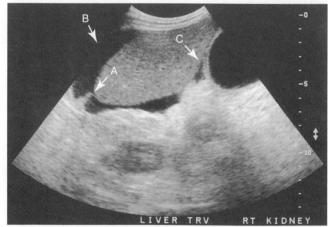

FIG. 18.4 Transverse sonogram of the right upper quadrant.

24. Arrow B is most consistent with which of the following conditions?
    a. hemothorax
    b. pleural effusion
    c. subphrenic ascites
    d. subhepatic ascites

25. Which of the following peritoneal spaces is identified by arrow C?
    a. lesser sac
    b. Morison pouch
    c. subhepatic space
    d. right paracolic gutter

Using Figure 18.5, answer question 26.

26. Ascites is identified in which of the following peritoneal spaces?
    a. space of Retzius
    b. subhepatic space
    c. paracolic gutter
    d. retrovesical pouch

Using Figure 18.6, answer question 27.

27. An abnormality is identified in which of the following regions?
    a. pleural space
    b. subhepatic space
    c. subphrenic space
    d. Morison pouch

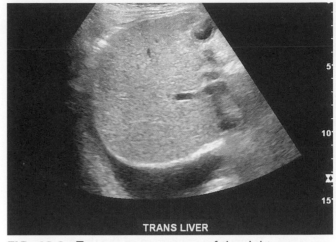

TRANS LIVER

FIG. 18.6   Transverse sonogram of the right upper quadrant.

Using Figure 18.7, answer question 28.

28. A fluid collection is identified in which of the following regions?
    a. retropubic space
    b. pouch of Douglas
    c. space of Retzius
    d. paracolic gutter

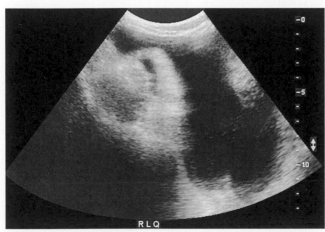

RLQ

FIG. 18.5   Sonogram of the right lower quadrant.

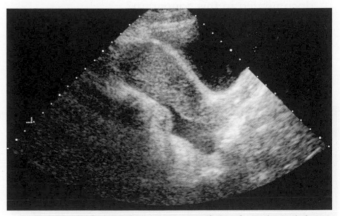

FIG. 18.7   Sagittal sonogram of the female pelvis.

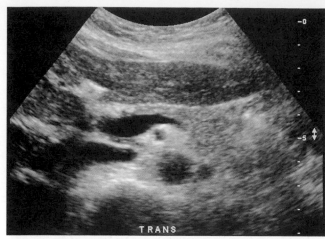

FIG. 18.8   Transverse sonogram of the upper abdomen.

Using Figure 18.8, answer question 29.

29. Which of the following peritoneal spaces is located in this sonogram?
    a. lesser sac
    b. subhepatic space
    c. pararenal space
    d. subphrenic space

Using Figure 18.9, answer question 30.

30. Which of the following invasive procedures is documented in this sonogram?
    a. cyst aspiration
    b. core-needle biopsy
    c. stent placement
    d. fine-needle aspiration

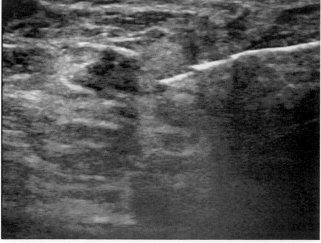

FIG. 18.9   Sonogram of an invasive procedure.

31. Which of the following functions is considered the responsibility of the peritoneum?
    a. production of lymphocytes
    b. production of antibodies
    c. secretion of serous fluid to reduce organ friction
    d. serves as a barrier between the subphrenic and subhepatic spaces

32. Which of the following is not considered a vital sign?
    a. pulse
    b. pallor
    c. respiration
    d. blood pressure

33. The subphrenic space is divided into right and left sides by the:
    a. coronary ligament
    b. falciform ligament
    c. ligamentum venosum
    d. crura of the diaphragm

34. The lungs are separated into hemispheres by which of the following structures?
    a. heart
    b. sternum
    c. pleural cavity
    d. pleural membrane

35. Which of the following acoustic windows is generally used in noncardiac imaging of the chest?
    a. subcostal
    b. intercostal
    c. intracostal
    d. suprasternal

36. Omental cysts generally develop adjacent to which of the following structures?
    a. liver and right kidney
    b. pancreas and stomach
    c. spleen and diaphragm
    d. umbilicus and urinary bladder

37. Which of the following patient positions is utilized for a paracentesis procedure?
    a. prone
    b. supine
    c. decubitus
    d. 30 degrees oblique

38. The prevesical space is located in which of the following regions?
    a. pelvis
    b. chest
    c. umbilical
    d. left upper quadrant

39. Palsy of the phrenic nerve is associated with:
    a. pleural effusion
    b. subphrenic ascites
    c. pericardial effusion
    d. diaphragmatic paralysis

40. Which of the following structures has the potential to seal off infections within the peritoneal cavity?
    a. greater omentum
    b. mesentery
    c. peritoneum
    d. lesser omentum

41. The inferior portion of the peritoneum is formed by which of the following structures?
    a. pouch of Douglas
    b. space of Retzius
    c. greater omentum
    d. vesicouterine pouch

42. Which of the following peritoneal spaces serves as a conduit between the upper abdominal cavity and pelvis?
    a. lesser sac
    b. Morison pouch
    c. paracolic gutters
    d. subhepatic space

43. Hemoperitoneum may be associated with which of the following conditions?
    a. cirrhosis
    b. cholecystitis
    c. necrotic neoplasm
    d. pyelonephritis

44. Failure of the mesentery to fuse is a congenital anomaly associated with development of a(n):
    a. omental cyst
    b. mesentery cyst
    c. umbilical hernia
    d. Meckel diverticulum

45. Which of the following terms is most likely used to describe the sonographic appearance of mesenteric lymphomatous?
    a. target sign
    b. sandwich sign
    c. keyboard sign
    d. doughnut sign

46. Which of the following structures encloses the inferior esophagus?
    a. lesser sac
    b. mesentery
    c. lesser omentum
    d. greater omentum

47. Which of the following is the best protection against the spread of pathogens?
    a. wearing gloves
    b. wearing a mask
    c. wearing a gown
    d. frequent handwashing

48. An accumulation of fluid and pus in the peritoneal cavity describes:
    a. chylous ascites
    b. peritonitis
    c. exudative ascites
    d. transudative ascites

49. Which of the following invasive procedures removes a small piece of tissue for microscopic analysis?
    a. biopsy
    b. lumpectomy
    c. laparoscopy
    d. fine-needle aspiration

50. When localizing a fluid collection for a paracentesis procedure, the sonographer must:
    a. increase transducer pressure
    b. remain parallel to the floor
    c. increase the transducer frequency
    d. remain perpendicular to the floor

ABDOMEN MOCK EXAM

1. Which of the following structures is used as a sonographic landmark in locating the gallbladder fossa?
   a. main portal vein
   b. main lobar fissure
   c. intersegmental fissure
   d. ligamentum venosum

2. Which of the following conditions is the most common cause of acute pancreatitis?
   a. alcohol abuse
   b. biliary disease
   c. hyperlipidemia
   d. parathyroid disease

3. Gerota fascia provides a protective covering around which of the following organs?
   a. liver
   b. spleen
   c. kidney
   d. prostate

4. Increased pressure within the portosplenic venous system will most likely lead to which of the following conditions?
   a. fatty infiltration
   b. intestinal angina
   c. portal hypertension
   d. portal vein thrombosis

5. Normal diameter of the main portal vein in the adult patient should not exceed:
   a. 0.3 cm
   b. 0.5 cm
   c. 1.3 cm
   d. 2.0 cm

6. The integrity of which of the following structures is evaluated with the Thompson test?
   a. calf muscles
   b. rotator cuff
   c. Achilles tendon
   d. carpal tunnel nerve

7. A small hyperechoic pancreas is identified on ultrasound. This is most suspicious for which of the following abnormalities?
   a. islet cell tumor
   b. cystic fibrosis
   c. chronic pancreatitis
   d. fatty infiltration

8. Which of the following structures is a part of the endocrine system?
   a. liver
   b. spleen
   c. pancreas
   d. gallbladder

9. Which of the following is a sonographic finding of an echinococcal cyst?
   a. target lesions
   b. cystic masses
   c. complex masses
   d. septated cystic mass

10. A predisposing risk factor associated with the development of cholangiocarcinoma may include a history of:
    a. hepatitis
    b. cholecystitis
    c. appendicitis
    d. ulcerative colitis

11. A synovial cyst located in the medial popliteal fossa describes a:
    a. Hunter cyst
    b. Baker cyst
    c. Caroli cyst
    d. Thompson cyst

12. Liver length should be measured:
    a. at midclavicular level
    b. at the level of the right anterior lobe
    c. medial to the right kidney
    d. at the level of the right posterior lobe

13. An ultrasound is requested to rule out Budd-Chiari syndrome. The sonographer should thoroughly evaluate which of the following organs?
    a. liver
    b. spleen
    c. kidneys
    d. adrenal glands

14. Which of the following structures divide the left lobe of the liver into two segments?
    a. left portal vein and ligamentum of Teres
    b. left hepatic vein and ligamentum venosum
    c. left hepatic vein and ligamentum of Teres
    d. main portal vein and ligamentum venosum

15. Cholecystokinin is stimulated after food reaches the:
    a. cecum
    b. stomach
    c. esophagus
    d. duodenum

16. The gallbladder is located on the posterior surface of the liver and:
    a. medial to the inferior vena cava
    b. anterior to the main lobar fissure
    c. medial to the right kidney
    d. superior to the main lobar fissure

17. The most important measurement when evaluating for pyloric stenosis is the:
    a. length of the pyloric canal
    b. transverse diameter of the pyloric canal
    c. thickness of the pyloric muscle
    d. anterior posterior diameter of the pyloric canal

18. A patient presents with a history of severe back pain, weight loss, and painless jaundice. An abnormality in which of the following organs is most likely to correlate with these symptoms?
    a. liver
    b. spleen
    c. pancreas
    d. gallbladder

19. "Current jelly" stool is a clinical finding in which of the following abnormalities?
    a. appendicitis
    b. Crohn disease
    c. pyloric stenosis
    d. intussusception

20. Which of the following structures surrounds the liver?
    a. Gerota's fascia
    b. greater omentum
    c. surgical capsule
    d. Glisson's capsule

21. Which of the following conditions is associated with Mirizzi syndrome?
    a. biliary atresia
    b. pancreatic neoplasm
    c. gallbladder neoplasm
    d. impacted stone in the cystic duct

22. A spaghetti-like echogenic tubular structure within a bile duct is a sonographic finding associated with:
    a. ascariasis
    b. clonorchiasis
    c. hydatid disease
    d. schistosomiasis

23. Gallbladder wall thickening is *not* a sonographic finding in:
    a. benign ascites
    b. nonfasting patients
    c. hyperalbuminemia
    d. congestive heart failure

24. The Whipple procedure is a surgical resection of which of the following organs?
    a. liver
    b. spleen
    c. pancreas
    d. gallbladder

25. A fluid collection caused by extravasated bile is termed a:
    a. biloma
    b. seroma
    c. hematoma
    d. lymphocele

26. Spontaneous separation of the intima and media layers of an artery describes a(n):
    a. rupture
    b. aneurysm
    c. dissection
    d. pseudoaneurysm

27. Which of the following peritoneal spaces most commonly demonstrates ascites?
    a. lesser sac
    b. paracolic gutter
    c. subphrenic space
    d. subhepatic space

28. Which of the following structures lies within the anterior pararenal space?
    a. spleen
    b. kidneys
    c. pancreas
    d. adrenal glands

29. The crura of the diaphragm are located:
    a. anterior to the inferior vena cava and abdominal aorta
    b. posterior to the inferior vena cava and abdominal aorta
    c. anterior to the inferior vena cava and posterior to the abdominal aorta
    d. posterior to the inferior vena cava and anterior to the abdominal aorta

30. Splenomegaly is a consistent finding in which of the following pathologies?
    a. polycystic disease
    b. hepatic vein thrombosis
    c. portal hypertension
    d. hepatocellular carcinoma

31. Carcinoma in which of the following structures can directly extend into the gallbladder?
    a. spleen
    b. lung
    c. kidney
    d. stomach

32. Enlargement of the gallbladder caused by obstruction of the common bile duct by a distal external neoplasm is termed:
    a. Bouveret sign
    b. Mirizzi syndrome
    c. Courvoisier sign
    d. Budd-Chiari syndrome

33. Which of the following structures define the superior and inferior borders of the retroperitoneum?
    a. diaphragm and pelvic rim
    b. pancreas and urinary bladder
    c. crura of the diaphragm and symphysis pubis
    d. posterior peritoneum and the posterior abdominal wall muscles

34. Elevation in prostatic specific antigen (PSA) is suspicious for:
    a. prostatitis
    b. hydronephrosis
    c. prostatic carcinoma
    d. benign prostatic hypertrophy

35. Thrombosis involving the hepatic veins describes which of the following conditions?
    a. Mirizzi syndrome
    b. Caroli disease
    c. Budd-Chiari syndrome
    d. Couinaud syndrome

36. A sonogram of the right upper quadrant demonstrates a calculus lodged in the cystic duct. This finding is a predisposing factor for developing:
    a. cholangitis
    b. acute cholecystitis
    c. adenomyomatosis
    d. portal vein thrombosis

37. Which of the following structures may be mistaken for an extrarenal pelvis?
    a. renal vein
    b. adrenal cyst
    c. fetal lobulation
    d. hypertrophied column of Bertin

38. An irregular complex, solitary liver mass in a febrile patient is most suspicious for a(n):
    a. hepatoma
    b. cystadenoma
    c. amebic abscess
    d. echinococcal cyst

39. Which of the following terms is more commonly used to describe an enlarged or dilated vein?
    a. varix
    b. venule
    c. aneurysm
    d. perforator

40. Which of the following conditions most commonly causes the formation of a hepatic abscess?
    a. hepatitis
    b. cholelithiasis
    c. acute pancreatitis
    d. ascending cholangitis

41. Which of the following structures is located in the anterolateral portion of the pancreatic head?
    a. splenic vein
    b. common bile duct
    c. gastroduodenal artery
    d. portosplenic confluence

42. A sonogram demonstrates an echogenic thyroid mass with a prominent hypoechoic peripheral halo. This mass is most suspicious for which of the following neoplasms?
    a. goiter
    b. lipoma
    c. adenoma
    d. carcinoma

43. Which of the following organs is responsible for manufacturing heparin?
    a. liver
    b. spleen
    c. pancreas
    d. adrenal gland

44. The length of a normal adult spleen should not exceed:
    a. 8 cm
    b. 10 cm
    c. 13 cm
    d. 17 cm

45. Which type of aneurysm is most commonly associated with a bacterial infection?
    a. true aneurysm
    b. mycotic aneurysm
    c. ectatic aneurysm
    d. dissecting aneurysm

46. The stomach produces which of the following enzymes?
    a. gastrin
    b. pepsin
    c. amylase
    d. cholecystokinin

47. Which of the following conditions is associated with rebound pain at McBurney point?
    a. pancreatitis
    b. cholecystitis
    c. appendicitis
    d. Crohn disease

48. Which of the following is the best defense against the spread of disease?
    a. wearing gloves
    b. wearing a mask
    c. wearing a gown
    d. frequent hand washing

49. Which of the following is the most common clinical symptom associated with portal vein thrombosis?
    a. jaundice
    b. weight loss
    c. lower extremity edema
    d. severe abdominal pain

50. Which of the following structures indicates the neck of the urinary bladder?
    a. trigone
    b. hypogastric artery
    c. urethral orifice
    d. superior vesical artery

Using Figure 1, answer questions 51 and 52.

51. A retroperitoneal ultrasound is ordered to follow up on previously documented hydronephrosis of the right kidney. An image of the right kidney demonstrates a small hyperechoic focus (arrow). This focus is most suspicious for a renal:
    a. calculus
    b. carcinoma
    c. hemangioma
    d. angiomyolipoma

52. Regarding the patient's previous history of hydronephrosis, the sonographer's technical impression on this current image should include:
    a. Grade 1 hydronephrosis
    b. Grade 2 hydronephrosis
    c. Grade 3 hydronephrosis
    d. Grade 4 hydronephrosis

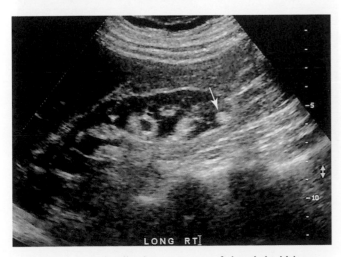

FIG. 1 Longitudinal sonogram of the right kidney.

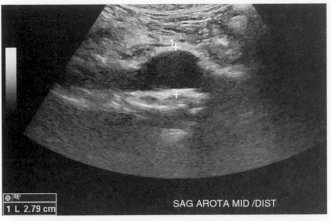

FIG. 2 Sagittal sonogram of the distal abdominal aorta.

Using Figure 2, answer question 53.

53. The sonogram of the distal abdominal aorta is most consistent with a(n):
    a. pseudoaneurysm
    b. ectatic aneurysm
    c. dissecting aneurysm
    d. abdominal aortic aneurysm

Using Figure 3, answer question 54.

54. Which of the following vascular structures does the arrow identify?
    a. right renal vein
    b. main portal vein
    c. right renal artery
    d. proper hepatic artery

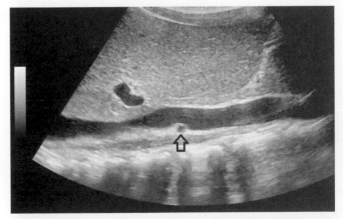

FIG. 3 Longitudinal sonogram of the right upper quadrant.

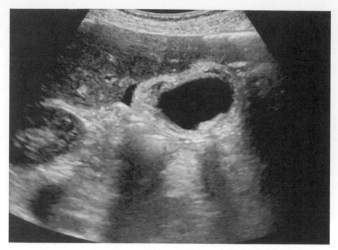

FIG. 4 Transverse sonogram of the gallbladder.

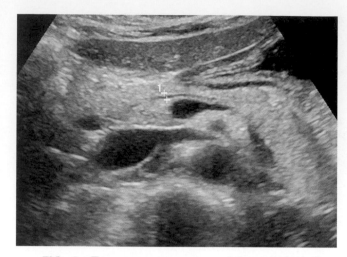

FIG. 6 Transverse sonogram of the pancreas.

Using Figure 4, answer question 55.

55. The pathology identified in this sonogram is most suspicious for:
    a. porcelain gallbladder
    b. Mirizzi syndrome
    c. acute cholecystitis
    d. gallbladder carcinoma

Using Figure 5, answer question 56.

56. The finding(s) in this sonogram is most suspicious for a(n):
    a. hydrocele
    b. ascites
    c. inguinal hernia
    d. epididymal cyst

Using Figure 6, answer question 57.

57. The calipers are measuring which of the following structures?
    a. splenic vein
    b. splenic artery
    c. pancreatic duct
    d. common bile duct

Using Figure 7, answer question 58.

58. The arrow is most likely identifying which of the following?
    a. adenoma
    b. hepatoma
    c. normal liver parenchyma
    d. focal nodular hyperplasia

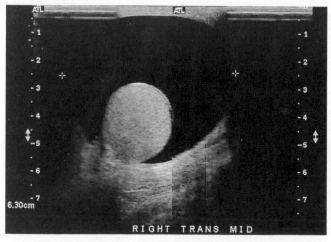

FIG. 5 Transverse sonogram of the scrotum.

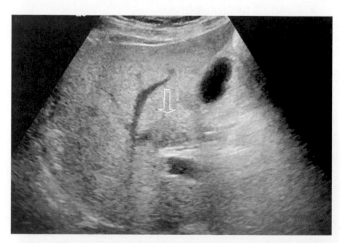

FIG. 7 Transverse sonogram of the liver.

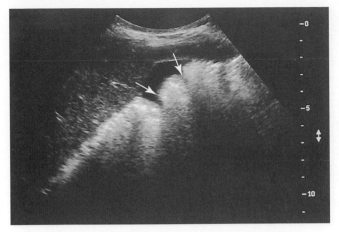

FIG. 8 Sonogram of the transverse colon.

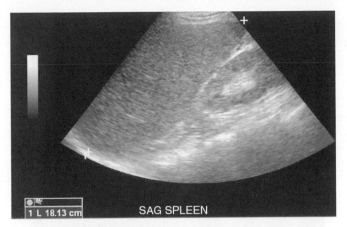

FIG. 10 Sagittal sonogram of the left upper quadrant.

Using Figure 8, answer question 59.

59. Which of the following structures do the arrows identify?
    a. rugae
    b. haustra
    c. polyps
    d. diverticulum

Using Figure 9, answer question 60.

60. An incidental finding is identified in this sonogram of the spleen. This sonogram is most suspicious for a(n):
    a. adenoma
    b. lipoma
    c. metastatic lesion
    d. cavernous hemangioma

Using Figure 10, answer questions 61 and 62.

61. A patient presents with a history of alcohol abuse. Which of the following splenic pathologies is most likely identified in this sonogram?
    a. infarction
    b. polysplenia
    c. lymphoma
    d. splenomegaly

62. With this pathological finding, the sonographer should evaluate for:
    a. pancreatitis
    b. cholelithiasis
    c. biliary obstruction
    d. venous collaterals

Using Figure 11, answer question 63.

63. Which of the following pathologies is identified in this sonogram of the right upper quadrant?
    a. cholangitis
    b. Courvoisier sign
    c. choledocholithiasis
    d. cholangiocarcinoma

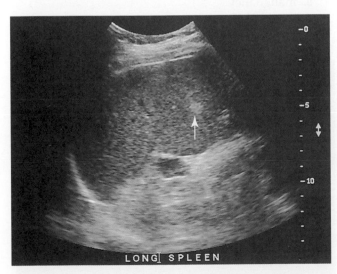

FIG. 9 Longitudinal sonogram of the spleen.

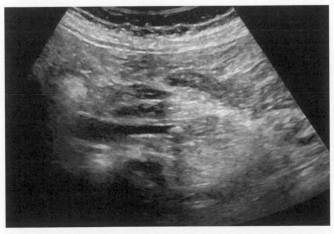

FIG. 11 Sagittal sonogram of the right upper quadrant.

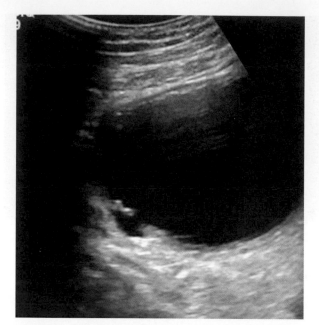

FIG. 12 Transverse sonogram of the urinary bladder.

Using Figure 12, answer question 64.

64. An abnormal finding identified in this sonogram is most consistent with a:
   a. hydroureter
   b. ureterocele
   c. bladder carcinoma
   d. bladder diverticulum

Using Figure 13, answer questions 65 and 66.

65. A patient presents with a history of uncontrolled hypertension and painless hematuria. On the basis of the clinical history, the sonogram is most suspicious for a:
   a. complex renal cyst
   b. malignant neoplasm
   c. necrotic angiomyolipoma
   d. hypertrophied column of Bertin

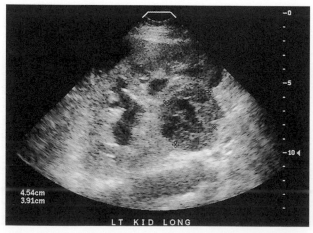

FIG. 13 Longitudinal sonogram of the left kidney.

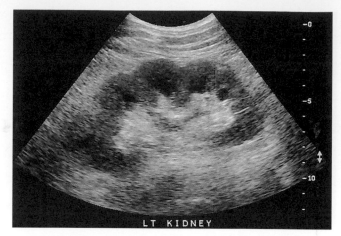

FIG. 14 Sagittal sonogram of the left kidney.

66. Which of the following conditions is also identified in this sonogram?
   a. renal failure
   b. multiple renal cysts
   c. hydronephrosis
   d. renal vein thrombosis

Using Figure 14, answer question 67.

67. Which of the following congenital anomalies is identified in this image of the left kidney?
   a. renal ptosis
   b. fetal lobulation
   c. dromedary hump
   d. junctional parenchymal defect

Using Figure 15, answer questions 68 and 69.

68. Which of the following is identified by the arrows?
   a. scrotal pearl
   b. malignancy
   c. microcalcifications
   d. tubular ectasia of the rete testis

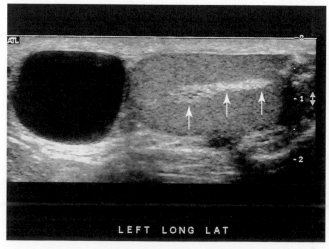

FIG. 15 Sonogram of the left scrotal sac.

69. A large anechoic structure is demonstrated in the superior portion of the left scrotum. This structure most likely represents a:
   a. scrotal cyst
   b. hydrocele
   c. testicular cyst
   d. epididymal cyst

Using Figure 16, answer questions 70 and 71.

70. Which of the following congenital anomalies is most likely identified in this sonogram of the right kidney?
   a. horseshoe kidney
   b. fetal lobulation
   c. renal duplication
   d. crossed fused ectopia

71. On the basis of the cortical thickness, which of the following abnormalities is most likely identified in this single image of the right kidney?
   a. pyelonephritis
   b. acute tubular necrosis
   c. chronic renal disease
   d. medullary sponge disease

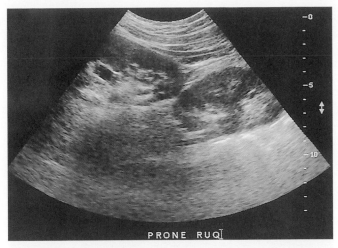

FIG. 17   Sonogram of the right upper quadrant.

Using Figure 17, answer question 72.

72. Which of the following congenital anomalies is most likely demonstrated in this sonogram?
   a. renal ptosis
   b. horseshoe kidney
   c. sigmoid kidney
   d. renal duplication

Using Figure 18, answer question 73.

73. Which of the following abnormalities is the most likely cause of the sonographic finding(s) in this image of the distal calf?
   a. cellulitis
   b. muscle tear
   c. multiple lipomas
   d. superficial thrombophlebitis

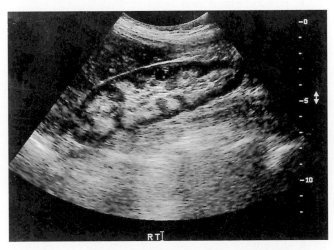

FIG. 16   Sagittal sonogram of the right kidney.

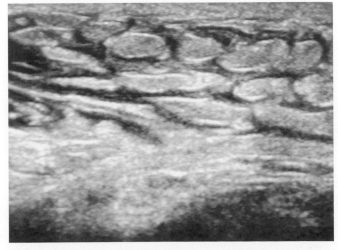

FIG. 18   Sagittal sonogram of the distal calf.

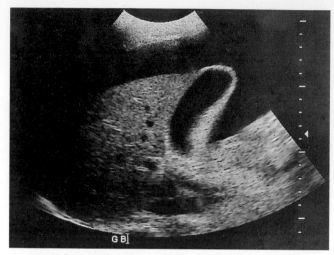

FIG. 19 Sonogram of the right upper quadrant.

Using Figure 19, answer questions 74 and 75.

74. Which of the following peritoneal spaces demonstrate a fluid collection?
    a. subphrenic space and Morison pouch
    b. subphrenic and subhepatic spaces
    c. subphrenic space and lesser sac
    d. subhepatic space and Morison pouch

75. The sonographer's technical impression of the gallbladder should state:
    a. cholelithiasis
    b. acute cholecystitis
    c. hydropic gallbladder
    d. probable noninflammatory wall thickening

76. Which of the following structures separates the caudate lobe from the left lobe of the liver?
    a. left portal vein
    b. falciform ligament
    c. main lobar fissure
    d. ligamentum venosum

77. A questionable mass is identified in the anterior portion of the right lobe of the liver. Which of the following structures border this region?
    a. left hepatic and right hepatic veins
    b. right portal and right hepatic veins
    c. middle hepatic and right hepatic veins
    d. right hepatic and main portal veins

78. A mass displacing the renal calyces is documented on a recent intravenous pyelogram. A sonogram over this area demonstrates a smooth circular anechoic renal mass. This mass is most suspicious for:
    a. a simple cyst
    b. a cystadenoma
    c. an extrarenal pelvis
    d. hydronephrosis

79. When hydronephrosis is encountered, the sonographer should evaluate the urinary bladder for evidence of a(n):
    a. infection
    b. obstruction
    c. duplication
    d. inflammation

80. Which of the following structures is most likely located adjacent to an omental cyst?
    a. stomach
    b. left kidney
    c. umbilicus
    d. gallbladder

81. To aid in demonstrating posterior acoustic shadowing, the sonographer should:
    a. decrease the image depth
    b. decrease the dynamic range
    c. increase the transducer frequency
    d. decrease the number of focal zones

82. A patient presents with a mass in the lateral aspect of the neck. An anechoic structure is demonstrated just beneath the jawline. Which of the following cystic structures is most likely identified?
    a. lingual cyst
    b. parotid gland cyst
    c. thyroglossal cyst
    d. brachial cleft cyst

83. Extension of pancreatic inflammation into the surrounding tissues is termed a(n):
    a. abscess
    b. pseudocyst
    c. hemorrhage
    d. phlegmon

84. The inferior vena cava is considered enlarged after the diameter exceeds:
    a. 1.7 cm
    b. 2.5 cm
    c. 3.0 cm
    d. 3.7 cm

85. Which of the following organs is associated with an elevation of aldosterone?
    a. testes
    b. thyroid
    c. pancreas
    d. adrenal gland

86. An incidental finding of a round, homogeneous, solid mass medial to the splenic hilum is identified The mass is most likely a(n):
    a. gastric neoplasm
    b. accessory spleen
    c. adrenal adenoma
    d. visceral lymph node

87. Which of the following vascular structures is commonly mistaken as the pancreatic duct?
    a. splenic artery
    b. splenic vein
    c. gastric artery
    d. gastroduodenal artery

88. Cortical thickness of the normal adult kidney should measure a minimum of:
    a. 0.7 cm
    b. 1.0 cm
    c. 1.5 cm
    d. 2.0 cm

89. Which of the following conditions is associated with a complete failure of the adrenocortical function?
    a. Cushing disease
    b. Addison disease
    c. Caroli disease
    d. Graves' disease

90. The main renal arteries arise from the lateral aspect of the aorta approximately 1.5 cm inferior to the:
    a. celiac axis
    b. portosplenic confluence
    c. caudate lobe of the liver
    d. superior mesenteric artery

91. Which of the following blood values is most commonly associated with internal hemorrhage?
    a. platelets
    b. leukocytes
    c. hematocrit
    d. hemoglobin

92. Which of the following is an abnormal flow characteristic of the hepatic veins?
    a. pulsatile
    b. hepatopetal
    c. multiphasic
    d. spontaneous

93. Which of the following organs is associated with the "olive sign"?
    a. liver
    b. stomach
    c. appendix
    d. gallbladder

94. Which of the following patient positions is typically used during a thoracentesis?
    a. prone
    b. sitting
    c. decubitus
    d. Trendelenburg

95. Which of the following structures is most commonly mistaken as a renal neoplasm?
    a. psoas muscle
    b. extrarenal pelvis
    c. junctional parenchymal defect
    d. hypertrophied column of Bertin

96. Which of the following laboratory tests will most likely elevate in cases of nonobstructive jaundice?
    a. serum albumin
    b. indirect bilirubin
    c. alkaline phosphatase
    d. conjugated bilirubin

97. Which region of the gallbladder is located most superiorly?
    a. body
    b. neck
    c. fundus
    d. phrygian cap

98. Which of the following conditions is associated with an increased risk in developing a thyroid malignancy?
    a. Graves disease
    b. de Quervain syndrome
    c. Hashimoto disease
    d. Addison disease

99. Which of the following invasive procedures removes a small piece of living tissue for microscopic analysis?
    a. core biopsy
    b. paracentesis
    c. fine-needle biopsy
    d. cyst aspiration

100. A pancreatic pseudocyst is most commonly located in which of the following regions?
    a. lesser sac
    b. subphrenic space
    c. pararenal space
    d. Morison pouch

101. A patient presents to the emergency department with severe left upper quadrant pain. Laboratory values demonstrate an elevation in serum lipase. An abdominal ultrasound is ordered to rule out:
    a. cirrhosis
    b. splenomegaly
    c. biliary disease
    d. hepatic malignancy

102. Which of the following anatomical variants demonstrates an outward bulge to the lateral renal cortex?
    a. fetal lobulation
    b. dromedary hump
    c. junctional parenchymal defect
    d. hypertrophied column of Bertin

103. A congenital anomaly associated with the fusion of both kidneys within the same body quadrant describes:
    a. a cake kidney
    b. a renal ptosis
    c. a horseshoe kidney
    d. crossed fused ectopia

104. A patient with a recent history of angioplasty presents with a pulsatile inguinal mass. A fluid collection adjacent to the common femoral artery is identified. Color and spectral Doppler demonstrates turbulent blood flow within the fluid collection. On the basis of the clinical history, the sonographic findings are most consistent with a(n):
    a. femoral hernia
    b. hematoma
    c. pseudoaneurysm
    d. arteriovenous malformation

105. Which of the following vascular structures should be documented when evaluating for an inguinal hernia?
    a. internal iliac artery
    b. inferior epigastric artery
    c. superior epigastric artery
    d. saphenofemoral junction

106. Which of the following tasks is a function of the spleen?
    a. regulate serum electrolytes
    b. remove foreign material from the blood
    c. convert excess amino acids into glucose
    d. maintain homeostasis of calcium concentration

107. An abnormality of the gallbladder wall exhibiting a "comet tail" artifact describes:
    a. pneumobilia
    b. adenomyomatosis
    c. porcelain gallbladder
    d. gallbladder carcinoma

108. A transplant kidney is more commonly placed in which of the following regions?
    a. left lower quadrant
    b. periumbilical area
    c. right lower quadrant
    d. right upper quadrant

109. Which of the following descriptions most accurately portrays the sonographic appearance and location of a Meckel diverticulum?
    a. hyperechoic mass located near the anal canal
    b. isoechoic mass located near the ileocecal valve
    c. anechoic or complex mass, slightly to the right of the umbilicus
    d. complex mass, slightly inferior to the ligamentum venosum

110. Which of the following terms describes a noninflammatory degenerative change in a tendon?
    a. tenalgia
    b. tendonitis
    c. tenodynia
    d. tendinosis

111. Within 5 years, the risk for rupture of an abdominal aortic aneurysm measuring 5 cm in diameter is:
    a. 5%
    b. 15%
    c. 25%
    d. 75%

112. Before the bifurcation, the last major visceral branch of the abdominal aorta is the:
    a. lumbar artery
    b. hypogastric artery
    c. median sacral artery
    d. inferior mesenteric artery

113. Which of the following abnormalities commonly coexists in patients with a popliteal aneurysm?
    a. synovial cyst
    b. deep vein thrombosis
    c. congestive heart failure
    d. abdominal aortic aneurysm

114. Which of the following peritoneal spaces is located superior to the liver?
    a. lesser sac
    b. prevesical space
    c. subphrenic space
    d. Morison pouch

115. A patient arrives for an abdominal ultrasound owing to a history of hepatitis B. Which of the following abnormalities is the clinician likely to exclude?
    a. cirrhosis
    b. fatty infiltration
    c. portal hypertension
    d. hepatocellular carcinoma

116. The majority of metastatic lesions in the liver originate from which of the following sites?
    a. lung
    b. breast
    c. colon
    d. pancreas

117. The common bile duct passes through which of the following structures before entering the duodenum?
    a. ampulla of Oddi
    b. duct of Wirsung
    c. ampulla of Vater
    d. foramen of Winslow

118. Which of the following conditions is the most common cause of hypothyroidism?
    a. Graves disease
    b. de Quervain syndrome
    c. Hashimoto disease
    d. Bouveret syndrome

119. The pyramidal lobe of the thyroid gland arises from the:
    a. inferior aspect of a thyroid lobe
    b. superior aspect of the isthmus
    c. anterior aspect of the thyroid gland
    d. posterior aspect of the isthmus

120. Under normal conditions, which of the following arteries supply the majority of blood to the brain?
    a. vertebral arteries
    b. external carotid arteries
    c. internal carotid arteries
    d. middle cerebral arteries

121. Which of the following abnormalities involves the distal ureter and the urinary bladder?
    a. ureterocele
    b. diverticulum
    c. urachal sinus
    d. bladder polyp

122. Postvoid residual in a normal adult urinary bladder should not exceed:
    a. 5 mL
    b. 20 mL
    c. 50 mL
    d. 100 mL

123. Malignant neoplasms involving the colon are more commonly located in which of the following regions?
    a. anus
    b. cecum
    c. rectum
    d. sigmoid colon

124. Which of the following vascular structures courses posterior to the superior mesenteric artery?
    a. splenic vein
    b. splenic artery
    c. left renal vein
    d. superior mesenteric vein

125. On ultrasound, visualization of a needle during an invasive procedure is attained in a plane:
    a. parallel to the needle path
    b. perpendicular to the needle path
    c. medial to the needle path
    d. perpendicular to the examination table

Using Figure 20, answer questions 126 and 127.

126. The sonographic findings are most suspicious for which of the following abnormalities?
    a. candidiasis
    b. liver metastasis
    c. cirrhosis
    d. focal nodular hyperplasia

127. A round anechoic mass is identified in the medial portion of the liver. Which of the following structures does this anechoic mass most likely represent?
    a. gallbladder
    b. hepatic cyst
    c. hepatic abscess
    d. choledochal cyst

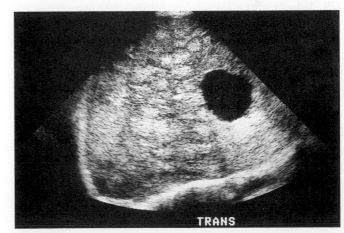

FIG. 20 Transverse sonogram of the liver.

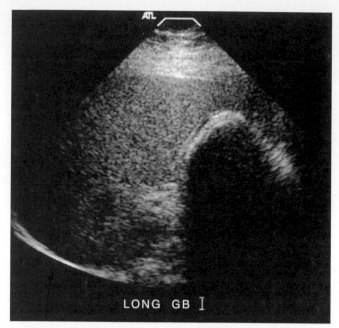

FIG. 21   Sagittal sonogram of the right upper quadrant.

Using Figure 21, answer question 128.

128. This sonographic finding is characteristic of the:
   a. target sign
   b. WES sign
   c. olive sign
   d. keyboard sign

Using Figure 22, answer question 129.

129. Which of the following intrahepatic structures does the arrow identify?
   a. falciform ligament
   b. main lobar fissure
   c. ligamentum of Teres
   d. ligamentum venosum

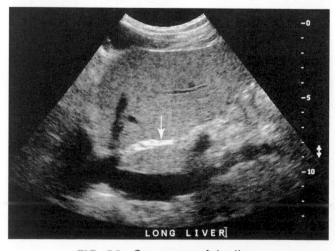

FIG. 22   Sonogram of the liver.

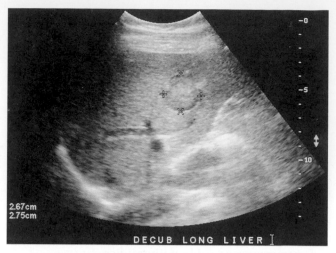

FIG. 23   Sagittal sonogram of the liver.

Using Figure 23, answer question 130.

130. An annual screening examination of the upper abdomen is ordered on an asymptomatic patient with a history of hepatitis B. On the basis of the clinical history, this sonogram is most suspicious for a(n):
   a. abscess
   b. hepatoma
   c. metastatic lesion
   d. cavernous hemangioma

Using Figure 24 (and Color Plate 7), answer question 131.

131. Which of the following conditions is most likely identified in this sonogram of the left biliary tree?
   a. Berry syndrome
   b. Caroli disease
   c. Klatskin disease
   d. Budd-Chiari syndrome

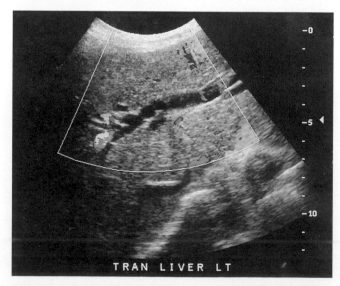

FIG. 24   Transverse sonogram of the liver (see Color Plate 7).

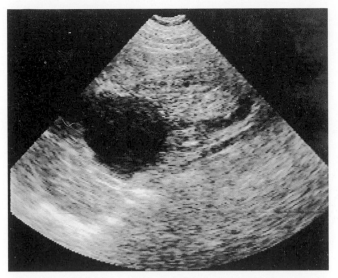

FIG. 25 Sagittal sonogram of the right upper quadrant.

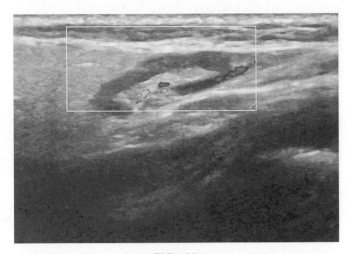

FIG. 27

Using Figure 25, answer question 132.

132. The sonographic characteristics of this mass are most consistent with a(n):
   a. renal cyst
   b. renal abscess
   c. malignant neoplasm
   d. adrenal hemorrhage

Using Figure 26, answer question 133.

133. Which of the following abnormalities is most likely identified in this transverse sonogram of the abdominal aorta?
   a. aortic rupture
   b. aortic dissection
   c. mycotic aneurysm
   d. aneurysm with intraluminal thrombus

Using Figure 27, answer question 134

134. Which of the following structures is most consistent with these sonographic findings?
   a. lipoma
   b. lymph node
   c. hematoma
   d. thrombosed vein

Using Figure 28, answer question 135.

135. An image of the left kidney in a pediatric patient demonstrates which of the following conditions?
   a. pyelonephritis
   b. mild hydronephrosis
   c. multiple peripelvic cysts
   d. normal neonatal kidney

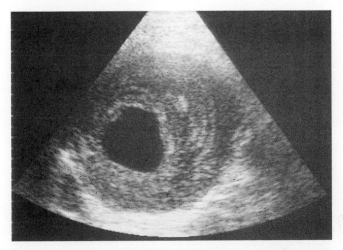

FIG. 26 Transverse sonogram of the abdominal aorta.

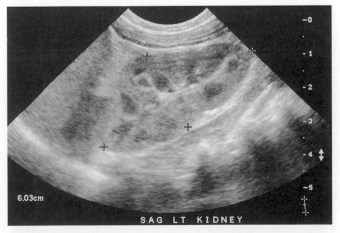

FIG. 28 Sagittal sonogram of a pediatric kidney.

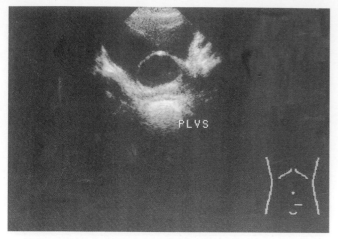

FIG. 29   Transverse sonogram of the urinary bladder.

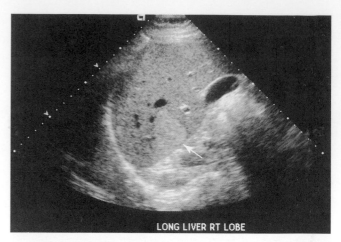

FIG. 31   Longitudinal sonogram of the liver.

Using Figure 29, answer question 136.

136. An incidental finding is identified in the urinary bladder. Which of the following abnormalities does this finding most likely represent?
 a. ureterocele
 b. hydroureter
 c. bladder diverticulum
 d. catheter balloon

Using Figure 30, answer question 137.

137. An older patient presents with a history of epigastric pain. A calculus is identified in the neck of the gallbladder. The echogenic foci are suspicious for tumefactive sludge or:
 a. adenomyomatosis
 b. metastatic lesions
 c. chronic cholecystitis
 d. gallbladder carcinoma

Using Figure 31, answer question 138.

138. An ultrasound examination of the abdomen is ordered on a thin female patient to evaluate a liver mass demonstrated on a CT scan. Which of the following pathologies does the arrow most likely identify?
 a. hepatoma
 b. adenoma
 c. cavernous hemangioma
 d. focal area of fatty infiltration

Using Figure 32, answer question 139.

139. Which of the following imaging artifacts is identified in this sonogram?
 a. mirror image
 b. reverberation
 c. focal banding
 d. edge shadowing

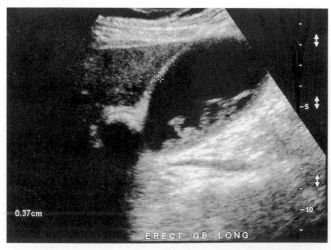

FIG. 30   Longitudinal sonogram of the gallbladder.

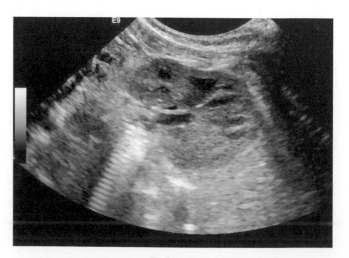

FIG. 32

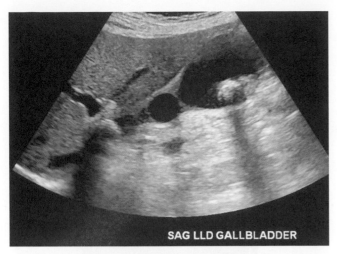

FIG. 33 Left lateral decubitus sonogram of the gallbladder.

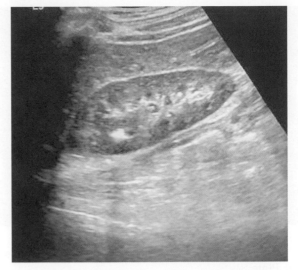

FIG. 34 Sagittal sonogram of the right kidney.

Using Figure 33, answer questions 140 and 141.

140. Which of the following structures is demonstrated in the region of the gallbladder neck?
   a. calculus
   b. surgical clip
   c. junctional fold
   d. Hartmann cap

141. This finding is most likely associated with which of the following?
   a. normal anatomical variant
   b. previous history of an abdominal surgery
   c. increased risk for developing cholelithiasis
   d. increased risk for developing acute cholecystitis

Using Figure 34, answer question 142.

142. Which of the following abnormalities is identified in this sagittal image of the right kidney?
   a. hamartoma
   b. nephrolithiasis
   c. angiomyolipoma
   d. arterial calcification

Using Figure 35, answer questions 143 and 144.

143. The sonographic findings in this image are most consistent with which of the following abnormalities?
   a. adenomas
   b. cholelithiasis
   c. metastatic lesions
   d. tumefactive sludge

144. Which of the following sonographic techniques will be most helpful in narrowing the differential considerations in this case?
   a. decubitus position
   b. ingestion of a fatty meal
   c. increasing the transducer frequency
   d. increased transducer pressure over the gallbladder

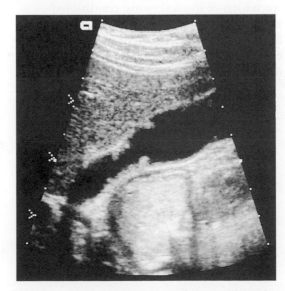

FIG. 35 Supine sonogram of the gallbladder.

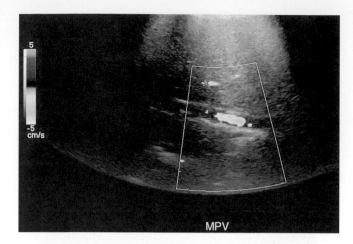

FIG. 36 Color Doppler image of the porta hepatis (see Color Plate 8).

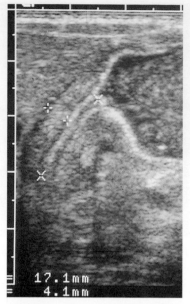

FIG. 37 Transverse sonogram.

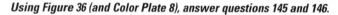

Using Figure 36 (and Color Plate 8), answer questions 145 and 146.

145. Which of the following abnormalities is demonstrated in this sonogram of the main portal vein?
   a. hepatopetal flow
   b. hepatofugal flow
   c. portal vein thrombosis
   d. Budd – Chiari syndrome

146. This abnormality is a sonographic finding for which of the following conditions?
   a. cirrhosis
   b. steatosis
   c. chronic hepatitis
   d. portal hypertension

Using Figure 37, answer question 147.

147. These sonographic findings are most suspicious for which of the following conditions?
   a. gastritis
   b. volvulus
   c. pyloric stenosis
   d. normal pyloric canal

Using Figure 38, answer question 148.

148. Which of the following abnormalities is identified in this sonogram of the pancreas?
   a. pseudocyst
   b. cystic fibrosis
   c. acute pancreatitis
   d. malignant neoplasm

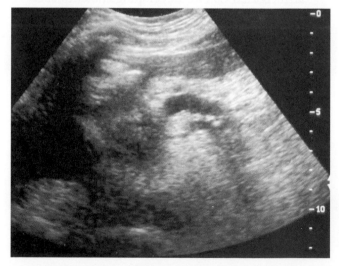

FIG. 38 Transverse sonogram of the pancreas.

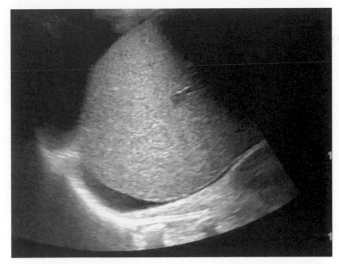

FIG. 39   Sagittal sonogram of the upper abdomen.

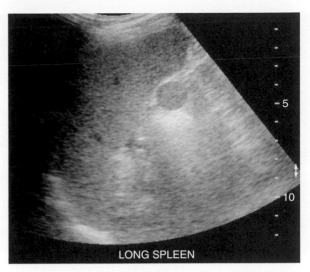

LONG SPLEEN

FIG. 41

Using Figure 39, answer question 149.

149. Which of the following ligaments is demonstrated in this sonogram of the upper abdomen?
   a. falciform
   b. venosum
   c. coronary
   d. hepatorenal

Using Figure 40, answer question 150.

150. Fluid collections are identified in which of the following regions?
   a. bilateral pleural spaces
   b. bilateral subphrenic spaces
   c. bilateral paracolic gutters
   d. subhepatic space and lesser sac

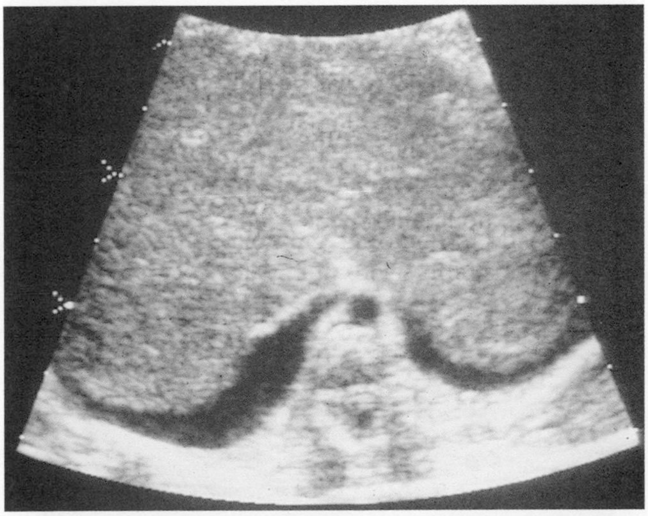

Using Figure 41, answer question 151.

151. Which of the following is identified in this sonogram of the left upper quadrant?
   a. an accessory spleen
   b. an adrenal adenoma
   c. renal cell carcinoma
   d. a retroperitoneal neoplasm

Using Figure 42, answer question 152.

152. Which of the following abnormalities is demonstrated in this post void image of the urinary bladder?
   a. polyp
   b. sludge
   c. carcinoma
   d. diverticulum

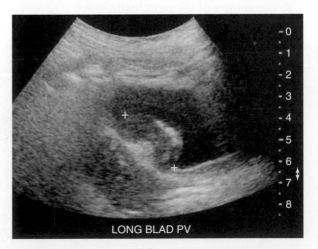

LONG BLAD PV

FIG. 42

FIG. 40   Transverse sonogram of the upper abdomen.

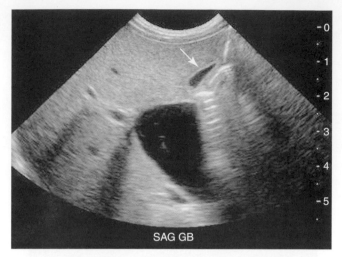

SAG GB

FIG. 43

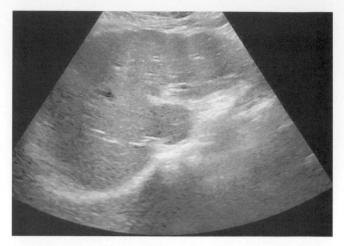

FIG. 45

Using Figure 43, answer question 153.

153. An asymptomatic 1-month-old infant presents with a history of jaundice. The arrow is pointing to the gallbladder. Based on this clinical history, the sonogram most likely demonstrates which of the following?
  a. biloma
  b. hepatic cyst
  c. portal vein varix
  d. choledochal cyst

Using Figure 44, answer question 154.

154. A patient presents with a history of vague right upper quadrant pain. Based on this clinical history, the sonogram most likely demonstrates which of the following pathologies?
  a. pseudocyst
  b. phlegmon
  c. chronic pancreatitis
  d. carcinoma of the pancreatic head

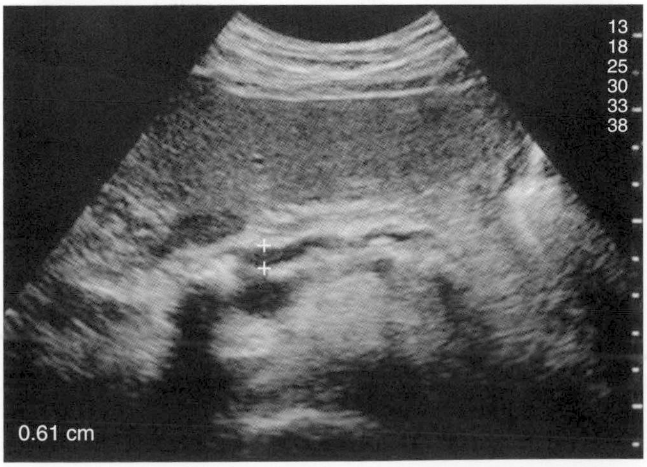

Using Figure 45, answer question 155.

155. A patient with a history of alcohol abuse arrives for an abdominal ultrasound. Based on this clinical history, the sonogram most likely demonstrates which of the following pathologies?
  a. cirrhosis
  b. steatosis
  c. metastatic liver disease
  d. focal nodular hyperplasia

Using Figure 46, answer questions 156 and 157.

156. The sonogram most likely demonstrates a(n):
  a. ureterocele
  b. ureteral stent
  c. stone in the distal ureter
  d. stone in the urinary bladder

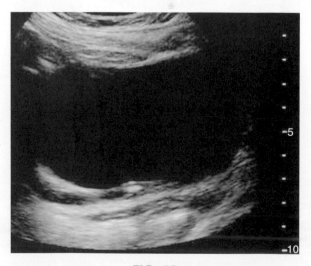

FIG. 46

0.61 cm

FIG. 44

157. What is most likely associated with this diagnosis?
   a. cholelithiasis
   b. hydronephrosis
   c. renal abscess
   d. nephrocalcinosis

Using Figure 47, answer question 158.

158. A febrile 30-year-old male patient presents to the emergency department complaining of fatigue and nausea for the previous 3 days. Laboratory tests show marked elevation in AST, ALT, and bilirubin levels. Based on this clinical history, the sonogram most likely demonstrates which of the following pathologies?
   a. candidiasis
   b. acute hepatitis
   c. hepatic steatosis
   d. peliosis hepatitis

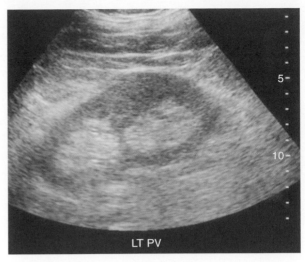

LT PV

FIG. 48

Using Figure 48, answer question 159.

159. The sonogram of the left kidney most likely demonstrates which of the following?
   a. dromedary hump
   b. renal duplication
   c. renal cell carcinoma
   d. hypertrophied column of Bertin

Using Figure 49, answer question 160.

160. A patient with a history of left testicular carcinoma presents with left upper quadrant pain. Based on this clinical history, the sonographic finding is most suspicious for which of the following pathologies?
   a. lymphadenopathy
   b. renal vein thrombosis
   c. metastatic disease
   d. bowel diverticulum

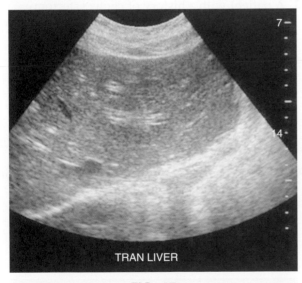

TRAN LIVER

FIG. 47

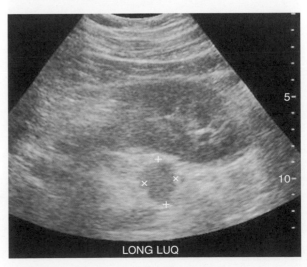

LONG LUQ

FIG. 49

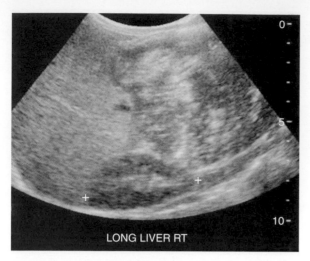

FIG. 50

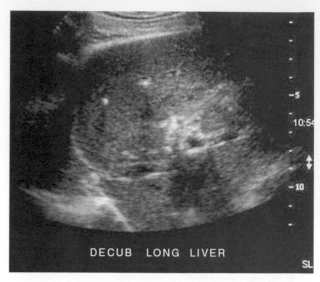

DECUB LONG LIVER

FIG. 52

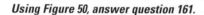

Using Figure 50, answer question 161.

161. A 13-month-old presents with a history of a palpable abdominal mass. Based on these findings, the sonogram is most suspicious for a(n):
   a. hematoma
   b. neuroblastoma
   c. bowel obstruction
   d. nephroblastoma

Using Figure 51, answer question 162.

162. A This sonogram of the anterior neck most likely demonstrates a(n):
   a. brachial cleft cyst
   b. thyroglossal cyst
   c. parathyroid cyst
   d. obstructed salivary gland

Using Figure 52, answer question 163.

163. A patient with a history of cholecystectomy arrives for an abdominal ultrasound.. Based on this clinical history, the sonogram most likely demonstrates:
   a. pneumobilia
   b. biliary calculi
   c. surgical clips
   d. calcified hepatic artery

Using Figure 53, answer question 164.

164. This transverse sonogram is most suspicious for which of the following abnormalities?
   a. hematoma
   b. urachal cyst
   c. diastasis rectus abdominis
   d. abdominal wall hernia

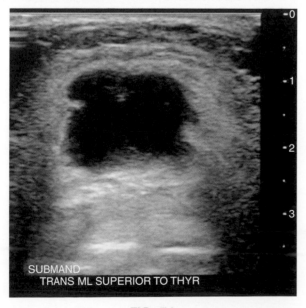

SUBMAND
TRANS ML SUPERIOR TO THYR

FIG. 51

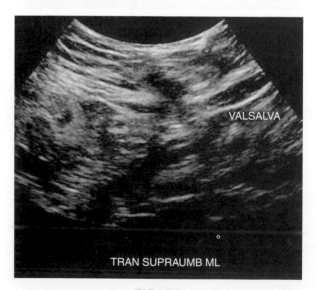

VALSALVA

TRAN SUPRAUMB ML

FIG. 53

165. The head of the pancreas surrounds the duodenum in which of the following anomalies?
    a. phlegmon
    b. ectopic pancreas
    c. annular pancreas
    d. pancreas divisum

166. Nonshadowing, low-amplitude echoes layering in the dependent portion of the gallbladder describe:
    a. gallstones
    b. biliary sludge
    c. adenomyomatosis
    d. tumefactive sludge

167. Which portion of the pancreas is located most superiorly in the abdomen?
    a. tail
    b. head
    c. neck
    d. body

168. Which of the following conditions is an inherited disorder?
    a. biliary atresia
    b. hyperaldosteronism
    c. polycystic kidney disease
    d. multicystic renal dysplasia

169. Renal dialysis patients have a predisposing factor for developing a renal:
    a. abscess
    b. lipoma
    c. calculus
    d. carcinoma

170. Which of the following approaches is used to evaluate for hip effusion in a pediatric patient?
    a. medial
    b. lateral
    c. anterior
    d. posterior

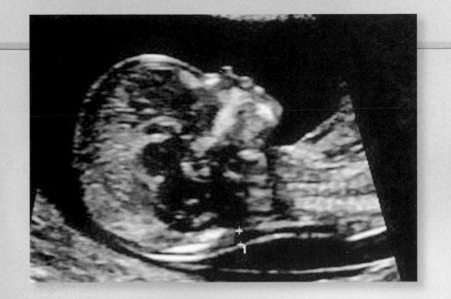

Obstetrics and Gynecology

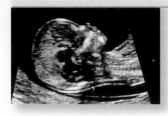

CHAPTER 19

Pelvic Anatomy

KEY TERMS

adnexa   region including the fallopian tube and ovary.

false pelvis   region of the pelvis located above the pelvic brim.

fimbriae ovarica   the one fimbriae attached to the ovary.

iliopectineal line   an imaginary line from the superior border of the sacrum to the superior margin of the pubis symphysis that divides the true and false pelvis.

ligament   extension of a double layer of peritoneum between visceral organs.

menarche   onset of menstrual cycles.

menopause   cessation of menses.

mesovarian   posterior portion of the peritoneum that attaches to the ovary.

mesosalpinx   upper fold of the broad ligament that drapes over the fallopian tube.

perineum   the surface region in both males and females between the pubic symphysis and the coccyx; area below the pelvic floor.

premenarche   time before the onset of menstrual cycles.

puberty   refers to the process of physical changes by which a child's body becomes an adult body capable of reproduction.

true pelvis   region of the pelvis found below the pelvic brim.

PELVIC ANATOMY (Fig. 19.1)

- Pelvis begins at the iliac crests and ends at the symphysis pubis.
- Divided into the true and false pelvis by the iliopectineal line.

True Pelvis

- Also known as pelvic cavity, lesser pelvis.
- Most inferior portion of the body cavity.
- Located inferior to the pelvic brim.
- Muscles and ligaments form a pelvic floor.
- Anterior boundary—symphysis pubis.
- Posterior boundary—sacrum and coccyx.
- Posterolateral wall—piriformis and coccygeus muscles.
- Anterolateral wall—hip bone and obturator internus muscles.
- Lateral boundaries—fused ilium and ischium.
- Pelvic floor—levator ani and coccygeus muscles.
- Contains—female reproductive system, urinary bladder, distal ureters, and bowel.

False Pelvis

- Located superior to the pelvic brim.
- Anterior boundary—abdominal wall.
- Posterior boundary—flanged portions of the iliac bones and base of the sacrum.
- Lateral boundaries—abdominal wall.
- Contains—loops of bowel.

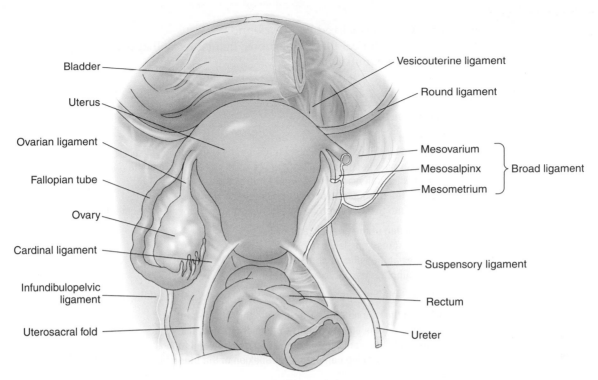

FIG. 19.1 Female pelvic anatomy.

Pelvic Muscles

PELVIC MUSCLE	DESCRIPTION	LOCATION	SONOGRAPHIC APPEARANCE
Levator ani	Name given to a group of muscles 1. puborectalis 2. iliococcygeus 3. pubococcygeus Forms the pelvic floor along with the piriformis muscles Supports and positions the pelvic organs	Most caudal structures within the pelvic cavity Medial to the obturator internus muscles Posterior to the vagina and cervix	Low-level, mildly curved linear echoes posterior to the vagina Hypoechoic compared with the normal uterus
Iliopsoas	Formed by the psoas major and iliacus muscles Lateral landmark of the true pelvis	Course anterior and lateral through the false pelvis Descend until attaching to the lesser trochanter of the femur	Low-level gray echoes with a distinct central hyperechoic focus Abut the lateral walls of the urinary bladder
Piriformis	Arise from the anterior sacrum Form part of the pelvic floor Course through the greater sciatic notch	Posterior to the uterus, ovaries, vagina, and rectum Anterior to the sacrum Course diagonally to the obturator internus muscle	Low-level linear echoes Hypoechoic compared with the normal uterus
Psoas major	Arises from the lumbar spine Descends into the false pelvis	Course laterally and anteriorly into the false pelvis Exits posterior to the inguinal ligament	Low-level echogenicity Round in shape in the transverse plane Imaged in the lower abdomen and upper pelvis lateral to the vertebrae
Obturator internus	Anterolateral margins of the true pelvis Surround the obturator foramen Extend through the sciatic foramen to attach to the greater trochanter	Posterior and medial to the iliopsoas muscles Level of the vagina Lateral to the ovaries	Low-level linear echoes abutting the lateral walls of the urinary bladder

Pelvic Ligaments

- Not routinely visualized by ultrasound.
- With intraperitoneal fluid collections, ligaments will appear as hyperechoic, moderately thin, linear structures.

Pelvic Ligaments

PELVIC LIGAMENT	DESCRIPTION
Broad	Wing-like double fold of peritoneum Drapes over the fallopian tubes, uterus, ovaries, and blood vessels Extends from the lateral walls of the uterus to the sidewalls of the pelvis Provides a small amount of support for the uterus Creates the retrouterine and vesicouterine pouches Divided into the mesometrium, mesosalpinx, and mesovarium segments
Cardinal	Continuation of the broad ligament Extends across the pelvic floor Attaches at the isthmus portion of the uterus Firmly supports the cervix
Ovarian	Extends from the cornua of the uterus to the medial aspect of the ovary
Round	Arises in the uterine cornua, anterior to the fallopian tubes Extends from the uterine fundus to the pelvic sidewalls Helps to maintain anteflexion of the uterine body and fundus Excessive stretching can permit retroflexion of the uterine body and fundus Contracts during labor
Suspensory	Also known as infundibulopelvic ligament Extends from the lateral portion of the ovary to the pelvic sidewall
Uterosacral	Extends from the upper cervix to the lateral margins of the sacrum Firmly supports the cervix

Pelvic Vasculature

VESSEL	LOCATION	INFORMATION

Arcuate vessels	Prominent vascular structures in the outer one third of the myometrium	Branch of the uterine artery
		Radial arteries arise from the arcuate arteries
		Radial artery branches:
		  Spiral arteries supply blood to the functional layer of the endometrium and respond to hormonal changes
		  Straight arteries supply blood to the basal layer of the endometrium
		Constriction of the spiral arteries cause menstruation to occur
		Larger-caliber vessels are typically arcuate veins

Internal iliac arteries	Posterior to the uterus and ovaries Follows a posterior course and enters the true pelvis near the sacral prominence	Aka: hypogastric arteries Supply the bladder, uterus, vagina, and rectum Give rise to the uterine arteries
Ovarian arteries	Arise from the lateral margins of the abdominal aorta, slightly inferior to the renal arteries Course medial within the suspensory ligaments	Primary blood supply to the ovaries Connect with the uterine arteries
Ovarian veins	Course within the suspensory ligaments	Right ovarian vein empties directly into the inferior vena cava Left ovarian vein empties into the left renal vein
Uterine arteries	Branch of the internal iliac arteries Medial in the levator ani muscles Ascend in a tortuous course lateral to the uterus within the broad ligament	Supply the cervix, vagina, uterus, ovaries, and fallopian tubes Course lateral and terminate at the confluence with the ovarian artery

Pelvic Spaces

- The peritoneum drapes over the uterus and fallopian tubes, dividing the pelvis into anterior and posterior sections.
- A potential space or cul-de-sac is created when the peritoneum folds.
- Not uncommon to visualize a small amount of free fluid in the retrouterine pouch.
- Masses within the space of Retzius will displace the urinary bladder posteriorly.
- Masses within the vesicouterine pouch will displace the urinary bladder anteriorly.
- Fluid or blood from an ectopic pregnancy ruptured graafian follicle, or hemorrhagic ovarian cyst accumulates in these spaces.

Pelvic Spaces

PELVIC SPACE	LOCATION
Retrouterine Pouch Posterior cul de sac Pouch of Douglas	Anterior to the rectum Posterior to the uterus Most inferior and dependent space in the pelvic cavity Most common site for fluid to accumulate
Space of Retzius Retropubic space Prevesical space	Anterior to the urinary bladder Posterior to the symphysis pubis
Vesicouterine Pouch Anterior cul de sac	Anterior to the uterus Posterior to the urinary bladder May contain bowel

FEMALE REPRODUCTIVE SYSTEM (Fig. 19.2)

Vagina

- Collapsed tube consisting of an outer muscular layer and an inner mucosal layer.
- Extends from the vulva to the cervix.
- Sides of the vagina are enclosed between the levator ani muscles.
- Half of the vagina lies above and the other half below the pelvic brim.
- Supplied by the vaginal and uterine arteries (branches of the internal iliac arteries) and empties into the internal iliac veins.

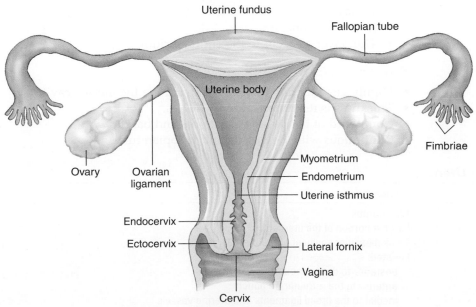

FIG. 19.2 Female reproductive anatomy.

Location of the Vagina

- Anterior to the rectum and anus.
- Posterior to the urinary bladder, urethra, and peritoneum.
- Inferior (caudal) to the cervix of the uterus.
- Medial to the levator ani muscles.

Sonographic Appearance of the Vagina

- Vaginal walls demonstrate low-level homogeneous echoes.
- Vaginal canal demonstrates a central hyperechoic linear echo pattern.

UTERUS

- Hollow, pear-shaped organ.
- Derived from the fused caudal portion of the paired, hollow müllerian ducts.
- Median septum of the fused ducts reabsorbs resulting in a single cavity.
- Muscular organ covered by peritoneum, except below the anterior cervical os.
- Supported by the levator ani muscles, cardinal ligaments, and uterosacral ligaments.
- Uterine growth begins at approximately 7 to 8 years of age, accelerates during puberty, and continues to grow until approximately 20 years of age.

Tissue Layers of the Uterus

Perimetrium

- Serosal or external surface.
- Part of the parietal peritoneum.
- May be difficult to distinguish on ultrasound.

Myometrium

- Thickest layer of the uterus.
- Composed of a three-layer thick, smooth muscle supported by connective tissue containing large blood vessels.
- **Outer layer:**
  - Adjacent to the serosa.
  - Separated from the intermediate layer by the arcuate vessels.
- **Intermediate layer:**
  - Thickest of the three layers.
- **Inner layer:**
  - Junctional zone.
  - Thin layer adjacent to the endometrium.

Endometrium

- Highly vascular mucous membrane lining the uterine cavity.
- Thickness is related to hormone levels.
- Composed of two layers: functional and basal.
- Contiguous with the vagina and fallopian tubes.

Regions of the Uterus	
REGION	**DESCRIPTION**
Body	Aka: corpus
	Largest portion of the uterus
	Thick muscular segment of the uterus
	Located:
	posterior to the vesicouterine pouch
	anterior to the retrouterine pouch
	medial to the broad ligaments and uterine vessels

Regions of the Uterus—(cont'd)

REGION	DESCRIPTION

Cervix	Proximal and inferior portion of the uterus located between the vagina and uterine isthmus
	Projects into the vaginal canal
	More fibrous and less flexible
	Anchored at the angle of the bladder by the parametrium
	Divided into the:
	    Internal cervical os - junction of the endocervical canal and endometrial canal at the uterine
	      isthmus
	    External cervical os – junction of the cervical canal with the vaginal canal
	    Endocervix – portion of the cervix surrounding the cervical canal
	    Exocervix – outer layer of the cervix contiguous with the vagina
	Peritoneal reflection is not demonstrated anterior to the cervix

Cornua	Lateral funnel-shaped horns of the uterus Located between the uterine fundus and the interstitial portion of the fallopian tube
Endometrial cavity	Consists of a superficial functional layer and a deep basal layer Functional layer sheds with menses Basal layer regenerates new endometrium and remains intact during menses. Thickness is dependent on hormone levels
Fundus	Dome-shaped widest, most distal and superior portion of the uterus Position may vary with bladder filling Located superior to the insertion of the fallopian tubes
Isthmus	"Narrow waist" of the uterus Termed *lower uterine segment during pregnancy* Located between the cervix and body of the uterus

Location of the Uterus

- Anterior to the rectum and piriformis muscles.
- Posterior to the urinary bladder, space of Retzius, and symphysis pubis.
- Medial to the ovaries, fallopian tubes, obturator internus muscles, and external iliac vessels.

Normal Sonographic Appearance of the Uterus

- Homogeneous mid-to-low level echogenic structure surrounding a hyperechoic endometrial cavity.
- Slight difference in echogenicity of the uterine layers with the outer and inner layers slightly hypoechoic to the intermediate layer.
- Uterine arteries demonstrate as anechoic tubular structures with a high-resistance flow pattern.
- Resistive index of the arcuate arteries range between 0.86 ± 0.04 (reproductive) and 0.89 ± 0.06 (postmenopause).

Normal Sonographic Appearance of the Endometrium

- Outer basal layer appears hypoechoic.
- Inner functional layer typically appears hyperechoic.
- Thickness varies with menstrual phase or status but should not exceed 14 mm.

Measuring the Uterus (Fig. 19.3)

- Length is measured from the fundus to the external cervical os.
- Height (thickness) is measured perpendicular to the length of the widest portion of the uterine body.
- Width is measured at the widest portion of the uterine body in the short axis.

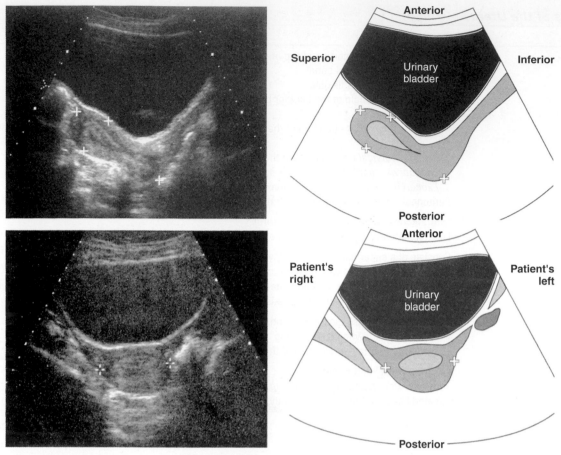

FIG. 19.3 Uterine measurements.

Measuring the Endometrium (Fig. 19.4)

- Anterior–posterior thickness is measured in the **sagittal plane**.
- Measured from echogenic interface to echogenic interface (functional layer).
- Thin hypoechoic area (basal layer) is not included in the measurement.
- Fluid within the endometrial cavity is not included in the measurement.

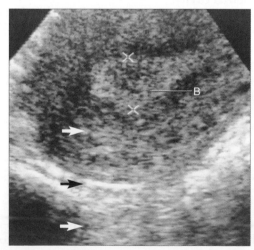

FIG. 19.4 Sonogram endometrium measurement. Note posterior acoustic enhancement *(arrows)*.

Uterine Size

MENSTRUAL STATUS	LENGTH (cm)	HEIGHT (cm)	WIDTH (cm)	CERVIX/CORPUS RATIO
Premenarche	2.0-4.0	0.5-1.0	1.0-2.0	2:1
Menarche	6.0-8.0 nulliparous 8.0-10.0 parous	3.0-5.0 nulliparous 3.0-5.0 parous	3.0-5.0 nulliparous 5.0-6.0 parous	1:2
Postmenopausal	3.5-6.5	2.0-3.0	4.0-6.0	1:1

- Postpartum uterus remains enlarged for 4 to 8 weeks following delivery.

Uterine Positions

- Flexion – refers to the relationship between the body of the uterus and the internal cervical os.
- Reversion – refers to the relationship between the cervix and the vagina.

POSITION (EMPTY BLADDER)	DESCRIPTION
Anteflexion	Uterine body and fundus bend significantly anterior until the fundus points inferior resting on the cervix
Anteversion	Uterine body and fundus are tipped anteriorly. Cervix forms an angle ≤ 90 degrees with the vaginal canal Most common uterine position
Dextroflexion	Uterine body is displaced or flexed to the right of the cervix Transverse imaging plane is best to evaluate whether uterus is dextroflexed
Levoflexion	Uterine body is displaced or flexed to the left of the cervix Transverse imaging plane is best to evaluate whether uterus is levoflexed
Retroflexion	Uterine body and fundus bend significantly posterior until the fundus is pointed inferior adjacent to the cervix Cervix and vagina are linear oriented. Transvaginal imaging is best to evaluate a retroflexed uterus
Retroversion	Uterine body and fundus are tipped posteriorly Cervix forms an angle <90 degrees with the vaginal canal Transvaginal imaging is best to evaluate a retroverted uterus

Congenital Uterine Anomalies

- Congenital anomalies result from improper fusion of the müllerian ducts or incomplete absorption of the septum between them.
- Coexisting renal anomalies occur in 20% to 30% of cases.

Congenital Anomalies of the Uterus

ANOMALY	ETIOLOGY	CLINICAL FINDINGS	SONOGRAPHIC FINDINGS	DIFFERENTIAL CONSIDERATIONS
Agenesis	Failure of the caudal müllerian ducts to develop fallopian tubes are present	Amenorrhea	Absent uterus	Hysterectomy Unicornuate uterus
Arcuate	Septum between the müllerian ducts is almost completely reabsorbed causing a slight indention of the superior endometrium by a thickened fundal myometrium	Asymptomatic Infertility Recurrent second trimester miscarriage	Normal external uterine contour Slight separation of the superior endometrium Heart-shaped appearance of the superior endometrium	Leiomyoma Synechiae Endometrial polyp

Continued

Congenital Anomalies of the Uterus—(cont'd)

ANOMALY	ETIOLOGY	CLINICAL FINDINGS	SONOGRAPHIC FINDINGS	DIFFERENTIAL CONSIDERATIONS
Bicornuate	Partial fusion of the müllerian ducts Two uteri in the superior portion of the uterus Two superior endometrial cavities	Asymptomatic Infertility Spontaneous abortion	Deep notch in the fundus Two distinct endometriums separated by a small amount of myometrium	Fibroid Septate uterus
Didelphys	Complete failure of the müllerian ducts to fuse	Asymptomatic Infertility Spontaneous abortion Vaginal septation	Wide separation between two distinct uterine fundi (transverse plane) Two separate cervix Possible septated vagina	Pelvic muscles Pedunculated fibroid
Septate	Complete fusion of the müllerian ducts with failure to completely reabsorb the septum Two uterine cavities and one uterine fundus Most common type of müllerian duct anomaly	Asymptomatic High incidence of infertility Recurrent first trimester miscarriage	Normal uterine contour Flat, convex, or small indentation (<1 cm) of the fundal contour (visualized best in the coronal plane) Two closely separated endometrial cavities containing fibrous or myometrial tissue Endometrial cavities are usually symmetrical	Fibroid Adenomyosis Endometrial polyp
Subseptus	Complete fusion of the müllerian ducts with partial failure to completely reabsorb the septum	Asymptomatic Infertility Multiple spontaneous abortions	Normal uterine contour May demonstrate a slight indentation of fundal contour Thin separation within the endometrial cavity by fibrous or myometrial	Fibroid Adenomyosis Endometrial polyp
Unicornuate	Unilateral development of the paired müllerian ducts	Asymptomatic Hypomenorrhea Infertility	Small uterine size Lateral uterine position Rudimentary horn may be visualized	Uterine didelphys

OVARIES

- Paired, elliptical-shaped endocrine glands located lateral to the uterus.
- Smooth surface in early life, becoming markedly pitted after years of ovulation.
- Without hormone replacement therapy, ovaries decrease in size after menopause.
- Attached to the posterior surface of the broad ligament by the mesovarium.
- The only organs in the abdominopelvic cavity not lined by peritoneum.
- Dual blood supply through the ovarian and uterine arteries.

Anatomy of the Ovaries

- The ovary is composed of an outer cortex and a central medulla.
  - *Cortex* consists of follicles and is covered with the tunica albuginea.
  - *Medulla* is composed of connective tissue and contains nerves, blood vessels, lymph vessels, and smooth muscle at the hilus region.
  - *Tunica albuginea* (outer layer) is surrounded by a thin layer of germinal epithelium.

- Each ovary is connected by:
  - Mesovarium ligament to the broad ligament.
  - Uteroovarian ligament to the inferior portion of the uterus.
  - Suspensory ligament to the pelvic sidewall.
  - The medial, lateral, and posterior borders of each ovary are not attached.

Physiology of the Ovaries

Function

- Produce ova.
- Produce hormones.
  - Estrogen—secreted by the follicle.
  - Progesterone—secreted by the corpus luteum.

Location of the Ovaries

- Intraperitoneal within the adnexa of the true pelvis.
- Uterine location influences the position of the ovaries.
- Generally located at the level of the uterine cornua.
- Medial to the external iliac vessels.
- Anterior to the internal iliac vessels and ureter.
- Lateral to the uterus.
- Posterior to the fallopian tubes, external iliac vessels, and broad ligament.

Normal Sonographic Appearance of the Ovary

- Ovoid low-to-medium-level echogenic structure.
- Isoechoic to hypoechoic compared with the normal uterus.
- Hypoechoic periphery representing the tunica albuginea.
- Anechoic follicle(s) demonstrating posterior enhancement may be present.
- Resistance of the ovarian arteries depends on the menstrual cycle.
- During menses and the early proliferative phases, the ovarian artery demonstrates a high resistance with a low flow velocity.
- Resistive index normally ranges from 0.4 to 0.8.
- Pulsatility index normally ranges from 0.6 to 2.5.

Measuring of the Ovaries (Fig. 19.5)

- Measure the length of the long axis.
- Anteroposterior dimension is measured perpendicular to the length.
- Width is measured in the transverse or coronal plane.

Ovarian Size

Menarche

- 2.5 to 5.0 cm in length.
- 1.5 to 3.0 cm in width.
- 0.6 to 2.2 cm in height.

Ovarian Volume

- Volume varies with age, menstrual status, body habitus, pregnancy status, and phase of menstrual cycle.
- Lowest volume during the luteal phase.
- Highest volume during the periovulatory phase.
- Larger volume at birth a result of maternal hormones.
- Stable volumes up to age 5 years.
- Volume peaks in the third decade.
- Begins to decline in the fifth decade.

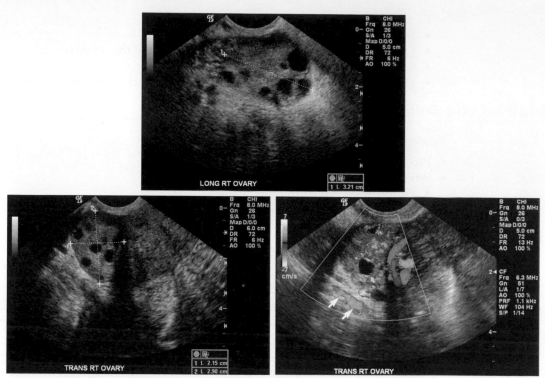

FIG. 19.5 Measurement of the ovaries. The arrows identifying iliac vessel.

Ovarian Volumes	
Premenarche	1.0 cm³ (0-5 yrs of age)
	1.2 cm³ (6-8 yrs of age)
	2.1 cm³ (9-10 yrs of age)
	2.5-3.0 cm³ (11-13 yrs of age)
Menstruating	9.8 cm³
Postmenopause	5.8 cm³

$$\text{Ovarian volume (cm}^3) = \frac{\text{Length} \times \text{Width} \times \text{Height}}{2} \text{ or } \left(\text{Length} \times \text{Width} \times \text{Height}\right) \times 0.523$$

Anatomical Ovarian Variant

L-Shaped Ovary
- Normal ovarian variant giving the appearance of two "arms."
- Lesions in one "arm" may appear exophytic or extrinsic to the ovary.

Congenital Ovarian Anomalies

Agenesis
- Associated with an abnormal karyotype.

Unilateral Ovary
- Rare occurrence.

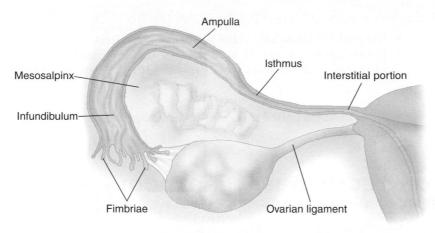

FIG. 19.6 Fallopian tubes (oviduct).

FALLOPIAN TUBES (Oviduct) (Fig. 19.6)

- Paired muscular tubes.
- Derived from the nonfused cranial portion of the müllerian ducts.
- Contained in the superior portion of the broad ligament and covered by peritoneum.
- Composed of an outer layer of peritoneum (serosa), middle muscular layer, and an internal mucosal layer.

Physiology of the Fallopian Tubes

Function

- Attract and transfer ova from the surface of the ovary to the endometrial cavity.
- Tubal peristalsis helps move the fertilized ovum into the endometrium.

Divisions of the Fallopian Tube	
SEGMENT	**DESCRIPTION**
Interstitial	Proximal portion of the fallopian tube that passes through the cornua of the uterus Narrowest and shortest portion
Isthmus	Immediately adjacent to the uterine wall Short, straight, narrow portion of the tube
Ampulla	Widest, longest, and most coiled portion Region where fertilization most commonly occurs Most common area of ectopic pregnancies
Infundibulum	Funnel-shaped distal portion of the tube Terminates at the fimbrial processes One fimbriae is attached to the ovary (fimbriae ovarica) Opens into the peritoneal cavity adjacent to the ovary

Location of the Fallopian Tubes

- Situated in the superior free margin of the broad ligament.
- Superior to the uteroovarian ligaments, round ligaments, and blood vessels.
- Course posterior and lateral from the cornua of the uterus curving anterior and medial to the corresponding ovary.
- Open into the peritoneal cavity.

Sonographic Appearance of the Fallopian Tube

- Normal fallopian tube is not routinely visualized.
- Interstitial segment may be visualized under normal conditions appearing as a long echogenic tenuous structure extending laterally from the uterine wall.

Size

- 7-cm to 12-cm coiled muscular tubes composed of smooth muscle and lined by a mucosa.
- 8 to 10 mm in diameter.

EXAMINATION TECHNIQUES, PROTOCOLS, AND IMAGE OPTIMIZATION

Preparation

- Preparation varies with type of imaging approach.

Transabdominal

- Requires bladder distention to extend superior to the uterine fundus.
  - Adult – Drink 28 to 32 oz of water 1 hour before examination.
  - If catharized, fill bladder to 375 mL.
  - Children – Fluid intake is adjusted according to age and weight.
  - Infants – No preparation.

Purpose of Bladder Distention

- Displaces uterus posteriorly and bowel laterally.
- Provides an acoustic window to visualize pelvic structures.
- Provides an anatomical and anechoic reference point.
- Overdistention may compress and distort pelvic structures.

Endovaginal and Translabial

- Urinary bladder should be emptied.

Contraindications for Endovaginal Imaging

- Any patient who does not or can not willingly consent to the examination.
- Premenarchal or virginal patients.
- Atrophy or narrowing of the vaginal canal.
- If the pain becomes too severe, terminate examination.

Transducer Selection

- Use the highest frequency possible to obtain optimal resolution for penetration depth.
  - Adults – 3.5 to 5.0 MHz transabdominal.
  - 4.0 to 8.0 MHz endovaginal.
  - 3.5 to 5.0 MHz translabial.
  - Children and small adults - 4.0 to 7.0 MHz.
  - Obese patients – 2.0 MHz may be required for transabdominal imaging.
- Curvilinear transducers provide a wider field of view.
- Sector or vector transducers have a smaller footprint.

Patient Positioning

- Supine position – transabdominal.
- Lithotomy position – endovaginal and translabial.
- Right and left posterior oblique may reposition overlying bowel gas.

Examination Protocol

- Unless contraindicated, a complete gynecological examination includes transabdominal and endovaginal imaging.

Transabdominal and Endovaginal

- Transabdominal approach should be the first and sometimes the only examination performed.
- Urinary bladder and iliac vessels are imaging landmarks.
- Systematic approach in the sagittal, coronal, and transverse planes carefully examining, imaging, and documenting all areas of the female pelvis including:
  - Uterus.
  - Endometrium.
  - Adnexae.
  - Pelvic spaces.
- Length, height, and width measurements of the uterus.
  - Length – measure from top of uterus to inferior border of cervix.
  - Height – measure at the widest portion of the uterine fundus.
  - Width - measure at the widest portion of the uterine fundus.
- Endometrial thickness measurement.
  - Measure anterior posterior (AP) endometrium in the **sagittal plane.**
  - Measure functional layer from echogenic surface to echogenic surface.
  - Thin hypoechoic basal layer is not included in measurement.
  - Fluid within the endometrial cavity is not included in the measurement.
- Length, height, and width measurements of the right and left ovaries.
- Document color Doppler and/or spectral analysis of ovarian vascularity.
- Document color Doppler of the uterine vascularity may be included.
- Abnormalities should be documented and when applicable measured in two imaging planes. Color and/or spectral Doppler evaluation of the abnormality should be included.

Image Optimization

- Place gains settings to display normal uterine myometrium as a medium shade of gray with adjustments to reduce artifactually produced echoes within the arcuate vessels.
- Focal zone(s) should be placed at or below the area of interest. The use of multiple focal zones increases detail resolution and decreases temporal resolution.
- Sufficient imaging depth to visualize structures immediately posterior to the area of interest.
- Harmonic imaging and decreasing system compression (dynamic range) can be used to reduce artifactual echoes in obese and gassy patients.
- Spatial compounding can be used to improve visualization of structures posterior to highly attenuating structures.
- Doppler settings should be adjusted for the different flow states of the female pelvis.
- Doppler angle should be 60 degrees or less with a sample volume smaller than the vessel interrogating.
- The use of multiple patient positions may redistribute overlying bowel gas.

ADVANTAGES AND DISADVANTAGE OF VARIOUS IMAGING APPROACHES

Transabdominal

Advantage

- Allows a wider field of view visualizing the entire pelvis and superficial structures.
- Use lower frequencies enabling better visualization of deep structures.

Disadvantage

- Decrease in image resolution due to lower transducer frequencies.
- Requires a full urinary bladder which is uncomfortable for the patient.

Endovaginal

Advantage

- Increase in resolution due to higher transducer frequencies.
- Closer proximity to the uterus and ovaries – a benefit with obese patients and those with a retroverted or retroflexed uterus.
- Requires an empty urinary bladder.

Disadvantage

- Limited field of view.
  - Large pelvic mass or enlarged uterus may be out of field of view.
  - Superiorly or laterally placed ovaries may be out of field of view.
- Adequate landmarks may be limited making orientation more difficult.

Translabial

Advantage

- Alternative to endovaginal imaging.
- Adequate anatomical landmarks may be limited making orientation more difficult.

Disadvantage

- Limited field of view.
- Rectal gas and the symphysis pubis may obscure image.

Helpful Hints

- Vector or sector transducer can aid in visualization of the pelvic structures when bladder is under distended.
- Anterior pressure over the adnexal region can move interfering bowel gas.
- Remember the location of the ovaries can range from the level of the cervix to superior to the uterus.

INDICATIONS FOR NON-GRAVID FEMALE PELVIS ULTRASOUND

- Pelvic pain.
- Pelvic or uterine mass.
- Abnormal uterine bleeding.
- Menorrhagia.
- Dysmenorrhea.
- Bloating.
- Family history of gynecological carcinoma.

URINARY BLADDER

Anatomy

- *Apex*—superior portion of the bladder.
- *Neck*—inferior portion of the bladder continuous with the urethra.
- *Trigone*—inflexible region between the apex and neck of the bladder; area where the ureters enter the bladder.
- Normal bladder wall thickness is 3 mm when distended.
- Normal bladder wall thickness is 5 mm when empty.
- Normal bladder wall is thicker in infants than in adults.
- Ureters enter the bladder wall at an oblique angle approximately 5 cm above the bladder outlet.
- Postvoid residual normally should not exceed 20 mL in adult patients.

Normal Sonographic Appearance

- Anechoic, fluid-filled structure located in the pelvic midline.
- Ureteric orifices appear as small echogenic protuberances on the posterior aspect of the bladder.
- Bladder wall thickness is dependent on distention of urinary bladder but should not exceed 5 mm.

Congenital Abnormalities of the Urinary Bladder

CONGENITAL ABNORMALITY	ETIOLOGY	CLINICAL FINDINGS	SONOGRAPHIC FINDINGS	DIFFERENTIAL CONSIDERATIONS
Bladder diverticulum	Bladder wall muscle weakness causing herniation of the mucosa through the muscular wall	Asymptomatic Urinary tract infection Pelvic pain May be associated with bladder obstruction or chronic inflammation	Anechoic pedunculation of the urinary bladder Neck of diverticulum is small May enlarge when bladder contracts	Ovarian cyst Fluid-filled bowel Ascites
Bladder ureterocele	Congenital obstruction of the ureteric orifice	Asymptomatic Urinary tract infection	Hyperechoic septation seen within the bladder at the ureteric orifice Demonstrated when urine enters the bladder	Artifact Bladder tumor Catheter balloon

Pathology of the Urinary Bladder

BLADDER PATHOLOGY	ETIOLOGY	CLINICAL FINDINGS	SONOGRAPHIC FINDINGS	DIFFERENTIAL CONSIDERATIONS
Bladder calculus	Urinary stasis Migrate from the kidney(s)	Asymptomatic Hematuria Urinary frequency and urgency	Hyperechoic focus(i) within the urinary bladder Posterior acoustic shadowing Mobile with patient position change	Intestinal air Calcified vessel
Cystitis	Infection Female prevalence	Dysuria Urinary frequency Leukocytosis Hematuria	Focal or diffuse increase in bladder wall thickness Mobile internal echoes	Bladder sludge
Bladder sludge	Debris in the bladder	Asymptomatic	Homogeneous low-level echoes Mobile with patient position change	Cystitis Hematuria
Bladder malignancy **Risk Factors** Elderly Male prevalence Analgesic abuse Tobacco use Excessive coffee consumption Recurrent UTI	Transitional cell carcinoma	Painless hematuria Frequent urination Dysuria	Polypoid echogenic bladder mass Irregular margins Immobile with patient position change Internal vascular blood flow May demonstrate irregular bladder wall thickening	Benign tumor Bladder sludge Ureterocele Metastatic tumor
Bladder adenoma	Papilloma	Asymptssomatic Frequent urination	Echogenic intraluminal mass Smooth margins Immobile with patient position change Internal vascular flow	Malignant tumor Bladder sludge Ureterocele

PELVIC ANATOMY REVIEW

1. Which pelvic ligament extends from the cornua of the uterus to the medial aspect of the ovary?
   a. round
   b. broad
   c. cardinal
   d. ovarian

2. Prominent anechoic structures near the periphery of the uterus most likely represent:
   a. adenomyosis
   b. arcuate vessels
   c. nabothian cysts
   d. physiological cysts

3. Which segment of the fallopian tube may be visualized under normal conditions?
   a. isthmus
   b. ampulla
   c. interstitial
   d. infundibular

4. The region including the ovary and fallopian tube is termed the:
   a. oviduct
   b. adnexa
   c. fimbriae ovarica
   d. space of Retzius

5. Which segment of the fallopian tube connects with the uterus?
   a. ampulla
   b. isthmus
   c. interstitial
   d. infundibulum

6. The flanged portions of the iliac bones form the:
   a. lateral border of the true pelvis
   b. posterior border of the true pelvis
   c. inferior border of the true pelvis
   d. posterior border of the false pelvis

7. The fallopian tubes are:
   a. covered by perineum.
   b. contained in the inferior portion of the round ligament.
   c. derived from the nonfused caudal portion of the müllerian ducts.
   d. contained in the superior portion of the broad ligament.

8. When measuring endometrial thickness, calipers are placed from:
   a. superior interface to inferior interface
   b. echogenic interface to echogenic interface
   c. echogenic interface to hypoechoic interface
   d. hypoechoic interface to hypoechoic interface

9. The ovary is attached to the pelvic sidewall by the:
   a. broad ligament
   b. round ligament
   c. ovarian ligament
   d. suspensory ligament

10. Failure of the müllerian ducts to fuse will most likely result in:
    a. uterine septate
    b. uterine agenesis
    c. bicornuate uterus
    d. uterine didelphys

11. Which of the following correctly measures endometrial thickness?
    a. anterior–posterior dimension in the coronal plane
    b. transverse dimension in the coronal plane
    c. anterior–posterior dimension in the sagittal plane
    d. anterior–posterior diameter in the transverse plane

12. Which of the following most accurately describes the perimetrium?
    a. The perimetrium lines the uterine cavity
    b. The perimetrium is composed of smooth muscle
    c. The serosal surface of the uterus is termed the *perimetrium*
    d. The perimetrium is composed of connective tissue and large blood vessels

13. Secondary blood supply to the ovaries is through the:
    a. arcuate arteries
    b. uterine arteries
    c. ovarian arteries
    d. hypogastric arteries

14. The vesicouterine pouch is located:
    a. posterior to the uterus and anterior to the rectum
    b. anterior to the uterus and posterior to the urinary bladder
    c. posterior to the symphysis pubis and anterior to the uterus
    d. anterior to the symphysis pubis and posterior to the rectus abdominis

15. In premenarche, the size of the uterine cervix is expected to be:
    a. half the size of the corpus
    b. equal to the uterine corpus
    c. twice as large as the corpus
    d. equal to the uterine fundus

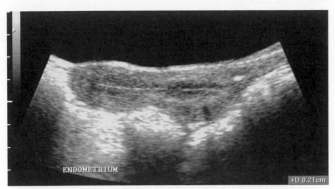

FIG. 19.7   Sagittal sonogram of the uterus.

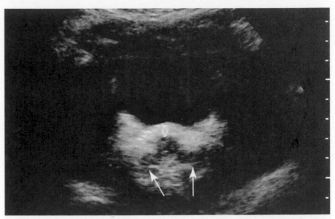

FIG. 19.9   Transverse sonogram at the level of the vagina (v).

Using Figure 19.7, answer question 16.

16. This sagittal image of the uterus most likely represents a:
   a. septate uterus
   b. bicornuate uterus
   c. menarche uterus
   d. postmenopausal uterus

Using Figure 19.8, answer question 17.

17. In this sagittal sonogram, the uterus is lying in which of the following positions?
   a. anteversion
   b. retroflexion
   c. anteflexion
   d. retroversion

Using Figure 19.9, answer question 18.

18. Which pelvic muscles are the arrows identifying?
   a. iliopsoas
   b. levator ani
   c. uterosacral
   d. obturator internus

Using Figure 19.10, answer questions 19 and 20.

19. A perimenopausal patient presents with a history of pelvic fullness and pain. A sagittal sonogram displays a fluid collection in the:
   a. prevesical space
   b. space of Retzius
   c. pouch of Douglas
   d. vesicouterine pouch

20. The position of the uterus is:
   a. anteverted
   b. anteflexed
   c. retroflexed
   d. retroverted

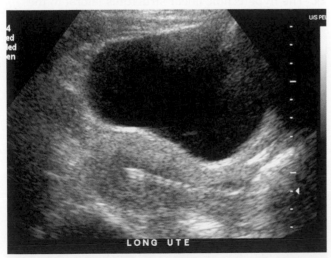

FIG. 19.8   Sagittal sonogram of the uterus.

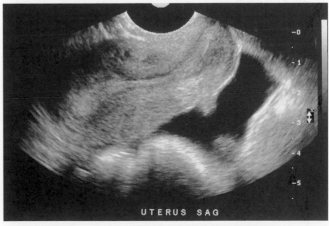

FIG. 19.10   Endovaginal sonogram.

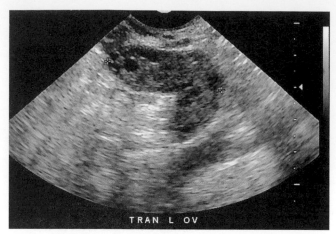

FIG. 19.11 Sonogram of the left ovary.

Using Figure 19.11, answer question 21.

21. The ovary is most likely demonstrating a(n):
   a. pyosalpinx
   b. ectopic pregnancy
   c. benign neoplasm
   d. anatomical variant

Using Figure 19.12, answer question 22.

22. The sonogram is *most suspicious* for a(n):
   a. arcuate uterus
   b. septate uterus
   c. uterine didelphys
   d. bicornuate uterus

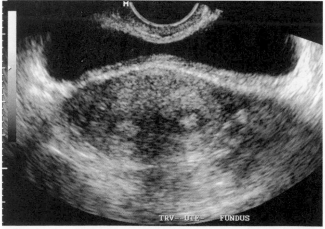

FIG. 19.12 Transverse sonogram at the level of the uterine fundus.

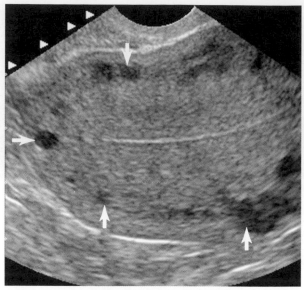

FIG. 19.13 Sagittal sonogram.

Using Figure 19.13, answer question 23.

23. The arrows in the sonogram are most likely identifying:
   a. leiomyomas
   b. adenomyosis
   c. arcuate vessels
   d. uterine arteries

Using Figure 19.14, answer question 24.

24. The hyperechoic linear structures lateral to the uterus most likely represent the:
   a. fallopian tubes
   b. broad ligaments
   c. round ligaments
   d. ovarian ligaments

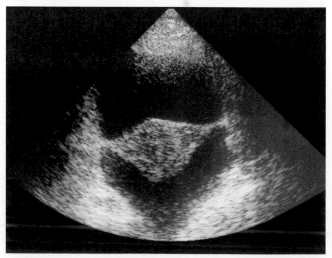

FIG. 19.14 Transverse sonogram of the uterus.

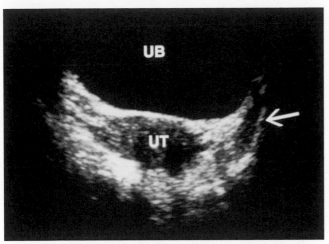

FIG. 19.15 Transverse sonogram of the uterus.

Using Figure 19.15, answer question 25.

25. The hypoechoic structure identified by the arrow most likely represents the:
    a. pelvis bone
    b. levator ani muscle
    c. piriformis muscle
    d. obturator internus muscle

Using Figure 19.16, answer question 26.

26. The coronal sonogram most likely identifies:
    a. arcuate uterus
    b. didelphys uterus
    c. septate uterus
    d. bicornuate uterus

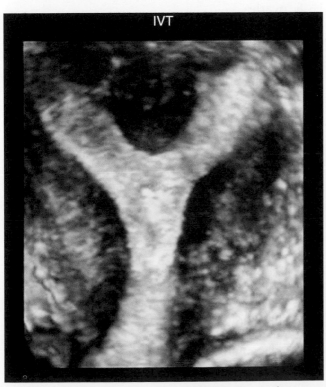

FIG. 19.16 3D rendering of the endometrium

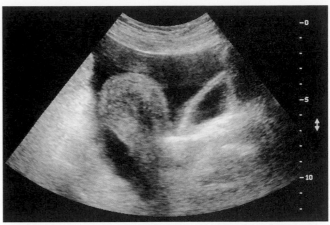

FIG. 19.17 Sagittal sonogram (on CD).

Using Figure 19.17, answer question 27.

27. Identification of free fluid in the pelvis is located in the:
    a. prevesical and retrouterine spaces
    b. retrouterine and retropubic spaces
    c. vesicouterine and retrouterine spaces
    d. retrouterine, vesicouterine, and retropubic spaces

Using Figure 19.18, answer question 28.

28. The position of the uterus in this sagittal sonogram is termed:
    a. anteflexion
    b. levoflexion
    c. retroflexion
    d. retroversion

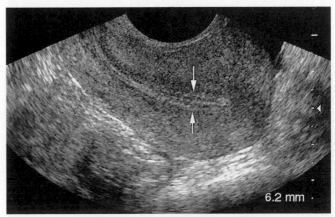

FIG. 19.18 Endovaginal sonogram.

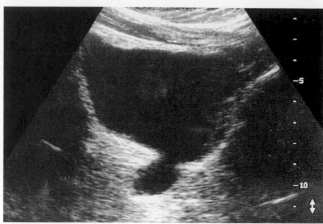

FIG. 19.19 Transverse sonogram of the urinary bladder (on CD).

Using Figure 19.19, answer question 29.

29. The abnormality demonstrated in this sonogram is most consistent with a(n):
   a. ureterocele
   b. hydroureter
   c. ovarian cyst
   d. bladder diverticulum

Using Figure 19.20, answer question 30.

30. The sonogram is most likely demonstrating:
   a. septate uterus
   b. arcuate uterus
   c. didelphys uterus
   d. bicornuate uterus

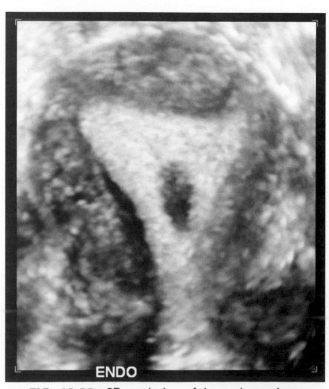

FIG. 19.20 3D rendering of the endometrium.

31. Which of the following attaches to the ovary?
   a. peritoneum
   b. broad ligament
   c. tunica albuginea
   d. ovarian ligament

32. Ovarian volume is lowest during the:
   a. luteal phase
   b. ovulatory phase
   c. menstrual phase
   d. periovulatory phase

33. The fallopian tube divides into which of the following segments?
   a. fimbria, isthmus, cornua, ampulla
   b. isthmus, ampulla, cornua, interstitial
   c. ampulla, infundibulum, fimbria, isthmus
   d. interstitial, isthmus, ampulla, infundibulum

34. Visualization of pelvic ligaments appears on sonography as:
   a. hypoechoic ovoid structures
   b. hyperechoic linear structures
   c. hyperechoic tubular structures
   d. hypoechoic tortuous structures

35. The cornua of the uterus is located between the:
   a. corpus and fundus of the uterus
   b. corpus and cervix of the uterus
   c. uterine fundus and fallopian tube
   d. uterine corpus and fallopian tube

36. The spiral artery provides the primary blood supply to which of the following pelvic structures?
   a. vagina
   b. ovaries
   c. endometrium
   d. fallopian tubes

37. Congenital uterine anomalies are associated with coexisting anomalies of the:
   a. ovaries
   b. kidneys
   c. oviducts
   d. adrenal glands

38. Which uterine anomaly most likely demonstrates a slight indentation of the fundal contour?
   a. septate
   b. didelphys
   c. bicornuate
   d. unicornuate

39. It is common to visualize a small amount of free fluid in the:
   a. prevesical space
   b. space of Retzius
   c. retrouterine space
   d. vesicouterine space

40. The section of time previous to the onset of menstruation is termed:
    a. puberty
    b. menarche
    c. premenarche
    d. perimenopause

41. Which of the following is a surface region located below the pelvic floor?
    a. mesentery
    b. omentum
    c. perineum
    d. peritoneum

42. Which congenital uterine anomaly does not distort the normal contour of the fundus?
    a. arcuate
    b. unicornuate
    c. didelphys
    d. bicornuate

43. Partial fusion of the caudal müllerian ducts will most likely result in an anomaly of the:
    a. uterus
    b. ovary
    c. vagina
    d. fallopian tube

44. The pelvis is divided into the true and false pelvis by the:
    a. iliac bones
    b. broad ligaments
    c. iliopectineal line
    d. iliopsoas muscles

45. The pelvic floor is formed by pelvic:
    a. bones and muscles
    b. bones and ligaments
    c. organs and ligaments
    d. ligaments and muscles

46. The uterosacral ligament extends from the lateral margins of the sacrum to the:
    a. cornua
    b. superior cervix
    c. inferior fundus
    d. inferior vagina

47. The innermost layer of the myometrium is termed the:
    a. basal zone
    b. functional zone
    c. junctional zone
    d. albuginea zone

48. In the menarche patient, the endometrial thickness should not exceed:
    a. 8 mm
    b. 10 mm
    c. 14 mm
    d. 20 mm

49. Which of the following structures is *not* lined by the peritoneum?
    a. cervix
    b. ovary
    c. bowel
    d. oviduct

50. Ovarian volume is the highest during the:
    a. luteal phase
    b. follicular phase
    c. menstrual phase
    d. periovulatory phase

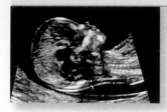

CHAPTER 20

Physiology of the Female Pelvis

KEY TERMS

amenorrhea absence of menstruation.

corpus albicans scar from previous corpus luteum.

corpus luteum a fluid structure formed from the graafian follicle after ovulation; produces progesterone.

cumulus oophorus protrusion within the graafian follicle containing the oocyte.

dysmenorrhea painful menses.

dyspareunia abnormal pain during sexual intercourse due to a spasm. Associated with endometriosis and hormonal changes in post menopause and lactating women.

estrogen hormone secreted by the follicle, promoting growth of the endometrium.

follicle functional or physiological ovulatory cyst consisting of an ovum surrounded by a layer of cells.

follicle-stimulating hormone hormone that stimulates growth and maturation of the graafian follicle(s).

graafian follicle mature follicle containing a cumulus mass with a single oocyte.

luteinizing hormone hormone that stimulates ovulation.

menopause the last menstrual cycle.

menorrhagia abnormally heavy or long menses.

menstrual cycle monthly cyclic changes in the female reproductive system typically 28 days in length.

mittelschmerz term used to describe pelvic pain preceding ovulation.

oligomenorrhea time between monthly menstrual cycles that exceeds 35 days.

ovulation explosive release of an ovum from a ruptured graafian follicle.

perimenopausal transition period occurring several years before menopause.

polymenorrhea time between monthly menstrual cycles that is fewer than 21 days.

precocious puberty an unusually early onset of puberty.

progesterone hormone that helps to prepare and maintain the endometrium.

NORMAL PHYSIOLOGY

- The onset of menstruation generally occurs between 11 and 13 years of age.
- Cessation of menstruation usually occurs around 50 years of age.
- The length of a menstrual cycle ranges between 21 and 35 days (average 28 days).
- Rupture of a graafian follicle should occur each cycle.
- Menstruation depends on the functional integrity of the hypothalamus, pituitary gland, and ovarian axis.

LABORATORY VALUES

Estradiol

- Normal levels:
  - Follicular: 30 to 100 pg/mL.
  - Ovulatory: 200 to 400 pg/mL.
  - Luteal: 50 to 140 pg/mL.
- Primarily reflects the activity of the ovaries.
- During pregnancy, estradiol levels will steadily rise.
- Small amounts are present in the adrenal cortex and arterial walls.

Estrogen

- Normal levels 5 to 100 μg/24 h (urine).
- Primary female sex hormone.
- Naturally occurring estrogens include estradiol, estriol, and estrone.
- Primarily produced by developing follicles and the placenta.
- Follicle-stimulating hormone (FSH) and luteinizing hormone (LH) stimulate the production of estrogen in the ovaries.
- Low levels of estrogen stimulate FSH.
- High levels of estrogen inhibit FSH production and promotes LH secretions.
- The breasts, liver, and adrenal glands produce a small amount of estrogen.
- Functions include: it promotes formation of female secondary sex characteristics, accelerates growth in height and metabolism, reduces muscle mass, stimulates endometrial growth and proliferation, and increases uterine growth.

Follicle-Stimulating Hormone (FSH)

- Normal levels:
  - Premenopause: 4 to 25 mU/mL.
  - Postmenopause: 4 to 30 mU/mL.
- Initiates follicular growth and stimulates the maturation of the graafian follicle(s).
- Secreted by the anterior pituitary gland.
- Levels are normally low in childhood and slightly higher after menopause.
- Levels decline in the late follicular phase and demonstrate a slight increase at the end of the luteal phase.

Follicle-Stimulating Hormone–Releasing Factor

- Becomes active before puberty.
- Produced by the hypothalamus.
- Released into the bloodstream, reaching the anterior pituitary gland.

Luteinizing Hormone (LH)

- Normal levels:
  - Follicular: 2 to 10 μ/L.
  - Midcycle peak: 15 to 65 μ/L.
  - Luteal: 10 to 12 μ/L.
  - Postmenopause: 1.3 to 2.1 mg/dL.
- Essential in both males and females for reproduction.
- Secreted by the anterior pituitary gland.
- Increasing estrogen levels stimulate LH production.
- A surge in LH levels triggers ovulation and initiates the conversion of the residual follicle into a corpus luteum. The corpus luteum produces progesterone to prepare the endometrium for possible implantation.
- LH surge typically lasts only 48 hours.

Luteinizing Hormone-Releasing Factor (LHRF)

- Becomes active before puberty.
- Produced by the hypothalamus.
- Released into the bloodstream, reaching the anterior pituitary gland.

Progesterone

- Normal levels:
  - Follicular: 0.1 to 1.5 ng/mL.
  - Luteal: 2.5 to 28.0 ng/mL.
- Levels are low in childhood and postmenopause.
- Produced in the adrenal glands, corpus luteum, brain, and placenta.
- Increasing amounts of progesterone are produced during pregnancy.

- Levels are low during the preovulatory phase, increase after ovulation, and remain elevated during the luteal phase.
- High levels of progesterone inhibit production within the pituitary gland.
- Functions include: preparing the endometrium for possible implantation or starting the next menstrual cycle.

ENDOMETRIUM

- Endometrial thickness should not exceed 14 mm.
- Thickness of the postmenopausal endometrium without hormone replacement therapy should not exceed 8 mm, and it is consistently benign when measuring 5 mm or less.
- Fluid within the endometrial cavity is not included in the measurement of the endometrial thickness.

PREMENARCHE

- Time before the onset of menses.
- Follicular cysts may be present.
- Cervix to corpus ratio is 2:1.

Precocious Puberty

- Early pubic hair, breast, or genital development may result from natural early maturation or from several other conditions.
- Pubic hair or genital enlargement in boys before 9 years.
- Breast development in boys before appearance of pubic hair and testicular enlargement.
- Pubic hair before 8 years or breast development in girls before 7 years.
- Menstruation in girls before 10 years.
- Elevated hormone levels indicate the possible presence of a hypothalamus, gonad, or adrenal gland neoplasm.
- Induces early bone maturation and reduces eventual adult height.
- Adult-shaped uterus; ovarian volume greater than 1 cm^3.
- Functional ovarian cysts are often present.

Precocious Pseudopuberty

- Early breast development.
- Adrenal or ovarian mass can secrete excess estrogen.
- Uterine cervix is larger than the fundus.
- Normal ovaries without functional follicles.

MENARCHE

- Onset of menstruation (Fig. 20.1).

Menstrual Phase of the Endometrium

DESCRIPTION	SONOGRAPHIC APPEARANCE
Menstruation occurs from days 1–5 Functional layer undergoes necrosis from a decrease in estrogen and progesterone levels	**Early Phase** Hypoechoic central line during menstruation measuring 4–8 mm **Late Phase** Thin, discrete, hyperechoic line postmenstruation measuring 2–3 mm

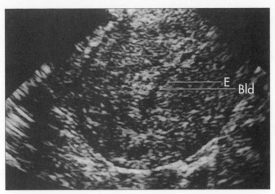

FIG. 20.1 Menstrual phase. (Hagen-Ansert SL: *Textbook of diagnostic ultrasonography,* ed 7, St Louis, 2011, Mosby/Elsevier.)

Proliferation Phase of the Endometrium

DESCRIPTION	SONOGRAPHIC APPEARANCE
Proliferation phase overlaps the postmenstruation phase and occurs from days 5–14 Increasing estrogen levels regenerates the functional layer Coincides with the follicular phase of the ovary	**Early Phase** (Fig. 20.2) Days 5–9 Thin, bright echogenic line measuring 4–8 mm **Late Phase** (Fig. 20.3) Days 10–14 (Preovulatory) A triple-line appearance measuring around 6 10 mm Thick hypoechoic functional layer and hyperechoic basal layer

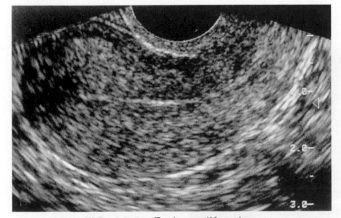

FIG. 20.2 Early proliferation.

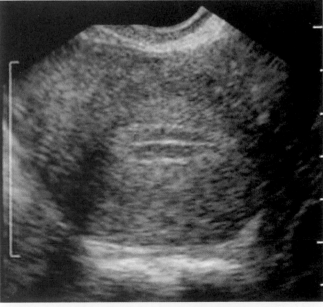

FIG. 20.3 Late proliferation.

Secretory Phase of the Endometrium

DESCRIPTION	SONOGRAPHIC APPEARANCE
Also known as postovulatory or premenstrual phase (Figs. 20.4 and 20.5) Days 15–28 Functional layer continues to thicken Progesterone level increase stimulates changes in endometrium	Functional layer appears hyperechoic Basal layer appears hypoechoic May demonstrate posterior acoustic enhancement Greatest thickness in this phase measuring 7–14 mm

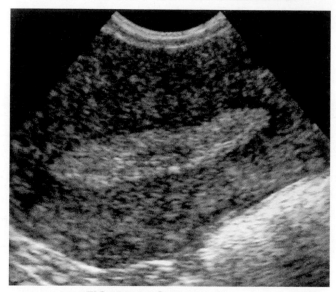

FIG. 20.4 Secretory phase.

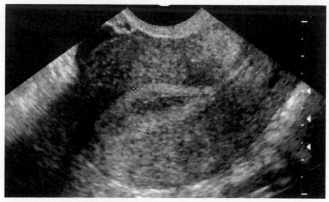

FIG. 20.5 Secretory phase.

OVARIES

- At birth, each ovary contains approximately 200,000 primary follicles.
- Secretion of FSH stimulates follicular development.
- Follicles will fill with fluid and secrete increasing amounts of estrogen.
- Typically, 5 to 11 follicles will begin to develop, with one reaching maturity each cycle.
- 80% of patients will demonstrate a nondominant follicle.
- Visualization of a cumulus oophorus indicates follicular maturity, with ovulation typically occurring within 36 hours.
- Increases in estrogen production from the graafian follicle stimulate production of LH in the anterior pituitary gland.
- LH usually reaches its peak 10 to 12 hours before ovulation.
- A surge in LH accompanied by a smaller FSH surge triggers ovulation.

Follicular Phase of the Ovary

DESCRIPTION	SONOGRAPHIC APPEARANCE
Begins at the start of menstruation	**Early Phase— Days 1–5** (Fig. 20.6)
Ends at ovulation	Multiple small anechoic functional cysts
Variable length but generally 14 days	5–11 small follicles typically begin to develop
FSH stimulates the growth of primary follicles	**Late Phase—Days 6–13** (Fig. 20.7)
Between days 5 and 7, a dominant secondary follicle is determined	Preovulatory phase
	Graafian follicle reaches 2.0–2.4 cm in diameter before ovulation
Dominant follicle will grow 2–3 mm/day	Visualization of a cumulus oophorus increases the probability that
Estrogen levels increase	ovulation will occur within the next 36 hours.

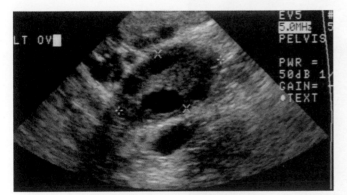

FIG. 20.6   Early follicular.

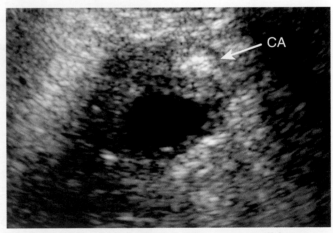

FIG. 20.7   Late follicular. CA = corpus albicans

Ovulatory Phase of the Ovary

DESCRIPTION	SONOGRAPHIC APPEARANCE
Occurs at the rupture of the graafian follicle—Day 14 (Figs. 20.8 and 20.9) Pelvic pain increases over the ovulatory ovary (Mittelschmerz)	Additional nondominant follicles of varying sizes are visualized in 80% of cases Irregular-shaped cystic structure Minimal amount of cul-de-sac fluid

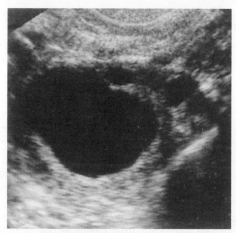

FIG. 20.8   Preovulatory.

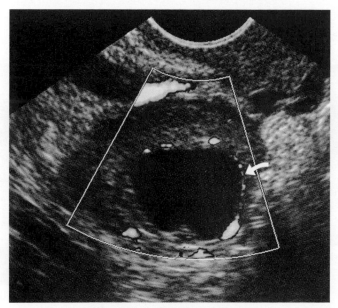

FIG. 20.9   Graafian follicle.

Luteal Phase of the Ovary

DESCRIPTION	SONOGRAPHIC APPEARANCE

Begins postovulation—Days 15–28
Constant 14-day lifespan
Corpus luteum grows for 7–8 days, secreting some estrogen and an increasing amount of progesterone
If the ovum is fertilized, the corpus luteum will continue to secrete progesterone
If fertilization does not occur, the corpus luteum regresses after approximately 9 days, and progesterone levels will decrease
	90% of ruptured follicles will disappear postovulation
	Nondominant follicles of varying size
	Amount of cul-de-sac fluid reaches peak volume in the early luteal phase (Fig. 20.10)
	Corpus Luteal Cyst
	  Small, irregular anechoic structure
	  Thick, hyperechoic wall margins
	  May contain internal echoes (hemorrhage)
	  Anechoic mass demonstrates peripheral hypervascularity (ring of fire) (Fig. 20.11)

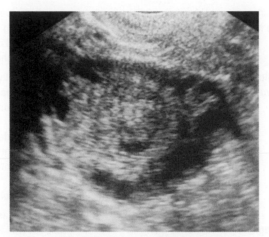

FIG. 20.10   Early luteal.

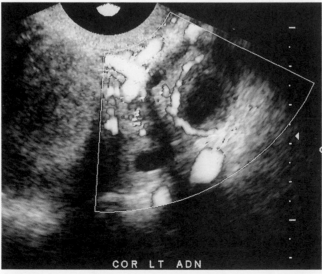

COR LT ADN

FIG. 20.11   Late luteal.

Physiological Ovarian Cysts

NEOPLASM	ETIOLOGY	CLINICAL FINDINGS	SONOGRAPHIC FINDINGS	DIFFERENTIAL CONSIDERATIONS
Corpus luteal cyst	Formed by the ruptured graafian follicle May take 6–12 weeks to resolve May persist to approximately 16 weeks when pregnant	Asymptomatic Pelvic pain	Small, irregular, cystic ovarian mass Hyperechoic, thin to thick walls May contain internal low-level echoes Hypervascular periphery (ring of fire) Small amount of anechoic free fluid in the cul-de-sac Generally unilateral	Ectopic pregnancy
Corpus albicans	Scar from previous corpus luteum	Asymptomatic	Hyperechoic focus(i) within the ovary	Cystic teratoma
Functional cyst Aka: follicular cyst	Benign cyst that responds to hormonal stimulation	Asymptomatic Pelvic pain	Anechoic ovarian mass measuring <3 cm Smooth wall margins Posterior enhancement	Paraovarian cyst Hydrosalpinx Bladder diverticulum
Hemorrhagic cyst	Rupture of a blood vessel at ovulation	Severe acute pelvic pain Nausea/vomiting Low-grade fever	Complex or hypoechoic ovarian mass Thin septations may be present Fluid in cul-de-sac with swirling internal echoes with rupture (blood) No internal blood flow	Ovarian torsion Cystadenoma Ectopic pregnancy Theca lutein cyst
Simple cyst	**Premenarche** Follicular in origin resulting from excessive hormones **Menarche** Failure of a dominant follicle to rupture **Postmenopausal** Follicular in origin	Asymptomatic Pelvic pain Irregular menses	Anechoic mass Smooth wall margins Posterior enhancement Most measure <5.0 cm and regress with subsequent menses	Serous cystadenoma Paraovarian cyst Hydrosalpinx Bladder diverticulum

POSTMENOPAUSE

- Cessation of menstruation for months.
- Approximately 15% of cases will demonstrate a simple ovarian cyst.
- Simple ovarian cysts less than 5.0 cm in diameter are most likely benign.

With Hormone Replacement Therapy

- Includes both estrogen and progesterone.
- Endometrium varies in thickness but should measure <5 mm if on continuous hormone replacement therapy (HRT) and up to 8 mm if sequential HRT.
- Atrophy of the ovaries is not as prevalent.

Without Hormone Replacement Therapy

- Uterus generally decreases in length and width.
- Endometrial thickness typically measures 4 to 5 mm and should not exceed 8 mm in asymptomatic patients or 5 mm in patients with vaginal bleeding.
- Ovaries atrophy and may be difficult to visualize.
- Decreases in estrogen can shorten the vagina and decrease cervical mucus.

CONTRACEPTION

Contraceptive Devices

TYPE OF CONTRACEPTION	DESCRIPTION	SONOGRAPHIC FINDINGS
Oral contraceptives	Inhibits ovulation and LH surge Changes endometrial lining and cervical mucus Contain estrogen and progesterone	Ovulatory phase should not occur Nondominant follicles may be present Endometrium appears as a thin echogenic line (similar to early proliferative phase)
Depot-medroxyprogesterone acetate	Inhibits ovulation and thickens cervical mucus Intramuscular injection every 3 months	Ovulatory phase should not occur Endometrium appears as a thin echogenic line
Fallopian tube microinserts Aka: Essure®	Spring-like coils inserted into the interstitial and isthmus portion of the fallopian tubes Tissue grows into coils in about 3 months blocking the sperm from reaching the ovum	Bilateral echogenic linear structures located lateral to the uterine cornua
Levonorgestrel implants	Inhibits ovulation and thickens cervical mucus Thin capsule is placed under the skin typically in the medial upper arm Lasts 5 years	Implant appears as a hyperechoic linear structure Ovulatory phase should not occur Endometrium appears as a thin echogenic line

Intrauterine device (IUD)	Foreign body is placed in the endometrial cavity at the level of the fundus and superior corpus
	Paraguard—copper T-shape
	Mirena—plastic T-shape that releases levonorgestrel
	
	Risk Factors
	  Infection
	  Perforation
	  Attachment to the basal layer
		Series of hyperechoic linear T-shaped echoes
		Located in the center of the endometrium at the level of the fundus and superior corpus
		Copper IUD—hyperechoic entrance and exit reflections with marked posterior acoustic shadowing
		Plastic IUD—not as reflective and with less posterior shadowing compared with metal IUD
		Ovulation and formation of a corpus luteum continue with nonhormonal IUD (e.g., Paraguard)

Vaginal ring Aka: Nuva® ring	Flexible ring inserted into the vagina Releases hormones to prevent pregnancy May be left in for 21 days	Hyperechoic ring in the superior portion of the vaginal canal near the external cervical os May appear as hyperechoic linear structures in the superior portion of the vaginal canal near the external cervical os

PHYSIOLOGY OF THE FEMALE PELVIS REVIEW

1. Progesterone levels increase in the:
   a. secretory phase
   b. follicular phase
   c. ovulatory phase
   d. menstrual phase

2. Which of the following endometrial phases demonstrates the thinnest dimension?
   a. early menstrual
   b. early secretory
   c. late proliferation
   d. early proliferation

3. Which of the following hormones reflects the activity of the ovaries?
   a. estradiol
   b. progesterone
   c. luteinizing hormone
   d. follicle-stimulating hormone

4. An asymptomatic postmenopausal patient displays a 3.0-cm simple ovarian cyst. This finding is considered:
   a. rare
   b. benign
   c. emergent
   d. malignant

5. If fertilization does not occur, the corpus luteum will:
   a. decrease in size and estrogen levels will increase
   b. increase in size and estrogen levels will decrease
   c. increase in size and progesterone levels will increase
   d. decrease in size and progesterone levels will decrease

6. The endometrium demonstrates a triple-line appearance between days:
   a. 1 to 5
   b. 6 to 9
   c. 10 to 14
   d. 14 to 21

7. A hyperechoic focus within a mature follicle most likely represents a:
   a. morula
   b. cumulus oophorus
   c. blastocyst
   d. corpus albicans

8. Visualization of a corpus luteal cyst indicates:
   a. ovulation is imminent
   b. ovulation has occurred
   c. fertilization has occurred
   d. ovulatory hemorrhage has occurred

9. Dysmenorrhea is a term used to describe:
   a. heavy menses
   b. painful menses
   c. pain during ovulation
   d. pain during sexual intercourse

10. Luteinizing hormone is secreted by the:
    a. ovary
    b. hypothalamus
    c. adrenal gland
    d. anterior pituitary gland

11. Which of the following structures produces small amounts of estrogen?
    a. spleen
    b. kidney
    c. pancreas
    d. adrenal gland

12. Which of the following hormones stimulates ovulation?
    a. estrogen
    b. progesterone
    c. luteinizing hormone
    d. follicle-stimulating hormone

13. Fluid within the endometrial cavity is:
    a. produced by the granulosa cells
    b. suspicious for endometrial hyperplasia
    c. not included in the endometrial measurement
    d. highly suspicious for endometrial malignancy

14. Mittelschmerz is associated with:
    a. pregnancy
    b. ovulation
    c. hemorrhage
    d. menstruation

15. Pain during sexual intercourse is termed:
    a. dysuria
    b. dysmenorrhea
    c. dyspareunia
    d. menorrhagia

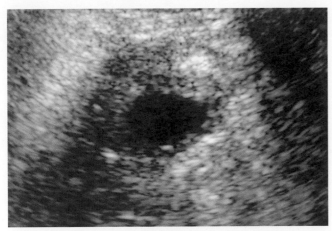

FIG. 20.12 Sonogram of the ovary.

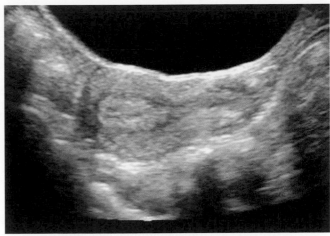

FIG. 20.13 Sagittal image of the uterus.

Using Figure 20.12, answer questions 16 and 17.

16. A patient presents with a history of intermittent lower quadrant pain. Her last menstrual period was 1 week earlier, and she denies the use of hormone contraceptives. Based on this clinical history, the anechoic areas most likely represent:
    a. corpus albicans
    b. functional cysts
    c. graafian follicles
    d. corpus luteal cysts

17. Hyperechoic foci within the ovary are most suspicious for:
    a. cystic teratoma
    b. corpus albicans
    c. hemorrhagic cysts
    d. cumulus oophorus

Using Figure 20.13, answer question 18.

18. Which endometrial phase is most likely demonstrated in this endovaginal sonogram?
    a. luteal
    b. secretory
    c. menstrual
    d. proliferative

Using Figure 20.14, answer question 19.

19. A patient presents with a history of right lower quadrant pain. Her last menstrual period was 7 days earlier. On the basis of this clinical history, the anechoic mass most likely represents a:
    a. simple cyst
    b. graafian follicle
    c. corpus luteal cyst
    d. serous cystadenoma

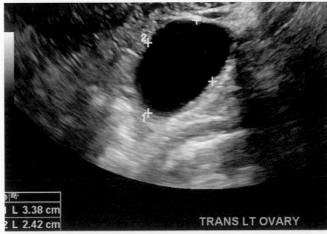

L 3.38 cm
L 2.42 cm
TRANS LT OVARY

FIG. 20.14 Transverse sonogram.

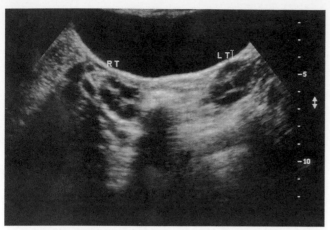

FIG. 20.15 Transabdominal sonogram.

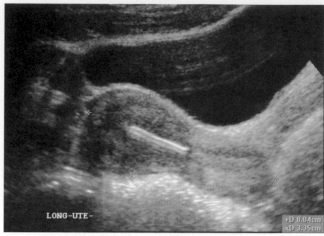

FIG. 20.17 Transabdominal sonogram.

Using Figure 20.15, answer question 20.

20. The ovaries in this sonogram coincide with which of the following uterine phases?
  a. late follicular
  b. early follicular
  c. late proliferation
  d. early proliferation

Using Figure 20.16, answer question 21.

21. Which of the following endometrial phases is most likely displayed in this sagittal sonogram of the uterus?
  a. late secretory
  b. early menstrual
  c. early secretory
  d. early proliferative

Using Figure 20.17, answer question 22.

22. A patient presents with a history of irregular menses. A transabdominal sonogram of the uterus demonstrates:
  a. endometritis
  b. Asherman syndrome
  c. endometrial hyperplasia
  d. an intrauterine contraceptive device

Using Figure 20.18, answer question 23.

23. The sonogram demonstrates a sagittal image of a(n):
  a. menarche uterus
  b. unicornuate uterus
  c. premenarche uterus
  d. postmenopausal uterus

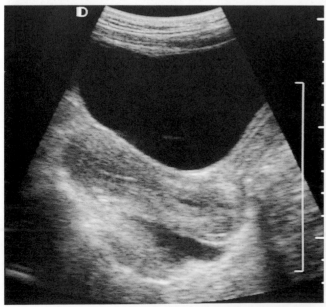

FIG. 20.16 Sagittal sonogram.

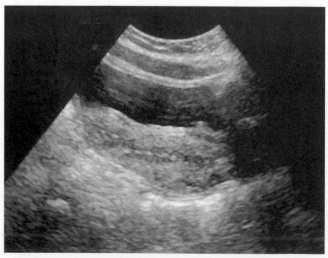

FIG. 20.18 Sagittal sonogram of the right ovary.

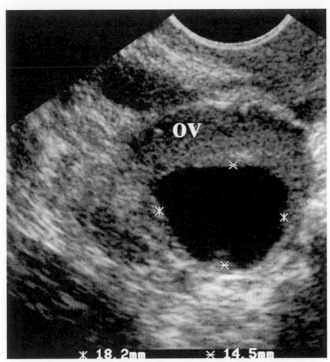

FIG. 20.19 Sonogram of the right ovary.

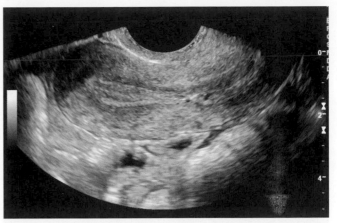

FIG. 20.20 Sagittal sonogram.

Using Figure 20.19, answer questions 24 and 25.

24. A 25-year-old patient presents with an 18-mm anechoic ovarian mass. This is most consistent with a:
   a. simple cyst
   b. graafian follicle
   c. corpus albicans
   d. serous cystadenoma

25. The echogenic focus demonstrated on the posterior wall just anterior to the caliper is most suspicious for:
   a. hemorrhage
   b. blood vessel
   c. serous debris
   d. cumulus oophorus

Using Figure 20.20, answer questions 26 and 27.

26. Which of the following endometrial phases is most likely displayed in the sagittal sonogram?
   a. early secretory
   b. late follicular
   c. early proliferation
   d. late proliferation

27. The sonographic appearance of this endometrium is termed:
   a. shotgun sign
   b. decidual reaction
   c. triple-line pattern
   d. double decidua sign

Using Figure 20.21 (and Color Plate 9), answer question 28.

28. A 28-year-old patient presents with a sudden onset of right lower quadrant pain. Her last menstrual period was approximately 3 weeks earlier. This duplex sonogram is most suspicious for a(n):
   a. graafian follicle
   b. ectopic pregnancy
   c. corpus luteal cyst
   d. nondominant follicle

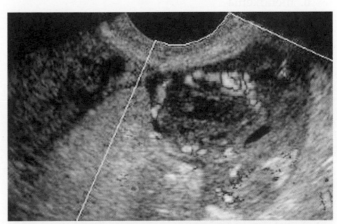

FIG. 20.21 Endovaginal sonogram (see Color Plate 9).

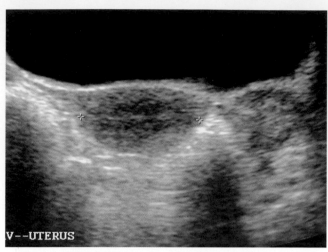

FIG. 20.22　Transverse sonogram.

Using Figure 20.22, answer question 29.

29. The endometrial phase in this patient is most consistent with:
    a. late secretory
    b. late menstrual
    c. early menstrual
    d. late proliferation

Using Figure 20.23, answer question 30.

30. Which of the following ovarian masses will most likely coincide with this endometrial phase?
    a. simple cyst
    b. graafian follicle
    c. theca lutein cyst
    d. corpus luteal cyst

31. A patient complains of heavy menstrual cycles. This is most consistent with:
    a. menoxenia
    b. dyspareunia
    c. menorrhagia
    d. dysmenorrhea

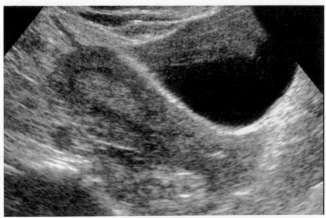

FIG. 20.23　Transabdominal sonogram.

32. Levels of follicle-stimulating hormone begin declining in the:
    a. late secretory phase
    b. late follicular phase
    c. early secretory phase
    d. early follicular phase

33. During the ovulatory phase, normal estradiol levels range between:
    a. 50 and 100 pg/mL
    b. 10 and 200 pg/mL
    c. 100 and 200 pg/mL
    d. 200 and 400 pg/mL

34. Which of the following ovarian phases coincides with the proliferation phase of the endometrium?
    a. luteal
    b. secretory
    c. follicular
    d. ovulatory

35. Corpus albicans appears on ultrasound as a(n):
    a. anechoic mass
    b. isoechoic mass
    c. hypoechoic mass
    d. hyperechoic mass

36. Endometrial thickness of an asymptomatic postmenopausal patient denying hormone replacement therapy should not exceed:
    a. 2 mm
    b. 5 mm
    c. 8 mm
    d. 10 mm

37. Which of the following hormone levels can be slightly higher after menopause?
    a. estrogen
    b. progesterone
    c. luteinizing hormone
    d. follicle-stimulating hormone

38. Which of the following describe the sonographic appearance of the endometrium during the late proliferation phase?
    a. thick, hyperechoic functional layer and a hyperechoic basal layer
    b. thin, hyperechoic functional layer and a hypoechoic basal layer
    c. thick, hyperechoic functional layer and a hypoechoic basal layer
    d. thick, hypoechoic functional layer and a hyperechoic basal layer

39. Acute pelvic pain during the periovulatory phase is termed:
    a. Murphy sign
    b. Mittelschmerz
    c. McBurney sign
    d. tip of the iceberg

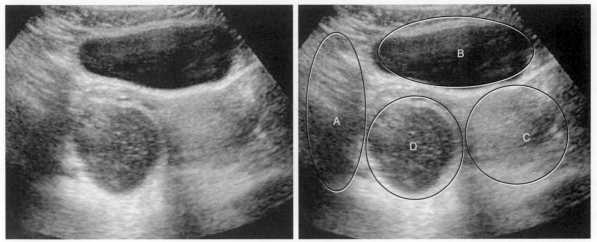

FIG. 20.24 Transabdominal transverse sonogram.

40. Which of the following hormones help to prepare the endometrium for implantation of the blastocyst?
 a. estrogen
 b. estradiol
 c. progesterone
 d. luteinizing hormone

41. Estrogen is primarily secreted by the:
 a. thyroid glands
 b. corpus luteum
 c. pituitary gland
 d. graafian follicle

42. The length of a normal menstrual cycle ranges between:
 a. 14 and 28 days
 b. 21 and 28 days
 c. 21 and 35 days
 d. 28 and 40 days

43. An early onset of puberty may be the result of a(n):
 a. renal neoplasm
 b. ovarian neoplasm
 c. thyroid gland neoplasm
 d. pituitary gland neoplasm

44. Regeneration of the endometrium occurs as a result of:
 a. increases in estrogen levels
 b. decreases in estrogen levels
 c. increases in progesterone levels
 d. decreases in progesterone levels

45. The endometrium displays the greatest thickness during the:
 a. follicular phase
 b. secretory phase
 c. menstrual phase
 d. proliferation phase

Using Figure 20.24, answer question 46.

46. An adolescent patient presents with a history of severe acute right lower quadrant pain. Her last menstrual period was 2 to 3 weeks earlier. Based on this clinical history, which of the following circles demonstrates the mostly likely cause of this patient's pelvic pain?
 a. A
 b. B
 c. C
 d. D

47. If fertilization occurs, the corpus luteum will continue to secrete:
 a. estrogen
 b. estradiol
 c. progesterone
 d. human chorionic gonadotropin

48. Which of the following describes the expected appearance of the endometrium in a patient using oral contraceptives?
 a. thin echogenic line
 b. thin hypoechoic line
 c. triple-line appearance
 d. thick and hyperechoic

49. An intrauterine device should be located:
 a. lateral to the uterine cornua in the corpus portion of the endometrium
 b. in the corpus portion of the endometrium
 c. in the fundal/cornual portion of the uterus
 d. in the superior corpus and fundal portion of the endometrium

50. Decreases in estrogen in postmenopausal patients can decrease cervical mucus and can also:
 a. shorten vaginal length
 b. increase cervical length
 c. thicken the vaginal walls
 d. thicken the endometrial cavity

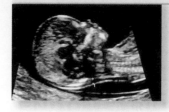

CHAPTER 21

Uterine and Ovarian Pathology

KEY TERMS

adenomyoma a tumor of the uterus characterized by a mass of smooth muscle containing endometrial tissue and glands.

adenomyosis benign invasive growth of endometrium into the myometrium. Found in approximately 70% of hysterectomies.

arteriovenous fistula vascular complex of arteries and veins without an intervening capillary system.

Asherman syndrome intrauterine adhesions ablating the endometrial lining.

Gartner duct cyst small cyst within the vagina.

hematocolpos blood accumulation in the vagina.

hematometra blood accumulation in the uterus.

hematometrocolpos blood accumulation in the uterus and vagina.

hyperplasia proliferation of the endometrial lining.

intramural leiomyoma mass distorting the myometrium; most common location.

leiomyoma most common benign gynecological tumor of the myometrium.

Meigs syndrome combination of pleural effusion, ascites, and an ovarian mass that resolve after surgery.

submucosal leiomyoma mass distorting the endometrium; least common but most likely to cause symptoms.

subserosal leiomyoma mass found on the serosal surface of the uterus.

tamoxifen antiestrogen medication used in treating breast cancer.

Tip of the Iceberg a term used to describe the sonographic appearance of a dense ovarian dermoid tumor.

Descriptive Terms for Pelvic Pathology

MASS CHARACTERISTIC	DESCRIPTIVE TERMS
Overall composition	Anechoic, echogenic, complex Hypoechoic, hyperechoic Homogeneous, heterogeneous
Internal characteristics	Unilocular, multilocular Fluid—fluid levels Mural nodules, internal debris
Wall definition	Thin, thick Smooth, irregular Well defined, ill defined
Doppler characteristics	Lack of vascular flow Hypervascular, hypovascular High resistance, low resistance

UTERINE PATHOLOGY

- Intramural leiomyomas are the most common uterine neoplasm.

Pathology of the Cervix

PATHOLOGY	ETIOLOGY	CLINICAL FINDINGS	SONOGRAPHIC FINDINGS	DIFFERENTIAL CONSIDERATIONS
Carcinoma	Epithelial neoplasm Third most common gynecological malignancy in the United States **Risk Factors** Human papilloma virus (HPV) Early sexual activity Multiple sex partners Use of oral contraceptives Smoking	Asymptomatic Vaginal discharge or bleeding Palpable mass Weight loss Intermenstrual or postcoital bleeding	Hypoechoic or heterogeneous retrovesical mass Irregular margins Dilated ureter Anechoic or hypoechoic endometrial fluid collection	Leiomyoma Complex cervical cyst Polyp
Nabothian cyst	Obstructed inclusion cyst(s) Chronic cervicitis	Asymptomatic	Round, anechoic structure Multiple or solitary Usually <2.0 cm in diameter May contain internal echoes Posterior enhancement	Leiomyoma Arcuate vessel Retained products of conception

Pathology of the Uterus

PATHOLOGY	ETIOLOGY	CLINICAL FINDINGS	SONOGRAPHIC FINDINGS	DIFFERENTIAL CONSIDERATIONS
Adenomyosis	Ectopic endometrial tissue within the myometrium **Risk Factors** Multiparity Elevated estrogen levels Aggressive curettage	Asymptomatic Pelvic pain or cramping Uterine enlargement Uterine tenderness Menorrhagia Dysmenorrhea	Diffuse uterine enlargement Smooth uterine contour Inhomogeneous myometrium Poorly defined anechoic areas within the myometrium Ill-defined endometrium Pseudo-thickening of the endometrium Striated edge shadows (venetian-blind) without focal myometrial mass Posterior uterine wall most commonly affected Adenomyoma – hypoechoic mass with ill-defined walls.	Degenerating fibroid Endometrial neoplasm

Continued

Pathology of the Uterus—(cont'd)

PATHOLOGY	ETIOLOGY	CLINICAL FINDINGS	SONOGRAPHIC FINDINGS	DIFFERENTIAL CONSIDERATIONS
Leiomyoma Also called fibroid or myoma **Intramural** Distorts the myometrium Confined to the myometrium Most common **Pedunculated** Attached to the uterus by a stalk Appears extrauterine **Submucosal** Distorts the endometrium Impedes the endometrium Most symptomatic **Subserosal** Located under the perimetrium Distorts uterine contour	Most common benign neoplasm of the uterine myometrium Estrogen dependent. May increase in size during pregnancy May decrease in size after menopause Prevalence in African Americans	Asymptomatic Menorrhagia Pelvic pain or pressure Uterine enlargement Irregular bleeding Urinary frequency Infertility	Diffuse uterine enlargement Uterine mass with a variable echo pattern ranging from hypoechoic to hyperechoic Well defined walls Lobulated uterine contour Heterogeneous mass with associated necrosis or hemorrhage Often multiple Diffuse uterine enlargement Calcifications may be present Low flow velocity on spectral Doppler May cause hematometra when located in the cervix	Ovarian neoplasm Leiomyosarcoma
Leiomyosarcoma	Derived from the smooth muscle of the uterus Rare	Asymptomatic Vaginal bleeding	Heterogeneous uterine mass Irregular margins	Leiomyoma Endometrial carcinoma

Endometrial Abnormalities

ABNORMALITY	ETIOLOGY	CLINICAL FINDINGS	SONOGRAPHIC FINDINGS	DIFFERENTIAL CONSIDERATIONS
Asherman syndrome	Adhesions from a previous deep curettage or endometrial infection	Asymptomatic Amenorrhea Dysmenorrhea Hypomenorrhea Infertility	Inability to distinguish an endometrial cavity Bright echoes within the endometrial cavity	Normal early proliferative phase Uterine mass compressing endometrial cavity
Carcinoma	Unknown Associated with estrogen stimulation Adenocarcinoma is most common **Risk Factors** Obesity Diabetes Anovulatory cycles Nulliparity Postmenopause	Abnormal bleeding	Focal irregularity of the endometrium Myometrial distortion Thickened endometrium Complex endometrial mass	Endometrial hyperplasia Endometrial polyp

Endometrial Abnormalities—(cont'd)

ABNORMALITY	ETIOLOGY	CLINICAL FINDINGS	SONOGRAPHIC FINDINGS	DIFFERENTIAL CONSIDERATIONS
Endometritis	Pelvic inflammatory disease Postpartum complication Postprocedural complication Vaginitis	Pelvic pain Fever Leukocytosis	Normal findings Thick and irregular endometrium Pronounced endometrium Enlarged, inhomogeneous uterus Hypervascular endometrium and myometrium	Normal uterus Adenomyosis Leiomyoma
Hematometra	Imperforated hymen Cervical stenosis Vagina neoplasm	Pelvic pain Amenorrhea Hypomenorrhea Pelvic mass	Large hypoechoic midline uterine mass Posterior enhancement Minimal or lack of visible myometrial tissue	Submucosal leiomyoma Endometrioma Retained products of conception
Hyperplasia	Unopposed estrogen Tamoxifen therapy Polycystic ovarian syndrome Obesity	Asymptomatic Abnormal bleeding Common cause of abnormal uterine bleeding in pre- and post-menopausal women Less common during reproductive years	Prominent thickening of the endometrium with or without cystic changes Premenopausal thickness >14 mm Postmenopausal thickness >5 mm in symptomatic women or >8 mm in asymptomatic women	Endometrial carcinoma Endometrial polyp
Polyp	Overgrowth of endometrial tissue Contains glands, stroma, and blood vessels Unresponsive to progesterone	Asymptomatic Abnormal bleeding Infertility More common in peri- and postmenopausal women	Focal areas of echogenic endometrial thickening Round or ovoid echogenic mass within the endometrial cavity Isoechoic to endometrium in the secretory phase Hyperechoic to the endometrium in the late proliferation phase May contain cystic areas Color Doppler may demonstrate flow within the stalk Multiple polyps found in approx. 20% of cases	Endometrial carcinoma Endometrial hyperplasia Submucosal leiomyoma
Tamoxifen effect	Side effects of antiestrogen medication	Asymptomatic Abnormal bleeding	Normal-appearing endometrium Thickening of the endometrial cavity Complex appearance to the endometrial cavity	Endometrial hyperplasia Endometrial polyp Endometrial carcinoma Submucosal leiomyoma

OVARIAN PATHOLOGY

- The majority of ovarian masses, removed from premenopausal patients, are benign.
- Cystic teratoma (dermoid) is the most common primary ovarian neoplasm.

Cystic Ovarian Pathology

PATHOLOGY	ETIOLOGY	CLINICAL FINDINGS	SONOGRAPHIC FINDINGS	DIFFERENTIAL CONSIDERATIONS
Cystadenocarcinoma	Epithelial neoplasm	Palpable pelvic mass Unexplained weight gain Pelvic pain	Multilocular, complex mass Ill-defined wall margins Mural nodules Ascites	Cystadenoma Cystic teratoma Tuboovarian abscess
Cystic teratoma Also called dermoid	Arises from the wall of a follicle Germ cell tumor Contains fat, hair, skin, and teeth Most common benign tumor of the ovary	Asymptomatic Abdominal pressure Mild to acute pelvic pain Palpable pelvic mass	"Tip of the Iceberg"— solid mass with diffusely bright internal echoes with or without shadowing Complex mass Thick, irregular margins Calcifications Commonly located superior to the uterine fundus	Endometrioma Hemorrhagic cyst Serous cystadenoma Ectopic pregnancy
Mucinous cystadenoma	Epithelial neoplasm	Pelvic pain Rapid increase in pelvic mass Irregular menses Bloating	Multilocular anechoic mass Thick, smooth wall margins May contain debris Generally unilateral	Endometrioma Tuboovarian abscess Theca lutein cyst Cystadenocarcinoma
Polycystic ovarian syndrome	Endocrine imbalance causing chronic anovulation Imbalance of luteinizing hormone (LH) and follicle-stimulating hormone (FSH)	Irregular menses Hirsutism Infertility Obesity	Bilateral round, enlarged ovaries Presence of ten or more follicles per ovary Multiple, small peripheral follicles Ovarian volume greater than 10^3	Normal functional cysts
Serous cystadenoma	Epithelial neoplasm Second most common benign tumor of the ovary	Rapid increase of a pelvic mass Pelvic pain Irregular menses Bloating	Large unilocular or multilocular anechoic mass Smooth, thin-walled margins May contain internal debris and septae Generally unilateral	Hydrosalpinx Theca lutein cysts Hyperstimulation syndrome
Surface epithelial cyst	Arise from the cortex of the ovary	Asymptomatic Pelvic pain	Small cluster of cysts	Polycystic ovarian disease Cystadenoma
Theca lutein cysts	Associated with high level of human chorionic gonadotropin Gestational trophoblastic disease Ovarian hyperstimulation syndrome	Asymptomatic Hyperemesis Abdominal bloating Associated with high level of human chorionic gonadotropin (hCG)	Multilocular cystic structure Bilateral condition	Cystadenoma Hydrosalpinx

Solid Ovarian Neoplasms

NEOPLASM	ETIOLOGY	CLINICAL FINDINGS	SONOGRAPHIC FINDINGS	DIFFERENTIAL CONSIDERATIONS
Brenner tumor	Benign tumor arising from fibroepithelial tissue Estrogenic in nature Associated with Meigs syndrome	Asymptomatic Unilateral pelvic pain or fullness	Small, hypoechoic, solid ovarian mass Well-defined wall margins Does *not* demonstrate posterior acoustic enhancement May demonstrate necrosis	Fibroma Pedunculated fibroid Thecoma
Carcinoma	Epithelial or germ cell neoplasm **Risk Factors** Late menopause High-fat diet Infertility Nulliparity Family history of breast or ovarian carcinoma	Asymptomatic Vague abdominal pain Palpable pelvic mass Elevated CA125 (80%) Vague GI symptoms Bloating	Predominantly solid, hypoechoic ovarian mass Irregular ovarian margins May appear complex Internal blood flow Resistive index <1.0 suggests malignancy	Endometrioma Metastatic lesion Granulosa cell tumor
Dysgerminoma	Malignant germ cell neoplasm Most common ovarian malignancy in childhood	Asymptomatic Precocious puberty Pelvic pain Palpable pelvic mass Associated with alpha-fetoprotein (AFP) and hCG levels Spreads to the lymphatics	Predominantly solid, homogeneous mass Irregular margins May appear complex Lymphadenopathy Unilateral (90%)	Cystadenocarcinoma Metastatic lesion
Fibroma	Rare, benign stromal tumor Associated with Meigs syndrome	Asymptomatic Pelvic pain or fullness Urinary or intestinal disturbance Menopause	Solid, hypoechoic adnexal mass (identical to a leiomyoma) Dense mass May demonstrate posterior shadowing Ascites 5-10 cm in size Unilateral (90%)	Pedunculated fibroid Cystic teratoma Thecoma Brenner tumor
Granulosa cell tumor	Hormonal tumor	Increase in estrogen Palpable mass Irregular bleeding	Solid, homogeneous adnexal mass May appear complex Thickening of the endometrium	Pedunculated fibroid
Thecoma	Benign stromal tumor Produces estrogen	Pelvic pain or pressure Menopause	Hypoechoic mass Prominent posterior shadowing May demonstrate calcifications	Fibroma Teratoma Brenner tumor

Vascular Ovarian Abnormalities

ABNORMALITY	ETIOLOGY	CLINICAL FINDINGS	SONOGRAPHIC FINDINGS	DIFFERENTIAL CONSIDERATIONS
Arteriovenous fistula	Pelvic surgery Pelvic trauma Gestational trophoblastic disease Malignancy	Menorrhagia Anemia Often diagnosed postabortion and postpartum	Multiple serpingous anechoic structures within the myometrium Abundant blood flow within the anechoic structures Intramural uterine mass Mosaic pattern on color Doppler Flow reversal and areas of aliasing High-velocity, low-resistance arterial flow coupled with high-velocity venous flow with an arterial component on spectral analysis	Adenomyosis Trophoblastic gestation Retained products of conception
Ovarian torsion	Partial or complete rotation of the ovary on its pedicle Commonly associated with an adnexal mass	Severe or consistent pelvic pain Nausea/vomiting Palpable pelvic mass	Decreased or absent venous and arterial blood flow to the ovary (venous outflow is first to be compromised) Enlarged, round, heterogeneous ovarian mass Free fluid Coexisting adnexal mass	Normal ovary Hemorrhagic cyst Cystic teratoma

UTERINE AND OVARIAN PATHOLOGY REVIEW

1. Abnormal accumulation of blood within the vagina is termed:
   a. hydrometra
   b. hematometra
   c. hydrocolpos
   d. hematocolpos

2. Risk factors associated with developing endometrial carcinoma include:
   a. anorexia, multiparity, hypertension
   b. obesity, diabetes mellitus, nulliparity
   c. hypertension, obesity, thyroid disease
   d. multiparity, thyroid disease, hormone replacement therapy

3. Hypervascularity within the endometrium is a characteristic finding in:
   a. endometritis
   b. adenomyosis
   c. Asherman syndrome
   d. endometrial hyperplasia

4. The most common ovarian malignancy occurring in childhood is a:
   a. fibroma
   b. thecoma
   c. dysgerminoma
   d. Brenner tumor

5. Which of the following is a common clinical symptom associated with adenomyosis?
   a. amenorrhea
   b. lower back pain
   c. urinary frequency
   d. uterine tenderness

6. A 50-year-old patient presents with a history of abdominal distention. In the left adnexa, a 10-cm, multilocular mass is identified. This mass most likely represents:
   a. a cystadenoma
   b. a cystic teratoma
   c. theca lutein cysts
   d. polycystic disease

7. The most common location for a uterine leiomyoma to develop is:
   a. serosal
   b. subserosal
   c. intramural
   d. submucosal

8. Inability to distinguish the endometrial cavity is a sonographic finding in:
   a. infertility
   b. tamoxifen therapy
   c. Asherman syndrome
   d. polycystic ovarian disease

9. Ovarian torsion is commonly associated with a coexisting:
   a. uterine mass
   b. hydrosalpinx
   c. adnexal mass
   d. ectopic pregnancy

10. Tamoxifen therapy is most likely to affect which of the following structures?
    a. cervix
    b. ovaries
    c. myometrium
    d. endometrium

11. A reproductive-age patient demonstrates a complex adnexal mass with diffusely bright internal echoes. These sonographic findings most likely describe a:
    a. dysgerminoma
    b. cystic teratoma
    c. hemorrhagic cyst
    d. cystadenocarcinoma

12. The most common location of a cystic teratoma is:
    a. lateral to the cervix
    b. anterior to the fundus
    c. superior to the fundus
    d. adjacent to the isthmus

13. Obstruction of an inclusion cyst results in a(n):
    a. nabothian cyst
    b. cystic teratoma
    c. endometrial polyp
    d. serous cystadenoma

14. A fibroid is most likely to cause irregular uterine bleeding in which location?
    a. cervical
    b. subserosal
    c. intramural
    d. submucosal

15. Polycystic ovarian disease can result from:
    a. high levels of hCG
    b. unopposed estrogen
    c. an endocrine imbalance
    d. follicular hyperstimulation

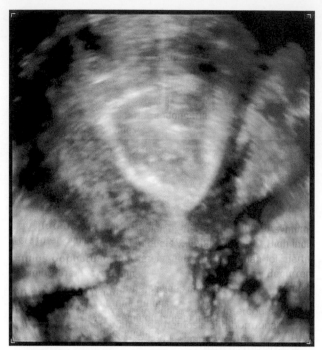

FIG. 21.1 3-D rendering of the endometrium.

Using Figure 21.1, answer question 16.

16. The finding in this sonogram of an asymptomatic patient receiving antiestrogen therapy is most suspicious for:
    a. a leiomyoma
    b. adenomyosis
    c. Asherman syndrome
    d. an endometrial polyp

Using Figure 21.2, answer question 17.

17. The finding in this sonogram, in a patient with a history of amenorrhea is most suspicious for:
    a. hematometra
    b. hematocolpos
    c. septate uterus
    d. endometrial hyperplasia

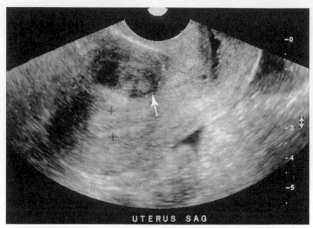

FIG. 21.3 Endovaginal sonogram.

Using Figure 21.3, answer questions 18 and 19.

18. The arrow in this sonogram is most likely identifying a(n):
    a. endometrioma
    b. adenomyoma
    c. subserosal leiomyoma
    d. submucosal leiomyoma

19. Free fluid is identified in which of the following pelvic recesses?
    a. prevesical space
    b. retropubic space
    c. retrouterine space
    d. vesicouterine space

Using Figure 21.4, answer question 20.

20. A 30-year-old patient presents with a history of left lower quadrant discomfort. Based on this clinical history, this sonogram is most suspicious for a(n):
    a. endometrioma
    b. cystic teratoma
    c. ovarian carcinoma
    d. tuboovarian abscess

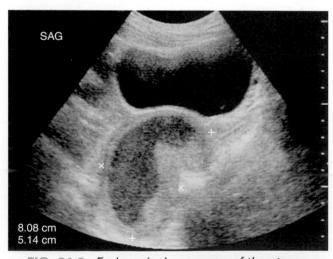

SAG

8.08 cm
5.14 cm

FIG. 21.2 Endovaginal sonogram of the uterus.

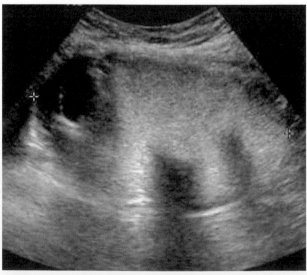

FIG. 21.4 Sonogram of the left lower quadrant.

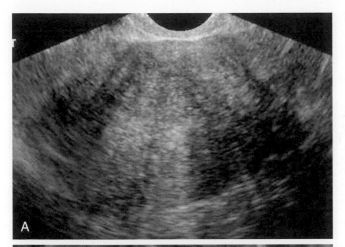

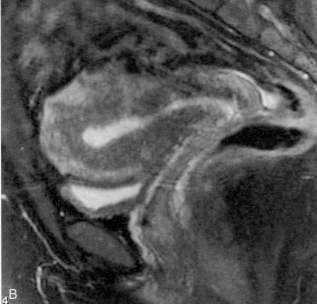

FIG. 21.5   **(A)** Coronal sonogram of the uterus. **(B)** MRI of the same uterus

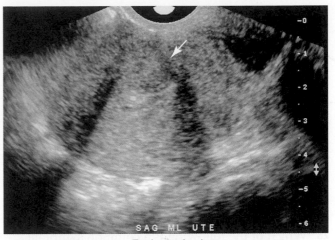

FIG. 21.6   Endovaginal sonogram.

Using Figure 21.6, answer questions 23 and 24.

23. The arrow in this sonogram is most likely identifying which of the following?
   a. leiomyoma
   b. adenomyosis
   c. endometrial polyp
   d. endometrial carcinoma

24. Which clinical finding is most likely associated with this pathology?
   a. amenorrhea
   b. menorrhagia
   c. dysmenorrhea
   d. postmenopausal bleeding

Using Figure 21.7, answer questions 25 and 26.

25. An asymptomatic patient presents with a history of an enlarged uterus. Based on this clinical history, the demonstrated pathology most likely represents a(n):
   a. endometrioma
   b. subserosal fibroids
   c. intramural fibroids
   d. submucosal fibroids

Using Figure 21.5 A and B, answer questions 21 and 22

21. This sagittal sonogram most likely displays:
   a. endometritis
   b. adenomyosis
   c. endometriosis
   d. Asherman syndrome

22. Which of the following is a clinical symptom associated with this finding?
   a. fever
   b. dysmenorrhea
   c. amenorrhea
   d. dyspareunia

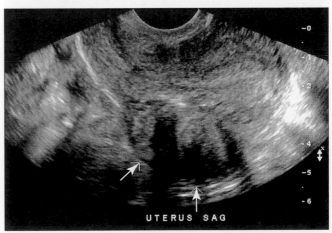

FIG. 21.7   Endovaginal sonogram.

26. This abnormality is located on the:
    a. anterior surface of a retroverted uterus
    b. posterior surface of a retroverted uterus
    c. anterior surface of a retroflexed uterus
    d. posterior surface of an anteverted uterus

Using Figure 21.8, answer questions 27 and 28.

27. The sonographic findings are most suspicious for which of the following pathologies?
    a. surface epithelial cysts
    b. polycystic ovarian disease
    c. overstimulation syndrome
    d. normal physiological cysts

28. Which of the following is a common symptom associated with this pathology?
    a. pelvic pain
    b. dysmenorrhea
    c. irregular menses
    d. abdominal distention

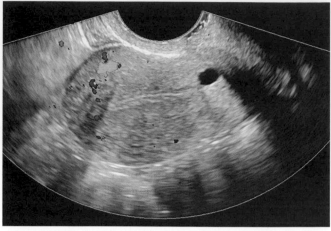

FIG. 21.9 Endovaginal sagittal sonogram.

Using Figure 21.9, answer question 29.

29. A sagittal image of the uterus most likely displays a(n):
    a. nabothian cyst
    b. endometrial polyp
    c. cervical malignancy
    d. gartner duct cyst

Using Figure 21.10, answer question 30.

30. A patient presents with a history of irregular menses and a large pelvic mass. Based on this clinical history, the sonographic finding is most suspicious for:
    a. surface epithelial cyst
    b. a mucinous cystadenoma
    c. polycystic ovarian disease
    d. overstimulation syndrome

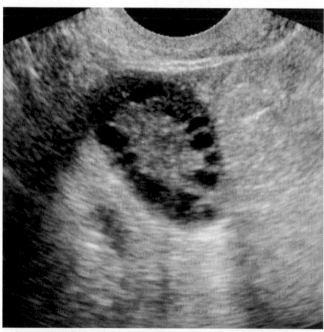

FIG. 21.8 Sonogram of the right ovary.

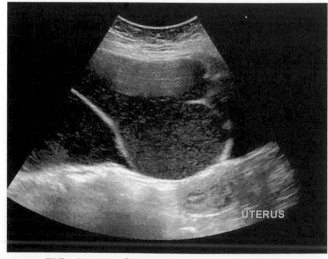

FIG. 21.10 Sonogram of the left adnexa.

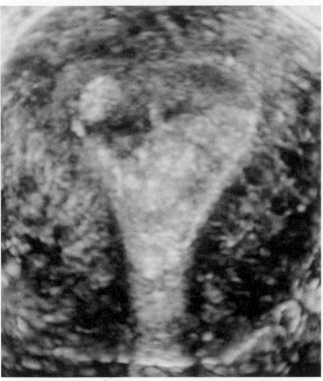

FIG. 21.11 3-D rendering of the endometrium.

Using Figure 21.11, answer question 31.

31. A three-dimensional image of the uterus shows a:
a. bicornuate uterus
b. hypoechoic endometrial mass
c. hyperechoic endometrial mass
d. normal-appearing endometrial cavity

32. Which of the following describe the typical sonographic appearance of Asherman syndrome?
a. diffuse uterine enlargement
b. discrete hypoechoic myometrial mass
c. inability to distinguish an endometrial cavity
d. hypoechoic irregularity to the endometrial cavity

33. A coexisting adnexal mass is commonly associated with which of the following ovarian pathologies?
a. cystadenoma
b. dysgerminoma
c. cystic teratoma
d. ovarian torsion

34. Hirsutism is a clinical symptom of:
a. endometriosis
b. hematometrocolpos
c. Asherman syndrome
d. polycystic ovarian disease

35. A rapid increasing pelvic mass is most suspicious for a(n):
a. leiomyoma
b. cystadenoma
c. endometrioma
d. cystic teratoma

36. A small cluster of ovarian cysts is a common sonographic finding associated with:
a. theca lutein cysts
b. cystadenocarcinoma
c. surface epithelial cysts
d. polycystic ovarian disease

37. Which of the following fibroid locations is most likely to cause menorrhagia?
a. cornual
b. intramural
c. subserosal
d. submucosal

38. Which of the following ovarian neoplasms demonstrates sonographic characteristics similar to a leiomyoma?
a. thecoma
b. fibroma
c. dysgerminoma
d. cystic teratoma

39. Multiple serpentine vascular structures within the myometrium in a patient complaining of abnormal bleeding following a recent dilation curettage procedure is most suspicious for which of the following abnormalities?
a. adenomyosis
b. endometriosis
c. arteriovenous fistula
d. Asherman syndrome

40. Sonographic appearance of ovarian carcinoma is generally described as a(n):
a. irregular hypoechoic ovarian mass
b. smooth hyperechoic ovarian mass
c. irregular hypoechoic adnexal mass
d. irregular hyperechoic ovarian mass

41. If a patient displays an endometrial thickness of 2.0 cm, it is considered:
a. suspicious for adenomyosis
b. within normal limits in a menarche patient
c. suspicious for proliferation of the endometrium
d. within normal limits regardless of menstrual status

42. Which of the following ovarian abnormalities may contain skin and hair?
    a. dysgerminoma
    b. cystic teratoma
    c. granulosa cell tumor
    d. mucinous cystadenoma

43. Multiparity is a risk factor associated with which of the following abnormalities?
    a. adenomyosis
    b. endometriosis
    c. nabothian cyst
    d. polycystic ovarian disease

44. Which of the following ovarian neoplasms will most likely demonstrate posterior acoustic shadowing?
    a. fibroma
    b. thecoma
    c. dysgerminoma
    d. Brenner tumor

45. A patient presents with a history of an intramural leiomyoma. An intramural leiomyoma:
    a. alters the perimetrium
    b. distorts the endometrium
    c. distorts the myometrium
    d. extends into the endometrium

46. A Gartner cyst is located within the:
    a. uterus
    b. cervix
    c. vagina
    d. oviduct

47. A patient presents with a history of postmenopausal bleeding. A heterogeneous intrauterine mass is identified on sonography. On the basis of the clinical history, the sonographic findings are most suspicious for:
    a. adenomyosis
    b. endometrioma
    c. leiomyosarcoma
    d. endometrial hyperplasia

48. Which of the following is the most common benign ovarian neoplasm?
    a. fibroma
    b. cystoadenoma
    c. cystic teratoma
    d. endometrioma

49. An ill-defined, multilocular, complex ovarian mass is most suspicious for:
    a. cystadenoma
    b. theca lutein cysts
    c. cystadenocarcinoma
    d. granulosa cell tumor

50. An ovarian mass combined with a pleural effusion and ascites resolving after surgery is known as:
    a. Meigs syndrome
    b. Turner syndrome
    c. Asherman syndrome
    d. Stein-Leventhal syndrome

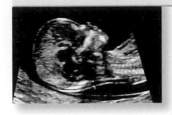

CHAPTER 22

Adnexal Pathology and Infertility

KEY TERMS

endometrioma   a collection of extravasated endometrial tissue.

endometriosis   a condition occurring when functional endometrial tissue invades the peritoneal cavity.

human chorionic gonadotropin (hCG)   a substitute for luteinizing hormone used in fertility assistance to trigger ovulation.

hydrosalpinx   dilatation of the fallopian tube with fluid.

Meckel diverticulum   an anomalous sac protruding from the ileum; caused by an incomplete closure of the yolk stalk.

pelvic inflammatory disease (PID)   a general classification for inflammatory conditions of the cervix, uterus, ovaries, fallopian tubes, and peritoneal surfaces.

salpingitis   inflammation within the fallopian tube.

synechia   scarring caused by previous dilation and curettage or spontaneous abortion; demonstrated as hyperechoic band of echoes within the endometrial cavity.

Adnexal Pathology

PATHOLOGY	ETIOLOGY	CLINICAL FINDINGS	SONOGRAPHIC FINDINGS	DIFFERENTIAL CONSIDERATIONS
Endometriosis	Ectopic location of functional endometrial tissue Attaches to the fallopian tubes, ovaries, colon, and bladder	Asymptomatic Dysmenorrhea Pelvic pain Irregular menses Dyspareunia Infertility	Difficult to visualize with sonography Obscure organ boundaries Fixation of the ovaries posterior to the uterus Endometrioma	Adhesions Bowel interference
Endometrioma	Focal collection of functional ectopic endometrial tissue Mesothelial in origin Typically located in the broad ligament. Termed "chocolate cyst"	Asymptomatic Pelvic pain Metromenorrhagia Dysmenorrhea Dyspareunia Palpable pelvic mass Infertility	Hypoechoic, homogeneous adnexal mass Thick, well-defined wall margins Diffuse, low-level echoes with or without solid components No internal blood flow Fluid/Fluid level Mass will not regress in size on serial sonograms	Hemorrhagic cyst Pedunculated fibroid Cystic teratoma Paraovarian cyst
Krukenberg tumors	Metastatic lesions Primary lesion from gastric carcinoma Other primary structures may include large intestines, breast, or appendix	Asymptomatic Abdominal pain Bloating	Bilateral adnexal or ovarian masses Oval or lobulated margins Hypoechoic areas within the mass Posterior enhancement Ascites Generally bilateral	Ovarian carcinoma Degenerating fibroid Tuboovarian abscess Cystic teratoma Endometrioma
Paraovarian cyst	Mesothelial in origin Typically located in the broad ligament Not associated with a history of pelvic inflammation, surgery, or endometriosis	Asymptomatic Pelvic pain Palpable pelvic mass	Round or ovoid anechoic adnexal mass Separate from ipsilateral ovary Thin, smooth wall margins Stable size on serial sonograms	Cystadenoma Hydrosalpinx Ovarian cyst Meckel diverticulum Peritoneal inclusion cyst Urinary bladder

Continued

Adnexal Pathology—(cont'd)

PATHOLOGY	ETIOLOGY	CLINICAL FINDINGS	SONOGRAPHIC FINDINGS	DIFFERENTIAL CONSIDERATIONS
Pelvic inflammatory disease	Bacterial infection Diverticulitis Appendicitis Sexual transmitted disease Postpartum infection	Abdominal pain Fever Vaginal discharge Urinary frequency	Normal pelvic appearance Thick and hypervascular endometrium Complex tubular adnexal mass Ill-defined multilocular adnexal mass Usually bilateral	Normal pelvis Loops of bowel Endometriosis Ectopic pregnancy
Peritoneal inclusion cyst	Adhesions trap fluid normally produced by the ovary Previous abdominal surgery Trauma Pelvic inflammatory disease Endometriosis	Asymptomatic Lower abdominal pain Palpable mass	Septated fluid collection surrounding an ovary Fluid is usually anechoic but may contain internal echoes Vascular flow can be demonstrated in septae Unilocular peritoneal cyst Do not regress in size May become very large in size	Ascites Paraovarian cyst Hydrosalpinx

Pathology of the Fallopian Tubes

PATHOLOGY	ETIOLOGY	CLINICAL FINDINGS	SONOGRAPHIC FINDINGS	DIFFERENTIAL CONSIDERATIONS
Carcinoma	Dysplasia Carcinoma in situ	Pelvic pain Abnormal bleeding Pelvic mass	Sausage-shaped complex adnexal mass Papillary projections	Tubo-ovarian abscess Loops of bowel
Hydrosalpinx	Pelvic inflammatory disease Endometriosis Postoperative adhesions	Asymptomatic Pelvic fullness Infertility	Anechoic tubular adnexal mass Thin wall margins Absence of peristalsis and internal vascular flow	Fluid-filled loop of bowel Dilated ureter External iliac vein Ovarian cyst Omental cyst
Pyosalpinx	Bacterial infection Diverticulitis Appendicitis	Asymptomatic Low-grade fever Pelvic fullness	Complex tubular adnexal mass Wall thickness ≥5 mm Irregular wall margins Mass attenuates the sound	Bowel loops Ovarian neoplasm Iliac vessel Hydroureter
Salpingitis	Pelvic infection	Pelvic pain Fever Dyspareunia Leukocytosis	Nodular, thick tubular adnexal mass Complex adnexal mass Posterior enhancement	Loops of bowel Endometriosis
Tubo-ovarian abscess	Pelvic infection Sexually transmitted disease	Severe pelvic pain Fever Leukocytosis Nausea/Vomiting	Complex multilocular adnexal mass Ill-defined wall margins Total breakdown of the normal adnexal anatomy	Endometriosis Ectopic pregnancy Hemorrhagic cyst

INFERTILITY

- Infertility is suggested when conception does not occur within 1 year.
- Caused by male or female reproductive abnormalities.
- Most common cause of female infertility is ovulatory disorders.
  - Polycystic ovarian disease.
  - Luteinizing unruptured follicle syndrome.
  - Luteal phase inadequacy.
- Fibroids are responsible for 15% of infertility cases.
- Other causes include oviduct disease, congenital uterine anomalies, endometrial pathology, cervical mucus abnormality, nutritional factors, metabolic disorders, and synechiae.

METHODS OF ASSISTED REPRODUCTIVE TECHNOLOGIES (ART)

- There are several methods of fertility assistance.

Ovarian Induction Therapy

- Medications are injected or taken orally to stimulate follicular development.
- Stimulates the pituitary gland to increase secretion of follicle-stimulating hormone.
- Follicular growth is monitored by periodic ultrasound examinations.
- Estradiol levels are monitored for timing of intramuscular injection of hCG to induce ovulation.

In Vitro Fertilization (IVF)

- Mature ova are aspirated with ultrasound guidance.
- Fertilization is accomplished in a laboratory setting.
- Lupron® or Synarel® is administered to temporarily stop ovarian function.
- Endometrium is prepared to accept embryo.
- Embryo(s) are transferred into the endometrium.

Gamete Intrafollicular Transfer (GIFT)

- Requires ovulation stimulation and retrieval of oocytes.
- The oocytes are mixed with sperm and then are transferred into the fallopian tube.

Zygote Intrafallopian Transfer (ZIFT)

- Zygote is transferred into the fallopian tube.

ULTRASOUND EVALUATION OF THE UTERUS

- Ultrasound is used to assess the structural anatomy of the uterus and endometrium.
- Uterus is evaluated for congenital anomalies or abnormalities.
- A septate uterus has a high incidence of infertility and can be amended with surgery.

ULTRASOUND MONITORING OF THE ENDOMETRIUM

- Full luteal function is expected with an endometrial thickness of 11 mm or greater during the midluteal phase.
- An endometrial thickness <8 mm is associated with a decrease in fertility.
- Lack of spiral artery or subendometrial vascular flow is associated with pregnancy loss.

ULTRASOUND MONITORING OF THE OVARIES

Baseline Study Before Therapy

- Assess for the presence of an ovarian cyst or dominant follicles.

During Induction Therapy

- Monitor the size and number of follicles per ovary.
- Count and measure only the follicles greater than 1.0 cm in diameter.
- Optimal follicle size before ovulation is 1.5 to 2.0 cm in diameter.
- Correlate estradiol level with size and number of follicles.

COMPLICATIONS OF ART

Ectopic Pregnancy

- More common in patients with a history of infertility.

Multiple Gestations

- Most common with in vitro technique (25% of cases).

Ovarian Hyperstimulation Syndrome

- Caused by high levels of hCG.
- Clinical findings include lower abdominal or back pain, abdominal distention, nausea/vomiting, hypotension, and leg edema.
- Theca lutein cysts.
- Multicystic ovarian enlargement >5 cm in diameter.
- Additional sonographic findings may include ascites and pleural effusion.

ADNEXAL PATHOLOGY AND INFERTILITY REVIEW

1. Krukenberg tumors are a result of:
   a. endometriosis
   b. hyperstimulation
   c. metastatic disease
   d. Asherman syndrome

2. A cystic structure located in the inferior broad ligament is most suspicious for a(n):
   a. hydrosalpinx
   b. endometrioma
   c. paraovarian cyst
   d. serous cystadenoma

3. Which of the following most accurately describes endometriosis?
   a. proliferation of the endometrial lining
   b. collection of ectopic endometrial tissue
   c. ectopic endometrial tissue located in the myometrium
   d. functional endometrial tissue invading the peritoneal cavity

4. Infertility is suggested when conception does not occur within:
   a. 6 months
   b. 9 months
   c. 12 months
   d. 24 months

5. Which of the following complications is commonly associated with in vitro fertilization?
   a. hyperstimulation
   b. ectopic pregnancy
   c. multiple gestations
   d. spontaneous abortion

6. A 25-year-old woman presents with high-grade fever, pelvic pain, and leukocytosis. An ill-defined, complex mass is identified in the left adnexa. Based on this clinical history, the sonographic finding is most suspicious for:
   a. salpingitis
   b. pyosalpinx
   c. endometritis
   d. tubo-ovarian abscess

7. A patient presents with lower abdominal pain and a palpable pelvic mass. A septated fluid collection surrounds a normal-appearing right ovary. The patient has a previous history of a ruptured appendix. Based on this clinical history, the sonographic finding is most suspicious for which of the following pathologies?
   a. endometriosis
   b. tubo-ovarian abscess
   c. mucinous cystadenoma
   d. peritoneal inclusion cyst

8. With the gamete intrafollicular transfer technique, the:
   a. embryos are transferred to the endometrial cavity
   b. zygotes are transferred to the endometrial cavity
   c. oocytes and sperm are transferred to the fallopian tube
   d. oocytes and sperm are transferred to the endometrial cavity

9. Monitoring of which hormone is routine during ovarian induction therapy?
   a. estrogen
   b. estradiol
   c. progesterone
   d. follicle-stimulating hormone

10. Metastatic lesions in the adnexa are more commonly associated with a primary malignancy of the:
    a. respiratory system
    b. genitourinary tract
    c. reproductive organs
    d. gastrointestinal tract

11. Which of the following abnormalities is most likely a consequence of pelvic inflammatory disease?
    a. adenomyosis
    b. hydrosalpinx
    c. endometriosis
    d. paraovarian cyst

12. During the midluteal phase, full luteal function is expected if the endometrial thickness is at least:
    a. 4 mm
    b. 8 mm
    c. 11 mm
    d. 14 mm

13. Which fertility assistance program inserts oocytes and sperm into the fallopian tube?
    a. in vitro fertilization
    b. zygote intrafallopian transfer
    c. gamete intrafollicular transfer
    d. oocyte and sperm fallopian transfer

14. Which of the following complications is most likely associated with ovulation induction therapy?
    a. ectopic pregnancy
    b. multiple gestations
    c. spontaneous abortion
    d. hyperstimulation syndrome

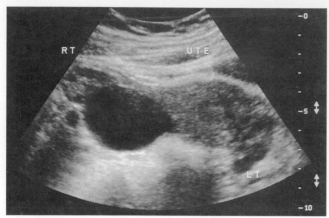

FIG. 22.1 Sonogram of the left adnexa.

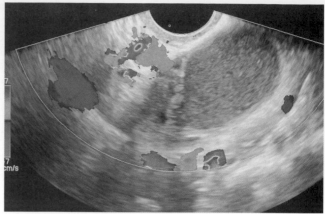

FIG. 22.2 Coronal sonogram of the left adnexa.

15. Hyperstimulation of the ovaries during induction therapy will likely result in:
   a. theca lutein cysts
   b. polycystic disease
   c. corpus luteal cysts
   d. hemorrhagic cysts

Using Figure 22.1, answer questions 16 and 17.

16. Differential considerations for this pelvic mass would most likely include:
   a. hydrosalpinx versus simple cyst
   b. simple cyst versus paraovarian cyst
   c. hydrosalpinx versus endometrioma
   d. paraovarian cyst versus endometrioma

17. Suggested follow-up care on this patient would most likely include:
   a. surgical intervention
   b. infertility assessment
   c. sonogram in 6 to 8 weeks
   d. sonogram in 2 to 3 weeks

Using Figure 22.2, answer question 18.

18. A patient presents with a history of dyspareunia and irregular menstrual cycles. A mass is identified adjacent to a normal-appearing ovary. Based on this clinical history, the sonographic finding is *most* suspicious for:
   a. endometrioma
   b. cystic teratoma
   c. hemorrhagic cyst
   d. pedunculated leiomyoma

Using Figure 22.3, answer questions 19 and 20.

19. A patient presents with a past history of an infection following an appendectomy. The anechoic area in this sonogram is most suspicious for a(n):
   a. hydroureter
   b. hydrosalpinx
   c. paraovarian cyst
   d. external iliac vein

20. The ovary most likely demonstrates a:
   a. hemorrhagic cyst
   b. suspicious solid mass
   c. normal anatomical variant
   d. suspicious isoechoic mass

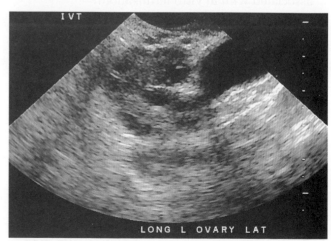

FIG. 22.3 Sagittal sonogram of the left adnexa.

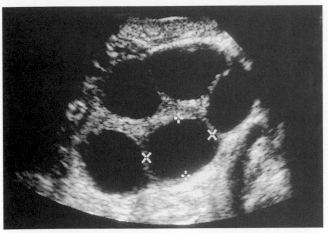

FIG. 22.4   Sonogram of the ovary.

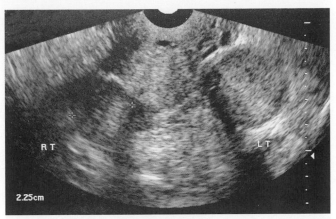

FIG. 22.6   Coronal sonogram.

Using Figure 22.4, answer question 21.

21. The sonogram most likely demonstrates:
    a. hypostimulation syndrome
    b. normal physiological cysts
    c. polycystic ovarian disease
    d. medically stimulated follicles

Using Figure 22.5, answer questions 22 and 23.

22. A patient presents with a history of endometriosis. Endometriosis is a result of:
    a. previous pelvic inflammatory disease
    b. endometrial tissue within the myometrium
    c. an accumulation of ectopic endometrial tissue
    d. endometrial tissue within the peritoneal cavity

23. The adnexal mass is most likely a(n):
    a. endometrioma
    b. cystic teratoma
    c. hemorrhagic cyst
    d. ectopic pregnancy

Using Figure 22.6, answer question 24.

24. A postmenopausal patient presents with a metastatic liver disease. Based on this clinical history, the sonographic findings are most suspicious for:
    a. endometriomas
    b. ovarian carcinoma
    c. pedunculated fibroids
    d. Krukenberg tumors

Using Figure 22.7, answer question 25.

25. An asymptomatic patient presents with a history of a palpable pelvic mass on physical examination. Based on this clinical history, the sonographic finding(s) is most suspicious for a:
    a. hydrosalpinx
    b. corpus luteal cyst um
    c. paraovarian cyst
    d. physiological cyst

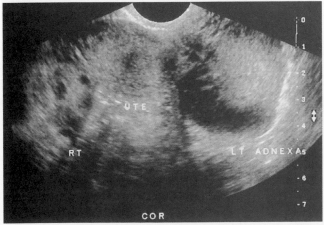

FIG. 22.5   Coronal sonogram.

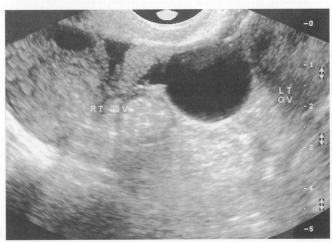

FIG. 22.7   Coronal sonogram.

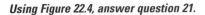

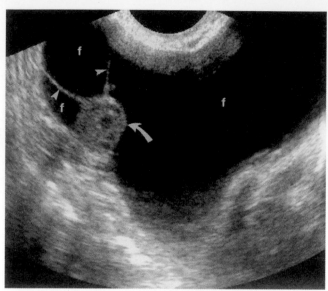

FIG. 22.8 Sonogram of the adnexa.

Using Figure 22.8, answer question 26.

26. A patient presents with a past history of a ruptured appendix. A sonogram demonstrates the ovary (curved arrow) surrounded by anechoic fluid. Based on the clinical history, the sonographic findings are most suspicious for a(n):
    a. paraovarian cyst
    b. serous cystadenoma
    c. tubo-ovarian abscess
    d. peritoneal inclusion cyst

Using Figure 22.9, answer question 27.

27. A menarche patient presents with a history of severe pelvic pain and fever. A urine pregnancy testing produced a negative result. Based on this clinical history, the sonographic findings are most suspicious for a(n):
    a. endometrioma
    b. ectopic pregnancy
    c. tubo-ovarian abscess
    d. carcinoma of the fallopian tube

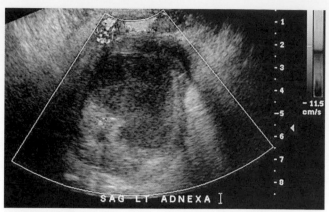

FIG. 22.9 Sagittal sonogram of the left adnexa.

Using Figure 22.10, answer question 28.

28. A patient presents with a history of infertility. The sonographic findings in this coronal sonogram are most suspicious for:
    a. adenomyosis
    b. subseptate uterus
    c. bicornuate uterus
    d. submucosal leiomyoma

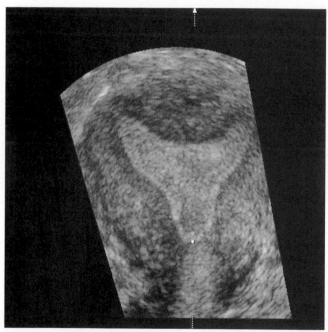

FIG. 22.10 Coronal sonogram.

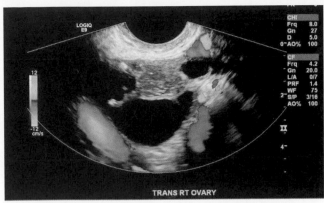

FIG. 22.11   Transverse right adnexa.

Using Figure 22.11, answer question 29.

29. The findings in this sonogram are most suspicious for a:
    a. hydroureter
    b. hydrosalpinx
    c. tubo-ovarian abscess
    d. peritoneal inclusion cyst

Using Figure 22.12, answer question 30.

30. An additional sonographic finding commonly associated with this abnormality is:
    a. ascites
    b. hydrosalpinx
    c. endometrioma
    d. ectopic pregnancy

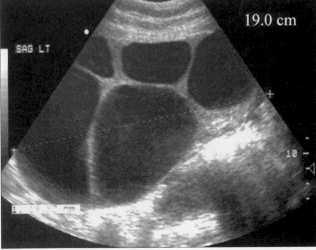

FIG. 22.12   Sonogram of a medically stimulated ovary.

31. Pelvic inflammatory disease is best described as a(n):
    a. sexually transmitted disease
    b. specific inflammatory process of the ovaries
    c. general classification of inflammatory conditions
    d. specific inflammatory condition of the fallopian tubes

32. During ovarian induction therapy, follicles are only measured when exceeding:
    a. 0.5 cm
    b. 1.0 cm
    c. 2.0 cm
    d. all follicles are measured

33. Which of the following is *not* likely to cause infertility?
    a. leiomyoma
    b. septate uterus
    c. nabothian cyst
    d. endometrial polyp

34. On serial examinations, a paraovarian cyst will:
    a. slowly resolve
    b. remain unchanged
    c. rapidly increase in size
    d. vary according to the ovulatory phase

35. A common symptom of endometriosis is:
    a. amenorrhea
    b. menorrhagia
    c. dysmenorrhea
    d. urinary frequency

36. Which of the following most accurately describes the sonographic appearance of a peritoneal inclusion cyst?
    a. complex ovarian cyst
    b. large unilocular adnexal mass
    c. small cluster of ovarian cysts
    d. septated fluid collection surrounding an ovary

37. A common sonographic finding associated with an endometrioma is a(n):
    a. irregular, hypoechoic ovarian mass
    b. well-defined anechoic ovarian mass
    c. heterogeneous, complex adnexal mass
    d. hypoechoic, homogeneous adnexal mass

38. Inflammation within the fallopian tube is termed:
    a. adnexitis
    b. salpingitis
    c. pyosalpinx
    d. hydrosalpinx

39. With ovarian induction therapy, intramuscular injection of what hormone triggers ovulation?
    a. progesterone
    b. luteinizing hormone
    c. follicle-stimulating hormone
    d. human chorionic gonadotropin

40. Scarring within the endometrium caused by invasive procedures is termed:
    a. albicans
    b. synechiae
    c. hyperplasia
    d. adenomyosis

41. Fixation of the ovaries posterior to the uterus is a sonographic finding associated with:
    a. adenomyosis
    b. endometriosis
    c. tubo-ovarian abscess
    d. pelvic inflammatory disease

42. A total breakdown of the normal adnexal anatomy is a sonographic finding associated with:
    a. pyosalpinx
    b. endometriosis
    c. Krukenberg tumors
    d. tubo-ovarian abscess

43. Which of the following is an acquired cause of infertility?
    a. endometritis
    b. bicornuate uterus
    c. Meigs syndrome
    d. Gartner duct cyst

44. Which of the following best describes the sonographic appearance of uterine synechiae?
    a. thick, irregular endometrium
    b. hypoechoic endometrial mass
    c. irregular hypoechoic myometrial masses
    d. bright band of echoes within the endometrium

45. Assessment for the presence of an ovarian cyst or dominant follicle is scheduled:
    a. before in vitro fertilization
    b. after gamete intrafollicular transfer
    c. before gamete intrafollicular transfer
    d. before initiating ovarian induction therapy

46. Which of the following is *not* a sonographic finding in pelvic inflammatory disease?
    a. normal-appearing pelvis
    b. complex tubular adnexal mass
    c. focal hypoechoic adnexal mass
    d. thick and hypervascular endometrium

47. Which of the following most accurately describes an endometrioma?
    a. overgrowth of endometrial tissue
    b. a collection of ectopic endometrial tissue
    c. ectopic location of active endometrial tissue
    d. ectopic endometrial tissue within the myometrium

48. A patient presents with a history of a leiomyoma. Which location will most likely cause infertility?
    a. serosal
    b. subserosal
    c. intramural
    d. submucosal

49. A nodular tubular adnexal mass demonstrating posterior acoustic enhancement is most suspicious for:
    a. salpingitis
    b. pyosalpinx
    c. hydrosalpinx
    d. endometrioma

50. A large multicystic ovarian mass, in an ovarian-stimulated patient, is most suspicious for:
    a. a corpus luteum
    b. polycystic ovarian disease
    c. multicystic ovarian disease
    d. ovarian hyperstimulation syndrome

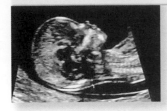

CHAPTER 23

Assessment of the First Trimester

KEY TERMS

abortion   first-trimester pregnancy loss. Aka: miscarriage.

amnion   extraembryonic membrane that lines the chorion and contains the fetus and amniotic fluid.

angiogenesis   formation of blood vessels.

blastocyst   consists of an outer trophoblast and an inner cell mass.

bradycardia   fetal heart rate of 110 beats per minute or less.

chorion   outermost of the fetal membranes; formed by the embryonic mesoderm and a double layer or trophoblasts; ultimately shrinks and is obliterated by the amnion between 12 and 16 weeks.

decidua   name applied to the endometrium during pregnancy.

decidua basalis   portion of the endometrium on which the implanted conceptus rests.

decidua capsularis   decidua that covers the surface of the implanted conceptus.

decidua parietalis   decidua exclusive of the area occupied by the implanted conceptus; Aka: decidua vera.

discriminatory zone   the threshold amount of hCG present at which there should be sonographic evidence of a gestational sac.

double decidua sign   composed of the decidua capsularis and decidua parietalis; thick hyperechoic rim surrounding a sonolucency; indicative of an intrauterine pregnancy.

elective abortion   intentional termination of a pregnancy.

embryo   term used for a developing zygote through the tenth week of gestation.

embryological age   length of time based from conception.

embryonic phase   gestational weeks 6 through 10.

empty amnion sign   visualization of the amniotic cavity without the presence of an embryo.

gestational age   length of time calculated from the first day of the last menstrual period.

gestational sac   fluid-filled structure normally found in the uterus, containing the pregnancy.

gravidity   refers to the number of times a woman has been pregnant including the current pregnancy, if applicable.

hematopoiesis   formation of blood cells.

intrauterine pregnancy (IUP)   pregnancy located within the uterus.

morula   solid mass of cells formed by cleavage of a fertilized ovum.

nuchal translucency   the sonographic appearance of subcutaneous accumulation of fluid behind the fetal neck in the first trimester of pregnancy; increases associated with chromosomal and other abnormalities.

parity   refers to the number of live births.

pseudogestational sac   centrally located endometrial fluid collection demonstrated with a coexisting ectopic pregnancy.

recurrent spontaneous abortion   two consecutive or three total spontaneous abortions.

spontaneous abortion   pregnancy loss caused by natural or unanticipated events.

tachycardia   fetal heart rate exceeding 180 beats per minute. May be a result of fetal movement and maternal and fetal disorders.

threatened abortion   bleeding in the first trimester.

yolk sac (YS)   provides nutrients to the embryo and is the initial site of alpha-fetoprotein.

EARLY EMBRYOLOGY (Fig. 23.1)

- Fertilization to implantation—approximately 5 to 7 days.
  - Ovum and sperm join in the distal fallopian tube, forming a zygote.
  - Cells of the zygote multiply, forming a cluster termed the *morula*.
  - Fluid rapidly enters the morula, forming a blastocyst.
  - The blastocyst implants into the endometrium.
- After implantation—trophoblastic growth continues.
  - Maternal vessels erode, establishing a circulation on the maternal side of the forming placenta (chorion basalis).
  - Trophoblastic tissue covers the entire embryo, developing into the fetal side of the forming placenta (chorion frondosum).

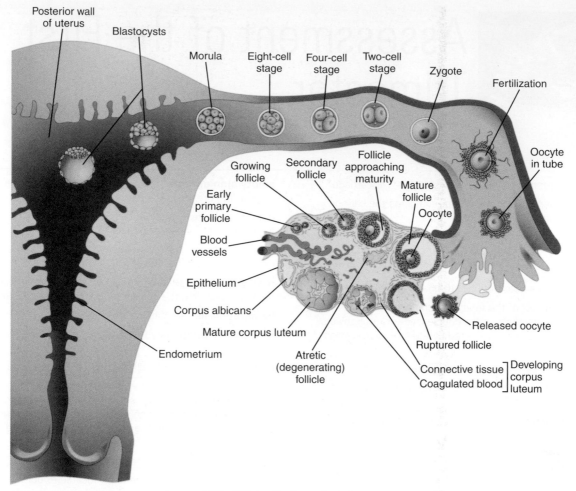

FIG. 23.1 Early embryology.

- Human chorionic gonadotropin (hCG) is secreted by the trophoblastic tissue.
- Organogenesis is the main feature during the embryonic period and generally completed by the tenth gestational week.
- Nearly all congenital malformations, except of genitalia originate before or during the embryonic period.
- Most pregnancy failures occur around 8 weeks gestation.

BLASTOCYST DEVELOPMENT (Fig. 23.2)

- Amnion begins.
- Secondary yolk sac begins.
- Chorionic villi evenly surround the blastocyst.
- Embryo is located between the amnion and yolk sac (Fig. 23.2, *A*).
- Embryo folds into the amnion.
- Amnion attaches to the anterior portion of the embryo.
- Yolk sac becomes "pinched" near the embryo, forming the body stalk.
- Chorionic villi become more prolific near the implantation site (Fig. 23.2, *B*).
- Amnion begins to fill more of the chorionic cavity.
- Yolk sac is pushed into the chorionic cavity.
- Umbilical cord begins to develop about the seventh to eighth gestational week.
- Areas of the chorion away from the implantation site become smooth (Fig. 23.2, *C*).
- Amnion fuses to the smooth chorion.
- Embryo or fetus lies within the amniotic cavity.
- Chorionic villi and decidua basalis have formed a placenta (Fig. 23.2, *D*).

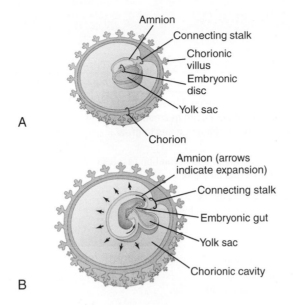

A

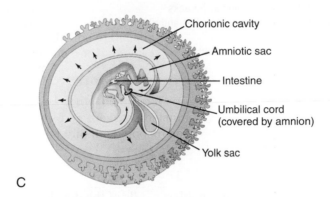

B

C

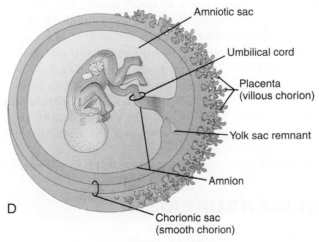

D

FIG. 23.2 Blastocyst development.

ANATOMY

First-Trimester Anatomy

STRUCTURE	DESCRIPTION	NORMAL SONOGRAPHIC FINDINGS
Abdominal wall	Physiological herniation of the fetal bowel into the umbilical cord around the eighth gestational week Herniation allows room for the intestines to grow and rotate. Bowel returns into abdomen, and herniation resolves by the eleventh gestational week	Umbilical herniation contiguous with the umbilical cord Abnormal if persists after 12 weeks gestation
Cardiovascular system	First system to function in the embryo Four heart chambers are formed by the eighth gestational week	Cardiac motion as early as 5.5 weeks
Cranium	Primitive brain consists of: Prosencephalon—forebrain Mesencephalon—midbrain Rhombencephalon—hindbrain	Prominent cystic space in the posterior portion of the brain (rhombencephalon) Ossification of the cranium begins the ninth gestational week
Skeletal system	Vertebral bodies and ribs are forming at 6 weeks Arms and legs are forming at 7 weeks Ossification of the vertebral bodies and rib cartilage at 9 weeks Long bones form during the 10th week	Spine appears as parallel echogenic linear structures in the center of the embryo or fetus Long bones appear as hyperechoic linear structure(s) within the soft tissue of the extremities

LABORATORY VALUES

Human Chorionic Gonadotropin (hCG)

- Produced by the trophoblastic cells of the developing chorionic villi and circulates in maternal blood and urine.
- Normally doubles every 48 hours during the first 6 weeks of pregnancy.
- There are two quantitative laboratory (blood) tests to detect the amount of beta hCG in maternal blood.
  - Second International Standard (2nd IS).
  - International Reference Preparation (IRP).
    - Twice the value of 2nd IS.
- Discriminatory zone for 2nd IS is 500 to 1200 miU/mL for endovaginal imaging.
- Discriminatory zone for IRP is 1000 to 2000 miU/mL for endovaginal imaging.
- Peaks at the tenth gestational week, then begins to decline, leveling out around 18 weeks gestation.
- Urine pregnancy test is a qualitative test to check for the presence of hCG.

FIRST-TRIMESTER MEASUREMENTS

Mean Sac Diameter (MSD)

- Establishes gestational age before visualization of an embryonic disc.
- Measures the length, height, and width of the inner-to-inner borders of the gestational sac.

$$MSD(mm) = \frac{Length(mm) + Height(mm) + Width(mm)}{3}$$

Crown–Rump Length (CRL)

- Measured until the twelfth gestational week.
- Most accurate method of dating a pregnancy.
- Sagittal measurement of the embryo or fetus from the top of the head to the bottom of the rump.
- Lower extremities are not included in the measurement.
- Length increases approximately 1 mm/day.

Nuchal Translucency

- First-trimester screening for chromosomal abnormalities.
- The gestation should be 11 weeks, 0 days, to 13 weeks, 6 days.
- Normal thickness is considered less than 3 mm.
- Scanning technique:
  - Midsagittal section of the fetus, spine-down, with the neck in a neutral position.
  - Magnify so that only the fetal head and upper thorax should be included in the image.
  - Skin and amnion should be clearly separate from nuchal translucency.
  - Measurement calipers should be placed inner to inner borders and perpendicular to the long axis of the fetus.
  - More than one measurement must be taken, and the maximum one is to be recorded.
- Pitfalls include poor fetal position, maternal obesity, and mistaking the amnion for the fetal skin.

EXAMINATION TECHNIQUES, PROTOCOLS, AND IMAGE OPTIMIZATION

Preparation

- Preparation varies with type of imaging approach.

Transabdominal

- Requires bladder distention.
  - Adult – Drink 28 to 32 oz of water, finishing 1 hour before examination.
  - If catharized, fill bladder to 375 mL.

Purpose of Bladder Distention

- Displaces uterus posteriorly and bowel laterally.
- Provides an acoustic window to visualize pelvic structures.
- Provides an anatomical and anechoic reference point.
- Overdistention may compress and distort gestational sac.

Endovaginal and Translabial

- Urinary bladder should be emptied.

Contraindications for Endovaginal Imaging

- Any patient who does not or cannot willingly consent to the examination.
- If the pain becomes too severe, terminate examination.

Transducer Selection

- Use the highest frequency possible to obtain optimal resolution for penetration depth.
  - Adults – 3.5 to 5.0 MHz transabdominal.
  - 4.0 to 8.0 MHz endovaginal.
  - 3.5 to 5.0 MHz translabial.
  - Obese patients – 2.0 MHz may be required for transabdominal imaging.

- Curvilinear transducers provide a wider field of view.
- Sector or vector transducers have a smaller footprint.

Patient Positioning

- Supine position – transabdominal.
- Lithotomy position – endovaginal and translabial.
- Left lateral decubitus, right and left posterior oblique may reposition overlying bowel gas.

Examination Protocol

- Conservative approach keeping the examination time as short as possible and for diagnostic purposes only.
- Transabdominal approach should be the first and sometimes the only examination performed.
- Urinary bladder and iliac vessels are imaging landmarks.
- Systematic approach in the sagittal, coronal/transverse planes carefully examining, imaging, and documenting all areas of the female pelvis including:
  - Uterus.
  - Endometrium.
  - Adnexae.
  - Pelvic spaces.
- Determine number and location of gestational sac(s).
- Measure length, height, and width measurements of the gestational sac (MSD).
- Measure crown-rump length of embryo/fetus if visualized.
- M-mode of embryo/fetal cardiac activity including beats per minute.
- *Do not use color or pulse Doppler during the first trimester to demonstrate cardiac activity.*
- Length, height, and width measurements of the right and left ovaries.
- Document color Doppler and/or spectral analysis of ovarian vascularity.
- Abnormalities should be documented and when applicable measured in two imaging planes. Color and/or spectral Doppler evaluation of the abnormality should be included.

Image Optimization

- Reduce system output power control by a minimum of -3dB or the lowest setting possible that allows a diagnostic image.
- Place gains settings to display normal uterus as a medium shade of gray with adjustments to reduce artifactually produced echoes within the arcuate vessels and gestational sac.
- Focal zone(s) should be placed at or below the area of interest. The use of multiple focal zones increases detail resolution and decreases temporal resolution.
- Sufficient imaging depth to visualize structures immediately posterior to the area of interest.
- Harmonic imaging and decreasing system compression (dynamic range) can be used to reduce artifactual echoes in obese and gassy patients.
- Spatial compounding can be used to improve visualization of structures posterior to highly attenuating structures.
- Doppler settings should be adjusted for the different flow states of the female pelvis.
- Doppler angle should be 60 degrees or less with a sample volume smaller than the vessel interrogating.
- The use of multiple patient positions may redistribute overlying bowel gas.

Helpful Hints

- Vector or sector transducer can aid in visualization of the uterus when bladder is under distended.
- To demonstrate the relationship of an adnexal mass from the ovary place external manual pressure over the area of concern to manipulate the ovary.

INDICATIONS FOR FIRST TRIMESTER ULTRASOUND

- Confirm intrauterine pregnancy.
- Confirm viability.
- Define vaginal bleeding.
- Rule out ectopic pregnancy.
- Estimate gestational age.
- Evaluate pelvic mass or pain.
- Abnormal serial hCG levels.

Sonographic Findings in the First Trimester

GESTATIONAL FINDING	DESCRIPTION	NORMAL SONOGRAPHIC FINDINGS	ABNORMAL SONOGRAPHIC FINDINGS
Gestational sac (GS)	Fluid-filled structure normally found in the uterus, containing the developing embryo First definitive sonographic finding to suggest early pregnancy Anechoic structure represents the chorionic cavity Echogenic rim represents decidual tissue and the developing chorionic villi	Round anechoic structure Surrounded by a thick hyperechoic rim (2 mm) Located in the mid- to upper portion of the uterus Eccentric location within the endometrium **Transabdominal** 5 mm mean sac diameter (MSD) about 5-6 weeks Double decidual sign evident with an MSD of 10 mm **Transvaginal** 2-3 mm about 4-5 weeks	Irregular or distorted GS Large GS without evidence of YS Abnormal uterine location Visualization of amnion without concomitant embryo **Transabdominal** Failure to identify a YS with an MSD >16 mm **Transvaginal** Failure to identify a YS with an MSD >8 mm
Yolk sac (YS)	Located in the chorionic cavity Earliest structure visualized in the gestational sac Used as a landmark to locate the embryo Functions: 1. transfer of nutrients 2. hematopoiesis 3. angiogenesis 4. formation of digestive tract Attached to the embryo by the vitelline duct Ultimately detaches from the embryo and remains within the chorionic cavity	Hyperechoic ring within the gestational sac Round or oval in shape *Inner-to-inner* border diameter should not exceed 6 mm **Transabdominal** Evident within an MSD of 16 mm **Transvaginal** Evident within an MSD of 8 mm	YS diameter exceeding 7 mm (inner-inner) **Transabdominal** Failure to identify a YS with an MSD >16 mm **Transvaginal** Failure to identify a YS with an MSD >8 mm
Embryo	Embryonic period extends from the sixth through the tenth gestational weeks	Initially a local thickening adjacent to the yolk sac Echogenic focus adjacent to the yolk sac **Transabdominal** Usually detected within an MSD of 25 mm **Transvaginal** Usually detected in an MSD of 16 mm	Embryo too small for gestational sac **Transabdominal** Failure to identify an embryo with cardiac activity in a GS >25 mm **Transvaginal** Failure to identify an embryo with cardiac activity in a GS >16 mm

Continued

Sonographic Findings in the First Trimester—(cont'd)

GESTATIONAL FINDING	DESCRIPTION	NORMAL SONOGRAPHIC FINDINGS	ABNORMAL SONOGRAPHIC FINDINGS
Amnion	Initially surrounds the newly formed amniotic cavity Attaches to the embryo at the umbilical cord insertion Expands with accumulation of amniotic fluid and growth of the embryo Obliterates the chorionic cavity by the sixteenth week	Thin hyperechoic line between the embryo and the yolk sac (chorion)	Visualization of the amnion without an embryo Thick hyperechoic amnion Large amniotic cavity compared with the size of the embryo
Cardiac activity	First system to function in the embryo	Cardiac activity should be identified by 6 weeks and as early as 5.5 weeks 100-115 beats per min before 6 weeks 120-160 beats per min after 6 weeks **Transabdominal** Should be evident with an MSD of 25 mm **Transvaginal** Should be evident with an MSD of 16 mm *or* Crown–rump length (CRL) exceeding 7 mm	Heart rates below 80 beats per min are associated with poor outcomes **Transabdominal** No cardiac activity in an embryo $\geq$9 mm Failure to identify cardiac activity in a GS $\geq$25 mm **Transvaginal** No cardiac activity in an embryo >7 mm Failure to identify cardiac activity in a GS >16 mm

- *Normal pregnancy progression may be determined with an additional examination scheduled 7 to 14 days after the initial ultrasound.*

Weekly Findings During the Normal First Trimester

GESTATIONAL WEEK	SONOGRAPHIC FINDINGS
Fourth	Thickening of the endometrium Mean sac diameter (MSD) = 2-3 mm
Fifth	MSD = 10 mm Yolk sac seen with vaginal imaging May visualize embryonic disc May visualize cardiac activity
Sixth	MSD = 15-20 mm gestational sac Yolk sac visualized C-shaped embryo measuring approximately 5 mm Cardiac activity should be present
Seventh	MSD = 30 mm Crown–rump length (CRL) = 1.0 cm Cardiac activity should be present Head constitutes one half of the embryo Limb buds appear
Eighth	CRL = 1.5 cm Embryo unfolds Head becomes dominant Midgut has herniated into the base of the umbilical cord Placenta location may be identified Spine may be visualized Amnion surrounding the embryo is more apparent

Weekly Findings During the Normal First Trimester—(cont'd)

GESTATIONAL WEEK	SONOGRAPHIC FINDINGS
Ninth	CRL = 2.3 cm Cranium begins to calcify Can differentiate the cerebral hemispheres Dominated by the lateral ventricles filled with the choroid plexus. Visualization of limb buds Early ossifications may be seen
Tenth	CRL approaches 3.0 cm Muscular movement has begun Hyperechoic choroid plexuses Cystic rhombencephalon demonstrated in the posterior fossa (8-11 weeks)
Twelfth	CRL reaches 5.5 cm Yolk sac no longer visualized Midgut has returned to the abdominal cavity Amnion is now abutting the chorion Fetus demonstrates a skeletal body Fluid is displayed in the fetal stomach Kidneys begin urine production

Abnormal First-Trimester Pregnancy

ABNORMALITY	DESCRIPTION	CLINICAL FINDINGS	SONOGRAPHIC FINDINGS	DIFFERENTIAL CONSIDERATIONS
Anembryonic Aka: Blighted ovum	Zygote develops into a blastocyst, but the inner cell mass fails to develop	Asymptomatic Serial beta hCG levels may remain normal initially and then may plateau or decline Small for dates No fetal heart tones	Empty gestational sac >25 mm (TA) >16 mm (TV) Absent yolk sac, amnion, and embryo	Missed abortion Pseudogestational sac
Complete abortion	Miscarriage	Bleeding Cramping Rapid decline in serial beta hCG levels	No evidence of intrauterine pregnancy Normal uterus and endometrium No adnexal masses	Ectopic pregnancy Early intrauterine pregnancy
Ectopic **Risk Factors** Pelvic infection Intrauterine device Oviduct scarring Infertility treatment Endometriosis Previous ectopic pregnancy Congenital anomalies of the uterus or fallopian tubes	Pregnancy in an abnormal location 95% are located in the fallopian tube, typically in the region of the ampulla Other areas may include ovary, cervix, peritoneum, broad ligament, and cornua of the uterus	Classic Triad 1. Pelvic pain 2. Abnormal vaginal bleeding 3. Palpable adnexal mass Abnormal rise in serial beta hCG levels Hypotension Cervical tenderness	No intrauterine pregnancy Centrally located endometrial fluid collection **Fallopian tube** Complex adnexal mass Increase in vascular flow surrounding adnexal mass may be demonstrated ("ring of fire") Cul-de-sac fluid May display as an extrauterine gestational sac with or without embryo **Cornual** Laterally placed gestational sac Myometrium incompletely surrounds the gestational sac Highly vascular location	Early intrauterine pregnancy or incomplete abortion with a corpus luteal cyst Pregnancy in one horn of a bicornuate uterus

Continued

Abnormal First-Trimester Pregnancy —(cont'd)

ABNORMALITY	DESCRIPTION	CLINICAL FINDINGS	SONOGRAPHIC FINDINGS	DIFFERENTIAL CONSIDERATIONS
Embryonic or fetal demise	Evidence of a nonliving embryo or fetus	Small for dates No fetal heart tones Spotting	Presence of an embryo or fetus No cardiac activity No fetal movement Overlapping of cranial bones	Incorrect dates
Gestational trophoblastic neoplasia	Abnormal proliferation of the trophoblast Hydatid swelling in a blighted ovum Trophoblastic changes in retained placental tissue	Bleeding Hyperemesis Dramatically elevated beta hCG levels Large for dates No fetal heart tones Low maternal AFP Preeclampsia	Moderately echogenic soft tissue uterine mass Small cystic structures within the mass Demonstrates vascular flow Bilateral theca lutein cysts May or may not demonstrate an adjacent fetus	Incomplete abortion Degenerating fibroid Adenomyosis
Heterotopic pregnancy	Extrauterine and intrauterine pregnancies Dizygotic pregnancy 1: 4000 pregnancies In-vitro fertilization	Pelvic pain Cramping Bleeding Hypotension	Intrauterine pregnancy Complex adnexal mass or extrauterine gestation Cul-de-sac fluid	Pregnancy in both horns of a bicornuate uterus Intrauterine pregnancy with coexisting complex corpus luteal cyst
Incomplete abortion	Retained products of conception	Asymptomatic Bleeding Cramping Abnormal rise in serial beta hCG levels	Thick, complex endometrium Intact gestational sac with nonviable embryo Irregular gestational sac with or without retained products of conception	Endometrial dysplasia Ectopic pregnancy
Pseudocyesis	False pregnancy Psychological condition	Nausea/vomiting Abdominal distention Amenorrhea Negative pregnancy test	Normal nongravid uterus Normal adnexa	Recent complete abortion
Subchorionic hemorrhage	Low-pressure bleed from implantation of blastocyst	Asymptomatic Vaginal spotting	Hypoechoic fluid collection between the gestational sac and uterine wall Becomes more anechoic with time No internal blood flow Variable size Resolves over time	Nonviable twin pregnancy Incomplete abortion Placenta abruption

Pelvic Masses During Early Pregnancy

MASS	DESCRIPTION	CLINICAL FINDINGS	SONOGRAPHIC FINDINGS	DIFFERENTIAL CONSIDERATIONS
Corpus luteum	Secretes progesterone before placental circulation Should be evident until approximately 12 weeks gestation	Asymptomatic Pelvic pain	Anechoic ovarian mass Thin to thick hyperechoic wall margins May contain internal low-level echoes Usually measure <5 cm in diameter Hypervascular periphery (ring of fire)	Ectopic pregnancy Endometrioma
Leiomyoma	Benign neoplasm of the uterine myometrium May increase in size with increases in hormones	Asymptomatic Pelvic pain Pelvic mass	Well-defined hypoechoic uterine mass May appear complex or heterogeneous Relationship to the cervix and placenta must be documented	Subchorionic hemorrhage Uterine contraction

ASSESSMENT OF THE FIRST-TRIMESTER REVIEW

1. Ectopic pregnancies are commonly located in the:
   a. ovary
   b. cervix
   c. fallopian tube
   d. uterine cornua

2. Which of the following structures implants into the endometrium?
   a. zygote
   b. morula
   c. embryo
   d. blastocyst

3. Which of the following structures secretes human chorionic gonadotropin?
   a. decidua basalis
   b. chorionic cavity
   c. decidua parietalis
   d. trophoblastic tissue

4. The optimal gestational age for measuring fetal nuchal translucency is from:
   a. 11 weeks and 0 days to 13 weeks and 6 days
   b. 10 weeks and 0 days to 12 weeks and 0 days
   c. 11 weeks and 6 days to 13 weeks and 0 days
   d. 11 weeks and 0 days to 12 weeks and 6 days

5. Which area of the embryo attaches to the amnion?
   a. calvaria
   b. nuchal fold
   c. thoracic cavity
   d. umbilical insertion

6. The mean sac diameter (MSD) measures gestational age before visualization of the:
   a. amnion
   b. embryo
   c. yolk sac
   d. fetal heart

7. Gestational weeks 6 through 10 constitute the:
   a. fetal phase
   b. first trimester
   c. conceptus phase
   d. embryonic phase

8. The decidua capsularis and decidua parietalis produce the:
   a. blastocyst
   b. decidua basalis
   c. double decidua sign
   d. pseudogestational sac

9. A rapid decline in serial hCG levels will most likely correlate with a(n):
   a. ectopic pregnancy
   b. spontaneous abortion
   c. anembryonic pregnancy
   d. heterotopic pregnancy

10. Which of the following is an abnormal finding in a first-trimester pregnancy?
    a. prominent cystic structure in the posterior brain
    b. visualization of the amnion without an embryo
    c. fetal heart rate of 100 beats per minute
    d. herniation of the fetal bowel into the umbilical cord

11. Subchorionic hemorrhage is a common consequence of:
    a. fertilization of the ovum
    b. implantation of the conceptus
    c. the expansion of the amniotic cavity
    d. the obliteration of the chorionic cavity

12. The decidua exclusive of the area occupied by the conceptus is termed decidua:
    a. basalis
    b. parietalis
    c. capsularis
    d. frondosum

13. Which of the following formulas calculates the mean sac diameter of the gestational sac?
    a. $Length + Height + Width$
    b. $\dfrac{Length + Width}{Height}$
    c. $\dfrac{Length + Height + Width}{3}$
    d. $\dfrac{Length \times Height \times Width}{3}$

14. Normally, the chorionic cavity should no longer be visible after how many gestational weeks?
    a. 10
    b. 12
    c. 16
    d. 20

15. Hyperemesis is a common clinical finding associated with:
    a. ectopic pregnancy
    b. embryonic demise
    c. trophoblastic disease
    d. heterotopic pregnancy

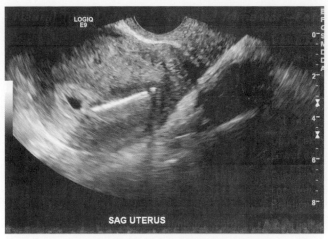

FIG. 23.3   Transvaginal sonogram.

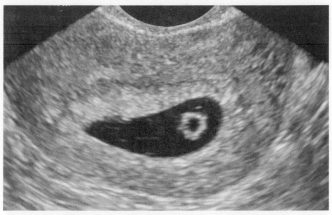

FIG. 23.4   Transvaginal sonogram.

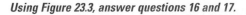

Using Figure 23.3, answer questions 16 and 17.

16. Which of the following is documented in this menarche patient?
    a. blighted ovum
    b. incomplete abortion
    c. pseudogestational sac
    d. early intrauterine pregnancy

17. Which of the following is also identified in this sonogram?
    a. hematometra
    b. incomplete abortion
    c. intrauterine device
    d. calcified uterine vessels

Using Figure 23.4, answer question 18.

18. A transvaginal sonogram of the superior uterus demonstrates a(n):
    a. embryonic demise
    b. anembryonic pregnancy
    c. amnion in an intrauterine pregnancy
    d. yolk sac in an intrauterine pregnancy

Using Figure 23.5, answer questions 19 to 21.

19. A patient presents with a history of rapidly increasing hCG levels. Based on this clinical history, the sonogram is most suspicious for:
    a. pseudocyesis
    b. heterotopic pregnancy
    c. retained products of conception
    d. gestational trophoblastic disease

20. With this abnormality, the adnexa are most likely to demonstrate:
    a. theca lutein cysts
    b. corpus luteal cysts
    c. solid ovarian masses
    d. complex adnexal masses

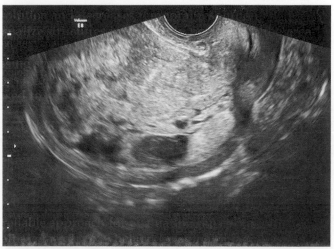

FIG. 23.5   Endovaginal sonogram of the uterus.

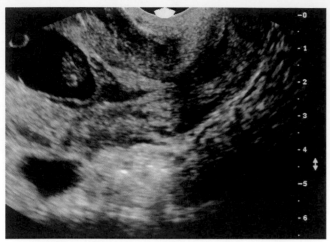

FIG. 23.6   Sagittal sonogram of the uterus.

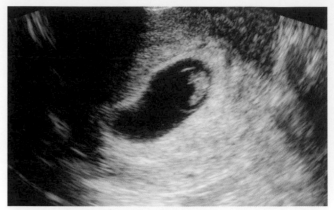

FIG. 23.8   Transvaginal sonogram.

21. The most common clinical symptom associated with this abnormality is:
    a. hyperemesis
    b. vaginal spotting
    c. pelvic cramping
    d. lower-extremity swelling

Using Figure 23.6, answer question 22.

22. The sonogram most likely demonstrates a(n):
    a. cornual pregnancy
    b. incompetent cervix
    c. subchorionic hemorrhage
    d. pregnancy in one horn of a bicornuate uterus

Using Figure 23.7, answer question 23.

23. This sonogram is most consistent with a(n):
    a. cornual pregnancy
    b. incomplete abortion
    c. intrauterine pregnancy
    d. subchorionic hemorrhage

Using Figure 23.8, answer question 24.

24. This gestational sac demonstrates a(n):
    a. large complex yolk sac
    b. embryo and the amnion
    c. abnormal twin gestation
    d. embryo and large yolk sac

Using Figure 23.9, answer questions 25 and 26.

25. What is the most likely diagnosis of this transvaginal sonogram?
    a. appendicitis
    b. corpus luteal cyst
    c. ectopic pregnancy
    d. pregnancy in one horn of a bicornuate uterus

26. Which clinical presentation is most likely associated with this diagnosis?
    a. leukocytosis
    b. elevated progesterone
    c. slowly rising hCG levels
    d. normal serial hCG levels

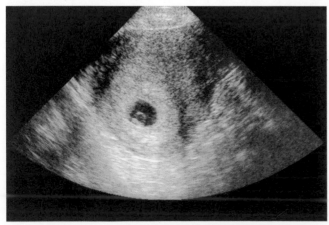

FIG. 23.7   Sagittal sonogram of the uterus.

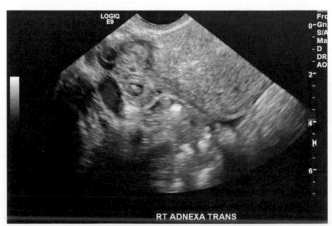

FIG. 23.9   Transvaginal sonogram.

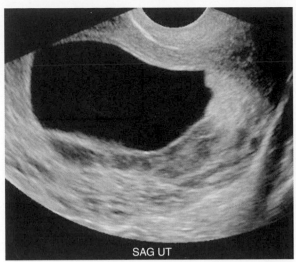

FIG. 23.10   Transvaginal sagittal sonogram of the first trimester.

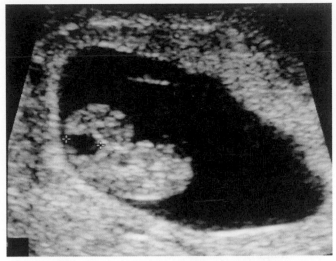

FIG. 23.12   First-trimester sonogram.

Using Figure 23.10, answer question 27.

27. This first trimester sonogram is most suspicious for a(n):
    a. fetal demise
    b. pseudogestational sac
    c. anembryonic pregnancy
    d. normal intrauterine pregnancy

Using Figure 23.11, answer question 28.

28. An afebrile patient presents with a history of a therapeutic abortion 2 weeks previously. She complains of continued vaginal spotting since the procedure. Based on this clinical history, the sonogram is most suspicious for:
    a. endometritis
    b. endometrial hyperplasia
    c. degenerating leiomyoma
    d. retained products of conception

Using Figure 23.12, answer question 29.

29. The sonogram of this first trimester fetus is most likely displaying a:
    a. subarachnoid cyst
    b. Dandy-Walker cyst
    c. normal prosencephalon
    d. normal rhombencephalon

Using Figure 23.13, answer question 30.

30. A hyperechoic linear structure located posterior to the fetus is most likely:
    a. a cystic hygroma
    b. the normal amnion
    c. a uterine synechiae
    d. a subchorionic hemorrhage

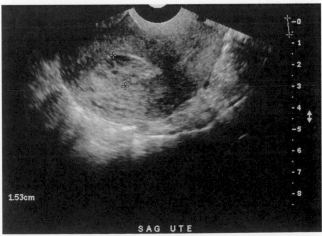

FIG. 23.11   Transvaginal sagittal sonogram of the uterus.

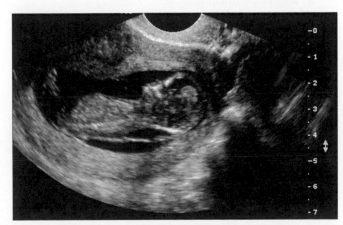

FIG. 23.13   First-trimester sonogram.

31. Subcutaneous accumulation of fluid behind the fetal neck measuring 3 mm in thickness is a(n):
    a. normal finding in the late first trimester
    b. abnormal finding in the late first trimester
    c. normal finding in the late second trimester
    d. abnormal finding regardless of gestational age

32. A patient presents with a positive pregnancy test and an hCG level of 750 mIU/mL 2nd IS. Based on this clinical history, which of the following best describes the expected sonographic findings?
    a. small gestational sac on transabdominal imaging
    b. possible small gestational sac on transvaginal imaging
    c. yolk sac within a gestational sac on transvaginal imaging
    d. gestational sac with viable embryo on transvaginal imaging

33. Normal human chorionic gonadotropin levels should:
    a. double every 24 hours
    b. double every 48 hours
    c. peak about the twentieth gestational week
    d. decrease and level out after the twelfth gestational week

34. On transvaginal imaging, in a normal pregnancy, cardiac activity must be identified within a gestational sac with a mean sac diameter of:
    a. 10 mm
    b. 16 mm
    c. 20 mm
    d. 25 mm

35. Presence of an embryo without visualization of the amnion is considered:
    a. a normal finding
    b. suspicious for fetal demise
    c. suspicious for amniotic band syndrome
    d. a precursor of an abdominal wall defect

36. Which of the following is an abnormal sonographic finding during the first trimester of pregnancy?
    a. failure to demonstrate an amnion adjacent to an embryo
    b. failure to demonstrate a yolk sac within a mean sac diameter of 10 mm when using the transvaginal approach
    c. failure to demonstrate a yolk sac within a mean sac diameter of 10 mm when using the transabdominal approach
    d. failure to demonstrate an embryo within a mean sac diameter of 20 mm when using a transabdominal approach

37. When measuring the mean sac diameter, the calipers should be placed from the:
    a. inner wall to inner wall
    b. inner wall to outer wall
    c. outer wall to outer wall
    d. superior wall to inferior wall

38. The secondary yolk sac:
    a. has no specific function
    b. is located in the chorionic cavity
    c. represents the developing chorionic villi
    d. secretes human chorionic gonadotropin

39. Initial visualization of the hyperechoic choroid plexuses is expected near the:
    a. eighth gestational week
    b. tenth gestational week
    c. fourteenth gestational week
    d. eighteenth gestational week

40. Which of the following ectopic locations is most life threatening to the patient?
    a. cervical
    b. ampullary
    c. interstitial
    d. peritoneal

41. Retained products of conception can be a contributing factor of:
    a. an ectopic pregnancy
    b. trophoblastic disease
    c. a heterotopic pregnancy
    d. ovarian hyperstimulation syndrome

42. An extrauterine and intrauterine pregnancy is termed a(n):
    a. mirror pregnancy
    b. interstitial pregnancy
    c. bicornuate pregnancy
    d. heterotopic pregnancy

43. Which of the following lines the chorion and contains the fetus?
    a. amnion
    b. decidua basalis
    c. chorion frondosum
    d. trophoblastic tissue

44. The term *embryo* is used to describe a developing zygote through the:
    a. fourth gestational week
    b. eighth gestational week
    c. tenth gestational week
    d. twelfth gestational week

45. A solid mass of cells formed by proliferation of a fertilized ovum is termed the:
   a. zygote
   b. morula
   c. blastocyst
   d. trophoblast

46. Chorionic villi are more prolific:
   a. adjacent to the yolk sac
   b. opposite the cervical os
   c. near the implantation site
   d. adjacent to the uterine fundus

47. Which of the following is the first system to function in the developing embryo?
   a. respiratory
   b. genitourinary
   c. cardiovascular
   d. gastrointestinal

48. A corpus luteum is most likely misdiagnosed as a(n):
   a. hydrosalpinx
   b. missed abortion
   c. ectopic pregnancy
   d. anembryonic pregnancy

49. The discriminatory zone determines:
   a. when angiogenesis occurs
   b. the location of the placenta
   c. when cardiac activity should be visualized
   d. when a gestational sac should be visualized

50. Which of the following is the most accurate method of measuring gestational age?
   a. yolk sac diameter
   b. mean sac diameter
   c. crown–rump length
   d. biparietal diameter

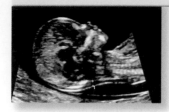

CHAPTER 24

Assessment of the Second Trimester

KEY TERMS

cavum septum pellucidi the space between the leaves of the septum pellucidum.

cephalic index a ratio of the cranium derived to determine the normality of the fetal head shape.

brachycephalic round shape to the fetal cranium; cephalic index 85%.

dolichocephalic elongated shape to the fetal cranium; cephalic index <70%.

ductus arteriosus a shunt in the fetal circulation that connects the main pulmonary artery with the descending aorta; allows most of the blood from the right ventricle to the aorta bypassing the lungs.

ductus venosus a shunt in the fetal circulation that enables oxygenated blood to pass into the heart bypassing the liver. Following birth, it becomes the ligamentum venosum.

falx cerebri a sickle-shaped fold of dura mater separating the two hemispheres of the cerebrum.

foramen ovale a shunt between the right and left atria that allows some blood to bypass the right ventricle.

maternal alpha-fetoprotein a blood test to assist in diagnosing certain fetal anomalies.

meconium a material that collects in the intestines of the fetus and forms the first stool of a newborn.

railway sign term describing the sonographic appearance of the fetal spine.

tentorium "tent" structure in the posterior fossa that separates the cerebellum from the cerebrum.

thalamus one of a pair of large oval nervous structures forming most of the lateral walls of the third ventricle of the brain and part of the diencephalon.

vermis cerebelli narrow median part of the cerebellum between the two lateral hemispheres.

SECOND TRIMESTER BIOMETRIC MEASUREMENTS

Biparietal Diameter

- Two-dimensional measurement.
- Thalamic view.
- Accurate predictor of gestational age before 20 weeks.
- Measured in a plane corresponding to the widest position of the head that passes through the third ventricle and thalami.
- Above the level of the orbits and cerebellum.
- Below the level of the ventricular atrium.
- Transverse axial plane is most common and includes the following landmarks:
  - Falx cerebri.
  - Third ventricle.
  - Thalamic nuclei.
  - Cavum septum pellucidi.
- Measure perpendicular to the falx, placing calipers from the outer margin of the upper cranium to the inner margin of the lower cranium.
- Measurement of the biparietal diameter (BPD) can be obtained from the head circumference plane.

Head Circumference

- Three-dimensional measurement.
- Reliable measurement independent of cranial shape.
- Measured in plane that must include the cavum septum pellucidi, third ventricle, thalami, and the tentorium.

- Measured parallel to the base of the skull, placing the calipers on the outer margins of the cranium.
- Measurement of the head circumference cannot always be obtained from the BPD plane.

Cephalic Index

- Three-dimensional measurement.
- Devised to determine the normality of the fetal head shape.
- Mean cephalic index is approximately 78% ± 4.4%.
- Abnormal when less than 74% or greater than 83%.

Abdominal Circumference

- Three-dimensional measurement.
- Predictor of fetal growth, not gestational age.
- Most difficult measurement to obtain.
- Cross-sectional measurement slightly superior to the cord insertion at the junction of the left and right portal veins (hockey stick) or demonstrates a short length of the umbilical vein, left portal vein, and fetal stomach.
- Place calipers on the outer margins of the skin edge.
- Measured at a level to include the liver.

Femur Length

- One-dimensional measurement.
- Long bone of choice because of ease of measurement.
- Normal femur demonstrates a straight lateral border and a curved medial border.
- Measured parallel to the femoral shaft placing calipers at the level of the femoral head cartilage and the distal femoral condyle.
- Cartilaginous epiphysis is not included.

LABORATORY VALUES

Alpha-Fetoprotein (AFP)

- Produced by the fetus.
- Found in the amniotic fluid and maternal serum.
- Normal values vary with gestational age.

Causes of High Alpha-Fetoprotein

- Underestimated gestational age; fetus older than expected.
- Multiple gestations.
- Open neural tube defect.
- Abdominal wall defect.
- Fetal – maternal hemorrhage.
- Renal anomalies.
- Fetal demise.

Causes of Low Alpha-Fetoprotein

- Overestimated gestational age; fetus younger than expected.
- Chromosomal abnormalities.
- Trophoblastic disease.
- Long-standing fetal demise.
- Chronic maternal hypertension or diabetes.

Quad Screen

- Screens AFP, unconjugated estradiol, free human chorionic gonadotropin (hCG), and inhibin A for chromosomal abnormalities.
- More commonly used in place of triple screen (AFP, unconjugated estriol, hCG).

EXAMINATION TECHNIQUES, PROTOCOLS, AND IMAGE OPTIMIZATION

Preparation

- Preparation varies with type of imaging approach.

Transabdominal

- Requires bladder distention.
  - Adult – drink 28 to 32 oz of water 1 hour before examination.
  - If catharized, fill bladder to 375 mL.

Endovaginal and Translabial

- Urinary bladder should be emptied.

Contraindications for Endovaginal Imaging

- Any patient who does not or cannot willingly consent to the examination.
- If the pain becomes too severe, terminate examination.

Transducer Selection

- Use the highest frequency possible to obtain optimal resolution for penetration depth.
  - Adults – 3.5 to 5.0 MHz transabdominal.
  - 4.0 to 8.0 MHz endovaginal.
  - 3.5 to 5.0 MHz translabial.
  - Obese patients – 2.0 MHz may be required for transabdominal imaging.
- Curvilinear transducers provide a wider field of view.
- Sector or vector transducers have a smaller footprint.

Patient Positioning

- Supine position – transabdominal.
- Lithotomy position – endovaginal and translabial.

Examination Protocol – Fetal Surveillance

- Conservative approach keeping the use of second trimester ultrasound for diagnostic purposes only and an examination time as short as possible.
- Begin examination with a quick survey the entire gravid uterus assessing fetal number, position, and viability.
- Assess fetal age using biometric measurements biparietal diameter (BPD), head circumference (HC), abdominal circumference (AC), femur length (FL).
- Evaluate and image the following:

Second Trimester—Fetal Surveillance

REGION	EVALUATE AND DOCUMENT

Cranial	Face
	    Profile – demonstrating the relationship of the forehead, nose, and chin
	    Coronal – demonstrating upper lip and nose
	Falx, third ventricle, thalami, and cavum septum pellucidi (BPD)
	Cerebellum/vermis – measurement of cerebellum may be included
	Cisterna magna – measurement may be included
	Atrium of the lateral ventricle – measurement should be included

Thorax	Four-chamber view of the heart Left and right ventricular outflow tracts – assess criss-cross relationship Motion mode tracing to include beats per minute Lung echogenicity Diaphragm

Second Trimester—Fetal Surveillance—(cont'd)

REGION	EVALUATE AND DOCUMENT
Abdomen	Stomach Kidneys – include length measurement of each kidney Bladder
Spine	Cervical, thoracic, lumbar, and sacral portions of the spine in the sagittal and transverse planes
Extremities	Upper extremities including hands Lower extremities including feet
Placenta	Echogenicity Location Relationship/distance to the cervix
Umbilical cord	Insertion into fetal abdomen Number of vessels within the cord and at insertion Color Doppler of hypogastric arteries at the level of the urinary bladder Insertion into the placenta may be included
Cervical os	Length – record the shortest of three measurements Relationship/distance to leading edge of the placenta
Amniotic fluid	Generally subjective observation in the second trimester Amniotic fluid volume (AFV) calculation may be included
Fetal position	Presentation of fetus in relationship to maternal anatomic planes
Pelvic structures	Uterus and ovaries Maternal urinary bladder

Image Optimization

- Reduce system output power control by a minimum of −3 dB (use OB presets).
- Place gains settings to display the myometrium hypoechoic to the normal placenta with adjustments to reduce artifactually produced echoes within the maternal urinary bladder.
- Focal zone(s) should be placed at or below the area of interest. The use of multiple focal zones increases detail resolution and decreases temporal resolution.
- Sufficient imaging depth to visualize structures immediately posterior to the area of interest.
- Harmonic imaging and decreasing system compression (dynamic range) can be used to reduce artifactual echoes in obese patients.
- Spatial compounding can be used to improve visualization of structures posterior to highly attenuating structures.
- Doppler settings should be adjusted for the different flow states of the fetus and adnexae.
- Doppler angle should be 60 degrees or less with a sample volume smaller than the vessel interrogating.

Helpful Hints

- Endovaginal imaging is most reliable approach for evaluating the cervix.
- Translabial may be used to evaluate the cervix when endovaginal imaging is contraindicated.
- A leading edge of placental tissue >2.0 cm from internal cervical os is associated with vaginal delivery.
- LVOT—from 4 chamber view angle transducer toward the fetal head.
- Coronal plane is the best scanning plane to image for cleft lip.

- Methods to help with poor fetal position:
  - Empty maternal urinary bladder.
  - Place patient in a right or left decubitus position.
  - Have patient walk around the examination room or ultrasound department.
  - Trendelenburg position may aid in achieving biometric head measurements with a cephalic fetal position.

INDICATIONS FOR A SECOND TRIMESTER ULTRASOUND

- Fetal surveillance.
- Fetal dating/growth.
- Fetal viability.
- Vaginal bleeding.
- Abdominal or pelvic pain.

FETAL ANATOMY

Fetal Circulation

- Oxygenated blood leaves the placenta and enters the fetus through the umbilical vein.
- After entering the abdomen, blood courses through the ductus venosum reaching the right atrium of the heart.
- Blood travels from the right to left atrium through the foramen ovale.
- Blood bypasses the lungs through the ductus arteriosus.
- From the left atrium to the left ventricle, blood ascends the aorta distributing blood to the fetal tissues.
- Approximately half of the blood leaves through the umbilical arteries and goes back to the placenta for reoxygenation.

Normal Cranial Anatomy

STRUCTURE	INFORMATION	SONOGRAPHIC APPEARANCE
Atrium of the lateral ventricle	Portion of the lateral ventricle where the body (central portion) occipital horn and temporal horn converge Located slightly superior to the level of the biparietal diameter (BPD) Evaluated for ventricular enlargement	Hyperechoic thin ventricle wall Hyperechoic choroid plexus Measured perpendicular to the ventricle walls from the glomus of the choroid plexus to the lateral ventricular wall Measurement should not exceed 10 mm throughout pregnancy Choroid plexus should almost fill the lateral ventricle
Cavum septum pellucidi	Presence excludes central nervous system anomalies Reservoir of cerebrospinal fluid between the frontal horns of the lateral ventricles. Found at the level of the BPD Located inferior to the anterior horns of the lateral ventricles Closes by 2 years of age	Small anechoic box located in the midline portion of the anterior brain Two hyperechoic parallel lines in the anterior midline portion of the brain
Cerebellum	Consists of a vermis and two lateral horns Located in the posterior fossa Assists in balance	Dumbbell-shaped echogenic structure located in the midline of the posterior fossa Adjunct measurement to determine fetal age—1 cm equals 1 gestational week

Normal Cranial Anatomy—(cont'd)

STRUCTURE	INFORMATION	SONOGRAPHIC APPEARANCE
Choroid plexus	Echogenic cluster of cells Important in the production of cerebrospinal fluid Not located in the anterior or occipital horns Choroid plexus cyst(s) are typically identified between 16 and 23 gestational weeks and should regress by 26 weeks' gestation	Hyperechoic structures located within each lateral ventricle Lie along the atrium of the lateral ventricle Cysts may be displayed within choroid
Cisterna magna	Fluid-filled space located between the undersurface of the cerebellum and medulla oblongata	Anterior – posterior diameter $\leq$10 mm Measured from the cerebellar vermis to the inside of the calvaria
Cranium	Begins ossification around the ninth gestational week Generally ovoid in shape	Hyperechoic outline surrounding the brain
Falx cerebri	Intrahemisphere fissure Separates the cerebral hemispheres	Echogenic midline linear structure
Nuchal fold	Soft-tissue thickness between the calvaria and posterior skin line Measured in the axial plane at a level to include the cerebellum, cistern magnum, and cavum septum pellucidi Measured from outer cranium to outer skin line Accurate between 15 and 21 gestational weeks Thickening associated with aneuploidy	Thickness <6 mm
Thalami	Provide synopsis between the cerebellum and posterior brain	Hypoechoic ovoid structures in the midportion of the brain located in each hemisphere Third ventricle is located between each individual thalamus

Normal Thoracic Anatomy

STRUCTURE	INFORMATION	SONOGRAPHIC APPEARANCE
Diaphragm	Muscle separating the thorax and abdominal cavities Courses anterior to posterior	Curvilinear hypoechoic structure compared with lungs and liver Abdominal contents lie inferior Chest contents lie superior
Heart	Occupies about one-third of the thorax Apex points toward the left side of the body at about a 45-degree angle Right ventricle lies most anterior – closest to chest wall Left atrium lies most posterior – closest to the spine	Four anechoic symmetrical chambers divided by uninterrupted septa which should only demonstrate an opening at the foramen ovale (atrial septum) LVOT – left ventricular connection with the aortic arch. RVOT – right ventricular connection with the main pulmonary artery (pulmonary trunk) 120–160 beats per minutes Hyperechoic focus within the ventricle is most likely the papillary muscle
Lungs	Serve as lateral borders to the heart Lie superior to the diaphragm	Moderately echogenic Homogeneous Increases in echogenicity as gestation progresses

Normal Abdominal Anatomy

STRUCTURE	INFORMATION	SONOGRAPHIC APPEARANCE
Bladder	Signifies genitourinary system is working The bladder fills and empties every 25–30 min, approximately Should be visualized by 13 gestational weeks	Round anechoic structure located centrally in the inferior pelvis Variable in size
Bowel	Meconium begins to accumulate in the small bowel Small bowel becomes visible in the late second trimester Large bowel becomes visible after 22 weeks' gestation	**Small Bowel** Moderately echogenic Hyperechoic compared with the normal liver Hypoechoic compared with bone Distinguished after 22 weeks **Large Bowel** Hypoechoic to the small bowel
Gallbladder	Visualization peaks around 20–32 gestational weeks Signifies the presence of the biliary tree	Elongated fluid-filled structure Located inferior and to the right of the umbilical vein
Kidneys	Urine formation begins near the end of the first trimester Should be identified by 12–13 weeks Consistently identified by 18–20 weeks	Isoechoic or hypoechoic structures located on each side of the spine Homogeneous, medium-gray elliptical structure on each side of the spine (sagittal plane) Homogeneous, medium-gray circular structure on each side of the spine(transverse plane) Renal pelvis contains a small amount of fluid <4 mm up to 33 weeks <7 mm from 33 weeks to term Abdominal/renal ratio is approximately 3:1
Liver	Largest organ in the fetal torso Reflects changes in fetal growth	Moderately echogenic structure Left lobe is larger than the right lobe Occupies most of the upper abdomen
Stomach	Reliably visualized by 13 gestational weeks Signifies normal swallowing sequence	Anechoic structure located in the left upper quadrant Size and shape will vary with recent swallowing Echogenic debris within the stomach may be demonstrated
Umbilical cord insertion	Smooth insertion into the anterior fetal abdomen superior to the urinary bladder Placental insertion generally located in the midportion of the placenta	Smooth abdominal wall at umbilical insertion (skin intact) Umbilical vein courses superiorly toward the liver Umbilical arteries arise from the hypogastric arteries on each side of the fetal bladder

Normal Musculoskeletal Anatomy

STRUCTURE	INFORMATION	SONOGRAPHIC APPEARANCE
Facial structures	**Sagittal view (profile) is useful in determining:** 1. Relationship of the nose to lips 2. Formation of the forehead 3. Formation of the chin 4. Presence of nasal bone **Coronal view is useful for visualizing:** 1. Orbital rings 2. Upper lip 3. Nasal septum 4. Maxilla and zygomatic arches **Tangential view is useful in determining:** 1. Craniofacial abnormalities	**Profile** The segments containing the forehead, the eyes, and nose, and the mouth and chin each form one-third of the face **Coronal** Upper lip and philtrum should be smooth and uninterrupted
Long bones	Ossification begins by 11 gestational weeks	Hyperechoic linear structure Foot length/femur length 1:1
Pelvis	Iliac wings ossify at 12 gestational weeks Ischium ossifies by 20 gestational weeks	Hyperechoic linear structure
Ribs	Rib cage should encompass more than one-half of the chest on either side	Hyperechoic curved linear structures
Spine	The spine widens near the base of the skull and tapers near the sacrum When evaluating the spine, the transducer must remain perpendicular to the spinous elements Ossification should be complete by 18 gestational weeks	**Coronal plane** 1. Three parallel hyperechoic lines **Sagittal plane** 1. Two ossification centers 2. Two curvilinear hyperechoic lines **Transverse plane** 1. Three equidistant ossification centers surrounding the neural canal 2. Spinal column appears as a closed circle **Skin line** 1. Echogenic smooth line posterior to the spine

Normal Placenta and Umbilical Cord

STRUCTURE	INFORMATION	SONOGRAPHIC APPEARANCE
Amniotic fluid (AF)	Surrounds and protects the fetus Provides important information on fetal renal and placental function Fetus becomes the major producer of AF through swallowing and urine production after 16 weeks	Subjective observation of the amount of amniotic fluid surrounding the fetus If appears abnormal calculate amniotic fluid index (AFI) Normal range—6 to 24 cm Swirling of fine echogenic particles (vernix)
Cervical os	Length of cervix determines competence Length is measured between the internal and external cervical os Normal length varies between 2.5 and 4.0 cm	Echogenic linear structure Hyperechoic central echoes Average length >3.0 cm
Placenta	Communication organ between the fetus and mother Supplies nutrition and products of metabolism to the fetus Location varies and may include anterior, posterior, fundal, right and left lateral or a combination (e.g., anterior fundal)	Echogenic disk-shaped mass of tissue Hyperechoic compared with the myometrium Leading placental edge measures >2.0 cm from the internal cervical os Smooth and tapered margins Thickness ≤4 cm before 24 weeks
Umbilical cord	Connecting lifeline between the fetus and placenta Consists of one vein and two arteries Umbilical vein enters the left portal vein Umbilical arteries arise from the internal iliac (hypogastric) arteries Normally inserts into the midportion of the placenta Bathed in Wharton jelly	Solid, coiled structure containing three anechoic vessels Twisting of the cord is normal **Umbilical Artery** Low resistance near the fetal insertion High resistance near the placental insertion **Umbilical Vein** Continuous low flow through systole and diastole Flow is directed from the placenta to the fetus

ASSESSMENT OF THE SECOND TRIMESTER REVIEW

1. Which portion of the fetal heart is located closest to the spine?
   a. left atrium
   b. right atrium
   c. left ventricle
   d. right ventricle

2. Abdominal circumference is measured at the level of the:
   a. liver
   b. spleen
   c. kidneys
   d. umbilical cord insertion

3. Cavum septum pellucidi is located in the:
   a. anterior portion of the fetal brain
   b. posterior portion of the fetal brain
   c. anterior portion of the fetal chest
   d. posterior portion of the fetal chest

4. In the late second trimester, anterior – posterior diameter of the normal renal pelvis should not exceed:
   a. 1 mm
   b. 4 mm
   c. 7 mm
   d. 10 mm

5. Which of the following structures is *not* identified in the biparietal diameter?
   a. thalami nuclei
   b. fourth ventricle
   c. cavum septum pellucidi
   d. falx cerebri

6. The umbilical arteries arise from which of the following vessels?
   a. spiral arteries
   b. internal iliac arteries
   c. external iliac arteries
   d. common iliac arteries

7. Visualization of the fetal gallbladder signifies:
   a. normal liver function
   b. a normal fetal karyotype
   c. the presence of the pancreas
   d. the presence of a biliary tree

8. Which of the following best describes the intention of the cephalic index?
   a. Gestational weight is determined by the cephalic index.
   b. The cephalic index primarily determines gestational age.
   c. Intrauterine growth restriction is determined by the cephalic index.
   d. The cephalic index helps to determine the normality of the fetal head shape.

9. Which of the following measurements is most widely used when determining gestational age in the second trimester?
   a. long bone length
   b. biparietal diameter
   c. cerebellar dimension
   d. abdominal circumference

10. Choroid plexus cysts should normally regress by:
    a. 12 weeks
    b. 16 weeks
    c. 26 weeks
    d. 28 weeks

11. Which of the following planes demonstrate the normal fetal spine as three parallel hyperechoic lines on ultrasound?
    a. axial
    b. sagittal
    c. coronal
    d. transverse

12. The normal length of the cervical os will vary, but it measures a minimum of:
    a. 2.0 cm
    b. 2.5 cm
    c. 3.0 cm
    d. 3.5 cm

13. Which of the following is not a fetal cardiac shunt?
    a. ductus venosus
    b. foramen ovale
    c. ductus arteriosus
    d. foramen Monro

14. Which of the following patient positions is preferred for translabial imaging?
    a. supine
    b. decubitus
    c. lithotomy
    d. Trendelenburg

15. Which of the following shunts blood between the atria of the fetal heart?
    a. foramen ovale
    b. ductus arteriosis
    c. foramen Monro
    d. ductus venosus

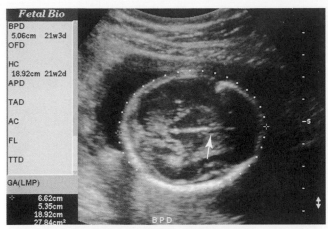

FIG. 24.1   Biparietal diameter.

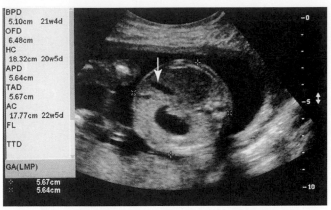

FIG. 24.3   Cross-sectional sonogram of the fetal abdomen.

Using Figure 24.1, answer question 16.

16. The arrow in this sonogram identifies the:
  a. thalami
  b. falx cerebri
  c. third ventricle
  d. cavum septum pellucidi

Using Figure 24.3, answer question 18.

18. The arrow identifies which of the following structures?
  a. hydroureter
  b. gallbladder
  c. umbilical vein
  d. right portal vein

Using Figure 24.2, answer question 17.

17. This coronal sonogram of a 26-week fetus most likely demonstrates a(n):
  a. abnormal thorax
  b. normal diaphragm
  c. abnormal stomach
  d. abnormal bowel pattern

Using Figure 24.4, answer questions 19 and 20.

19. Arrow *A* identifies the:
  a. vermis
  b. cerebellum
  c. sylvian fissure
  d. cisterna magna

20. Arrow *B* identifies the:
  a. cerebellum
  b. nuchal fold
  c. cisterna magna
  d. fourth ventricle

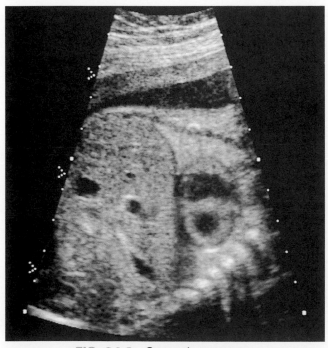

FIG. 24.2   Coronal sonogram.

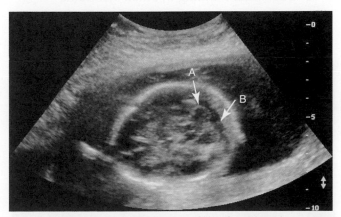

FIG. 24.4   Sonogram of the fetal head.

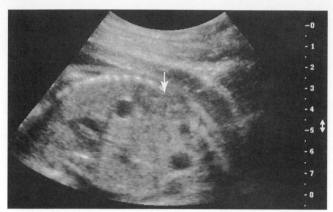

FIG. 24.5 Sonogram of the fetal abdomen.

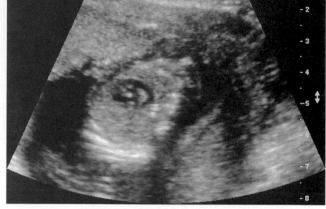

FIG. 24.7 Sonogram of the fetal chest.

Using Figure 24.5, answer question 21.

21. A sagittal image of the fetal abdomen (arrow) identifies a structure most consistent with a:
    a. normal right kidney
    b. normal left kidney
    c. left adrenal hemorrhage
    d. right adrenal hemorrhage

Using Figure 24.6, answer questions 22 and 23.

22. Which of the following fetal structures does the arrow most likely identify?
    a. urinary bladder
    b. umbilical varix
    c. hypogastric artery
    d. fluid-filled bowel loop

23. The echogenic focus within the fetal stomach is considered:
    a. a normal incidental finding
    b. suspicious for Turner syndrome
    c. a precursor to meconium peritonitis
    d. a consistent finding in Patau syndrome

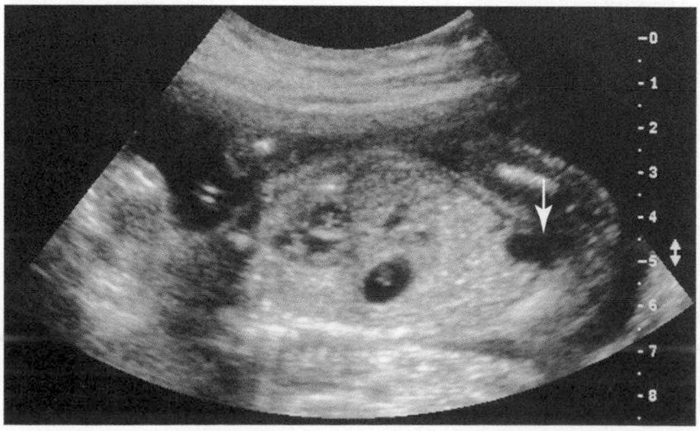

Using Figure 24.7, answer question 24.

24. The sonogram displays which of the following cardiac structures?
    a. aortic arch
    b. foramen ovale
    c. left ventricular outflow tract
    d. right ventricular outflow tract

Using Figure 24.8, answer question 25.

25. The calipers are measuring the:
    a. nuchal fold
    b. cerebellum
    c. cisterna magna
    d. lateral ventricle

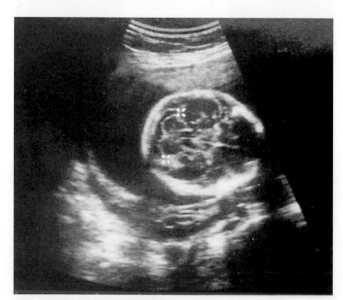

FIG. 24.8 Sonogram of the fetal head.

FIG. 24.6 Sagittal sonogram of the fetal body.

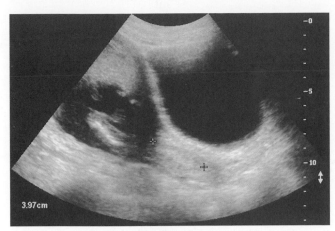

FIG. 24.9   Sagittal sonogram.

Using Figure 24.9, answer questions 26 and 27.

26. The relationship of the placenta to the internal cervical os is termed:
    a. low-lying placenta
    b. within normal limits
    c. marginal placenta previa
    d. incomplete placenta previa

27. This image displays the location of the placenta as:
    a. fundal
    b. anterior
    c. posterior
    d. right lateral

Using Figure 24.10, answer question 28.

28. The arrow identifies which of the following fetal structure?
    a. stomach
    b. renal cyst
    c. gallbladder
    d. renal pelvis

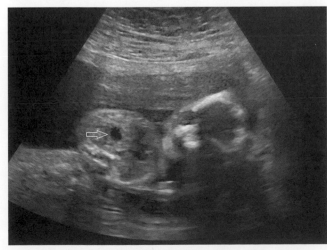

FIG. 24.10   Sonogram of the fetal abdomen.

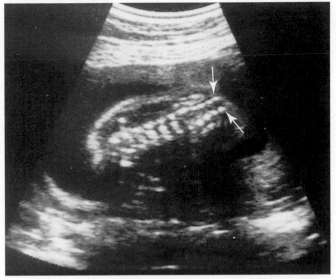

FIG. 24.11   Sonogram of the fetal spine.

Using Figure 24.11, answer question 29.

29. The arrows in this sonogram demonstrate a:
    a. coronal view of a sacral defect
    b. sagittal view of a normal coccyx
    c. coronal view of a normal sacrum
    d. sagittal view of a normal sacrum

30. In the transverse plane, the normal fetal spine appears on ultrasound as:
    a. two ossification centers lateral to the spinal canal
    b. three parallel hyperechoic lines surrounding the neural canal
    c. three parallel ossification centers surrounding the neural canal
    d. three equidistant ossification centers surrounding the spinal canal

31. Which landmark localizes the appropriate level for measuring the abdominal circumference?
    a. stomach
    b. gallbladder
    c. cord insertion
    d. junction of the left and right portal veins

32. Which of the following is a possible cause for elevated maternal alpha-fetoprotein?
    a. maternal diabetes
    b. abdominal wall defect
    c. chromosomal abnormalities
    d. overestimation of gestational age

33. The biparietal diameter measurement is taken at the level of the:
    a. falx cerebri
    b. third ventricle
    c. cisterna magna
    d. corpus callosum

34. Left ventricular outflow tract denotes the:
    a. ascending aorta
    b. papillary muscle
    c. descending aorta
    d. pulmonary artery

35. Which of the following provides important information about fetal renal function?
    a. renal size
    b. bladder volume
    c. renal pelviectasis
    d. amniotic fluid volume

36. Normal measurement of the atrium of the lateral ventricle atria should not exceed:
    a. 6 mm
    b. 8 mm
    c. 10 mm
    d. 12 mm

37. If the maternal alpha-fetoprotein level is decreased, the sonographer should carefully evaluate for:
    a. abdominal wall defects
    b. chromosomal abnormalities
    c. genitourinary abnormalities
    d. cardiovascular abnormalities

38. A small echogenic focus within the left ventricle of the fetal heart is most likely the:
    a. mitral valve
    b. foramen ovale
    c. pulmonary vein
    d. papillary muscle

39. Insertion of the umbilical cord into the abdominal wall of the fetus is located at a level:
    a. superior to the liver
    b. superior to the bladder
    c. superior to the adrenal glands
    d. inferior to the hypogastric arteries

40. Which of the following determines cervical competence?
    a. width
    b. height
    c. length
    d. thickness

41. Ossification of the cranium begins around the:
    a. eighth gestational week
    b. ninth gestational week
    c. eleventh gestational week
    d. thirteenth gestational week

42. Oxygenated blood enters the fetus through the:
    a. placenta
    b. umbilical vein
    c. chorionic villi
    d. umbilical arteries

43. Nuchal thickness is measured in a plane to include the:
    a. thalamic cerebri, falx cerebri, third ventricle
    b. cerebellum, cisterna magna, cavum septum pellucidi
    c. lateral ventricle atria, third ventricle, corpus callosum
    d. thalamic cerebri, fourth ventricle, cavum septum pellucidi

44. Sonographic appearance of a normal small bowel during the second trimester is described as:
    a. hyperechoic compared with bone
    b. hyperechoic compared with the liver
    c. hypoechoic compared with the spleen
    d. hypoechoic compared with the large bowel

45. Echogenic debris swirling within the amniotic cavity is:
    a. consistent with fetal demise
    b. a normal sonographic finding
    c. consistent with polyhydramnios
    d. suspicious for chromosomal anomalies

46. The fetus becomes the major producer of amniotic fluid in the:
    a. late first trimester
    b. early second trimester
    c. late second trimester
    d. early third trimester

47. Visualization of which brain structure excludes most central nervous system anomalies?
    a. falx cerebri
    b. third ventricle
    c. corpus callosum
    d. cavum septum pellucidi

48. The material collecting in the fetal intestines is termed:
    a. sludge
    b. vernix
    c. vermis
    d. meconium

49. Head circumference is measured at a level to include the:
    a. third ventricle and cisterna magna
    b. cavum septum pellucidi and tentorium
    c. peduncles and cavum septum pellucidi
    d. atrium of the lateral ventricle and cerebellum

50. Which of the following measurements is a good predictor of fetal growth?
    a. femur length
    b. biparietal diameter
    c. head circumference
    d. abdominal circumference

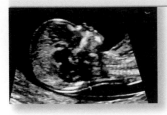

CHAPTER 25

Assessment of the Third Trimester

KEY TERMS

asymmetrical intrauterine growth restriction most common type of growth abnormality demonstrating normal cranial growth and a decrease in abdominal growth.

biophysical profile objective means for assessing fetal well-being.

hypertension systolic pressure ≥140 mm Hg or a diastolic pressure ≥90 mm Hg.

oligohydramnios amniotic fluid below the normal range for gestational age. Total volume <200 mL.

polyhydramnios amniotic fluid above the normal range for gestational age. Total volume >2000 mL.

postterm pregnancy gestation greater than 42 weeks.

macrosomia a condition in which accelerated fetal growth results in an infant with a birth weight greater than 4000 g in nondiabetic mother or greater than 4500 g in diabetic mother; associated with birth asphyxia and trauma.

symmetrical intrauterine growth restriction fetal growth abnormality resulting in a proportionally small fetus.

vernix caseosa fatty material found on the fetal skin and amniotic fluid late in pregnancy.

THIRD TRIMESTER

- Lungs, organs, and vessels are maturing in preparation for birth.

THIRD TRIMESTER MEASUREMENTS

- Biparietal diameter (BPD).
- Head circumference (HC).
- Abdominal circumference (AC).
- Femur length (FL).
- Amniotic fluid volume.
- Head circumference-to-abdominal circumference ratio (HC/AC).
  - During the early third trimester, the head circumference is slightly larger than the circumference of the abdomen.
  - During the late third trimester, with the increase of fetal body fat, the abdominal circumference is typically equal to or slightly larger than the head circumference.
- Estimated fetal weight.
  - Most commonly calculated using the biparietal diameter, femur length, and abdominal circumference.

EXAMINATION TECHNIQUES, PROTOCOLS, AND IMAGE OPTIMIZATION

Preparation

- Preparation varies with type of imaging approach.

Transabdominal

- Requires bladder distention.
  - Adult—drink 28 to 32 oz of water 1 hour before examination.
  - If catharized, fill bladder to 375 mL.

Endovaginal and Translabial

- Urinary bladder should be emptied.

Contraindications for Endovaginal Imaging

- Any patient who does not or cannot willingly consent to the examination.
- If the pain becomes too severe, terminate examination.

Transducer Selection

- Use the highest frequency possible to obtain optimal resolution for penetration depth.
  - Adults—3.5 to 5.0 MHz transabdominal.
  - 4.0 to 8.0 MHz endovaginal.
  - 3.5 to 5.0 MHz translabial.
  - Obese patients—2.0 MHz may be required for transabdominal imaging.
- Curvilinear transducers provide a wider field of view.
- Sector or vector transducers have a smaller footprint.

Patient Positioning

- Supine position—transabdominal.
- Lithotomy position—endovaginal and translabial.

Examination Protocol

- Begin examination with a quick survey the entire gravid uterus.
- Assess fetal age and growth using biometric measurements (BPD, HC, AC, FL).
- Evaluate and image the following:
  - Fetal presentation and viability.
  - Amniotic fluid volume.
  - Placenta location and grade.
  - Length of internal cervical os.
  - Fetal anatomy surveillance may be included.
- Abnormalities should be documented and when applicable measured in two imaging planes. Color and/or spectral Doppler evaluation of the abnormality should be included.

Image Optimization

- Reduce ultrasound system power control by a minimum of −3 dB.
- Place gain settings to display the normal placenta as a medium shade of grade.
- Focal zone(s) should be placed at or below the area of interest. The use of multiple focal zones increases detail resolution and decreases temporal resolution.
- Avoid placing focal zone at level of fetal bone.
- Sufficient imaging depth to visualize structures immediately posterior to the area of interest.
- Harmonic imaging and decreasing system compression (dynamic range) can be used to reduce artifactual echoes in obese patients.
- Spatial compounding can be used to improve visualization of structures posterior to highly attenuating structures.
- Doppler setting should be set for slow to moderate blood flow.

INDICATIONS FOR THIRD TRIMESTER ULTRASOUND

- Fetal growth.
- Amniotic fluid volume.
- Fetal well-being.
- Fetal presentation.
- Late prenatal care.
- Placenta location (refer to Chapter 28).
- Follow-up on previous ultrasound finding.

FETAL GROWTH

- Interval fetal growth can be determined with ultrasound examinations a minimum of 7 days apart.
- Distal femoral epiphysis (DFE) is visualized around 32 gestational weeks.
- Proximal tibial epiphysis (PTE) is visualized around 35 gestational weeks.

Decrease in Fetal Growth

Small for Gestational Age (SGA)

- Covers both normal and subnormal fetal growth.
- May be a result of incorrect dates or oligohydramnios.

Intrauterine Growth Restriction (IUGR)

- Results from insufficient oxygen and nutrition delivery to the fetus from the placenta (placental insufficiency).
- Defined as a fetal weight at or below the 10th percentile for gestational age.
- No single reliable criterion is available to diagnose intrauterine growth restriction.
- Serial examinations are necessary.
- Associated with maternal hypertension.
- Evaluation of the amniotic fluid volume, estimated fetal weight, and maternal blood pressure results in the most accurate diagnosis.
- The liver is one of the most severely affected fetal organs.
- Decrease in liver size results in a decrease in abdominal circumference.

Intrauterine Growth Restriction

TYPE	ETIOLOGY	CLINICAL FINDINGS	SONOGRAPHIC FINDINGS	DIFFERENTIAL CONSIDERATIONS
Asymmetric	Placental insufficiency (most common) Chromosomal abnormality Fetal infection Multiple gestations **Maternal Risk Factors** Hypertension (most common) Poor nutrition Alcohol and drug abuse	Small for dates Low maternal weight gain Hypertension Preeclampsia History of previous SGA infant	Lack of fetal growth on serial sonograms Decrease in abdominal circumference Normal head circumference and femur length Decrease in amniotic fluid volume Increase in HC/AC ratio Placentomalacia Grade 3 placenta **Umbilical Artery** Systolic – diastolic ratio of umbilical artery >3.0 after 30 weeks Absence or reversal of diastolic flow is considered critical **Umbilical Vein** Decrease in flow volume	Normal small fetus
Symmetric	Result of embryological insult Fetal infection Congenital malformations Living at a high altitude (low oxgen levels) Irradiation	Small for dates	Symmetrically small head and abdomen circumference Oligohydramnios	Incorrect menstrual dates Normal small fetus Skeletal dysplasia

Increase in Fetal Growth

Large for Gestational Age (LGA)

- Covers both normal and increased fetal growth.
- May be a result of incorrect dates, macrosomia, or polyhydramnios.

Macrosomia

- Fetal weight above 4000 g in nondiabetic mother or >4500 g in a diabetic mother or above the 90th percentile for gestational age.
- Fetuses of diabetic mothers are likely to display organomegaly, whereas fetuses of nondiabetic mothers will demonstrate normal growth.
- Fetuses of diabetic mothers demonstrate a higher mortality rate.

Macrosomia

CONDITION	ETIOLOGY	CLINICAL FINDINGS	SONOGRAPHIC FINDINGS	DIFFERENTIAL CONSIDERATIONS
Macrosomia	Maternal diabetes mellitus Maternal obesity Postterm pregnancy Multipariety Advanced maternal age History of previous LGA infant	Large for dates	Large abdominal circumference Decreased HC/AC ratio Estimated fetal weight >4000 g in nondiabetic mother or >4500 g in diabetic mother Polyhydramnios Placentomegaly	Normal large fetus Suboptimal fetal measurements

AMNIOTIC FLUID

- Normal volume of amniotic fluid varies with gestational age.
- Early in gestation, the major source of amniotic fluid is the amniotic membrane.
- As the embryo and placenta develop, fluid is produced by the placenta and fetus.
- After 16 gestational weeks, the fetus is the major producer of amniotic fluid.

Functions of the Amniotic Fluid

- Maintains intrauterine temperature.
- Allows fetus free movement within the amniotic cavity.
- Protects the developing fetus from injury.
- Prevents adherence of the amnion to the fetus.
- Promotes lung growth and development.

Amniotic Fluid Production

- Kidneys—primary source of production through urine production.
- Lungs—secretions from lungs.
- Umbilical cord.
- Amniotic membrane.

Amniotic Fluid Removal

- Gastrointestinal tract—primary source of removal through swallowing and fluid absorption in the intestines.
- Placenta—fetal blood perfuses across the placenta.
- Umbilical cord.
- Lungs.

Amniotic Fluid Volume

- Normal volume of amniotic fluid increases progressively until about 33 gestational weeks.

- During the late second and early third trimester, the amniotic fluid volume appears to surround the fetus.
- By the late third trimester, the amniotic fluid displays as isolated fluid pockets.
- Regulated by the production of fluid, removal of fluid, and fluid exchange within the lungs, membranes, and umbilical cord.
- Normal lung development depends on the exchange of amniotic fluid within the lungs.
- Oligohydramnios increases risk of fetal death and neonatal morbidity.

Measuring Amniotic Fluid Volume

- Transducer must remain perpendicular to the maternal coronal plane and parallel to the maternal sagittal plane.
- Measurement of fluid pocket must be free of umbilical cord or any fetal part.
- Too much transducer pressure can reduce the fluid pocket measurement.

Methods of Assessing Amniotic Fluid Volume

METHOD	DESCRIPTION	NORMAL SONOGRAPHIC FINDINGS	ABNORMAL SONOGRAPHIC FINDINGS
Amniotic fluid index (AFI)	Determined by dividing the uterus into four equal parts Measure deepest unobstructed pocket in each quadrant AFI is equal to the sum of all four quadrants	AFI >5 cm and <24 cm	AFI <5 cm or >24 cm
Single deepest pocket	Maximum vertical depth of any amniotic fluid pocket	Largest pocket >2 cm and <8 cm	Largest pocket <2 cm or >8 cm
Subjective assessment	Observing the amount of amniotic fluid during real-time examination Experience increases accuracy	Amount of amniotic fluid appears within normal limits for gestation	Amniotic fluid appears greater or less than expected for the gestational age

Abnormal Amniotic Fluid Volume

ABNORMALITY	ETIOLOGY	SONOGRAPHIC FINDINGS	DIFFERENTIAL CONSIDERATIONS
Oligohydramnios	**Fetal** Genitourinary tract abnormality Intrauterine growth restriction Post term pregnancy **Maternal** Premature rupture of membranes (most common) Hypertension Dehydration Placenta insufficiency	AFI below 5 cm Below the 5th percentile for gestational age Largest single pocket below 1 cm Poor fetal – fluid interface Total volume <200 mL	Lower limits of normal Premature rupture of membranes
Polyhydramnios	**Fetal Anomalies** Central nervous system Gastrointestinal tract Abdominal wall defects Cardiovascular defects **Maternal** Diabetes mellitus Cardiac disease Preeclampsia Rh isoimmunization Idiopathic	AFI above 24 cm Above the 95th percentile for gestational age Total volume exceeding 2000 mL Fetal anatomy is easy to visualize AFI above 24 cm associated with fetal anomalies May resolve spontaneously on serial examinations	Upper limits of normal

FETAL WELL-BEING

Biophysical Profile

- Indirectly tests for fetal hypoxia.
- Nonstress test findings, fetal tone, breathing, and body movements are markers of acute fetal hypoxia.
- Amniotic fluid volume is a marker of chronic fetal hypoxia.

Biophysical Profile

	DESCRIPTION	NORMAL FINDINGS	ABNORMAL FINDINGS
Biophysical profile	Objective means for assessing fetal well-being Fetus is observed for 30 min Five parameters are evaluated: 1. Fetal tone 2. Fetal movement 3. Fetal breathing movement 4. Amniotic fluid volume 5. Nonstress test or placenta grade Scoring of the parameters: 0 = does not exhibit 1 = partially exhibits 2 = exhibits fully	1. **Fetal Tone** One complete episode of flexion to extension and back to flexion 2. **Fetal Movement** Three separate fetal movements within 30 min 3. **Fetal Breathing Movement** Movement of the diaphragm ≥30 s 4. **Amniotic Fluid Volume** Amniotic pocket >2 cm or Amniotic fluid index >5 cm 5. **Nonstress Test** Exhibits two fetal heart accelerations within 20 min or Placental grade ≥2 Total points ≥8	1. **Fetal Tone** Incomplete or lack of flexion to extension and back to flexion 2. **Fetal Movement** Two or fewer separate fetal movements within 30 min 3. **Fetal Breathing Movement** No movement of the diaphragm or duration <30 s 4. **Amniotic Fluid Volume** An amniotic pocket <2 cm or Amniotic fluid index ≤5 cm 5. **Nonstress Test** Exhibits two or fewer fetal heart accelerations within 40 min or Placental grade = 3 Total points <6

FETAL PRESENTATION

- Relationship of the fetal head with the long axis of the uterus.
- Fetal position changes less frequently after 34 gestational weeks.
- Nonvertex fetal position after 34 weeks may be predictive of positional or placental problems.

Cephalic or Vertex

- Fetal head lies most inferior, closest to the cervical os.

Transverse

- Fetal head and body lie across the maternal abdomen.
- Check for signs of placenta previa.

Oblique

- Fetal head and body are lying at a 45-degree angle to the sagittal plane of the uterus.
- Document location of the fetal head.

Breech

- Fetal head is located in the superior portion of the uterus.
- Presenting part should be determined after 36 weeks' gestation.

Frank Breech

- Fetal buttocks are presenting with the feet near head.
- Hips flexed and knees extended.
- Most common.

Complete Breech

- Fetal buttocks are presenting with the knees bent and feet down.
- Both hips and knees are flexed.
- Least common.

Footling Breech

- Incomplete breech.
- Fetal foot is the presenting part.
- One or both hips and knees are extended.
- Greatest risk for prolapsed cord.

ASSESSMENT OF THE THIRD TRIMESTER REVIEW

1. The most common maternal factor associated with intrauterine growth restriction is:
   a. obesity
   b. hypertension
   c. diabetes mellitus
   d. oligohydramnios

2. Polyhydramnios demonstrates an amniotic volume index greater than:
   a. 5 cm
   b. 10 cm
   c. 15 cm
   d. 24 cm

3. The distal femoral epiphysis is consistently visualized by:
   a. 20 weeks
   b. 28 weeks
   c. 32 weeks
   d. 35 weeks

4. Oligohydramnios in the third trimester is most likely a result of:
   a. duodenal atresia
   b. diaphragmatic hernia
   c. infantile polycystic renal disease
   d. cystic adenomatoid malformation

5. The most common maternal cause of macrosomia is:
   a. anemia
   b. proteinuria
   c. hypertension
   d. diabetes mellitus

6. Which portion of the biophysical profile study is a chronic marker of fetal hypoxia?
   a. fetal tone
   b. fetal movement
   c. amniotic fluid volume
   d. maturity of the placenta

7. When measuring amniotic fluid volume, the transducer must remain:
   a. parallel to both the maternal sagittal and coronal planes
   b. perpendicular to both the maternal sagittal and coronal planes
   c. parallel with the maternal coronal plane and perpendicular to the sagittal plane
   d. perpendicular to the maternal coronal plane and parallel to the maternal sagittal plane

8. A pregnancy is postterm when the:
   a. fetus weighs more than 3000 g
   b. pregnancy is longer than 40 gweeks
   c. fetus weighs more than 4000 g
   d. pregnancy is longer than 42 weeks

9. Symmetrical intrauterine growth restriction is more commonly a result of:
   a. first trimester insult
   b. maternal hypertension
   c. placental insufficiency
   d. second trimester insult

10. Doppler of the umbilical artery evaluates fetal well-being using the:
    a. resistive index
    b. pulsatility index
    c. peak systolic velocity
    d. systolic – diastolic ratio

11. Macrosomia is defined as a newborn weight exceeding:
    a. 1000 g
    b. 2500 g
    c. 4000 g
    d. 5500 g

12. In a biophysical profile, which of the following will document fetal tone?
    a. movement of the fetal diaphragm
    b. three separate fetal movements in 30 seconds
    c. two fetal heart accelerations within 20 minutes
    d. complete episode of flexion to extension and back to flexion

13. Documentation of fetal position demonstrates a frank breech presentation. This means the fetal head is located in the superior portion of the uterus and the:
    a. buttocks are down with one foot presenting
    b. fetal feet are presenting with both legs extended
    c. buttocks are presenting with the feet near the head
    d. buttocks are presenting with the knees bent and feet down

14. Maternal hypertension is defined as a systolic pressure above:
    a. 100 mm Hg
    b. 140 mm Hg
    c. 175 mm Hg
    d. 180 mm Hg

15. Oligohydramnios is defined as an amniotic fluid index below:
    a. 2 cm
    b. 5 cm
    c. 10 cm
    d. 18 cm

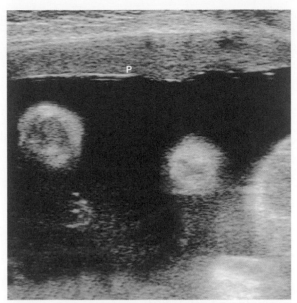

FIG. 25.1 Third trimester sonogram. (Norton M, Scoutt, L., Feldstein, V: Callen's Ultrasonography in Obstetrics and Gynecology 6e, Philadelphia, 2017, Elsevier.)

Using Figure 25.1, answer question 16.

16. This third trimester image is most suspicious for:
    a. macrosomia
    b. polyhydramnios
    c. oligohydramnios
    d. gastrointestinal distress

Using Figure 25.2, answer question 17.

17. Determine the fetal lie in this sonogram of the transverse gravid uterus:
    a. breech
    b. cephalic
    c. transverse head to maternal right
    d. position cannot be determined by a single image

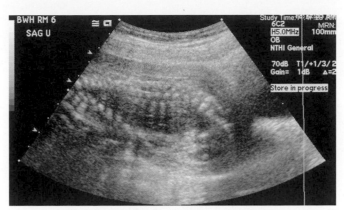

FIG. 25.3 Third trimester sonogram.

Using Figure 25.3, answer questions 18 and 19.

18. What does this third trimester sonogram demonstrate?
    a. oligohydramnios
    b. trophoblastic disease
    c. diaphragmatic hernia
    d. cystic adenomatoid malformation

19. Which of the following is the most likely cause for this diagnosis?
    a. fetal hydrops
    b. duodenal atresia
    c. multicystic renal dysplasia
    d. premature rupture of membrane

Using Figure 25.4, answer questions 20 and 21.

20. In addition to the gender of the fetus, this image reveals a(n):
    a. anterior placenta
    b. myelomeningocele
    c. skeletal dysplasia
    d. abnormal cord insertion

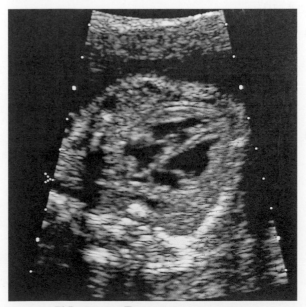

FIG. 25.2 Transverse sonogram.

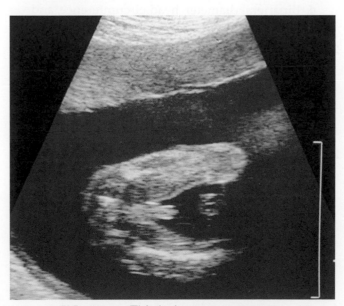

FIG. 25.4 Third trimester sonogram.

21. The fluid volume in this image is suspicious for:
    a. polyhydramnios
    b. oligohydramnios
    c. neural tube defects
    d. chromosomal anomalies

22. Which of the following is not an indication for a third trimester ultrasound?
    a. fetal growth
    b. fetal gender
    c. fetal viability
    d. fetal presentation

23. Comparison of the abdominal circumference to the head circumference during the early third trimester demonstrates a(n):
    a. equal head circumference compared with abdominal circumference
    b. abdominal circumference twice as large as the head circumference
    c. head circumference slightly larger than the abdominal circumference
    d. abdominal circumference slightly larger than the head circumference

24. Asymmetrical intrauterine growth restriction is usually a result of:
    a. preeclampsia
    b. gestational diabetes
    c. multifetal gestations
    d. placental insufficiency

25. Estimated fetal weight is most commonly calculated using which of the following biometric parameters?
    a. femur length and abdominal circumference
    b. abdominal circumference, femur length, and biparietal diameter
    c. head circumference, abdominal circumference, and femur length
    d. biparietal diameter, head circumference, and abdominal circumference

26. Intrauterine growth restriction most severely affects which fetal body organ?
    a. heart
    b. liver
    c. brain
    d. kidney

27. Assessing the total amount of amniotic fluid within the gestational sac using the sum of four equal quadrants is termed:
    a. pocket index
    b. total uterine volume
    c. amniotic fluid index
    d. amniotic fluid volume

28. The single most sensitive indicator of intrauterine growth restriction is:
    a. femur length
    b. head circumference
    c. abdominal circumference
    d. head circumference-to-abdominal circumference ratio

29. Which of the following conditions increases fetal risk of injury during vaginal delivery?
    a. macrosomia
    b. cephalic presentation
    c. lateral placental placement
    d. intrauterine growth restriction

30. Which technique is both valid and reproducible when assessing amniotic fluid volume?
    a. uterine volume
    b. amniotic fluid index
    c. single vertical pocket
    d. subjective assessment

31. Which of the following produces and removes amniotic fluid?
    a. kidneys
    b. placenta
    c. umbilical cord
    d. gastrointestinal tract

32. A biophysical profile examination of a 35-week fetus demonstrates a complete extension and flexion of lower extremities, four separate fetal movements, amniotic fluid volume of 10 cm, and a normal stress test. Fetal diaphragm or breathing motion is not identified. On the basis of these sonographic findings, the biophysical profile score would be:
    a. 2
    b. 5
    c. 8
    d. 10

33. The primary source of amniotic fluid removal is through the:
    a. liver
    b. kidneys
    c. bladder
    d. gastrointestinal tract

34. Which of the following correctly describes the expected sonographic findings with asymmetrical intrauterine growth restriction?
    a. decrease in head circumference and femur length
    b. decrease in abdominal circumference and femur length
    c. normal head circumference and decrease in abdominal circumference
    d. normal abdominal circumference and decrease in head circumference

35. Intrauterine growth restriction is defined as a fetal weight:
 a. below the 5th percentile for gestational age
 b. below the 10th percentile for gestational age
 c. at or below the 5th percentile for gestational age
 d. at or below the 10th percentile for gestational age

36. The best diagnostic accuracy of intrauterine growth restriction is offered when evaluating the:
 a. amniotic fluid volume, head circumference, and abdominal circumference
 b. placental maturity, umbilical artery, and amniotic fluid volume
 c. cephalic index, abdominal circumference, and placental maturity
 d. amniotic fluid volume, estimated fetal weight, and maternal blood pressure

37. A transverse fetal position in the late third trimester of pregnancy is most likely associated with:
 a. macrosomia
 b. placenta previa
 c. polyhydramnios
 d. intrauterine growth restriction

38. Which of the following fetal positions is at most risk for cord prolapse?
 a. oblique
 b. transverse
 c. frank breech
 d. incomplete breech

39. The biophysical profile is a sonographic method of evaluating fetal:
 a. weight
 b. movement
 c. well-being
 d. swallowing

40. Which of the following should be assessed in a fetus presenting with a genitourinary abnormality?
 a. fetal heart
 b. fetal growth
 c. fetal presentation
 d. amniotic fluid volume

41. Which of the following maternal conditions is most likely to result in a growth-restricted fetus?
 a. obesity
 b. diabetes
 c. drug abuse
 d. hypotension

42. Interval fetal growth can be determined with sonographic examinations performed a minimum of how many weeks apart?
 a. 1
 b. 3
 c. 5
 d. 7

43. Which of the following is *not* a function of the amniotic fluid?
 a. protects fetus from injury
 b. allows free fetal movement
 c. stores protein, calcium, and iron
 d. maintains intrauterine temperature

44. Which of the following is a sonographic finding in cases of asymmetrical intrauterine growth restriction?
 a. polyhydramnios
 b. short femur length
 c. normal biparietal diameter
 d. normal abdominal circumference

45. The primary source of amniotic fluid production is through the
 a. lungs
 b. kidneys
 c. umbilical cord
 d. amniotic membrane

46. The single most useful biometric parameter to assess fetal growth is the:
 a. femur length
 b. biparietal diameter
 c. head circumference
 d. abdominal circumference

47. The following term indicates that the fetal head is located in the uterine fundus:
 a. vertex
 b. breech
 c. oblique
 d. cephalic

48. A fetus presenting in the breech position during the third trimester may demonstrate a cranial shape that is termed:
 a. lemon sign
 b. dolichocephalic
 c. brachycephalic
 d. strawberry sign

49. If a fetus is lying perpendicular to the maternal sagittal plane, the fetal presentation is:
 a. vertex
 b. breech
 c. oblique
 d. transverse

50. Visualization of the proximal tibial epiphysis first occurs around:
 a. 24 weeks' gestation
 b. 28 weeks' gestation
 c. 32 weeks' gestation
 d. 35 weeks' gestation

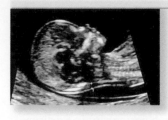

CHAPTER 26

Fetal Abnormalities

KEY TERMS

acromelia   shortening of the bones of the hands or feet.

aqueduct of Sylvius   a channel between the third and fourth ventricles of the brain.

banana sign   crescent shape to the cerebellum displayed with a coexisting neural tube defect.

corpus callosum   band of white matter tissue connecting the cerebral hemispheres; serves a function in both learning and memory.

Foramen of Monro   lies at the junction between the third ventricle and the paired lateral ventricles of the brain.

frontal bossing   protrusion or bulging of the forehead associated with hydrocephalus.

hydrocephalus   overt enlargement of the lateral ventricles secondary to an increase in intracranial pressure.

hypertelorism   abnormally widespread position of the orbits.

hypotelorism   abnormally close position of the orbits.

keyhole sign   appearance of the dilated bladder superior to the obstructed male urethra.

lemon sign   concavity to the front bones of the fetal cranium; associated with spina bifida.

macroglossia   an excessively large tongue.

mesomelia   shortening of the middle portion of a limb.

micromelia   shortening of all portions of a limb.

myelomeningocele   a developmental defect of the central nervous system in which a hernial sac containing a portion of the spinal cord, its meninges, and cerebrospinal fluid protrudes through a congenital cleft in the vertebral column.

nuchal thickness   distance between the calvaria and posterior skin line.

proboscis   protrusion of nasal tissue above the orbits.

rhizomelia   shortening of the proximal portion of a limb.

steer sign   enlargement and upper displacement of the third ventricle associated with agenesis of the corpus callosum.

ventriculomegaly   ventricular enlargement characterized by excessive cerebrospinal fluid within the ventricles.

vermis   structure located between the hemispheres of the cerebellum.

Cranial Abnormalities

ABNORMALITY	INFORMATION	SONOGRAPHIC FINDINGS	DIFFERENTIAL CONSIDERATIONS
Acrania	Abnormal migration of mesenchymal tissues Skull is absent Brain is present Elevated alpha-fetoprotein levels Coexisting spinal defects, clubfoot, cleft lip, and palate	Lack of hyperechoic bony calvaria Brain tissue development Prominent sulcal markings	Anencephaly Osteogenesis imperfecta
Agenesis of the corpus callosum	Failure of callosal fibers to form a normal connection May be partial or complete Associated with multiple anomalies	Dilation and elevation of the third ventricle Outward angling and wide separation of the frontal horns of the lateral ventricles (steer sign) Disproportionate enlargement of the occipital horns (colpocephaly) Absent cavum septum pellucidi	Holoprosencephaly

Cranial Abnormalities—(cont'd)

ABNORMALITY	INFORMATION	SONOGRAPHIC FINDINGS	DIFFERENTIAL CONSIDERATIONS
Arachnoid cyst	Congenital abnormality of the pia-arachnoid layer A result of trauma, infarction, or infection	Splaying of cerebellum hemispheres Normal vermis	Dandy-Walker cyst Prominent cisterna magna Vein of Galen aneurysm Improper technique
Arnold-Chiari type II malformation	Displacement of the cerebellar vermis, fourth ventricle, medulla oblongata through foramen of magna into the upper cervical canal	Compressed shape to the cerebellum (banana sign) Obliteration of the cisterna magna Ventriculomegaly Lemon-shaped cranium	Spina bifida
Dandy-Walker syndrome	Congenital malformation of the cerebellum with associated maldevelopment of the fourth ventricle Result of alcohol abuse, autosomal recessive disorder, or viral infection	Enlarged posterior fossa Splaying of the cerebellar hemispheres Complete or partial agenesis of the vermis Cisterna magna >1.0 cm in diameter Ventriculomegaly Enlarged fourth ventricle	Prominent posterior fossa Arachnoid cyst Vein of Galen aneurysm Artifact
Hydranencephaly	Destruction of the cerebral cortex resulting from vascular compromise or congenital infection (usually carotid area) Brain tissue is replaced by cerebrospinal fluid	Anechoic brain tissue Not associated with other abnormalities Presence of the falx cerebri Brainstem usually spared Choroid plexus may be displaced Variable presence of the third ventricle	Severe hydrocephalus Holoprosencephaly
Hydrocephalus (ventriculomegaly)	Increase in ventricular volume caused by outflow obstruction, decrease in cerebrospinal fluid (CSP) production, or overproduction of CSP Occipital horn dilates first	Ventriculomegaly is generally symmetrical **Mild Enlargement** Lateral ventricle measuring 10–15 mm **Severe Enlargement** Lateral ventricle measuring >15 mm Dangling of the choroid plexus Echogenic rim of solid brain tissue	Hydranencephaly Holoprosencephaly Improper technique
Holoprosencephaly	Group of disorders arising from abnormal development of the forebrain Strongly associated with Trisomy 13 **Alobar** Monoventricular cavity Most severe form **Semilobar** Monoventricular cavity Milder form **Lobar** Two large lateral ventricles Mildest form	**Alobar** Large central single ventricle Fused thalami Absence of cavum septum pellucidi, falx cerebri, corpus callosum, and third ventricle Normal cerebellum Hypotelorism Cyclopia Proboscis **Semilobar** Large central single ventricle Occipital and temporal horns may be present Variable development of the falx and interhemispheric fissure Associated with cleft lip and palate **Lobar** Two large lateral ventricles Absent cavum septum pellucid, and corpus callosum	Severe hydrocephalus Hydranencephaly

Continued

Cranial Abnormalities—(cont'd)

ABNORMALITY	INFORMATION	SONOGRAPHIC FINDINGS	DIFFERENTIAL CONSIDERATIONS
Lemon shape	May be a normal finding Associated with spina bifida	Bilateral indentation of the frontal bones	Dolichocephaly
Microcephaly	Overall reduction in brain size Chromosomal aberration Intrauterine infection Difficult to detect before 24 weeks	Small biparietal diameter (BPD) Small head circumference (HC) measuring more than 3 SD below normal Decreased HC/abdominal circumference (AC) ratio Sloping forehead	Anencephaly Encephalocele
Prosencephaly	A result of infarction or hemorrhage of the brain	Anechoic mass within an area of brain tissue Midline brain shift	Cystic leukomalacia
Strawberry shape	Associated with Trisomy 18	Flattened occiput diameter and narrowing of the frontal portion of the skull	Brachycephaly
Vein of Galen aneurysm	Cerebral arteriovenous malformation (AVM) Vein of Galen becomes dilated due to increased flow from the malformation Associated with cardiomegaly, ventriculomegaly, and nonimmune hydrops	Single fluid space close to midline (dilated veins) Variable in shape Turbulent vascular flow within associated AVM	Prominent or dilated third ventricle Agenesis of the corpus callosum

Neural Tube Defect

DEFECT	INFORMATION	SONOGRAPHIC FINDINGS	DIFFERENTIAL CONSIDERATIONS
Anencephaly	Failure of the cephalic end of the neural tube to close completely Portions of the midbrain and brainstem may be present Most common neural tube defect Elevated alpha-fetoprotein (AFP) levels Associated with malformations of the spine, face, feet, and abdominal wall	Absence of the cranial vault Bulging eyes (froglike face) Rudimentary brain tissue herniating from the defect Macroglossia Polyhydramnios Increase in fetal activity	Severe microcephaly Acrania Encephalocele Amniotic band syndrome
Caudal regression	Structural abnormality of the caudal end of the neural tube More common in patients with diabetes Associated with genitourinary, gastrointestinal, neural tube, and cardiovascular abnormalities	Absent sacrum Fused pelvis Short femurs	Skeletal dysplasia
Encephalocele	Normal AFP level Defect in the bony calvarium allows herniation of intracranial contents (brain tissue and cerebral spinal fluid) More commonly arises in the occipital region	Spherical fluid-filled or complex mass extending from the calvaria Bony calvarial defect	Cystic hygroma Cloverleaf skull deformity Amniotic band syndrome Microcephaly

Neural Tube Defect—(cont'd)

DEFECT	INFORMATION	SONOGRAPHIC FINDINGS	DIFFERENTIAL CONSIDERATIONS
Spina bifida	Failure of the neural tube to close completely **Occulta** Defect is covered by normal soft tissue Normal AFP level **Aperta** Defect is uncovered Elevated AFP level Associated with cleft lip and palate, cardiac defects, encephalocele, gastrointestinal anomalies, and clubfoot	**Coronal** Disappearance of the middle hyperechoic line Widening of the external hyperechoic lines **Sagittal** Posterior hyperechoic line and overlying soft tissues are absent **Transverse** Outward splaying of the lateral posterior ossification centers into a "U" or "V" shape Cystic or complex mass protruding from spinal defect Cerebellum takes on a crescent shape (banana sign) Frontal bones of the cranium are concave (lemon shaped)	Sacrococcygeal teratoma

Facial Abnormalities

ABNORMALITY	INFORMATION	SONOGRAPHIC FINDINGS	DIFFERENTIAL CONSIDERATIONS
Anophthalmia	Lack of fusion of the maxillary prominences with the nasal prominence on one or both sides Failure of the optic vesicle to form Associated with Goldenhar-Gorlin syndrome when unilateral	Absence of the globe or often the orbit Documented best on the transaxial view at the level of the orbits Important to document the presence of the ocular lens bilaterally	Poor fetal position Technical error
Cyclopia	Midline fusion of the orbits Associated with holoprosencephaly, cytomeglovirus, Trisomy 13, microcephaly, Williams syndrome	Single midline orbit Proboscis	Poor fetal position Technical error
Facial cleft	Failed fusion of the maxilla, primary and secondary palates Defect of the upper lip and palate Two thirds of cases include cleft palate Most common facial abnormality	Anechoic defect (gap) between the upper lip and nostrils Documented best on the coronal view Polyhydramnios Small stomach	Technical error
Hypotelorism	Orbits placed closer together than expected Most commonly associated with holoprosencephaly Also associated with Trisomy 13, microcephaly, and Williams syndrome	Abnormally small interocular distance for gestational age Documented best on the transaxial view slightly below the level of the BPD	Poor fetal position Technical error
Hypertelorism	Orbits placed wider apart than expected Associated with Trisomy 18, Noonan syndrome, Median cleft syndrome, craniosynostosis, and anterior cephalocele	Abnormally wide interocular distance for gestational age Documented best on the transaxial view slightly below the level of the BPD	Poor fetal position Technical error

Continued

Facial Abnormalities—(cont'd)

ABNORMALITY	INFORMATION	SONOGRAPHIC FINDINGS	DIFFERENTIAL CONSIDERATIONS
Macroglossia	Associated with Beckwith-Wiedemann and Down syndromes Persistent protrusion of the tongue	Persistent protrusion of the fetal tongue Documented best on the sagittal profile view Polyhydramnios	Normal tongue Umbilical cord
Micrognathia	Hypoplastic mandible Associated with Trisomy 18	Small receding chin and lower lip Documented best on the sagittal profile view Polyhydramnios Protrusion of the upper lip	Technical error Normal chin

Neck Abnormalities

ABNORMALITY	INFORMATION	SONOGRAPHIC FINDINGS	DIFFERENTIAL CONSIDERATIONS
Cystic hygroma	Developmental defect of the lymphatic system Associated with chromosomal abnormalities, fetal hydrops, and fetal heart failure	Thin-walled multiseptated cystic mass in the neck, axilla, or mediastinum No cranial defect Continuous with abnormal skin and subcutaneous tissues	Encephalocele Cystic teratoma Normal umbilical cord Pocket of amniotic fluid Nuchal edema
Nuchal edema	Thickening of the nuchal fold Associated with chromosomal abnormalities	Anechoic posterior cervical mass Midline septum	Cystic hygroma

Chest Abnormalities

ABNORMALITY	INFORMATION	SONOGRAPHIC FINDINGS	DIFFERENTIAL CONSIDERATIONS
Cystic adenomatoid malformation	Abnormal formation of the bronchial tree Replacement of normal pulmonary tissues with cysts May be associated with renal or gastrointestinal abnormalities	Simple or multiloculated cystic chest mass Mediastinal shift Diaphragm is visible and intact Fetal hydrops Polyhydramnios Usually unilateral	Diaphragmatic hernia Pleural effusion Pericardial fluid
Ectopia cordis	Partial or complete displacement of the heart outside of the thorax Associated with intracardiac anomalies and omphalocele	Small thorax Heart located outside of the thorax Extrathoracic pulsating mass	Acardiac twin Diaphragmatic hernia
Ebstein anomaly	Displacement of the septal and posterior leaflets of the tricuspid valves into the right ventricle Variable in degree Associated with maternal use of lithium	Visualized on the four-chamber heart Enlargement of the heart (especially right atrium) Regurgitation across the tricuspid valve with color and spectral Doppler Can be difficult to see if a mild form	Tetralogy of Fallot Ventricular septal defect

Chest Abnormalities—(cont'd)

ABNORMALITY	INFORMATION	SONOGRAPHIC FINDINGS	DIFFERENTIAL CONSIDERATIONS
Diaphragmatic hernia	Diaphragm fails to close allowing herniation of the abdominal cavity contents Associated with cardiac, renal, chromosomal, and central nervous system anomalies Two Forms **Bochdalek hernia** Posterolateral diaphragm defect Most common **Morgagni's hernia** Anterior diaphragm defect Rare	Stomach or liver located in the thorax Inability to visualize normal diaphragm Mediastinal shift Small abdominal circumference Polyhydramnios Usually unilateral Left-sided defect more common	Cystic adenomatoid malformation
Pleural effusion	Most commonly a malformation of the thoracic duct Associated with hydrops, infection, Turner syndrome, and chromosomal and cardiac abnormalities	Anechoic fluid collection in the fetal chest Fluid contours to surrounding lung and diaphragm Lung tissue appears echogenic	Diaphragmatic hernia Fetal hydrops
Tetralogy of Fallot	Most common form of cyanotic heart disease **Criteria** Subaortic ventricular septal defect Aortic valve overriding the defect Pulmonic stenosis Hypertrophy of the right ventricle in the third trimester	Four-chamber view can appear normal Ventricular septal defect Increase rotation of the heart Overriding aorta Ascending aorta will appear larger than pulmonary artery	Ebstein anomaly
Transposition of the great vessels	Aorta arises from the right ventricle and the pulmonary arteries arise from the left ventricle	Normal four-chamber view Two great vessels do not crisscross but arise parallel from the base of the heart	Technical error

Abnormalities of the Gastrointestinal Tract

ABNORMALITY	INFORMATION	SONOGRAPHIC FINDINGS	DIFFERENTIAL CONSIDERATIONS
Bowel atresia	Obstruction usually occurring in the inferior small bowel May be associated with meconium ileus and cystic fibrosis	Multiple anechoic structures within the fetal abdomen Polyhydramnios	Normal prominent loops of bowel Multicystic kidney
Duodenal atresia	Blockage of the duodenum usually near the ampulla of Vater Normal alpha-fetoprotein (AFP) level Associated with Trisomy 21, cardiac, urinary, and GI anomalies	Dilated stomach and proximal duodenum (double bubble) Polyhydramnios Not evident until after 20 weeks' gestation	Normal fluid-filled stomach Fluid-filled loop of bowel
Esophageal atresia	Congenital malformation of the foregut Associated with tracheoesophageal fistula (90%)	Absence of stomach Small stomach on serial examinations Possible polyhydramnios Polyhydramnios with intrauterine growth restriction	Normal esophagus

Continued

Abnormalities of the Gastrointestinal Tract—(cont'd)

ABNORMALITY	INFORMATION	SONOGRAPHIC FINDINGS	DIFFERENTIAL CONSIDERATIONS
Echogenic bowel	Associated with cystic fibrosis, intraamniotic hemorrhage, congenital infection, intrauterine growth restriction, and chromosomal abnormalities If isolated, normal fetal outcome	Echogenicity of the bowel is equal to bone	Meconium ileus
Meconium ileus	Impaction of thick meconium in the distal ileum Frequently associated with cystic fibrosis	Dilated ileum Ileum filled with echogenic material Colon is small and empty	Normal echogenic bowel
Meconium peritonitis	Bowel perforation caused by bowel atresia or meconium ileus	Abdominal calcification Bowel dilation Polyhydramnios	Gallstone Splenic calcification Congenital infection Hepatic necrosis

Abnormalities of the Genitourinary System

ABNORMALITY	INFORMATION	SONOGRAPHIC FINDINGS	DIFFERENTIAL CONSIDERATIONS
Extrophy of the bladder	Externalization of the bladder onto the anterior abdominal wall Also known as ectopia vesicae Caused by incomplete closure of the inferior part of the anterior abdominal wall Male prevalence	Cystic mass located in the inferior anterior abdominal wall Wide separation of the pubic bones Normal kidneys Normal amniotic fluid volume Low cord insertion Undescended testes or cleft clitoris	Umbilical cord Umbilical cord cyst
Hydronephrosis	Urinary tract obstruction	Pelviectasis ≥10 mm Ratio of the renal pelvis diameter to the anterior–posterior renal diameter >50%	Prominent renal pelvis Renal cyst
Infantile polycystic disease	Bilateral renal disease Autosomal recessive Lethal condition	Hyperechoic enlarged kidneys Extreme oligohydramnios No visible or small fetal bladder	Hyperechoic bowel Premature rupture of membranes
Multicystic dysplastic kidney	Kidney tissue is replaced by cysts Additional renal anomalies occur in up to 40% of cases	Renal tissue is replaced by noncommunicating multiple cysts Variable size Usually unilateral	Fluid-filled bowel loops Hydronephrosis
Posterior urethral valve obstruction	Occurs in males Presence of a membrane within the posterior urethra Urine is unable to pass through the urethra Results in overdistention of the urinary bladder Can cause severe damage to kidneys, ureters, and bladder	Dilated bladder Dilated posterior urethra (keyhole) Hydroureter Hydronephrosis Oligohydramnios	Normal fetal bladder Ureterovesical obstruction
Renal agenesis	Absence of one or both kidneys Pulmonary hypoplasia secondary to oligohydramnios Adrenal gland(s) may mimic kidneys Associated with facial anomalies	**Unilateral Agenesis** Absence of one kidney Enlarged contralateral kidney Fetal bladder visualized Normal amniotic fluid volume **Bilateral Agenesis** Absence of both kidneys No evidence of fetal bladder Severe oligohydramnios (noted after 16 weeks' gestation)	Infantile polycystic renal disease

Abnormalities of the Genitourinary System—(cont'd)

ABNORMALITY	INFORMATION	SONOGRAPHIC FINDINGS	DIFFERENTIAL CONSIDERATIONS
Renal cyst	Rare finding	Anechoic renal mass Round or oval Smooth, thin wall margins Posterior acoustic enhancement	Hydronephrosis Multicystic dysplastic kidney
Ureteropelvic junction obstruction (most common)	Obstruction between the renal pelvis and proximal ureter Results from an abnormal bend or kink in the ureter Male prevalence	Hydronephrosis Normal fetal bladder Normal amniotic fluid volume level Unilateral	Renal cyst Loop of bowel
Ureterovesical junction obstruction	Results from a urethral defect Ureterocele Ureter stenosis	Dilated renal pelvis and ureter (megaureter) Tortuous ureter Possible hydronephrosis secondary to distal obstruction Normal amniotic fluid volume when unilateral	Ureteropelvic junction obstruction Loop of bowel
Wilms' tumor (nephroblastoma)	Malignant mass	Echogenic solid renal mass	Adrenal hemorrhage

Fetal Body Wall Abnormalities

ABNORMALITY	INFORMATION	SONOGRAPHIC FINDINGS	DIFFERENTIAL CONSIDERATIONS
Gastroschisis	Defect involves all layers of the abdominal wall Markedly elevated alpha-fetoprotein (AFP) levels Not associated with chromosomal abnormalities Higher incidence in women younger than 20 years of age	Paraumbilical wall defect Typically to the right of a normal umbilical cord insertion Normal cord insertion Free-floating herniated small bowel within the amniotic cavity (no membranous sac) Bowel loops may appear thick and dilated Normal to low amniotic fluid volume	Ruptured omphalocele Normal umbilical cord
Omphalocele	Midline defect covered by the amnion and peritoneum Normal or elevated AFP level Associated with cardiac, genitourinary, gastrointestinal, central nervous system anomalies and chromosomal abnormalities Fetus with sac containing only bowel are at higher risk for chromosomal abnormalities	Midline anterior abdominal wall mass Membranous sac containing herniated viscera Umbilical cord enters mass	Umbilical hernia Fetal position

Continued

Fetal Body Wall Abnormalities—(cont'd)

ABNORMALITY	INFORMATION	SONOGRAPHIC FINDINGS	DIFFERENTIAL CONSIDERATIONS
Sacrococcygeal teratoma	Benign neoplasm protruding from the posterior wall of the sacrum and may extend into the pelvis and abdomen **Four Types** 1. Predominately external, with minimal presacral component 2. Predominantly external, with significant intrapelvic component 3. Predominantly internal, with abdominal extension 4. Entirely internal, with no external component Possible increase in AFP level Female prevalence (4:1)	Solid or complex mass protruding from the fetal rump Calcifications (bone fragments) Normal spine Bladder displacement Hydronephrosis Polyhydramnios	Myelomeningocele
Umbilical hernia	Less serious than omphalocele	Small anterior abdominal wall defect Normal cord insertion Typically contains peritoneum Rarely contains omentum or bowel	Omphalocele Fetal position

Skeletal Abnormalities

- Femur length 2 standard deviations below the mean for gestational age raises concern for a skeletal dysplasia or intrauterine growth restriction.

ABNORMALITY	INFORMATION	SONOGRAPHIC FINDINGS	DIFFERENTIAL CONSIDERATIONS
Achondrogenesis	Failure of the ossification process Lethal short limb dysplasia **Type I (Parenti – Fraccaro)** Autosomal recessive 20% of cases Thin ribs **Type II (Langer – Saldino)** Autosomal dominant 80% of cases Ribs appear thicker	Severe micromelia Bowing of long bones Short trunk Protruding abdomen and forehead Poor vertebral and cranial ossifications Small pelvis	Achondroplasia Osteogenesis imperfecta
Achondroplasia	Abnormal cartilage deposits at the long bone epiphysis Most common form of skeletal dysplasia Autosomal dominant	Macrocrania Micromelia Frontal bossing Depressed nasal ridge Hypoplastic thorax Ventriculomegaly	Achondrogenesis Osteogenesis imperfecta
Clubfoot	Developmental defect Abnormal relationship of the tarsal bones and the calcaneus 55% of cases are bilateral Polynesian and Middle Eastern descent prevalence	Forefoot is oriented in the same plane as the lower leg Persistent abnormal inversion of the foot at an angle perpendicular to the lower leg	Normal mobility of the fetal foot

Skeletal Abnormalities—(cont'd)

ABNORMALITY	INFORMATION	SONOGRAPHIC FINDINGS	DIFFERENTIAL CONSIDERATIONS
Osteogenesis imperfecta	Disorder of collagen production leading to brittle bones Types I–IV Type II is most lethal Before 24 weeks, demineralization of the bone or abnormal limb length or shape may not yet be apparent	**Type I** Bowing of long bones May demonstrate fractures Thick bones having a wrinkled appearance Head is of normal size **Type II (Most Severe)** Hypomineralization Significant bone shortening Narrow bell-shaped chest Multiple fractures of long bones, ribs, and spine Thin cranium **Type III** Occasional rib fractures Thin cranium Mild leg bowing **Type IV (Mildest)** Bowing of limbs Occasional rib and limb fractures Head is of normal size	Achondroplasia Achondrogenesis
Rocker bottom foot	Trisomy 18 Other chromosomal abnormalities Fetal syndromes	Prominent heel Convex sole	Normal foot
Thanatophoric dysplasia	Lethal skeletal dysplasia Male dominance	Severe rhizomelia Micromelia Bowing of limbs Cloverleaf skull deformity Macrocephaly Frontal bossing Depressed nasal bridge Hypertelorism Ventriculomegaly Thick soft tissue Narrow, bell-shaped chest Protuberant abdomen Narrow spinal canal Short fingers Polyhydramnios	Achondroplasia Osteogenesis imperfecta

FETAL ABNORMALITIES REVIEW

1. Ebstein anomaly is associated with a
   a. gastrointestinal anomaly
   b. cardiovascular anomaly
   c. genitourinary anomaly
   d. central nervous system anomaly

2. Demonstration of multiple unilateral renal cysts is most suspicious for:
   a. infantile polycystic disease
   b. multicystic dysplastic kidney
   c. cystic adenomatoid malformation
   d. ureteropelvic junction obstruction

3. "Double bubble" is a sonographic sign associated with:
   a. spina bifida
   b. hydronephrosis
   c. duodenal atresia
   d. esophageal atresia

4. Which of the following sonographic findings helps to differentiate Dandy-Walker syndrome from an arachnoid cyst?
   a. ventriculomegaly
   b. presence of a normal vermis
   c. absence of the third ventricle
   d. splaying of the cerebellar hemispheres

5. Dilation of the third ventricle is a sonographic finding associated with:
   a. anencephaly
   b. prosencephaly
   c. holoprosencephaly
   d. agenesis of the corpus callosum

6. Maternal alpha-fetoprotein levels in a pregnancy with gastroschisis will:
   a. markedly increase
   b. mildly increase
   c. remain normal
   d. mildly decrease

7. Which skeletal abnormality is most likely to demonstrate a cloverleaf skull?
   a. achondroplasia
   b. achondrogenesis
   c. osteogenesis imperfecta
   d. thanatophoric dysplasia

8. A crescent-shaped appearance to the cerebellum should signal the sonographer to give additional attention to which of the following fetal structures?
   a. heart
   b. lungs
   c. spine
   d. abdominal wall

9. Peritoneal calcifications with associated dilated loops of bowel and polyhydramnios visualized in a 30-week fetus most likely represent:
   a. intussusception
   b. arteriosclerosis
   c. hyperechoic bowel
   d. meconium peritonitis

10. Which of the following abnormalities is the most common neural tube defect?
    a. spina bifida
    b. anencephaly
    c. encephalocele
    d. cystic hygroma

11. Which of the following conditions is most likely associated with frontal bossing?
    a. anencephaly
    b. encephalocele
    c. hydrocephalus
    d. caudal regression

12. Which of the following abnormalities demonstrates a cranial defect?
    a. encephalocele
    b. cystic hygroma
    c. holoprosencephaly
    d. agenesis of the corpus callosum

13. Which of the following is a common sonographic finding with fetal facial abnormalities?
    a. duodenal atresia
    b. polyhydramnios
    c. diaphragmatic hernia
    d. ventricular septal defect

14. Demonstration of fetal bone fractures raises suspicion for which skeletal abnormality?
    a. achondroplasia
    b. achondrogenesis
    c. thanatophoric dysplasia
    d. osteogenesis imperfecta

15. A large single ventricular cavity is most suspicious for:
    a. microcephaly
    b. macrocephaly
    c. holoprosencephaly
    d. agenesis of the corpus callosum

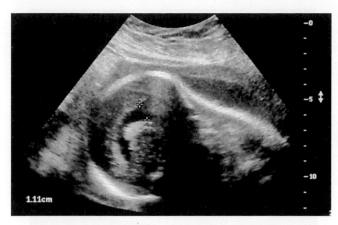

FIG. 26.1

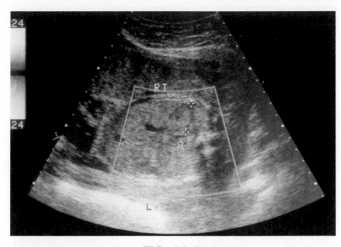

FIG. 26.3

Using Figure 26.1, answer question 16.

16. The sonographic finding in this image is most suspicious for:
    a. hydranencephaly
    b. ventriculomegaly
    c. holoprosencephaly
    d. agenesis of the corpus callosum

Using Figure 26.2, answer questions 17 and 18.

17. A sagittal image of the fetal body is most suspicious for:
    a. fetal demise
    b. chorioangioma
    c. myelomeningocele
    d. sacrococcygeal teratoma

18. Associated findings with this abnormality include:
    a. spinal defect
    b. cranial defect
    c. hydronephrosis
    d. polyhydramnios

Using Figure 26.3, answer questions 19 and 20.

19. During a late second-trimester screening examination, what does this image of the fetal abdomen most likely show:
    a. renal agenesis
    b. multicystic dysplasia
    c. infantile polycystic disease
    d. bilateral adrenal hemorrhage

20. Which of the following conditions will likely occur because of this abnormality?
    a. fetal hypoxia
    b. placentomegaly
    c. polyhydramnios
    d. oligohydramnios

Using Figure 26.4, answer question 21.

21. This sagittal image of the fetal abdomen most likely demonstrates:
    a. renal cyst
    b. hydronephrosis
    c. duodenal atresia
    d. diaphragmatic hernia

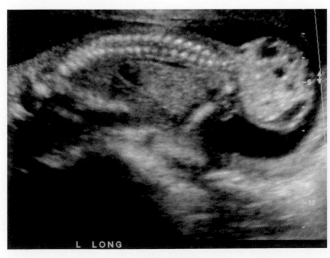

FIG. 26.2

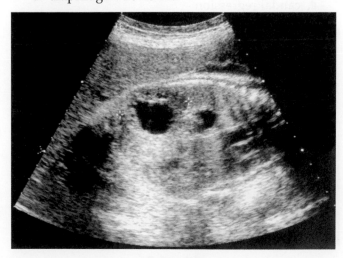

FIG. 26.4

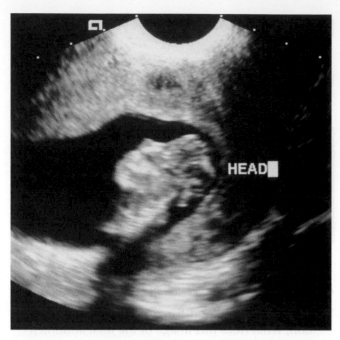

FIG. 26.5

Using Figure 26.5, answer question 22.

22. A patient arrives for an early second-trimester sonogram for gestational dating. An endovaginal image demonstrates a fetal abnormality that is *most* suspicious for:
   a. acrania
   b. anencephaly
   c. encephalocele
   d. holoprosencephaly

Using Figure 26.6, answer question 23.

23. This sagittal image of the lower spine is most suspicious for:
   a. spina bifida
   b. umbilical cord
   c. cystic hygroma
   d. caudal regression

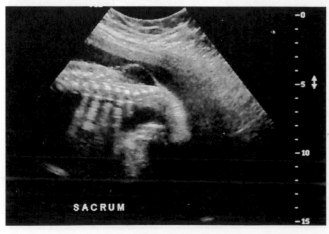

FIG. 26.6

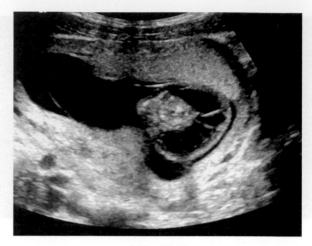

FIG. 26.7

Using Figure 26.7, answer questions 24 and 25.

24. What abnormality is most likely present in this image of the cranium?
   a. encephalocele
   b. nuchal edema
   c. cystic hygroma
   d. myelomeningocele

25. The etiology of this abnormality is typically:
   a. idiopathic
   b. Rh sensitivity
   c. autosomal recessive
   d. chromosomal

Using Figure 26.8, answer questions 26 and 27.

26. A patient presents for an ultrasound to determine gestational age. An image of this early second-trimester fetus is most suspicious for:
   a. acrania
   b. anencephaly
   c. microcephaly
   d. holoprosencephaly

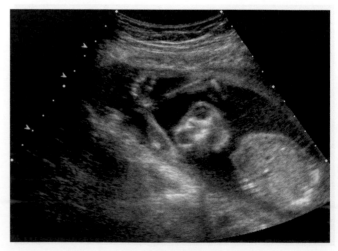

FIG. 26.8

27. Which of the following is most likely associated with this finding?
    a. fetal demise
    b. preeclampsia
    c. gestational diabetes
    d. elevated maternal alpha-fetoprotein

Using Figure 26.9, answer question 28.

28. This sagittal image of a second-trimester fetus is most suspicious for which of the following pathologies?
    a. pericardial effusion
    b. diaphragmatic hernia
    c. loculated pleural effusions
    d. cystic adenomatoid malformation

Using Figure 26.10, answer question 29.

29. This sonogram of an early second-trimester cranium is most suspicious for:
    a. hydrocephalus
    b. hydranencephaly
    c. holoprosencephaly
    d. agenesis of the corpus callosum

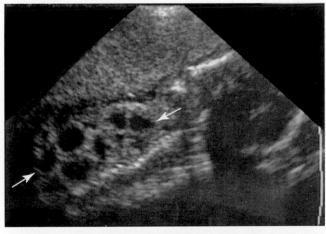

FIG. 26.9

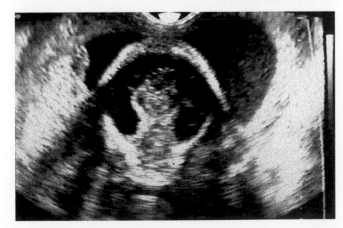

FIG. 26.10

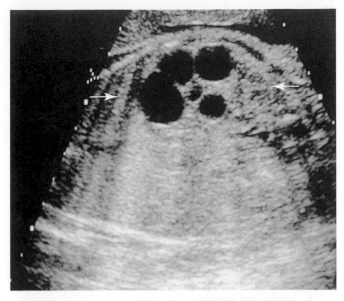

FIG. 26.11

Using Figure 26.11, answer question 30.

30. This oblique sonogram of the fetal abdomen most likely demonstrates:
    a. hydronephrosis
    b. duodenal atresia
    c. infantile polycystic disease
    d. multicystic dysplastic kidney

31. Lateral ventricular enlargement becomes ventriculomegaly after the diameter exceeds:
    a. 6 mm
    b. 8 mm
    c. 10 mm
    d. 12 mm

32. Caudal regression syndrome is more commonly found in patients with:
    a. proteinuria
    b. hypertension
    c. systemic lupus
    d. diabetes mellitus

33. Which of the following is the most common fetal neck mass?
    a. goiter
    b. hemangioma
    c. cystic hygroma
    d. myelomeningocele

34. Which of the following abnormalities is more commonly associated with proboscis?
    a. spina bifida
    b. ventriculomegaly
    c. holoprosencephaly
    d. diaphragmatic hernia

35. Which of the following abnormalities is *not* associated with pulmonary hypoplasia?
    a. duodenal atresia
    b. skeletal dysplasia
    c. diaphragmatic hernia
    d. infantile polycystic renal disease

36. A diagnosis of clubfoot may be made with persistent abnormal inversion of the:
    a. foot
    b. ankle
    c. foot parallel to the lower leg
    d. foot perpendicular to the lower leg

37. Opening in the layers of the abdominal wall with evisceration of the bowel describes which of the following abnormalities:
    a. gastroschisis
    b. omphalocele
    c. umbilical hernia
    d. intussusception

38. Which of the following is the most common *nonlethal* skeletal dysplasia?
    a. achondroplasia
    b. achondrogenesis
    c. diastrophic dysplasia
    d. thanatophoric dysplasia

39. Hydronephrosis in utero is most commonly caused by an obstruction:
    a. in the urethra
    b. in the distal ureter
    c. at the bladder inlet
    d. at the ureteropelvic junction

40. Herniated contents of an omphalocele are covered by a membrane consisting of:
    a. chorion and amnion
    b. amnion and peritoneum
    c. Wharton jelly and amnion
    d. peritoneum and Wharton jelly

41. The presence of a posterior fossa cyst and agenesis of the cerebellar vermis are characteristic findings of:
    a. arachnoid cyst
    b. holoprosencephaly
    c. Dandy-Walker malformation
    d. agenesis of the corpus callosum

42. Which of the following is *not* associated with hydrocephalus?
    a. spina bifida
    b. encephalocele
    c. myelomeningocele
    d. choroid plexus cysts

43. Anechoic regions within brain tissue are most suspicious for:
    a. arachnoid cyst
    b. hydranencephaly
    c. holoprosencephaly
    d. choroid plexus cysts

44. Outward angling of the frontal and lateral horn of the lateral ventricles is a sonographic finding in:
    a. ventriculomegaly
    b. hydranencephaly
    c. holoprosencephaly
    d. agenesis of the corpus callosum

45. The renal pelvis in a third-trimester fetus demonstrates an anterior–posterior diameter of 10 mm. This is considered:
    a. a megaureter
    b. mild hydronephrosis
    c. within normal limits
    d. moderate hydronephrosis

46. In the late second trimester, which sonographic finding consistently displays with renal agenesis?
    a. facial cleft
    b. omphalocele
    c. oligohydramnios
    d. skeletal dysplasia

47. The most common sonographic finding associated with multicystic renal dysplasia is:
    a. unilateral multicystic kidney
    b. bilateral multicystic kidneys
    c. unilateral enlarged hyperechoic kidney
    d. bilateral enlarged hyperechoic kidneys

48. Sonographic findings associated with osteogenesis imperfecta may not be apparent before:
    a. 12 weeks' gestation
    b. 18 weeks' gestation
    c. 24 weeks' gestation
    d. 28 weeks' gestation

49. Which classification of osteogenesis imperfecta is the most severe?
    a. type I
    b. type II
    c. type III
    d. type IV

50. A consistently small fetal stomach on serial sonograms is most suspicious for which abnormality?
    a. omphalocele
    b. duodenal atresia
    c. esophageal atresia
    d. diaphragmatic hernia

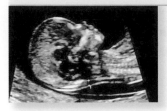

CHAPTER 27

Complications in Pregnancy

KEY TERMS

anasarca   severe generalized massive edema often seen with hydrops fetalis.

aneuploidy   the presence of an abnormal number of chromosomes and is almost always associated with abnormalities of physical and cognitive development.

clinodactyly   inward curving of the fifth finger associated with Down syndrome.

cubitus valgus   abnormal outward bending or twisting of the elbow.

eclampsia   gravest form of pregnancy-induced maternal hypertension characterized by seizures, coma, proteinuria, and edema.

ectopia cordis   a condition in which the ventral wall of the chest fails to close and the heart develops outside of the chest.

exencephaly   a condition where the skull is defective, causing exposure or extrusion of the brain.

fetus papyraceus   demise of a twin that is too large to reabsorb.

karyotype   picture of chromosomes and how they look structurally.

micrognathia   underdevelopment of the jaw, especially the mandible.

microphthalmia   abnormal smallness of one or both eyes.

polydactyly   congenital anomaly characterized by the presence of more than the normal number of digits.

preeclampsia   an abnormal condition characterized by the onset of acute hypertension after 24 weeks' gestation. Classic triad includes maternal edema, proteinuria, and hypertension.

premature rupture of membranes (PROM)   early rupture of the gestational sac with leakage of part or all of the amniotic fluid.

preterm labor   onset of labor before 37 weeks' gestation.

Rh disease   caused when the mother forms a corresponding antibody to the fetal blood, resulting in destruction of fetal red blood cells.

sandal toe deformity   increased distance between the first and second toes associated with Down syndrome.

Spalding sign   overlapping of the cranial bones associated with fetal demise.

syndactyly   congenital anomaly characterized by the fusion of the fingers or toes.

twin–twin transfusion syndrome (TTS)   the arterial blood of the donor twin pumps into the venous system of the receiving twin.

CHROMOSOMAL ABNORMALITIES

- Can be either numeric or structural.
- Occurs in approximately 0.9% of newborns.
- 95% of chromosomally abnormal conceptions are lost before term.

Chromosomal Abnormalities

ANOMALY	INFORMATION	SONOGRAPHIC FINDINGS ASSOCIATED WITH	DIFFERENTIAL CONSIDERATIONS

Edward syndrome	Trisomy 18
	80% of cases display a
	   clenched fist
	Decrease in alpha-fetoprotein
	   (AFP)
	1:8000 live births
	Overall poor prognosis
	95% spontaneously abort
	Female prevalence
		Cardiac defects
		Choroid plexus cysts
		Clenched hands
		Micrognathia
		Clubbed or rocker bottom feet
		Cleft lip and palate
		Renal anomalies
		Omphalocele
		Spina bifida
		Cystic hygroma
		Diaphragmatic hernia
		Two-vessel cord
		Intrauterine growth restriction (IUGR)
			Trisomy 13
			Triploidy

Continued

Chromosomal Abnormalities—(cont'd)

ANOMALY	INFORMATION	SONOGRAPHIC FINDINGS ASSOCIATED WITH	DIFFERENTIAL CONSIDERATIONS
Down syndrome	Trisomy 21 Most common Decrease in AFP levels 1:700 live births Coexisting anomalies dictate overall prognosis Approximately 30% of cases demonstrate duodenal atresia	Subtle anomalies Atrioventricular defect Ventricular septal defect Nuchal thickening Small or absent nasal bone Macroglossia Mild ventriculomegaly Duodenal atresia Pyelectasis Hyperechoic bowel Nonimmune hydrops Sandal toe deformity Clinodactyly Low-set ears Shorten limbs Femur length below the 10th percentile for gestational age Small humeral length	Beckwith-Wiedemann syndrome
Patau syndrome	Trisomy 13 90% of cases display cardiac defects Syndrome of midline defects 1:20,000 live births Overall poor prognosis Multiple anomalies, many involving the brain	Holoprosencephaly Microcephaly Cystic hygroma Absent or small eyes Facial clefts Cardiac defects Omphalocele Echogenic kidneys Diaphragmatic hernia Clubfoot Polydactyly IUGR Polyhydramnios	Meckel-Gruber syndrome
Triploidy	Three complete sets of chromosomes Most will abort spontaneously 1:5000 live births	Early onset IUGR Holoprosencephaly Hypertelorism Micrognathia Microphthalmia Ventriculomegaly Oligohydramnios 2 vessel cord Cardiac abnormalities Clubfeet Syndactyly	Trisomy 13 Trisomy 18
Turner syndrome	45 chromosomes, including a single X chromosome Elevated AFP levels Female fetus 1:5000 live births	Cystic hygroma Cardiac defects Renal anomalies Cubitus valgus Short femurs Nonimmune hydrops	Cephalocele Trisomy 13 Hydrops fetalis

FETAL SYNDROMES

- Demonstrate normal karyotype.
- *Malformation* refers to a defect of an organ that results from an intrinsically abnormal development process.
- *Deformation* refers to an abnormal form, shape, or position of a part caused by mechanical forces antenatally.
- *Disruption* is a defect of an organ resulting from the breakdown of previously normal tissue.
- *Sequence* refers to a pattern of multiple anomalies that result from a single anomaly or mechanical factor.

Fetal Syndromes

SYNDROME	INFORMATION	SONOGRAPHIC FINDINGS	DIFFERENTIAL CONSIDERATIONS
Amniotic band syndrome	Ruptured amnion sticks and entangles fetal parts Associated with fetal abnormalities and amputations	Thin hyperechoic linear structure floating within the amniotic cavity Fetal abnormalities	Synechia Amniotic chorionic separation Limb–body wall complex Placental shelf
Beckwith-Wiedemann syndrome	Classic triad of macrosomia, omphalocele, and macroglossia Normal karyotype Increases risk of developing Wilms' tumor, hemihypertrophy, renal anomalies, and hepatosplenomegaly	Hemihypertrophy Macroglossia Omphalocele	Down syndrome
Eagle-Barrett syndrome	Prune belly syndrome Hypotonic abdominal wall muscles Associated with dilated fetal bladder, small thorax, and imperforate anus	Hydronephrosis Megaureter Oligohydramnios Small thorax Large abdomen Cryptorchidism Hip dislocation Scoliosis	Urinary obstruction Urethral atresia
Limb-body wall complex	Rare complex malformation caused by the failure of closure of the ventral body wall Two or more of the following 　Limb defects 　Lateral wall defects (esp. left) 　Encephalocele 　Exencephaly 　Facial defects 　Scoliosis	Ventral wall defect Cranial anomalies Marked scoliosis Limb defects Short umbilical cord Amniotic bands	Amniotic band syndrome Trisomy 13
Meckel-Gruber syndrome	Lethal condition Occurs equally in males and females Autosomal recessive	Encephalocele Infantile polycystic kidneys Oligohydramnios Bladder not visualized Polydactyly	Trisomy 13 Infantile polycystic disease
Pentalogy of Cantrell	Congenital disorder characterized by two out of the following major defects 1. Cardiac defect 2. Abdominal wall defect 3. Diaphragmatic hernia 4. Defect of diaphragmatic pericardium 5. Ectopia cordis	Pulsating mass outside of the chest cavity Omphalocele Gastroschisis Diaphragmatic hernia	Beckwith-Wiedemann syndrome Acardiac twin

Continued

Fetal Syndromes—(cont'd)

SYNDROME	INFORMATION	SONOGRAPHIC FINDINGS	DIFFERENTIAL CONSIDERATIONS
VACTERL	Group of complex anomalies Associated with maternal diabetes and lead exposure	Vertebral defects Anal atresia Cardiac anomalies Transesophageal fistula Renal anomalies Limb anomalies Polyhydramnios Collapsed stomach	VATER Chromosomal abnormality
VATER	Group of complex anomalies Associated with maternal diabetes and lead exposure	Vertebral defects Anal atresia Tracheoesophageal fistula Renal anomalies Polyhydramnios Collapsed stomach	VACTERL Chromosomal abnormality

HYDROPS FETALIS

- An abnormal interstitial accumulation of fluid in the body cavities and soft tissues.
- Fluid accumulation may result in anasarca, ascites, pericardial effusion, pleural effusion, placentomegaly, and polyhydramnios.
- Hydrops may result from antibodies in the maternal circulation that destroy the fetal red blood cells (immune) or without evidence of blood group incompatibility (nonimmune).
- Sonography cannot differentiate immune from nonimmune hydrops.

Fetal Hydrops

HYDROPS	CLINICAL FINDINGS	SONOGRAPHIC FINDINGS	DIFFERENTIAL CONSIDERATIONS
Immune	Rh sensitivity	Scalp edema Pleural effusion Pericardial effusion Polyhydramnios Placentomegaly	Nonimmune hydrops Pleural effusion
Nonimmune	Large for dates	Anasarca Edema or fluid accumulation in at least two fetal sites Ascites Scalp edema Pleural effusion Pericardial effusion Polyhydramnios Placentomegaly Fetal tachycardia 200–240 bpm	Immune hydrops Pleural effusion

MULTIFETAL GESTATIONS

- 70% of pregnancies beginning with twins will deliver a singleton pregnancy.
- Monozygotic twins result from a single fertilized ovum.
- Dizygotic twins result from two separate ova.
- Majority of pregnancies are dizygotic.

- Dizygotic pregnancies are always dichorionic/diamniotic.
- Label each fetus with Twin A closest to the internal os.
- IUGR is the most common cause of discordant growth in a dichorionic multifetal gestation.
- Twin–twin transfusion syndrome is the most common cause of discordant growth in a monochorionic multifetal gestation.
- Abnormal growth.
  - 10% discrepancy in crown rump lengths.
  - 5 days or more difference in gestational age.
  - 20 mm or more difference in abdominal circumferences.

SONOGRAPHIC EVALUATION

- Number of embryos/fetuses.
- Presence or absence of dividing membrane(s).
- Number or placentas and locations.
- Biometric measurements.
- Fetal surveillance (same as singleton).
- Amniotic fluid volume.

Monozygotic Multifetal Gestations

TYPE	DESCRIPTION	SONOGRAPHIC FINDINGS	DIFFERENTIAL CONSIDERATIONS
Dichorionic/diamniotic (most common)	Zygote splits within 3–5 days of fertilization Four-layered membrane	Two or more individual gestational sacs and placentas Thick membrane with "V" shape called twin peak or lambda sign (λ)	Mirror-image artifact
Monochorionic/ diamniotic	Zygote splits 5–10 days after fertilization Three-layer membrane	Two or more individual gestational sacs with shared placenta Membrane attachment of one chorion creates a "T" shape Moderately thick membrane	Mirror-image artifact
Monochorionic/ monoamniotic	Zygote splits 10–14 days postfertilization	Two or more fetuses Single gestational sac No membrane	Technical difficulty in locating membrane

Multifetal Gestational Abnormalities

ABNORMALITY	DESCRIPTION	SONOGRAPHIC FINDINGS	DIFFERENTIAL CONSIDERATIONS
Acardiac twin Parabolic twinning	Monochorionic/diamniotic twin pregnancy Rare anomaly Twin reversed arterial perfusion (TRAP) syndrome Results from an artery-to-artery and a vein-to-vein anastomoses Results in reversed flow direction in the umbilical arteries and vein of the acardiac twin (recipient twin) Places a large cardiovascular burden on the normal twin	Partially imaged normal fetus and a large perfused tissue mass lacking an upper body **Acardiac Twin—Recipient** Poorly developed upper body Anencephaly Absent or rudimentary heart Limbs may be present but truncated Oligohydramnios **Normal Twin—Donor** May develop: Hydrops Cardiac failure Polyhydramnios	Twin–twin transfusion syndrome

Continued

Multifetal Gestational Abnormalities—(cont'd)

ABNORMALITY	DESCRIPTION	SONOGRAPHIC FINDINGS	DIFFERENTIAL CONSIDERATIONS
Conjoined twins	Monozygotic Incomplete division of embryonic disk Usually anterior and one body part	Inseparable fetal bodies and skin contours Limited or no fetal position change No membrane	Acardiac twin Normal twin pregnancy
Stuck twin	Poli-Oli sequence Monochorionic/diamniotic Usually manifests between 16 and 26 gestational weeks	One twin displays polyhydramnios One twin displays oligohydramnios	Acardiac twin Twin–twin transfusion syndrome
Twin–twin transfusion syndrome	Same-sex fetuses Single placenta The arterial blood of the donor twin pumps into the venous system of the recipient twin (arteriovenous anastomosis) Recipient twin ultimately receives too much blood (may be arterial to arterial anastomosis)	Fetal weight discordance of ≥20% **Donor twin** may display intrauterine growth restriction and oligohydramnios **Receiving twin** may acquire hydrops fetalis and polyhydramnios Thin membrane	Acardiac twin Poli-Oli syndrome
Vanishing twin	Early fetal demise of one embryo	Twin pregnancy Demised twin resolves Becomes singleton pregnancy	Succenturiate placenta Subchorionic hemorrhage

COMPLICATIONS IN PREGNANCY REVIEW

1. A clenched fetal fist is commonly associated with which of the following syndromes?
   a. Patau
   b. Down
   c. Edward
   d. Eagle-Barrett

2. Anasarca is a condition often seen in cases of:
   a. triploidy
   b. macrosomia
   c. fetal hydrops
   d. amniotic band syndrome

3. Which of the following is a sonographic finding associated with Beckwith-Wiedemann syndrome?
   a. megaureter
   b. micrognathia
   c. macroglossia
   d. cystic hygroma

4. Megaureter and oligohydramnios are sonographic findings associated with which fetal syndrome?
   a. Trisomy 18
   b. Eagle-Barrett
   c. Meckel-Gruber
   d. Beckwith-Wiedemann

5. Twin–twin transfusion syndrome generally demonstrates:
   a. fetal hydrops in the donor twin
   b. polyhydramnios in the amniotic cavity of the donor twin
   c. a minimum fetal weight discordance of 20%
   d. oligohydramnios in the amniotic cavity of the receiving twin

6. Duodenal atresia is typically documented in one third of cases of:
   a. fetal hydrops
   b. Down syndrome
   c. Edward syndrome
   d. Eagle-Barrett syndrome

7. Fetal papyraceus is a term used to describe:
   a. Rh disease
   b. twin–twin transfusion syndrome
   c. vanishing twin phenomenon
   d. demise of a twin too large to resolve

8. Which of the following most accurately describes twin–twin transfusion syndrome?
   a. venous blood from the donor twin is pumped into the arterial system of the receiving twin
   b. arterial blood from the donor twin is pumped into the arterial blood of the receiving twin
   c. venous blood of the receiving twin is pumped into the venous system of the donor twin
   d. arterial blood from the donor twin is pumped into the venous system of the receiving twin

9. Fusion of the fingers or toes is termed:
   a. talipes
   b. syndactyly
   c. polydactyly
   d. clinodactyly

10. Which of the following sonographic findings is *not* associated with Meckel-Gruber syndrome?
    a. polydactyly
    b. anencephaly
    c. oligohydramnios
    d. infantile polycystic disease

11. The most common cause of discordant growth in dichorionic multifetal gestation is:
    a. intrauterine growth restriction
    b. chromosomal abnormality
    c. twin–twin transfusion syndrome
    d. twin reversal arterial profusion

12. VACTERL is associated with:
    a. Trisomy 21
    b. maternal diabetes
    c. Pentalogy of Cantrell
    d. maternal hypertension

13. Which of the following syndromes is more commonly associated with clinodactyly?
    a. Patau
    b. Down
    c. Turner
    d. Edward

14. VATER demonstrates which of the following complex anomalies?
    a. ventriculomegaly, anal atresia, tranesophageal fistula, renal anomalies
    b. vertebral defects, anal atresia, transesophageal fistula, and renal anomalies
    c. vertebral defects, anal atresia, tracheoesophageal fistula, and renal anomalies
    d. ventriculomegaly, adrenal hemorrhage, tracheoesophageal fistula, radial agenesis

15. Trisomy 13 is also known as:
    a. Patau syndrome
    b. Down syndrome
    c. Turner syndrome
    d. Edward syndrome

Using Figure 27.1, answer question 16.

16. What is the most likely abnormality noted in this viable second trimester twin gestation?
    a. fetus papyraceous
    b. Pentalogy of Cantrell
    c. acardiac twin pregnancy
    d. twin–twin transfusion syndrome

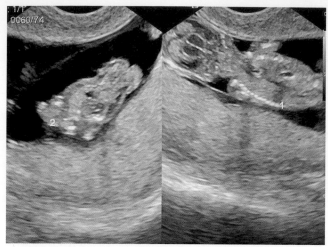

FIG. 27.1

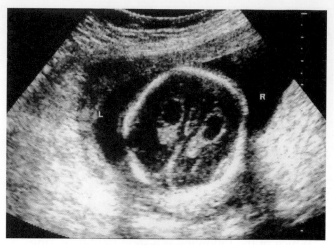

FIG. 27.3

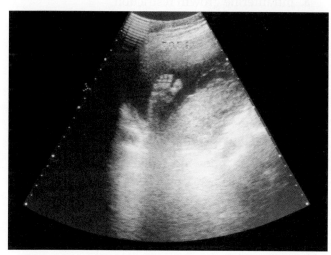

FIG. 27.2

Using Figure 27.2, answer questions 17 and 18.

17. A plantar image of the fetal foot shows a sonographic finding termed:
    a. sandal toe
    b. thumb toe
    c. rocker foot
    d. hammer toe

18. This sonographic finding is associated with:
    a. Trisomy 13
    b. Trisomy 18
    c. Trisomy 21
    d. Eagle-Barrett syndrome

Using Figure 27.3, answer questions 19 and 20.

19. A second-trimester fetus is demonstrating which of the following abnormalities?
    a. holoprosencephaly
    b. Dandy-Walker cysts
    c. bilateral hydrocephalus
    d. bilateral choroid plexus cysts

20. This can be associated with which of the following?
    a. Trisomy 13
    b. Trisomy 18
    c. Trisomy 21
    d. Meckel-Gruber syndrome

Using Figure 27.4, answer questions 21 and 22.

21. A cross-sectional sonogram at the level of the fetal neck/upper chest documents which of the following abnormalities?
    a. encephalocele
    b. fetal hydrops
    c. nuchal edema
    d. cystic hygroma

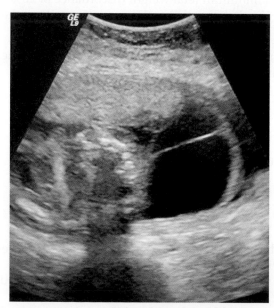

FIG. 27.4

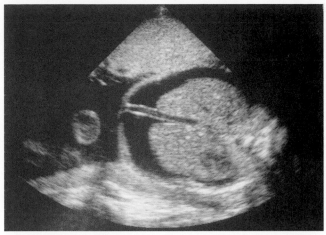

FIG. 27.5

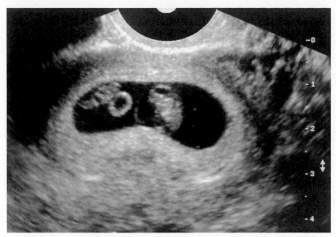

FIG. 27.7

22. This is a common sonographic finding associated with which chromosomal abnormality?
  a. trisomy 13
  b. Turner syndrome
  c. Edward syndrome
  d. Meckel-Gruber syndrome

Using Figure 27.5, answer question 23.

23. The sonographic findings are most suspicious for:
  a. gastroschisis
  b. omphalocele
  c. fetal hydrops
  d. pseudoascites

Using Figure 27.6, answer question 24.

24. A patient presents for an early second-trimester sonogram. A cross-sectional image shows two fetal abdomens. This image is most suspicious for:
  a. acardiac twin
  b. vanishing twin
  c. conjoined twins
  d. twin–twin transfusion syndrome

Using Figure 27.7, answer question 25.

25. A first-trimester sonogram demonstrates:
  a. diamniotic twins
  b. dichorionic twins
  c. monoamniotic twins
  d. monochorionic twins

Using Figure 27.8, answer questions 26 and 27.

26. The abnormality present in this 18-week gestation is most suspicious for which chromosomal anomaly?
  a. triploidy
  b. Trisomy 13
  c. Trisomy 18
  d. Trisomy 21

27. Which of the following abnormalities is associated with this syndrome?
  a. omphalocele
  b. microcephaly
  c. cystic hygroma
  d. duodenal atresia

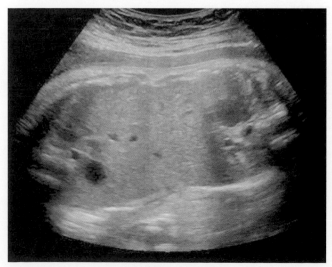

FIG. 27.6

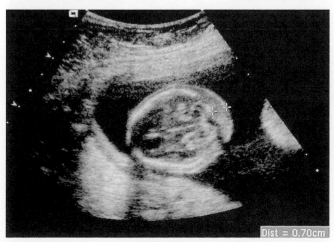

FIG. 27.8

Using Figure 27.9, answer questions 28 and 29.

28. What is the most likely chromosomal anomaly associated with this second-trimester fetus?
    a. triploidy
    b. Trisomy 13
    c. Trisomy 18
    d. Trisomy 21

29. Which of the following extremity malformations is associated with this condition?
    a. rocker bottom feet
    b. long bone fractures
    c. hypomineralization
    d. sandal toe deformity

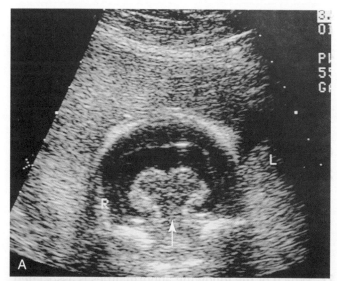

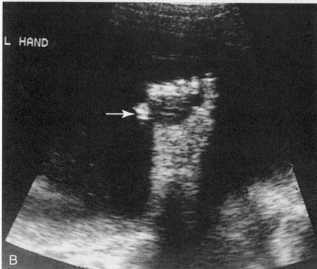

FIG. 27.9 A and B

30. Preeclampsia is a complication of pregnancy demonstrating:
    a. fetal ascites, pleural effusion, and scalp edema
    b. maternal hypertension, proteinuria, and edema
    c. gestational diabetes, hematuria, and hypertension
    d. maternal hypertension, grand mal seizures, and coma

31. Preterm labor is defined as the onset of labor before:
    a. estimated due date
    b. 40 weeks' gestation
    c. 38 weeks' gestation
    d. 37 weeks' gestation

32. Which of the following is likely to occur if a single zygote divides 7 days after fertilization?
    a. one amnion and one chorion
    b. two amnion and two chorion
    c. one amnion and two chorion
    d. two amnion and one chorion

33. Arteriovenous shunting within the placenta occurs with:
    a. vanishing twin
    b. fetal papyraceus
    c. twin–twin transfusion syndrome
    d. acardiac twin pregnancy

34. With twin–twin transfusion syndrome, the recipient twin is likely to acquire:
    a. macrosomia
    b. hydrops fetalis
    c. placentomalacia
    d. skeletal dysplasia

35. What sonographic finding confirms the presence of a diamniotic pregnancy?
    a. two yolk sacs
    b. two placentas
    c. two allantoic ducts
    d. two gestational sacs

36. Which of the following is *not* a sonographic finding in fetal hydrops?
    a. anasarca
    b. scalp edema
    c. pleural effusion
    d. umbilical vein varix

37. Fetal hydrops resulting from fetal tachycardia most commonly demonstrates a fetal heart rate of:
    a. 120 to 200 beats per minute
    b. 160 to 180 beats per minute
    c. 200 to 240 beats per minute
    d. 250 to 300 beats per minute

38. Twin gestation arising from two separate fertilized ova is termed:
    a. zygotic twins
    b. identical twins
    c. dizygotic twins
    d. diamniotic twins

39. Which of the following abnormalities increases the risk of fetal injury?
    a. uterine shelf
    b. amniotic bands
    c. amniotic sheets
    d. amniochorionic separation

40. Amniotic band syndrome may result in:
    a. polyhydramnios
    b. placenta accreta
    c. an acardiac twin
    d. fetal amputation

41. Which of the following syndromes demonstrates a normal karyotype and is associated with hemihypertrophy?
    a. Turner syndrome
    b. Eagle-Barrett syndrome
    c. Meckel-Gruber syndrome
    d. Beckwith-Wiedemann syndrome

42. A dizygotic gestation is expected to be:
    a. dichorionic/diamniotic
    b. monochorionic/diamniotic
    c. dichorionic/monoamniotic
    d. monochorionic/monoamniotic

43. The gravest form of pregnancy-induced maternal hypertension is termed:
    a. anasarca
    b. eclampsia
    c. preeclampsia
    d. gestational hypertension

44. Leakage of part or all of the amniotic fluid in a 32-week gestation is termed:
    a. TTS
    b. IUGR
    c. PROM
    d. TARP

45. A monochorionic twin pregnancy in which one develops without an upper body is termed:
    a. acardiac twin
    b. vanishing twin
    c. conjoined twin
    d. ectopia cordis

46. Which of the following syndromes is manifested by dilatation of the renal collecting system?
    a. Patau syndrome
    b. Pentalogy of Cantrell
    c. Eagle-Barrett syndrome
    d. Meckel-Gruber syndrome

47. Which of the following twin abnormalities demonstrates a venous-to-venous anastomosis?
    a. acardiac twin
    b. conjoined twin
    c. vanishing twin
    d. twin–twin transfusion syndrome

48. Which of the following is a common abnormality associated with Trisomy 13?
    a. clinodactyly
    b. macrocephaly
    c. holoprosencephaly
    d. hyperechoic bowel

49. Which of the following conditions displays ectopia cordis and gastroschisis?
    a. Patau syndrome
    b. Pentalogy of Cantrell
    c. Meckel-Gruber syndrome
    e. Beckwith-Wiedemann syndrome

50. Inward curving of the fifth finger is a clinical finding associated with:
    a. Patau syndrome
    b. Down syndrome
    c. Pentalogy of Cantrell
    d. Meckel-Gruber syndrome

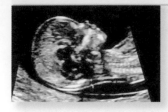

CHAPTER 28

Placenta and Umbilical Cord

KEY TERMS

abruptio placentae   premature detachment of the placenta from the maternal wall.

allantoic duct   elongated duct that contributes to the development of the umbilical cord.

basal plate   maternal surface of the placenta.

battledore placenta   cord insertion into the margin of the placenta.

Braxton-Hicks contraction   spontaneous uterine contraction occurring throughout pregnancy.

chorion frondosum   the portion of the chorion that develops into the fetal portion of the placenta.

chorionic leave   chorion around the gestational sac on the opposite side of implantation.

chorionic plate   fetal surface of the placenta.

chorionic villi   vascular projections from the chorion at the implantation and placental site.

circumvallate placenta   a placental condition in which the chorionic plate of the placenta is smaller than the basal plate.

nuchal cord   occurs when the cord is completely wrapped around the fetal neck at a minimum of two times.

molar pregnancy   abnormal proliferation of the trophoblastic cells in the first trimester.

placental abruption   premature separation of the normally implanted placenta from the uterus.

placenta accreta   growth of the chorionic villi superficially into the myometrium. Abnormal placental attachment to the myometrium that does not separate after delivery.

placenta increta   growth of the chorionic villi deep into the myometrium.

placenta percreta   growth of the chorionic villi through the myometrium.

placenta previa   placenta completely covers the internal cervical os.

placental migration   as the uterus enlarges and stretches, the attached placenta appears to "move" further from the lower uterine segment.

retroplacental complex   area behind the placenta composed of the decidua, myometrium, and uteroplacental vessels.

succenturiate placenta   additional placenta tissue (lobes) connected to the body of the placenta by blood vessels.

umbilical herniation   failure of the anterior abdominal wall to close completely at the level of the umbilicus.

vasa previa   occurs when the intramembranous vessels course across the cervical os.

Wharton jelly   mucoid connective tissue that surrounds the vessels within the umbilical cord.

PLACENTA

ANATOMY (Fig. 28.1)

- Develops from trophoblastic cells that make up the chorion.
- Formed by the decidua basalis and decidua frondosum.
- Separated from the uterine myometrium by the retroplacental complex.
- Blood supply to the intervillous spaces is supplied by the maternal spiral arteries.

PHYSIOLOGY

- Vital support organ for the developing fetus.
- Chorionic villus is the major functioning unit of the placenta and contains the intervillous spaces.
- Maternal blood enters the intervillous spaces.

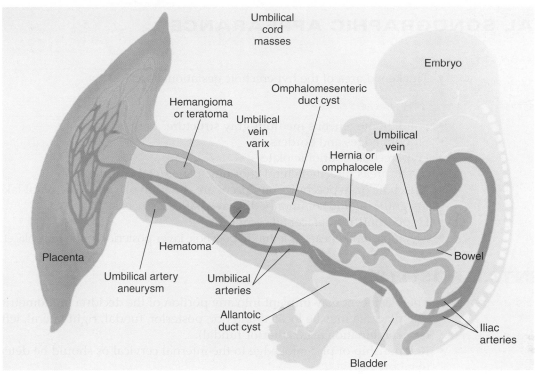

FIG. 28.1 Placental anatomy.

FUNCTIONS

Respiration

- Oxygen in maternal blood passes through the placenta into the fetal blood.
- Carbon dioxide returns through the placenta to the maternal blood.

Nutrition

- Nutrients pass from the maternal blood through the placenta to the fetal blood.

Excretion

- Waste products cross from the fetal blood through the placenta to the maternal blood.

Protection

- Provides a barrier between the mother and fetus, protecting the fetus from maternal immune rejection.

Storage

- Carbohydrates, proteins, calcium, and iron are stored in the placenta and released into the fetal circulation.

Hormone Production

- Produces human chorionic gonadotropin, estrogens, and progesterone.

SIZE

- Varies with gestational age.
- Generally, measures 2 to 3 cm in greatest thickness.
- Maximum thickness should not exceed 4.0 cm in the second trimester or 6.0 cm in the third trimester.

NORMAL SONOGRAPHIC APPEARANCE

First Trimester

- Thickened area of the hyperechoic gestational sac.

Second and Third Trimesters

- Solid, homogeneous medium-gray structure.
- Smooth edges and borders.
- Hyperechoic chorionic plate.
- Cystic areas directly behind chorionic plate (fetal vessels).
- Anechoic or hypoechoic sonolucent areas within placenta (placental lakes) are insignificant and commonly displayed after 25 weeks.
- Hypoechoic retroplacental complex.
- Myometrium appears as a thin hypoechoic layer posterior to the retroplacental complex.

PLACENTAL POSITION

- The blastocyst may implant into any portion of the decidua (endometrium).
- The placenta may be located anterior, posterior, fundal, right lateral, left lateral, or a combination (e.g., anterior fundal).
- Relationship of placental edge to the internal cervical os should be determined (e.g., previa)

PLACENTAL MATURITY AND GRADING

- Grading scale of 0 to 3.
- Grading dependent on echogenicity attributed to calcium and fibrous deposition with advancing age.
- Maternal hypertension, cigarette smoking, intrauterine growth restriction, and multifetal gestation may cause premature maturation.
- Premature maturation of the placenta suggests placental insufficiency.
- Delayed maturation is most commonly associated with maternal diabetes mellitus.

Grade 0

- No calcifications.
- Smooth basal and chorionic plates.
- First and early second trimester.

Grade 1

- Scattered calcifications throughout the placenta.
- Most common up until 34 gestational weeks.

Grade 2

- Demonstrates calcifications along the basal plate.
- Chorionic plate becomes slightly lobular.

Grade 3

- Marked calcifications and placental lakes.
- Distinct hyperechoic lobulations extending from the chorionic to basal plate.
- Usually not apparent before 35 weeks' gestation.

PLACENTA PREVIA

- Placental placement in front of the fetus relative to the birth canal.
- Primary cause of painless vaginal bleeding in the third trimester.

- Risk factors include advanced maternal age, multiparity, previous cesarean section, previous therapeutic abortion(s), uterine leiomyoma, or closely spaced pregnancies.
- Complications of placenta previa include premature delivery, life-threatening maternal hemorrhage, and increased risk of placenta accreta, stillbirth, and intrauterine growth restriction.
- Only 5% of cases diagnosed with placenta previa in the second trimester remain at term, a result of placental migration.
- Endovaginal technique most accurate in diagnosing placenta previa.
- Transperineal can also avoid fetal structures obscuring the internal cervical os.

PLACENTA PREVIA

- Measure distance from lower edge of placenta to the center of the internal cervical os.
- Distance greater than 2 cm is associated with vaginal delivery.

TYPE	CLINICAL FINDINGS	SONOGRAPHIC FINDINGS	DIFFERENTIAL CONSIDERATIONS
Complete	Painless vaginal bleeding Abnormal fetal position	Placenta covers the entire cervical os	Myometrial contraction Overdistention of the urinary bladder Uterine leiomyoma Improper technique
Partial (incomplete)	Painless vaginal bleeding	Placenta covers a portion of the cervical os	Myometrial contraction Overdistention of the urinary bladder Uterine leiomyoma Improper technique
Marginal	Asymptomatic Painless vaginal bleeding	Edge of the placenta abuts the cervical os	Myometrial contraction Overdistention of the urinary bladder Uterine leiomyoma Low-lying placenta
Low-lying	Asymptomatic	Edge of the placenta lies close but does not abut or cover the cervical os Within 2 cm of the internal os	Myometrial contraction Overdistention of the urinary bladder Uterine leiomyoma Marginal previa
Vasa previa	Bleeding Cord compression Prolapsed cord Transverse fetal lie	Fetal vessels cross over the internal os	Normal free-floating cord Velamentous cord Succenturiate placenta Myometrial contraction

Placental Abnormalities

ABNORMALITY	INFORMATION	SONOGRAPHIC FINDINGS	DIFFERENTIAL CONSIDERATIONS
Abruption	Premature placental detachment from the endometrial surface Disrupts placental maternal circulation Marginal abruption most common Clinical findings include severe pelvic pain, tense uterine wall, and vaginal bleeding Risk factors include maternal hypertension, cigarette smoking, diabetes, trauma, placenta previa, uterine leiomyoma, methamphetamine use, and short umbilical cord	Hypoechoic retroplacental mass Placental thickening Well-defined margins Elevation of placental edges Subamniotic or preplacental locations are rare	Normal retroplacental complex Amniochorionic separation Myometrial contraction Circumvallate placenta

Continued

Placental Abnormalities—(cont'd)

ABNORMALITY	INFORMATION	SONOGRAPHIC FINDINGS	DIFFERENTIAL CONSIDERATIONS
Accreta	**Accreta** Least invasive Chorionic villi of the placenta penetrate the decidua but do not invade the myometrium Attributed to complete or partial absence of the decidua basalis Risk factors include multiparity, placenta previa, prior uterine surgery, and previous cesarean section **Increta**—placenta penetrates the uterine myometrium **Percreta**—placental vessels penetrate the uterine myometrium and serosa May attach to adjacent organs	Carefully assess the hypoechoic placental/myometrial border **Accreta** Obscured or absent retroplacental complex Numerous placental lakes **Increta** Extension of villi into the myometrium **Percreta** Extension of villi outside of the uterus MRI can help diagnose cases that are equivocal	Adenomyosis Myometrial contraction Uterine leiomyoma
Amniochorionic separation	Amnion can be separated from the fetal surface of the placenta but cannot be separated from the umbilical insertion site Chorion can be separated from the endometrial lining but cannot be separated from the placental edge	Localized fluid between the fetal side of the placenta and the amniotic membrane Membrane may move	Placental abruption Normal venous lakes
Battledore placenta	Cord inserts into the end margin of the placenta Aka: marginal cord Associated with intrauterine growth restriction	Insertion of the cord into the end margin of the placenta Paddle appearance to the placenta	Normal cord lying adjacent to the placental margin Velamentous cord
Calcifications	Sign of maturing placenta Associated with maternal cigarette smoking or thrombotic disorders	Hyperechoic focus within the placental tissue Posterior acoustic shadowing	Molar pregnancy
Circumvallate placenta	Abnormal attachment of placental membranes to fetal placental surface Abnormal placental shape in which the membranes insert away from the placental edge toward the center Increases risk for abruption, intrauterine growth restriction, premature labor, and vaginal bleeding	Basal plate area is larger than the fetal surface of the placenta "Rolled up" placental edge Irregular fold or thickening of the placenta Upturned placental edge contains hypoechoic or cystic spaces Thick placental cord insertion	Abruption Amniotic shelf Synechiae
Fibrin deposits	More commonly located along the subchorionic region of the placenta Attributed to the regulation of intervillous circulation	Hypoechoic area beneath the chorionic plate of the placenta Triangular or rectangle in shape	Venous lake Subchorionic hematoma
Placental infarct	Result of ischemic necrosis Occurs in 25% of pregnancies No clinical risk when small	Hypoechoic focal placental mass Calcification may occur	Intervillous thrombosis/placental lakes
Placental lakes	Intervillous thrombosis Also called venous lakes Occurs in one third of pregnancies Insignificant unless found in the first trimester	Anechoic or hypoechoic area within the placenta Internal blood flow	Placental infarct

Placental Abnormalities—(cont'd)

ABNORMALITY	INFORMATION	SONOGRAPHIC FINDINGS	DIFFERENTIAL CONSIDERATIONS

Placentomalacia	Small placenta
	Associated with:
	  Eccentric cord insertion
	  Intrauterine growth restriction
	  Intrauterine infection
	  Chromosomal abnormality
	  Maternal diabetes mellitus
		Small overall placental size
		Anterior-posterior thickness
		  ≤1.5 cm
			Succenturiate placenta
			Placenta accreta, increta,
			  percreta
			Normal placenta with marked
			  polyhydramnios

Placentomegaly	Primary causes include maternal
	  diabetes mellitus, anemia, and
	  Rh sensitivity
	Associated with maternal anemia,
	  fetal hydrops, twin–twin transfusion
	  syndrome, fetal anomalies, and
	  intrauterine infection
		Maximum thickness
		  >4.0 cm before 24 weeks
		  >6.0 cm in third trimester
		Heterogeneous texture associated
		  with triploidy, molar pregnancy,
		  or hemorrhage
		Homogeneous texture associated
		  with anemia, fetal hydrops, and
		  Rh sensitivity
			Myometrial contraction
			Uterine leiomyoma
			Succenturiate placenta
			Placental abruption
			Intraplacental hemorrhage

Succenturiate placenta
 	
Aka: accessory placenta
	A result of the lack of the adjacent
	  chorionic villi to atrophy
	Increased risk of velamentous cord
	  and vasa previa
		Additional placental tissue adjacent
		  to the main placenta
		Connected to the body of the
		  placenta by blood vessels
			Myometrial contraction
			Leiomyoma

Placenta Neoplasms

NEOPLASM	INFORMATION	SONOGRAPHIC FINDINGS	DIFFERENTIAL CONSIDERATIONS

Chorioangioma	Arises from the chorionic
	  tissue of the amniotic surface
	  of the placenta
	Most common benign tumor
	  of the placenta
	May increase maternal serum
	  alpha-fetoprotein
	No clinical significance when
	  small
	Fetus may demonstrate distress
	  owing to vascular shunting
	  from the normal placenta to
	  the hemangioma when larger
		Well-circumscribed hypoechoic
		  or complex placental mass
		Placental enlargement
		Moderately vascular
		mass protruding from the
		  chorionic plate
		Usually occur at the umbilical
		  insertion site
		Polyhydramnios
		Fetal hydrops
		Intrauterine growth
		  restriction
			Myometrial contraction
			Uterine leiomyoma

Choriocarcinoma	Highly metastatic trophoblastic
	  tumor
	Metastases to the lungs, spleen,
	  kidneys, intestines, liver, and
	  brain.
		Hypoechoic or complex
		  intraplacental mass
		Possible theca lutein cysts
			Myometrial contraction
			Uterine leiomyoma

Gestational trophoblastic disease	Molar pregnancy
	Complete molar pregnancy
	  may develop into
	  choriocarcinoma
	Partial mole carries little
	  malignant potential
		Inhomogeneous uterine
		  texture
		Various-sized cystic structures
		  within the placenta
		No identifiable fetal parts
		  when complete molar
		  pregnancy
		Coexisting fetus with a
		  decrease in amniotic
		  fluid volume when partial
		  molar pregnancy
			Intraplacental hemorrhage
			Degenerating uterine
			  leiomyoma
			Prominent maternal venous
			  lakes

UMBILICAL CORD

- Essential link to the placenta.
- Normally inserts into the center of the placenta and midline portion of the anterior abdominal wall of the fetus (umbilicus).
- Umbilical vein carries oxygenated blood.
- Umbilical arteries return venous blood back to the placenta.

ANATOMY

- Formed by the fusion of the yolk stalk and body stalk (allantoic ducts).
- Amniotic membrane covers the umbilical cord and blends into the fetal skin at the umbilicus.
- Composed of one vein and two arteries surrounded by myxomatous connective tissue (Wharton jelly).

Umbilical Vein

- Formed by the confluence of the chorionic veins of the placenta.
- Enters the umbilicus and joins the left portal vein of the fetal liver.
- Carries oxygenated blood to the fetus.

Umbilical Arteries

- Umbilical arteries are contiguous with the hypogastric arteries on each side of the fetal urinary bladder.
- Exit at the umbilicus.
- Return deoxygenated (venous) blood from the fetus back to the placenta.
- Demonstrate low-resistance blood flow with continuous diastolic flow.
- Absent or reversal of diastolic flow is considered abnormal after 18 to 20 weeks, gestation.

SIZE

- Length of the umbilical cord is equal to the crown–rump length during the first trimester and continues to have the same length as the fetus throughout pregnancy.
- 40 to 60 cm in length during the second and third trimesters.
- Diameter of the umbilical cord usually measures <2.0 cm.
- Umbilical vein diameter normally measures <9 mm.
- Coiling of the umbilical cord is normal and thought to aid in resistance to compression.
- Whether the cord spirals left or right does not appear to have clinical significance.
- Develops approximately 40 spiral turns by birth.

Abnormalities of the Umbilical Cord

ABNORMALITY	INFORMATION	SONOGRAPHIC FINDINGS	DIFFERENTIAL CONSIDERATIONS
Cyst	Normal finding in the first trimester Associated with abdominal wall defects and genitourinary abnormalities	Nonvascular anechoic enlargement of the umbilical cord Generally located near the fetal end of the cord	True or false cord knot
False knots of the cord	Coiling of the blood vessels, giving the appearance of knots	Blood vessels folding over on themselves mimicking umbilical nodules	Normal coiling of the cord True cord knots

Abnormalities of the Umbilical Cord—(cont'd)

ABNORMALITY	INFORMATION	SONOGRAPHIC FINDINGS	DIFFERENTIAL CONSIDERATIONS
Hemangioma	Most common solid tumor of the umbilical cord Rare	Hyperechoic or complex umbilical cord mass Well defined wall margins Usually found near the placental end of the umbilical cord	Thrombosed umbilical vein
Long cord	Cord length >80 cm Associated with nuchal cord, polyhydramnios, cord knot, and vasa previa	Nuchal cord Polyhydramnios True umbilical cord knots	Gastroschisis Normal cord with polyhydramnios
Nuchal cord	Cord completely surrounds fetal neck with more than one loop Found in 25% of pregnancies Significant finding at term Fetus will turn in and out of the umbilical cord throughout the pregnancy	Two or more complete loops of cord around the fetal neck Flattening of the cord	One complete loop around the neck Prolapsed cord
Prolapsed cord	Cord precedes the fetus in the birthing process	Presence of the cord before the presenting fetal part	Vasa previa Nuchal cord
Short cord	Cord length <35 cm	Limited fetal movement Inadequate fetal descent Cord compression Oligohydramnios	Normal cord length
Single umbilical artery	Most common abnormality especially in multifetal gestations Umbilical cord may demonstrate both single and double umbilical arteries within the same cord Increases risk of intrauterine growth restriction and fetal anomalies	Two vessels of similar size within the umbilical cord Umbilical artery transverse diameter >4 mm Umbilical cord may appear straight, or noncoiled	Normal three-vessel cord
Thrombosis of the umbilical vessels	Primarily the umbilical vein Results from both primary and secondary causes Higher incidence in diabetic mothers	Absent or abnormal blood flow Hypoechoic enlargement of one or more umbilical vessels	Two-vessel cord
Varix of the umbilical vein	Focal dilatation of the umbilical vein Nearly always intraabdominal Associated with normal outcomes	Intraabdominal focal dilatation of the umbilical vein Located between the anterior abdominal wall and the fetal liver	Gallbladder Technical error
Velamentous cord insertion	Umbilical cord inserts into the membranes before entering the placenta Not protected by Wharton jelly Associated with preterm labor, abnormal fetal heart pattern, vasa previa, intrauterine growth restriction, low Apgar scores, and low birth weight.	Insertion of the umbilical cord into the membranes adjacent to the edge of the placental margin	Battledore placenta Normal cord adjacent to the placenta Succenturiate placenta

CERVICAL OS

- Cylindrical portion of the uterus, which enters the vagina and lies at right angles to it.
- Cervical canal extends from the internal os to the uterus; external os extends to the vagina.

Cervical Length

- Measures between 2.5 and 5.0 cm in length (usually > 3.0 cm).
- Measure the distance from the internal cervical os to the external cervical os.

Transabdominal Approach

- Partial to full urinary bladder.
- Entire echogenic cervical canal should be measured.
- Avoid overdistention.

Transvaginal Approach

- Empty urinary bladder.
- Entire echogenic cervical canal should be measured.
- Internal os should be flat or a "V-shaped" notch.
- External os is identified by an echogenic triangular area.
- Most reliable.

Transperineal Approach

- Empty or partially full urinary bladder.
- Entire echogenic cervical canal should be measured.
- Place sheathed transducer between labial and vaginal introitus.
- Cervix will be displayed horizontal and 90 degrees to the lower uterine segment.

Abnormality of the Cervix

ABNORMALITY	INFORMATION	SONOGRAPHIC FINDINGS	DIFFERENTIAL CONSIDERATIONS
Incompetent cervix (cervical insufficiency)	Cervical shortening Generally painless Decrease in cervical length of ≥6 mm on serial examinations increases risk of preterm labor **Risk Factors** include multiple pregnancies, history of premature labor, or previous history of cervical surgery Treatment Bed rest for cervical lengths 2.5 to 1.6 cm Cerclage used for cervical lengths < 1.6 cm	Cervical length <2.5 cm Beak like protrusion of the amniotic fluid at the internal os (funneling) Dilating of the cervical os >3–6 mm Obtain width and length of funneling Record shortest length of three measurements	Myometrial contraction Improper technique

PLACENTA AND UMBILICAL CORD REVIEW

1. Growth of the placenta into the superficial myometrium is termed placenta:
   a. previa
   b. increta
   c. accreta
   d. percreta

2. Placement of the placental margin within 2 cm of the internal cervical os is termed:
   a. low-lying placenta
   b. circumvallate placenta
   c. succenturiate placenta
   d. marginal placenta previa

3. The location of an umbilical vein varix is most frequently within the:
   a. placenta
   b. fetal liver
   c. fetal abdomen
   d. umbilical cord

4. The umbilical cord is covered by which of the following?
   a. amnion
   b. chorion
   c. meconium
   d. Wharton jelly

5. Insertion of the umbilical cord into the end margin of the placenta is termed a:
   a. battledore placenta
   b. velamentous placenta
   c. membranous placenta
   d. circumvallate placenta

6. Placenta accreta can be ruled out by observing a normal:
   a. chorionic plate
   b. retroplacental complex
   c. maternal urinary bladder
   d. homogeneous echo pattern

7. The cervical canal extends from the:
   a. internal os to the uterus
   b. external os to the uterus
   c. internal os to the vagina
   d. external os to the vagina

8. During the first trimester, the length of the normal umbilical cord is equal to the:
   a. gestational weeks
   b. mean sac diameter
   c. crown–rump length
   d. width of the gestational sac

9. Classic symptoms of placental abruption include:
   a. painless vaginal bleeding
   b. severe pelvic pain and vaginal bleeding
   c. mild abdominal pain and vaginal spotting
   d. severe pelvic pain without vaginal bleeding

10. Identification of arterial flow on each side of the fetal bladder verifies which of the following?
    a. two umbilical arteries
    b. normal femoral arteries
    c. normal aortic bifurcation
    d. duplicated hypogastric arteries

11. Extension of an anterior placenta into the maternal urinary bladder is a sonographic finding associated with:
    a. endometriosis
    b. placenta increta
    c. placenta previa
    d. placenta percreta

12. Which portion of the gestational sac develops into the fetal side of the placenta?
    a. chorion laeve
    b. chorion basalis
    c. chorion parietalis
    d. chorion frondosum

13. Which of the following describes a condition where the chorionic plate of the placenta is smaller than the basal plate?
    a. vasa previa
    b. battledore placenta
    c. succenturiate placenta
    d. circumvallate placenta

14. A true nuchal cord is defined as:
    a. one complete loop of the umbilical cord around the fetal neck
    b. two or more complete loops of the umbilical cord near the fetal neck
    c. two or more complete loops of the umbilical cord around the fetal neck
    d. thickening of the nuchal fold coexisting with one complete loop of the umbilical cord around the fetal neck

15. A placenta located immediately adjacent to the cervix is termed a(n):
    a. low-lying placenta
    b. battledore placenta
    c. marginal placenta previa
    d. incomplete placenta previa

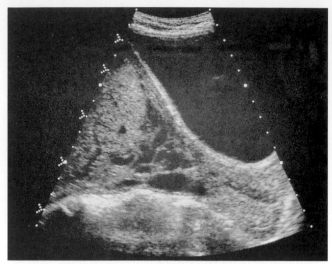

FIG. 28.2   Sagittal sonogram.

Using Figure 28.2, answer questions 16 and 17.

16. Which of the following conditions is most likely identified in this sagittal sonogram of the cervix?
 a. battledore placenta
 b. placenta previa
 c. placenta accreta
 d. velamentous cord insertion

17. Which clinical finding is more commonly associated with this condition?
 a. fetal tachycardia
 b. cephalic fetal lie
 c. small for gestational age
 d. painless vaginal bleeding

Using Figure 28.3, answer question 18.

18. Which of the following is the most accurate placental location?
 a. fundal
 b. anterior
 c. posterior
 d. right lateral

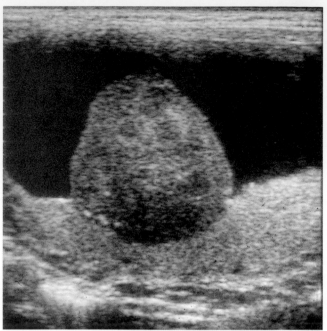

FIG. 28.4   Transverse sonogram.

Using Figure 28.4, answer question 19.

19. The sonogram is most likely identifying which of the following?
 a. chorioangioma
 b. uterine leiomyoma
 c. battledore placenta
 d. myometrial contraction

Using Figure 28.5, answer question 20.

20. This transverse image of the uterus is most likely demonstrating:
 a. battledore placenta
 b. succenturiate placenta
 c. myometrial contraction
 d. vanishing twin syndrome

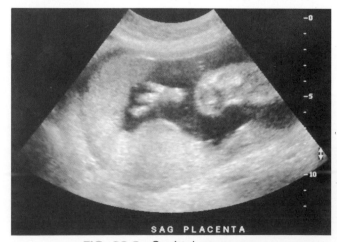

SAG PLACENTA

FIG. 28.3   Sagittal sonogram.

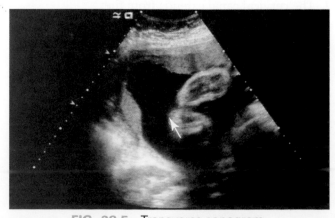

FIG. 28.5   Transverse sonogram.

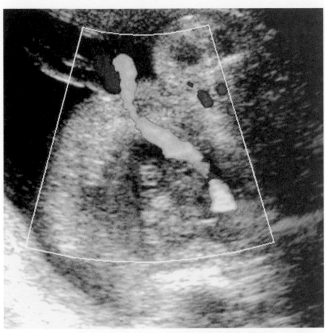

FIG. 28.6 (See Color Plate 10.)

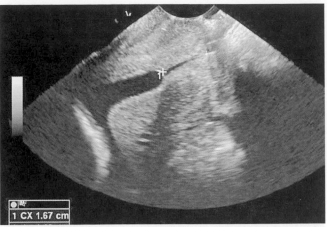

FIG. 28.7 Sagittal sonogram.

Using Figure 28.6 (and Color Plate 10), answer questions 21 and 22.

21. This duplex image identifies which of the following structures?
    a. umbilical varix
    b. velamentous cord
    c. single umbilical artery
    d. thrombosis of an umbilical artery

22. This finding is associated with:
    a. fetal demise
    b. premature labor
    c. multifetal gestations
    d. maternal diabetes mellitus

Using Figure 28.7, answer question 23.

23. The lower uterine segment in this sonogram is consistent with a(n):
    a. placenta previa
    b. placenta accreta
    c. myometrial contraction
    d. incompetent cervix

Using Figure 28.8, answer question 24.

24. A patient presents with severe lower abdominal pain and vaginal spotting. Based on the clinical history, the sonographic findings are most suspicious for:
    a. chorioangioma
    b. placenta accreta
    c. placenta abruption
    d. circumvallate placenta

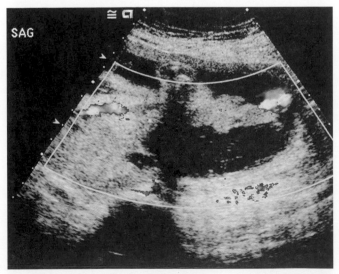

FIG. 28.8

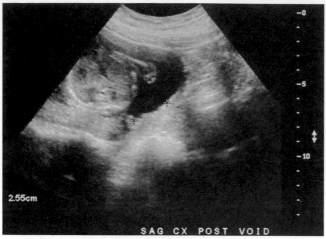

FIG. 28.9 Sagittal sonogram.

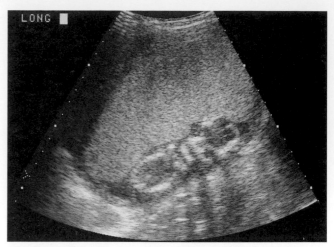

FIG. 28.11 Transverse sonogram.

Using Figure 28.9, answer question 25.

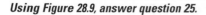

25. This postvoid transabdominal image of the cervix demonstrates:
    a. a low-lying placenta
    b. a cervix free of placenta
    c. marginal placenta previa
    d. incomplete placenta previa

Using Figure 28.10, answer questions 26 and 27.

26. A sagittal image of the cervix in a late second-trimester pregnancy demonstrates:
    a. placenta previa
    b. placental abruption
    c. an incompetent cervix
    d. a left lateral placenta

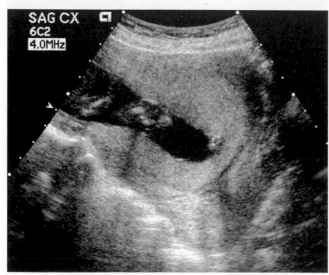

FIG. 28.10 Sagittal sonogram.

27. This patient most likely presents with:
    a. mild pelvic pain
    b. severe pelvic pain
    c. abdominal cramping
    d. painless vaginal bleeding

Using Figure 28.11, answer questions 28 and 29.

28. An image of an early second-trimester pregnancy demonstrates:
    a. placenta previa
    b. placentomegaly
    c. placentomalacia
    d. circumvallate placenta

29. Maternal causes for this abnormality include:
    a. hypertension
    b. diabetes mellitus
    c. previous cesarean section
    d. previous therapeutic abortions

30. Membranous insertion of the umbilical cord is termed a(n):
    a. vasa previa
    b. allantois cord
    c. velamentous cord
    d. battledore placenta

31. What is the most common cause of painless vaginal bleeding in the third trimester?
    a. placenta previa
    b. placenta accreta
    c. placenta abruption
    d. incompetent cervix

32. An eccentric insertion of the umbilical cord into the placenta is termed a:
    a. vasa previa
    b. velamentous cord
    c. battledore placenta
    d. circumvallate placenta

33. Placental implantation encroaching on the internal cervical os is termed:
   a. placenta increta
   b. marginal previa
   c. placenta accreta
   d. low-lying placenta

34. The vascular projections arising from the chorion are termed:
   a. chorionic villi
   b. chorionic leave
   c. chorionic venules
   d. myxomatous tissue

35. Which of the following conditions demonstrates extension of the chorionic villi into the myometrium?
   a. placenta increta
   b. placenta accreta
   c. placenta percreta
   d. battledore placenta

36. Coiling of the umbilical cord is associated with:
   a. a long cord
   b. a short cord
   c. a normal fetus
   d. chromosomal abnormalities

37. Which of the following is the most common placental location for deposits of fibrin to collect?
   a. basal plate
   b. subchorionic
   c. within a placental lake
   d. within the retroplacental complex

38. The primary cause of placentomegaly is:
   a. maternal hypertension
   b. twin–twin transfusion syndrome
   c. succenturiate placenta
   d. maternal diabetes mellitus

39. Complications of placenta previa include all of the following *except:*
   a. stillbirth
   b. macrosomia
   c. placenta accreta
   d. premature delivery

40. The presence of additional placental tissue adjacent to the main placenta is termed a(n):
   a. accessory placenta
   b. battledore placenta
   c. velamentous placenta
   d. circumvallate placenta

41. Which placenta most likely demonstrates an overall abnormal contour?
   a. battledore placenta
   b. velamentous placenta
   c. succenturiate placenta
   d. circumvallate placenta

42. Placentomalacia may result from which of the following conditions?
   a. Rh sensitivity
   b. maternal anemia
   c. twin–twin transfusion syndrome
   d. intrauterine growth restriction

43. The maternal side of the placenta is formed by the decidua:
   a. leave
   b. basalis
   c. parietalis
   d. frondosum

44. Placental thickness will vary with gestational age but generally measures:
   a. 1 to 2 cm
   b. 2 to 3 cm
   c. 4 to 5 cm
   d. 5 to 6 cm

45. Which of the following conditions is most likely to demonstrate a small placenta?
   a. Rh sensitivity
   b. maternal anemia
   c. maternal diabetes
   d. chromosomal anomalies

46. Which of the following occurs when intramembranous vessels course across the internal cervical os?
   a. vasa previa
   b. placenta accreta
   c. battledore placenta
   d. circumvallate placenta

47. Which of the following is associated with a nuchal cord?
   a. long cord
   b. short cord
   c. velamentous cord
   d. true knots of the cord

48. Which of the following describes a prolapsed umbilical cord?
   a. focal dilatation of an umbilical vessel
   b. the cord precedes the fetus in the birthing process
   c. the intramembranous vessels of the fetus precede the fetus
   d. the cord completely surrounds the fetal neck with one loop

49. A succenturiate placenta is at an increased risk for which of the following?
   a. velamentous cord
   b. placental abruption
   c. intervillous thrombosis
   d. amniochorionic separation

50. Direction of umbilical cord coiling is:
   a. abnormal if coiled left
   b. abnormal if coiled right
   c. of no clinical significance
   d. associated with fetal anomalies

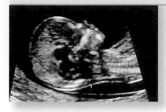

CHAPTER 29

Patient Care and Interventional Procedures

KEY TERMS

accountability   being required to answer for one's actions.

airborne pathogen   pathogens that remain infectious over long distances when suspended in air; pathogens transmitted by airborne route.

advance directive   a legal document describing one's health-care wishes if one is unable to communicate them.

Agency for Healthcare Research and Quality (AHRQ)   a government agency looking to improve the quality, safety, efficiency, and effectiveness of American health care.

autonomy   the right to make one's own independent decisions.

beneficence   bringing about good by maximizing benefits and minimizing possible harm.

Center for Disease Control (CDC)   federal agency that protects America from health, safety and security threats, both foreign and in the United States. Part of the U.S. health services.

code of conduct   the moral code, which guides professional conduct of duties and obligations.

contact pathogen   pathogens spread by direct or indirect contact with a patient or patient environment.

droplet pathogen   pathogens transmitted by respiratory droplets that are generated by a patient who is coughing, sneezing, or talking.

ethics   systems of valued behaviors and beliefs that govern proper conduct to ensure protection of individual's rights.

glutaraldehyde   a powerful solution commonly used to disinfect ultrasound transducers.

Health Insurance Portability and Accountability Act (HIPAA)   federal agency overseeing many health-care functions, the primary being patient confidentiality.

integrity   adherence to moral and ethical principles.

hysterosalpingogram   radiographic procedure where contrast material is injected through the endometrial cavity to evaluate uterine contour and fallopian tube patency.

The Joint Commission (JC)   an organization of health-care institutions devoted to improving, regulating, and accrediting its member institutions, with the goal of providing safe and efficient patient care, formerly the Joint Commission on Accreditation of Healthcare Organizations (JCAHO).

morality   the protection of cherished values that relate to how persons interact and live in peace.

patient-care partnership   standard describing patient's health-care rights.

personal protective equipment (PPE)   refers to wearable equipment that is intended to protect health-care worker from exposure or contact with infective pathogens.

veracity   truthfulness; honesty.

PATIENT CARE

Patient health-care rights include:
- High-quality medical care.
- A clean and safe environment.
- Involvement in his or her own care.
- Ability to express autonomy.
- Privacy protection of health-care information.

STANDARD PRECAUTIONS AND INFECTION CONTROL

- Previously termed *universal precautions.*
- Precautions compiled by the Centers for Disease Control and Prevention (CDC) and other federal agencies.
- To provide safety to both the patient and caregiver.
- Practiced two ways:
  1. General measures taken to keep health-care workers, patients, and the environment clean to prevent the spread of germs.
  2. Isolated precautions that are performed to confine disease-producing germs.

Standard Precautions for Use with All Patients*

- Standard precautions are not disease specific and apply to blood, all body secretions and excretions, nonintact skin, and mucous membranes.
- Proper hand washing before and after ALL patient contact.
- Use of gloves with ALL patient contact especially when touching body fluids, excretions, nonintact skin, mucous membranes, and contaminated items.
- Masks or face shields are to be worn if the face is likely to be splattered with contaminated body fluids and excretions.
- Fluid-resistant gowns are worn if clothing is likely to be splattered with contaminated body fluids or excretions.
- Patient-care equipment is properly cleaned after use and single-use items are discarded.
- Contaminated linen is placed in leakproof bags to prevent skin and mucous membrane exposure.
- All sharp instruments and needles are discarded in a puncture-resistant container. Center for Disease Control (CDC) recommends that needles be disposed of uncapped or a mechanical device be used for recapping

*Formerly universal precautions and body substance isolation.

Personal Protective Equipment (PPE)

- **Gloves**
  - Should cover the wrist.
  - Should only be used once and then discarded.
  - When removing gloves, ensure the inside part is on the outside.
  - Wash hands immediately after removing gloves.
- **Gowns**
  - Most protective clothing.
  - Should be long and large enough to cover your clothing.
  - Put gloves on after you have gowned.
- **Masks**
  - Used for airborne particle and droplet protection.
- **Eye and Face Shields**
  - Protect the mucous membranes of the face from pathogens.

Respiratory Hygiene/Cough Etiquette

- Targeted at patients and their family members with undiagnosed respiratory infections.
  1. Education of health-care facility staff, patients, and visitors.
  2. Post signs, in languages appropriate to the population served, with instructions to patients and family members with respiratory infections to cover their noses/mouths when sneezing or coughing, prompt disposal of used tissues, using surgical masks on the coughing person when tolerated.
  3. Availability of masks to patients and family members upon entry to facility.
  4. Proper hand washing after contact with respiratory secretions.
  5. Spatial separation, ideally greater than 3 feet of persons with respiratory infections in common waiting areas whenever possible.

Proper Hand Washing Technique

- Best protection to stop the spread of disease
  1. Wet your hands with clean, running water; turn off the tap; and apply soap.
  2. Lather your hands by rubbing them together. Be sure to lather the backs of your hands, between your fingers, and under your nails.
  3. Scrub your hands for at least 20 seconds.
  4. Rinse your hands well under clean, running water.
  5. Dry your hands using an air dryer or clean towel.

Transmission-Based Precautions

- Used when the route of transmission is not completely interrupted using standard precautions alone.
- Must be implemented while test results are pending based on the clinical presentation and likely pathogens.
- Gloves should be worn for ALL patient contact.

METHOD OF EXPOSURE	ILLNESS ASSOCIATED WITH:	GOWN	MASK/ FACE SHIELD	ROOM PRECAUTIONS	ROOM TURNOVER
Airborne	Chicken pox, Measles, Varicella zoster, Tuberculosis, Severe acute respiratory syndrome (SARS)	Only with likelihood of splattering of body fluids	Yes, unless immune to airborne illness. Patient may also be requested to wear a mask	Place patient in room with door closed as soon as possible (ASAP)	Clean any contaminated surface with disinfectant. Keep exam room closed for 4 hours. Clean any equipment used immediately after patient leave.
Contact	Gastrointestinal, respiratory, skin or wound infections, Chicken pox, Shingles, Rubella, Scabies, Lice, Hepatitis A, SARS, Multidrug resistant organisms	Yes, when working close to a patient or patient contact	Yes, if face is likely to be splattered with body fluids	Place patient in private room with door closed ASAP. In rooms with multiple patients, a distance of 3 feet or greater between patients is advised	Clean any contaminated surface with disinfectant. Clean any equipment used immediately after the patient leaves
Droplet	Influenza, Pneumonia, Meningitis, Pertussis, Rubella, Mump, Streptococcal disease, Rhinovirus, SARS	Yes, when working close to the patient and patient contact	Yes, if face is likely to be splattered with body fluids. Patient may also be required to wear a mask	Place patient in a private room ASAP. Door may remain open. In rooms with multiple patients, a distance of 3 feet or greater between patients is advised	Clean any contaminated surface with disinfectant

Emergency Situations

SITUATION	CAUSES	TREATMENT
Cardiac distress	Heart attack Respiratory arrest Medication interaction	Cardiopulmonary resuscitation (CPR) Automated external defibrillator (AED)
Choking	Obstruction	Abdominal thrusts
Respiratory distress	Heart attack Stroke Seizures Fainting	Open airway 1–2 ventilations lasting 1–2 s each
Syncope	Dehydration Postural hypotension Medications Diabetes mellitus Stroke Vasovagal reaction	Lay person supine with legs elevated If sitting, place head down between knees

TRANSDUCER CARE

- Following the manufacturer's recommendation, clean and disinfect transducers after each use.
- Probe covers are essential with transvaginal and translabial imaging.
- Glutaraldehyde is a powerful substance used as a high-level disinfectant for ultrasound transducers.
- Disinfection can also take place in an automated, closed system using a vaporized hydrogen peroxide solution as a high level disinfect for ultrasound transducers (e.g., Trophon®).
- Do not use heat sterilization technique to disinfect transducer or assembly.

SONOGRAPHER RESPONSIBILITIES

- Keep conversations low and private.
- Set screensavers to the lowest setting.
- Keep patient records private and out of public view.
- Maintain privacy of patient information from nonproviding personnel.
- Maintain a safe environment for patients and staff.
- Assess and evaluate patient information (e.g., medical chart, previous pertinent diagnostic imaging examinations).
- Perform quality ultrasound examinations following institution protocol, including necessary adaption when abnormalities are detected.
- Obtain and maintain appropriate professional credentials in areas of clinical practice.
- Dedication to life-long learning through continuing education, professional experience, and training.
- Remove patient identification from images used in publications or presentations.

SONOGRAPHER CODE OF ETHICS

- Scope of Practice - Clinical Standards and Code of Ethics for diagnostic medical sonographers have been developed and adopted by the Society of Diagnostic Medical Sonography (SDMS) and are available on their website http://sdms.org.

- Treat all patients, visitors, and colleagues with empathy and respect, honoring their autonomy and privacy.
- Be accountable for professional judgments and decisions.
- Provide patient care with equal respect for all.
- Respect and promote patient rights, provide patient care with respect for dignity and needs and acts as a patient advocate.
- Does not perform sonographic procedures without a medical order or indication, except for educational purposes.

PATIENT–SONOGRAPHER INTERACTION

- Sonographer–patient interaction is unique.
- Communication skills are an important aspect of the sonography profession.
- Keeping the patient relaxed, safe, and comfortable is the responsibility of the sonographer.

Patient–Sonographer Interaction

TIME FRAME	INTERACTION
Before examination	Review medical order Verify that proper examination is scheduled Review previous diagnostic studies, if available Review institution's examination protocol, if needed Address patient by his or her first and last name Introduce yourself to the patient and family Explain examination requested by the physician before beginning the scan Obtain patient history, including possible medication or latex allergies in a private environment Verify that patient name and identification number are correct on imaging screen Select the proper transducer frequency, limiting acoustic output in compliance with the as low as reasonably achievable (ALARA) principle
During examination	Perform ordered sonographic examination following institution protocol while • Maintaining patient modesty and privacy • Alleviating and addressing patient's concerns and questions • Performing basic patient care tasks as needed • Recognize and document sonographic characteristic of normal and abnormal tissues, structures, and blood flow • Perform measurements and calculations according to institutional protocol • Use professional judgment expanding on examination protocol as needed
After examination	Explain expected time frame for the patient's physician to receive a report Clean transducer(s), equipment, and keyboard Oral or written technical impression of real-time examination including any examination limitations to the reading physician.

INTERVENTIONAL PROCEDURES

Interventional Procedures—Gynecology

PROCEDURE	DESCRIPTION	TECHNIQUE

Abscess drainage	Percutaneous drainage	Percutaneous drainage
		Contents of abscess is aspirated and irrigated
		Catheter Placement
		A. Trocar technique
		  1. Catheter fits over a stiffen cannula
		  2. Sharp stylet is placed within cannula for insert
		  3. Catheter assembly is advanced under ultrasound guidance
		B. Seldinger technique
		  1. Guidewire is advanced through an aspiration needle and coiled within the abscess
		  2. Needle is removed
		  3. Dilators are introduced through guidewire
		  4. Once dilated, the catheter/cannula assembly is advanced into the abscess
		  5. Guidewire and inner cannula are removed while the catheter is advanced

Follicular aspiration	Used to retrieve mature oocytes for reproduction Retrival is occurs 30–34 h after administration of hCG	1. Use of transvaginal transducer with a needle guide attachment 2. Under ultrasound guidance an aspiration needle is inserted through the guide to the ovary 3. Using gentle suction, follicular fluid including the oocyte is aspirated 4. All of the fluid is removed, refilled, then reaspirated
Hysterosalpingogram (HSG)	Radiologic procedure Evaluates internal structures 1. Outlines extent of duplicated uterus 2. Localizes masses 3. Evaluates fallopian tube patency	Contrast media (iodine based) is injected into the uterine cavity Images are taken in real time using fluoroscopy Delayed x-ray images of the pelvis are generally included
Hysterosonogram	Installation of sterile saline solution into the endometrium to evaluate the endometrial cavity **Contraindications** 1. Positive pregnancy test 2. Pelvic inflammatory disease 3. Active menstrual bleeding	1. Sterile speculum is inserted by physician 2. Small catheter is inserted into the endometrial cavity to the level of the fundus 3. Speculum is removed 4. Injection of 10 to 15 mL of sterile saline into the endometrial cavity under ultrasound observation 5. Sagittal and coronal images to delineate the entire endometrial cavity

Intervention Procedures—Obstetrics

PROCEDURE	DESCRIPTION	SONOGRAHY CONTRIBUTIONS

Amniocentesis	Used to analyze fetal chromosomes in early pregnancy
	Typically, between 15 and 18 gestational weeks
	Can be performed as early as 12 gestational weeks
		Fetal survey to exclude congenital anomalies
		Assist in locating the optimal collection site away from:
		  Fetus
		  Umbilical cord
		  Central placenta
		  Uterine vessels
		Assess fetal well-being after procedure

Intervention Procedures—Obstetrics—(cont'd)

PROCEDURE	DESCRIPTION	SONOGRAHY CONTRIBUTIONS
Chorionic villi sampling	Performed between 10 and 12 gestational weeks Results available in 1 week	Determine the relationship between the lie of the uterus and cervix and the path of the catheter route Assess fetal viability and location Identify uterine masses Needle guidance during biopsy Assess fetal well-being after procedure
Cordocentesis	In utero sampling of umbilical cord blood for diagnostic and therapeutic purposes Indications 1. **Diagnostic** Rapid karyotyping Fetal infections Fetal hematocrit 2. **Therapeutic** Transfusion Drug infusion	Needle guidance during aspiration procedure Assess the fetus well-being after procedure
Embryoscopy	Permits direct viewing of the developing fetus	Assess fetal well-being after procedure
Intrauterine transfusion	Access into the fetal circulation through the umbilical vein Goal—correct anemia and suppress fetal erythropoiesis Umbilical artery puncture associated with vasospasm, bradycardia, and sudden death	Needle guidance during procedure Assess fetal well-being after procedure

PATIENT CARE AND TECHNIQUE REVIEW

1. An advance directive communicates to all health-care providers the:
   a. medical history of the patient
   b. health-care wishes of the patient
   c. emergency contacts of the patient
   d. food and drug allergies of the patient

2. Explaining the ultrasound examination is accomplished:
   a. during the examination
   b. when the patient inquires
   c. before an invasive procedure
   d. before beginning the examination

3. Maintaining privacy of patient medical information is a primary goal of the:
   a. Patient-Care Partnership
   b. Joint Review Committee
   c. Agency for Healthcare Research and Quality
   d. Health Insurance Portability and Accountability Act

4. Which of the following is *not* a responsibility of the sonographer?
   a. keep conversations low and private
   b. give technical report to the patient
   c. set screensavers to the lowest setting
   d. keep patient records out of public view

5. Which of the following is *not* a patient health-care right?
   a. high-quality medical care
   b. clean and safe environment
   c. subjugation of self-sufficiency
   d. involvement in his or her own medical care

6. On completion of the examination, the sonographer should:
   a. introduce himself or herself to the patient
   b. explain the examination to the patient
   c. obtain clinical information from the patient
   d. inform patient of expected time frame for examination results

7. Medical imaging transducers are cleaned and sterilized according to the:
   a. manufacturer's recommendations
   b. supervising sonographer's preference
   c. institution's infection control department
   d. Occupational Safety and Health Administration

8. Genetic testing by amniocentesis is typically performed between:
   a. 8 and 12 gestational weeks
   b. 10 and 12 gestational weeks
   c. 15 and 18 gestational weeks
   d. 18 and 20 gestational weeks

9. Which of the following procedures may use a Trocar technique?
   a. embryoscopy
   b. abscess drainage
   c. follicular aspiration
   d. chorionic villi sampling

10. Adherence to moral and ethical principles describes:
    a. ethics
    b. integrity
    c. morality
    d. beneficence

11. Which of the following is required of a medical facility to promote respiratory hygiene?
    a. availability of surgical face masks
    b. spatial spacing of patients a minimum of 2 feet apart
    c. availability of nonlatex gloves
    d. spatial spacing of patients a minimum of 4 feet apart.

12. Which of the following illnesses may be transmitted through the air?
    a. lice
    b. scabies
    c. hepatitis A
    d. tuberculosis

13. Which of the following require a patient to be placed in a private room with the door closed? '
    a. contact pathogens
    b. droplet pathogens
    c. airborne pathogens
    d. airborne and contact pathogens

14. When using the hand washing technique, hands should be scrubbed for a minimum of:
    a. 10 seconds
    b. 20 seconds
    c. 40 seconds
    d. 60 seconds

15. What is considered the best protection to stop the spread of disease?
    a. spatial separation
    b. wearing gloves
    c. wearing a surgical mask
    d. proper hand washing

16. Gloves should be worn with:
    a. all patients
    b. patients with pneumonia
    c. auto-immune suppressed patients
    d. patients with multidrug-resistant infections

17. Transmission of severe acute respiratory syndrome may occur through:
    a. airborne exposure
    b. airborne and contact exposure
    c. contact and droplet exposure
    d. droplet, contact and airborne exposure

18. Follicular aspiration occurs:
    a. on day 10 of the menstrual cycle
    b. 24 to 30 hours after administration of hCG
    c. on day 14 of the menstrual cycle
    d. 30 to 34 hours after administration of hCG

19. Chorionic villi sampling is typically performed between:
    a. 6 and 8 gestational weeks
    b. 8 and 10 gestational weeks
    c. 10 and 12 gestational weeks
    d. 12 and 14 gestational weeks

20. The goal of intrauterine transfusion is:
    a. to correct fetal anemia
    b. for rapid karyotyping
    c. to diagnose fetal infection
    d. to correct fetal hydrops

21. Which of the following is commonly used for high disinfection of ultrasound transducers?
    a. acetone
    b. Tegaderm
    c. glutaraldehyde
    d. hydrogen peroxide

22. Maximizing benefits and minimizing possible harm describes:
    a. ethics
    b. autonomy
    c. accountability
    d. beneficence

23. Contaminated linens are always:
    a. discarded only into the blue linen bins
    b. discarded only into the regular linen bins
    c. discarded only into the red linen bins
    d. placed into a leak proof bag and placed in appropriate linen bins

24. Coughing etiquette is mainly targeted at:
    a. visitors
    b. patients
    c. health-care workers
    d. patients and visitors

25. Which of the following characterizes veracity?
    a. honesty
    b. the right to make personal decisions
    c. minimizing possible harm to patients
    d. moral and ethical principles

26. General measures taken to keep health-care workers, patients, and the surrounding environment clean are commonly known as:
    a. patient care
    b. standard precautions
    c. universal precautions
    d. body substance isolation

27. A standard used to describe patient health-care rights is termed:
    a. universal precautions
    b. advanced directive
    c. health-care partnership
    d. patient-care partnership

28. Which of the following accurately describes transmission-based precautions (TBP)?
    a. TBP used to be termed universal precautions
    b. TBP must be implemented based on clinical presentation
    c. TBP must be implemented before standard precautions.
    d. TBP does not have to be implemented until test results are positive.

29. If a person faints, the sonographer should:
    a. lay the person supine and call 911
    b. lay the person down and elevate their head
    c. lay the person down with their head extended back
    d. lay the person down and elevate their legs

30. Which of the following is a responsibility of the sonographer?
    a. keep the patient relaxed
    b. keep the patient safe
    c. keep the patient comfortable
    d. all of the above

31. Ultrasound examinations should only be performed with an order and proper indication EXCEPT in cases of:
    a. fetal viability
    b. gender determination
    c. educational purposes
    d. infertility monitoring

32. Being accountable for professional judgments and decisions is an example of:
    a. standard precautions
    b. sonographer ethics
    c. patient-care partnership
    d. patient-sonographer interaction

33. Which of the following governs proper conduct?
    a. ethics
    b. justice
    c. autonomy
    d. accountability

34. What refers to a person's capacity to formulate, express, and carry out value-based preferences?
    a. ethics
    b. autonomy
    c. beneficence
    d. nonmaleficence

35. Clinical Standards and Code of Ethics specific for diagnostic medical sonographers has been developed and adopted by the:
    a. Society of Diagnostic Medical Sonographers
    b. American Registry in Diagnostic Medical Sonographers
    c. Joint Review Committee for Diagnostic Medical Sonography
    d. Commission on Accreditation of Allied Health Educational Programs

36. Washing hands before and after an examination are examples of:
    a. OSHA standards
    b. isolation techniques
    c. respiratory isolation
    d. standard precautions

37. Which of the following pathogens is spread through droplet exposure?
    a. lice
    b. scabies
    c. rubella
    d. hepatitis A

38. How do automated disinfectant systems decontaminate ultrasound transducers?
    a. steam with water
    b. vaporize with Tegaderm
    c. vaporize with acetone
    d. vaporize with hydrogen peroxide

39. Which of the following is a common cause of cardiac distress?
    a. seizures
    b. fainting
    c. vasovagal reaction
    d. medication interaction

40. Reviewing pertinent diagnostic studies should be completed:
    a. prior to beginning the examination
    b. at the conclusion of the examination
    c. during the examination when an abnormality is visualized
    d. during the examination when an abnormality is not visualized

41. Hysterosalpingogram is a(n):
    a. radiological procedure to evaluate the cervix
    b. ultrasound procedure to evaluate the endometrium
    c. radiological procedure to evaluate for fallopian tube patency
    d. computed tomography procedure to evaluate the myometrium

42. A health-care professional's duty to protect the privacy of patient information is termed:
    a. ethics
    b. integrity
    c. beneficence
    d. confidentiality

43. Which of the following is a therapeutic indication for cordocentesis?
    a. transfusion
    b. fetal infection
    c. fetal hematocrit
    d. rapid karyotype

44. The initials CDC stand for:
    a. Country Disease Control
    b. Center for Disease Control
    c. Chronic Diseases in the Country
    d. Center of Disease Consensus

45. Which of the following is NOT considered personal protective equipment?
    a. gloves
    b. gowns
    c. hair net
    d. face shields

46. Gloves should be long enough to cover the:
    a. hand
    b. wrist
    c. mid portion of the forearm
    d. lower third of the forearm

47. What is the proper method to remove gloves?
    a. inside portion is on the inside
    b. wash hands before removing gloves
    c. inside portion is on the outside
    d. there is no method to remove gloves

48. Which federal agency looks to improve the quality, safety, efficiency, and effectiveness of American health care?
    a. CDC
    b. OSHA
    c. HIPPA
    d. AHRQ

49. HIPAA stands for
  a. Health Insurance Privacy and Accountability Act
  b. Health Institution Portability and Accountability Act
  c. Health Institution Privacy and Accountability Act
  d. Health Insurance Portability and Accountability Act

50. Hepatitis A is an example which of the following exposures?
  a. droplet
  b. contact
  c. airborne
  d. airborne and contact

1. A cloverleaf-shaped cranium in a second trimester fetus is characteristic of:
   a. anencephaly
   b. fetal demise
   c. oligohydramnios
   d. skeletal dysplasia

2. Which genitourinary abnormality depends on fetal gender?
   a. infantile polycystic disease
   b. multicystic dysplastic kidney
   c. ureteropelvic junction obstruction
   d. posterior urethral valve obstruction

3. Which pelvic structure contains the uterine blood vessels and nerves?
   a. psoas muscles
   b. broad ligament
   c. ovarian ligaments
   d. suspensory ligaments

4. When the vascular space between the placenta and myometrium is absent, the sonographer should suspect:
   a. placenta accreta
   b. placenta abruptio
   c. circumvallate placenta
   d. umbilical vein thrombosis

5. Measurement of the biparietal diameter is taken at a level to include the:
   a. falx cerebri
   b. cisterna magna
   c. fourth ventricle
   d. thalamic cerebri

6. The best measuring method for evaluating gestational age is the:
   a. femur length
   b. biparietal diameter
   c. crown–rump length
   d. head circumference

7. Bilateral symmetric pelvic masses are most likely:
   a. pelvic muscles
   b. follicular cysts
   c. theca lutein cysts
   d. uterine leiomyomas

8. A localized hypoechoic adnexal mass is present on serial sonograms. Ovaries appear within normal limits. Based on this clinical history, the adnexal mass is most suspicious for a(n):
   a. dermoid cyst
   b. endometrioma
   c. parovarian cyst
   d. hemorrhagic cyst

9. Maintaining privacy of a patient's medical and personal information is a primary concern of the:
   a. Patient Care Partnership
   b. Joint Review Committee
   c. Agency for Healthcare Research and Quality
   d. Health Insurance Portability and Accountability Act

10. Which of the following is *not* evaluated during a fetal biophysical profile?
    a. nonstress test
    b. fetal swallowing
    c. diaphragm movement
    d. amniotic fluid volume

11. An echogenic endometrium with posterior acoustic enhancement is present during which of the following phases?
    a. follicular
    b. secretory
    c. menstrual
    d. proliferative

12. Normal serum maternal alpha-fetoprotein levels vary with:
    a. fetal weight
    b. fetal gender
    c. maternal age
    d. gestational age

13. A diamniotic/monochorionic multifetal pregnancy will demonstrate:
    a. one placenta and one gestational sac
    b. two placentas and one gestational sac
    c. one placenta and two gestational sacs
    d. two placentas and two gestational sacs

14. Symmetrical intrauterine growth restriction is most likely a result of:
    a. first trimester insult
    b. placental insufficiency
    c. maternal hypertension
    d. chromosomal abnormality

15. Which of the following structures shunts blood away from the fetal lungs?
    a. pulmonary vein
    b. coronary artery
    c. ductus venosus
    d. ductus arteriosus

16. Which of the following abnormalities demonstrates an arteriovenous anastomosis?
    a. acardiac twin
    b. twin–twin transfusion syndrome
    c. conjoined twins
    d. intrauterine growth restriction

17. Which rare benign ovarian neoplasm occurs most often in postmenopausal women?
    a. thecoma
    b. dysgerminoma
    c. Brenner tumor
    d. granulosa cell tumor

18. Hydranencephaly is an abnormality of the:
    a. vein of Galen
    b. third ventricle
    c. cerebral cortex
    d. cisterna magna

19. Common sonographic findings associated with Dandy-Walker syndrome include:
    a. macroglossia and omphalocele
    b. megaureter and oligohydramnios
    c. infantile polycystic disease and oligohydramnios
    d. enlarged posterior fossa and absence of the cerebellar vermis

20. A diffusely enlarged uterus demonstrating a inhomogeneous myometrium is most suspicious for:
    a. endometritis
    b. adenomyosis
    c. endometriosis
    d. subserosal fibroid

Using Figure 1, answer question 21.

21. Which of the following does the arrow identify?
    a. adenomyosis
    b. endometriosis
    c. refraction artifact
    d. pedunculating fibroid

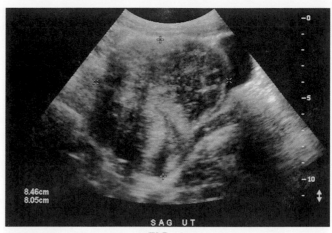

FIG. 2

Using Figure 2, answer question 22.

22. Differential considerations for this sonogram would include:
    a. leiomyomas or leiomyosarcomas
    b. cystic teratomas or endometriosis
    c. ovarian torsion or ectopic pregnancy
    d. endometrial hyperplasia or hematometra

Using Figure 3, answer question 23.

23. A menarche patient presents with a history of mild pelvic pain. Only one ovary is identified with certainty. Based on this history, the sonogram most likely identifies a(n):
    a. appendicitis
    b. endometrioma
    c. cystic teratoma
    d. hemorrhagic cyst

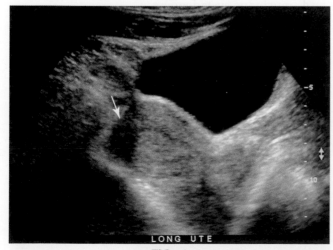

FIG. 1

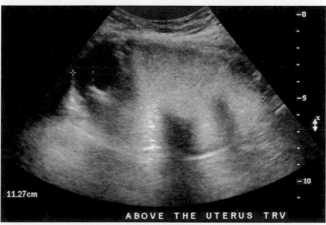

FIG. 3 Transverse sonogram.

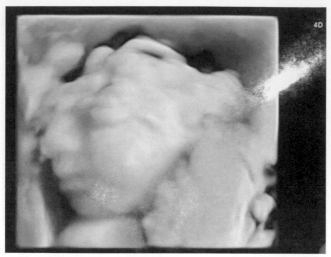

FIG. 4

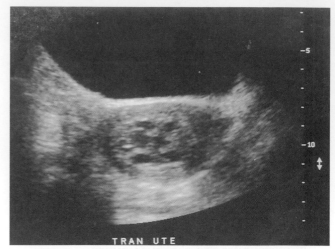

FIG. 6 Transverse sonogram of the uterus.

Using Figure 4, answer question 24.

24. This 3-D sonogram is most likely demonstrating:
   a. acrania
   b. anencephaly
   c. microcephaly
   d. hydranencephaly

Using Figure 5, answer question 25.

25. This sagittal image of the uterus documents:
   a. Asherman syndrome
   b. an intrauterine device
   c. endometrial hyperplasia
   d. intrauterine vascular calcifications

Using Figure 6, answer question 26.

26. An asymptomatic postmenopausal patient presents with a history of breast cancer and tamoxifen therapy. Based on this clinical history, the sonographic findings are most suspicious for:
   a. endometritis
   b. adenomyosis
   c. endometrial polyp
   d. degenerating fibroid

Using Figure 7, answer question 27.

27. A 15-year-old presents with a history of amenorrhea and pelvic fullness. Based on this clinical history, the sagittal sonogram is most suspicious for:
   a. hematometra
   b. endometrioma
   c. tuboovarian abscess
   d. mucinous cystadenoma

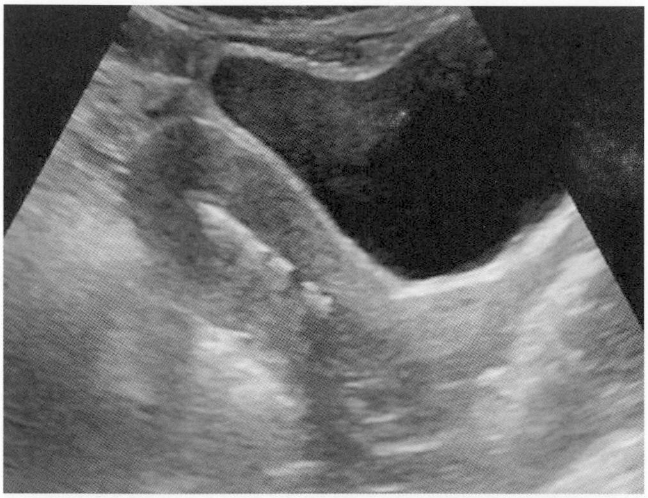

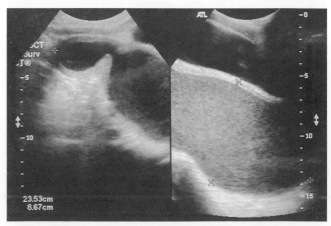

FIG. 5 Transabdominal sonogram.

FIG. 7 Sonogram of the pelvic midline.

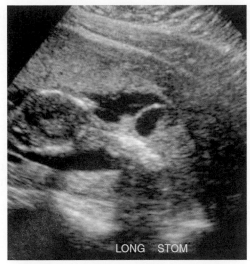

FIG. 8 Sonogram of the left ovary.

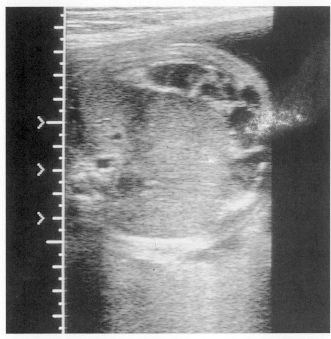

FIG. 10

Using Figure 8, answer question 28.

28. This sonogram of a second trimester fetus is most suspicious for:
    a. duodenal atresia
    b. transesophageal fistula
    c. diaphragmatic hernia
    d. cystic adenomatoid malformation

Using Figure 9, answer question 29.

29. This sonogram is most suspicious for which of the following abnormalities?
    a. cloverleaf skull
    b. encephalocele
    c. cystic hygroma
    d. normal umbilical cord

Using Figure 10, answer question 30.

30. This third trimester cross-sectional image of the fetal abdomen is suspicious for:
    a. megaureter
    b. fetal hydrops
    c. duodenal atresia
    d. meconium peritonitis

31. Which phase of the endometrium demonstrates the thinnest diameter?
    a. early secretory
    b. late menstrual
    c. early menstrual
    d. early proliferative

32. Normal embryonic herniation of the bowel permits development of the:
    a. diaphragm
    b. thoracic cavity
    c. umbilical cord
    d. abdominal organs

33. Which classification of osteogenesis imperfecta is most lethal?
    a. Type I
    b. Type II
    c. Type III
    d. Type IV

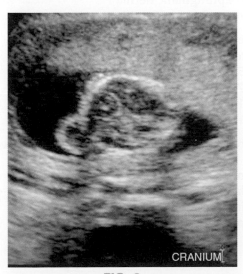

FIG. 9

34. Which leiomyoma location is most likely to cause heavy irregular uterine bleeding?
   a. serosal
   b. intramural
   c. subserosal
   d. submucosal

35. The landmark used to localize the correct level for measuring abdominal circumference is:
   a. kidneys
   b. stomach
   c. cord insertion
   d. left portal vein

36. Which of the following is transmitted through droplet exposure?
   a. shingles
   b. influenza
   c. tuberculosis
   d. hepatitis A

37. Normal nuchal translucency should not exceed:
   a. 2 mm
   b. 3 mm
   c. 5 mm
   d. 10 mm

38. Which obstetrical condition is an indication for immediate delivery?
   a. vasa previa
   b. placenta accreta
   c. placental abruption
   d. incompetent cervix

39. At what gestational age are chorionic villus sampling procedures commonly performed?
   a. 5 to 7 weeks
   b. 7 to 9 weeks
   c. 10 to 12 weeks
   d. 15 to 18 weeks

40. Which structure would you evaluate if a patient presents with a history of a gartner cyst?
   a. cervix
   b. vagina
   c. endometrium
   d. fallopian tube

41. Brightly echogenic bowel in the second trimester is most likely associated with which abnormality?
   a. bowel atresia
   b. meconium ileus
   c. Down syndrome
   d. Pentalogy of Cantrell

42. Clinodactyly refers to:
   a. the fusion of digits
   b. the absence of digits
   c. widespread digits
   d. the inward curvature of digits

43. In postmenopausal women, endometrial thickness is consistently benign when measuring:
   a. 5 mm or less
   b. 8 mm or less
   c. 10 mm or less
   d. 12 mm or less

44. Fluid within the endometrial cavity is:
   a. a pathological finding
   b. characteristic of an endometrial polyp
   c. not included in the endometrial measurement
   d. a sonographic finding in Asherman syndrome

45. The cervix-to-corpus ratio of a premenarche uterus is:
   a. 1:2
   b. 3:1
   c. 1:1
   d. 2:1

46. Enlargement of the third ventricle is a finding associated with:
   a. hydranencephaly
   b. Dandy-Walker syndrome
   c. agenesis of the corpus callosum
   d. Beckwith-Wiedemann syndrome

47. Which segment of the fallopian tube is potentially the most life-threatening in a ruptured ectopic pregnancy?
   a. isthmus
   b. ampulla
   c. interstitial
   d. infundibulum

48. If the fluid-filled fetal stomach is not visualized on serial sonograms, the sonographer should suspect:
   a. duodenal atresia
   b. esophageal atresia
   c. diaphragmatic hernia
   d. meconium peritonitis

49. The yolk sac is abnormal after the diameter exceeds:
   a. 5 mm
   b. 7 mm
   c. 10 mm
   d. 12 mm

50. In relation to the ovaries, the external iliac vessels are located:
   a. medial
   b. lateral
   c. inferior
   d. posterior

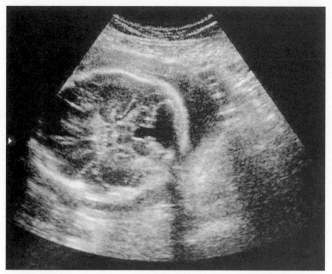

FIG. 11

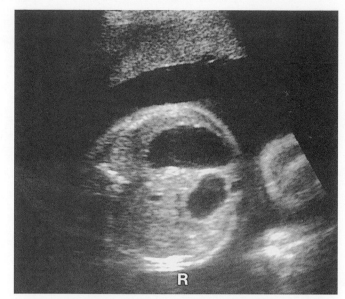

FIG. 12

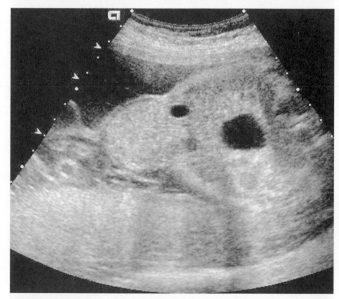

FIG. 13

Using Figure 11, answer question 51.

51. This late second trimester sonogram of the fetal cranium is most suspicious for which of the following abnormalities?
   a. arachnoid cyst
   b. hydrocephalus
   c. coexisting spina bifida
   d. Dandy-Walker syndrome

Using Figure 12, answer questions 52 and 53.

52. This cross-sectional abdominal image of a second trimester fetus shows an abnormality most suspicious for:
   a. omental cyst
   b. umbilical varix
   c. meconium ileus
   d. duodenal atresia

53. Which of the following most likely coexists with this abnormality?
   a. macrosomia
   b. fetal hydrops
   c. polyhydramnios
   d. intrauterine growth restriction

Using Figure 13, answer questions 54 and 55.

54. This image of the fetal abdomen most likely identifies which of the following abnormalities?
   a. gastroschisis
   b. omphalocele
   c. umbilical hernia
   d. abdominal teratoma

55. With this finding, maternal serum alpha-fetoprotein levels are expected to demonstrate a:
   a. significant decrease
   b. significant elevation
   c. normal or slightly elevated level
   d. normal or minimally decreased level

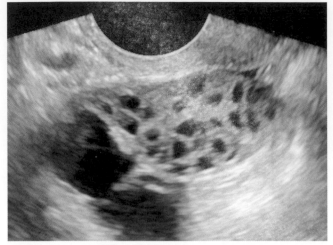

FIG. 14

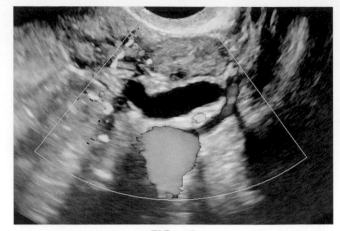

FIG. 16

Using Figure 14, answer question 56.

56. A 30-year-old patient presents with a history of infertility. Based on this history, the sonogram of the right ovary most likely displays which of the following abnormalities?
   a. theca lutein cysts
   b. dilated ovarian vessels
   c. polycystic ovarian syndrome
   d. ovarian hyperstimulation syndrome

Using Figure 15, answer question 57.

57. The arrow in this cross-sectional image of the fetal chest identifies which of the following?
   a. pleural effusion
   b. pericardial effusion
   c. diaphragmatic hernia
   d. transposition of the great vessels

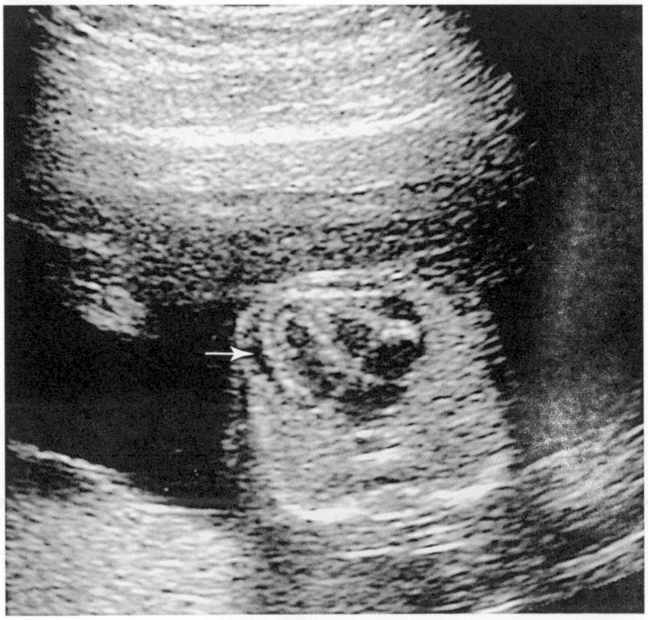

Using Figure 16, answer question 58.

58. This sonogram of the left adnexa is most suspicious for:
   a. hydrosalpinx
   b. ovarian torsion
   c. tuboovarian abscess
   d. ruptured ectopic pregnancy

Using Figure 17 (and Color Plate 11), answer question 59.

59. A 30-year-old patient presents with a history of dysmenorrhea. Bilateral ovaries appear within normal limits. Based on this clinical history, this sonogram of the left adnexa is most suspicious for:
   a. endometrioma
   b. cystic teratoma
   c. ovarian carcinoma
   d. paraovarian cyst

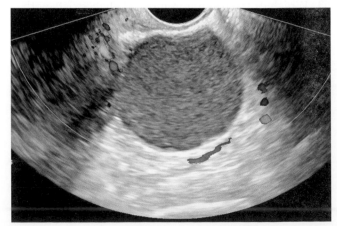

FIG. 17   Sonogram of the adnexa (see Color Plate 11).

FIG. 15

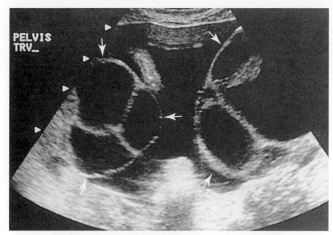

FIG. 18

Using Figure 18, answer questions 60 and 61.

60. This transverse sonogram in a patient undergoing ovulation induction therapy demonstrates which of the following?
    a. bilateral hydrosalpinx
    b. bilateral cystadenomas
    c. polycystic ovarian syndrome
    d. ovarian hyperstimulation syndrome

61. With this diagnosis, the sonographer should also evaluate the:
    a. kidneys for nephrolithiasis
    b. right upper quadrant for ascites
    c. urinary bladder for obstruction
    d. right upper quadrant for biliary obstruction

62. Twin peak sign is present with:
    a. dichorionic-diamniotic twin pregnancy
    b. monochorionic-diamniotic twin pregnancy
    c. dichorionic-monoamniotic twin pregnancy
    d. monochorionic-monoamniotic twin pregnancy

63. Which of the following is the best protection against the spread of disease?
    a. wearing gowns
    b. wearing gloves
    c. proper handwashing
    d. wearing face shields

64. Placenta previa is ruled out when the placental edge is located a minimum of what distance from the internal os?
    a. 1.0 cm
    b. 1.5 cm
    c. 2.0 cm
    d. 3.0 cm

65. Dangling of the choroid plexus is associated with:
    a. arachnoid cyst
    b. ventriculomegaly
    c. holoprosencephaly
    d. agenesis of the corpus callosum

66. A defect of the fetal lymphatic system typically results in development of a(n):
    a. facial cleft
    b. arachnoid cyst
    c. cystic hygroma
    d. diaphragmatic hernia

67. In a menarche patient, a multilayered appearance is present during which endometrial phase?
    a. late secretory phase
    b. late menstrual phase
    c. late proliferation phase
    d. early proliferation phase

68. Which vessel provides the best imaging landmark for locating the ovaries?
    a. internal iliac artery
    b. external iliac artery
    c. common iliac artery
    d. distal abdominal aorta

69. Which pelvic muscle is most frequently mistaken for the ovary?
    a. piriformis
    b. levator ani
    c. pubococcygeus
    d. obturator internus

70. Proliferation of the endometrium is a result of:
    a. estrogen
    b. progesterone
    c. luteinizing hormone
    d. human chorionic gonadotropin

71. What is the most specific measurement for determining intrauterine growth restriction and macrosomia?
    a. femur length
    b. cephalic index
    c. head circumference
    d. abdominal circumference

72. An extrauterine mass most commonly develops on which of the following structures?
    a. ovary
    b. fallopian tube
    c. large intestines
    d. broad ligament

73. A mature physiological cyst is termed a:
    a. corpus luteum
    b. graafian follicle
    c. corpus albicans
    d. cumulus oophorus

74. The levator ani muscles are at the level of the:
    a. vagina
    b. ovaries
    c. iliac vessels
    d. uterine corpus

75. Which of the following is not physiological in origin?
    a. nabothian cyst
    b. corpus albicans
    c. theca lutein cyst
    d. corpus lutein cyst

76. Encephaloceles are typically located in which region of the calvaria?
    a. frontal
    b. parietal
    c. temporal
    d. occipital

77. Which of the following is most likely to mimic anencephaly?
    a. acrania
    b. encephalocele
    c. arachnoid cyst
    d. holoprosencephaly

78. The most common neural tube defect is:
    a. anencephaly
    b. caudal regression
    c. spina bifida aperta
    d. spina bifida occulta

79. Holoprosencephaly is most often associated with which of the following syndromes?
    a. Patau
    b. Turner
    c. Edward
    d. Noonan

80. Which of the following is the result of a cranial defect?
    a. prosencephaly
    b. encephalocele
    c. cystic hygroma
    d. Dandy-Walker malformation

81. Which of the following abnormalities most likely demonstrates a normal maternal serum alpha-fetoprotein (MSAFP) level?
    a. anencephaly
    b. encephalocele
    c. spina bifida aperta
    d. multifetal gestation

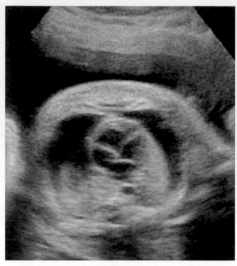

FIG. 19

Using Figure 19, answer question 82.

82. What anomaly is present in this image of the fetal chest?
    a. ectopia cordis
    b. pleural effusions
    c. pericardial effusion
    d. diaphragmatic hernia

Using Figure 20, answer question 83.

83. The arrow in this sonogram identifies which of the following?
    a. uterine fibroid
    b. battledore placenta
    c. succenturiate placenta
    d. myometrial contraction

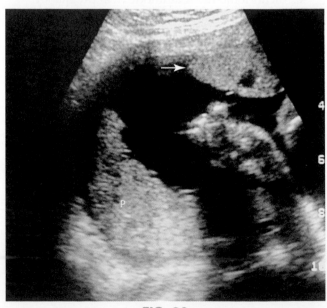

FIG. 20

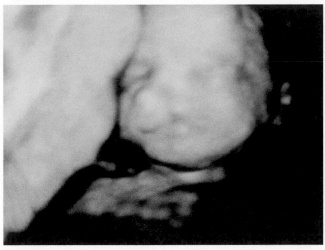

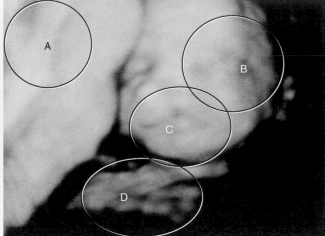

FIG. 21

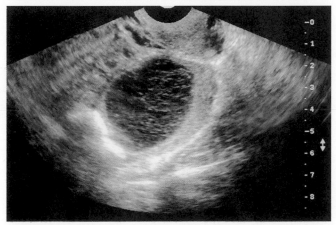

FIG. 22

Using Figure 21, answer questions 84 and 85.

84. Which of the following circled areas demonstrates a fetal anomaly?
   a. A
   b. B
   c. C
   d. D

85. This anomaly is most commonly associated with which of the following?
   a. spina bifida
   b. polyhydramnios
   c. oligohydramnios
   d. duodenal atresia

Using Figure 22, answer question 86.

86. A patient presents with a history of acute left lower quadrant pain. Her last menstrual period was approximately 3 weeks earlier. Based on this clinical history, the sonogram is most suspicious for:
   a. cystic teratoma
   b. theca lutein cyst
   c. graafian follicle
   d. hemorrhagic cyst

Using Figure 23, answer question 87.

87. This color Doppler image of the fetal pelvis is most suspicious for:
   a. an ovarian cyst
   b. the keyhole sign
   c. the umbilical vein
   d. one umbilical artery

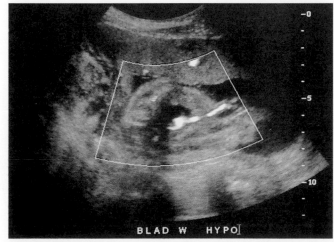

FIG. 23

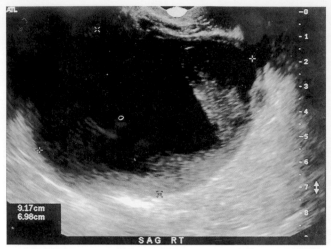

FIG. 24

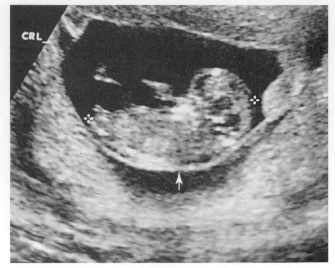

FIG. 26

Using Figure 24, answer question 88.

88. The sagittal image of the right adnexa is most suspicious for a:
   a. cystic teratoma
   b. theca lutein cyst
   c. serous cystadenoma
   d. polycystic ovarian disease

Using Figure 25, answer question 89.

89. Which of the following abnormalities is most likely displayed in this third trimester sonogram?
   a. urethral fistula
   b. nabothian cyst
   c. placenta accreta
   d. incompetent cervix

Using Figure 26, answer question 90.

90. The arrowhead most likely identifies a(n):
   a. normal amnion
   b. normal chorion
   c. normal nuchal translucency
   d. abnormal nuchal translucency

Using Figure 27, answer question 91.

91. This sonogram most likely demonstrates:
   a. a uterine contraction
   b. marginal placenta previa
   c. circumvallate placenta
   d. complete placenta previa

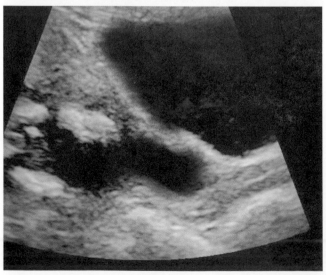

FIG. 25

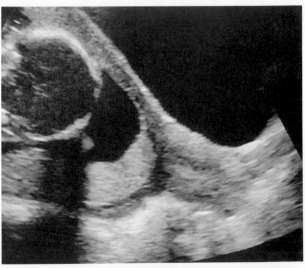

FIG. 27

92. Normal maximum placental thickness in a second trimester pregnancy should not exceed:
   a. 2 cm
   b. 3 cm
   c. 4 cm
   d. 5 cm

93. Which of the following is most likely associated with oligohydramnios?
   a. facial cleft
   b. duodenal atresia
   c. diaphragmatic hernia
   d. intrauterine growth restriction

94. Which chamber of the heart lies more anterior?
   a. left atrium
   b. right atrium
   c. left ventricle
   d. right ventricle

95. Which of the following fetal abnormalities is more commonly associated with diabetic patients?
   a. anencephaly
   b. caudal regression
   c. spina bifida aperta
   d. spina bifida occulta

96. Which hormone is responsible for inducing ovulation during a normal menstrual cycle?
   a. estrogen
   b. progesterone
   c. luteinizing hormone
   d. follicle-stimulating hormone

97. A cystic hygroma is often associated with which of the following?
   a. cranial defect
   b. maternal hypertension
   c. maternal diabetes mellitus
   d. chromosomal abnormality

98. Nabothian cysts are located in the:
   a. cervix
   b. vagina
   c. perineum
   d. broad ligament

99. Which portion of the fetal brain demonstrates ventriculomegaly first?
   a. third ventricle
   b. frontal horn of the lateral ventricle
   c. occipital horn of the lateral ventricle
   d. temporal horn of the lateral ventricle

100. Which abnormality is associated with trophoblastic disease?
   a. corpus albicans
   b. cystic teratomas
   c. theca lutein cysts
   d. mucinous cystadenomas

101. On day 20 of the menstrual cycle the endometrium displays a:
   a. triple line appearance
   b. thin discrete hyperechoic line
   c. hypoechoic functional layer and hyperechoic basal layer
   d. hyperechoic functional layer and hypoechoic basal layer

102. What forms the chorion?
   a. amnion
   b. decidua basalis
   c. decidua capsularis
   d. a double layer of trophoblasts

103. Thickness of the endometrium is dependent on:
   a. hormone levels
   b. the patient's age
   c. the dominant follicle
   d. the number of days between menses

104. A "chocolate cyst" is a term used to describe which of the following?
   a. dermoid cyst
   b. endometrioma
   c. corpus luteal cyst
   d. hemorrhagic cyst

105. Diffuse uterine enlargement demonstrating diffuse myometrial anechoic areas are sonographic findings consistent with:
   a. endometritis
   b. adenomyosis
   c. endometriosis
   d. Asherman syndrome

106. Transvaginally, in a sagittal plane, the urinary bladder should display on which portion of the screen?
   a. left lower
   b. right lower
   c. left upper
   d. right upper

107. Which laboratory value determines when the ovary is ready to ovulate?
   a. estradiol
   b. progesterone
   c. luteinizing hormone
   d. follicle-stimulating hormone

108. A 30-year-old patient with normal menses presents for an ultrasound on the tenth day of her cycle. The endometrial stripe is expected to demonstrate:
a. a thick, hypoechoic functional and basal layer
b. a thick, hypoechoic functional layer and a hyperechoic basal layer
c. a thin, hypoechoic functional layer and a thick, hyperechoic basal layer
d. a thick, hyperechoic functional layer and a thin, hypoechoic basal layer

109. Which of the following statements is true for a postmenopausal patient not receiving hormone replacement therapy?
a. Ovarian size remains the same.
b. Ovarian cysts are a common finding.
c. Decreases in estrogen can shorten the vagina.
d. Endometrial carcinoma is the most common cause of postmenopausal bleeding.

110. Which portion of the uterus is indistinct in the nongravid state?
a. cervix
b. corpus
c. fundus
d. isthmus

111. The suspensory ligament attaches the:
a. cervix to the sacrum
b. ovary to the pelvic sidewall
c. fallopian tube to the uterus
d. ovary to the cornua of the uterus

112. An anechoic tubular adnexal mass posterior and lateral to the uterus in an asymptomatic patient is most likely the:
a. hydrosalpinx
b. endometrioma
c. parovarian cyst
d. tuboovarian abscess

Using Figure 28, answer question 113.

113. This transverse image of a second trimester sacrum most likely demonstrates which of the following?
a. spina bifida
b. caudal regression
c. bladder exstrophy
d. sacrococcygeal teratoma

Using Figure 29, answer question 114.

114. A patient presents with a history of breast carcinoma and tamoxifen therapy. The endovaginal image of the uterus is most suspicious for which of the following abnormalities?
a. adenomyosis
b. endometriosis
c. endometrial polyp
d. endometrial hyperplasia

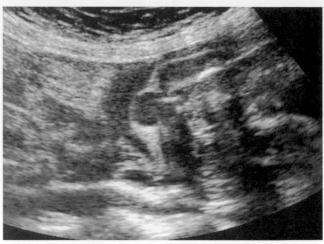

FIG. 28

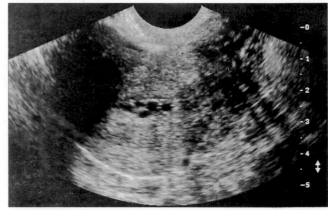

FIG. 29

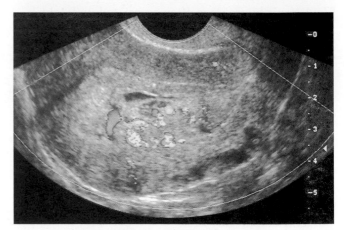

FIG. 30   (See Color Plate 12.)

Using Figure 30 (and Color Plate 12), answer question 115.

115. A patient presents with a history of vaginal spotting since a therapeutic abortion 3-weeks earlier. The transvaginal sonogram of the uterus is most suspicious for:
a. endometritis
b. trophoblastic disease
c. a pseudogestational sac
d. anembryonic pregnancy

502

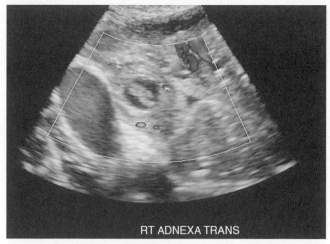

RT ADNEXA TRANS

FIG. 31

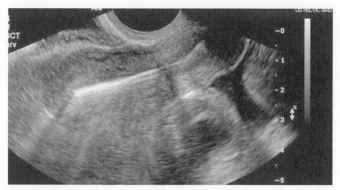

FIG. 33

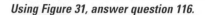

Using Figure 31, answer question 116.

116. A patient presents with a history of pelvic pain and a last menstrual period 6- weeks earlier. This sonogram of the right adnexa is most suspicious for a(n):
   a. dermoid cyst
   b. endometrioma
   c. ectopic pregnancy
   d. hemorrhagic corpus luteum

Using Figure 32, answer question 117.

117. A patient presents with a positive pregnancy test and an unsure last menstrual period. This sonogram of the uterus most likely shows a(n):
   a. molar pregnancy
   b. hematometra
   c. pseudogestational sac
   d. anembryonic pregnancy

Using Figure 33, answer question 118.

118. In which of the following pelvic spaces is free fluid located?
   a. space of Retzius
   b. Morison pouch
   c. pouch of Douglas
   d. vesicouterine space

Using Figure 34, answer question 119.

119. This image of the left ovary displays:
   a. theca lutein cysts
   b. normal functional cysts
   c. ovarian hyperstimulation
   d. polycystic ovarian disease

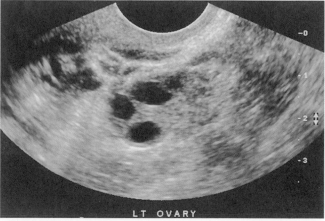

LT OVARY

FIG. 34

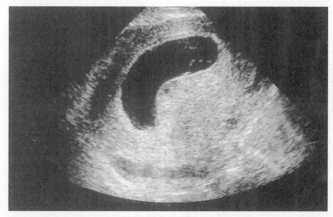

FIG. 32

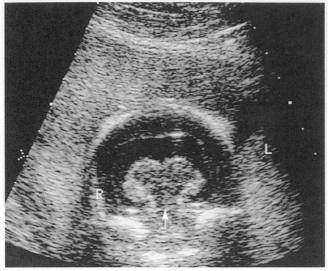

FIG. 35

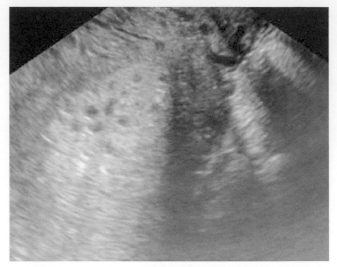

FIG. 36

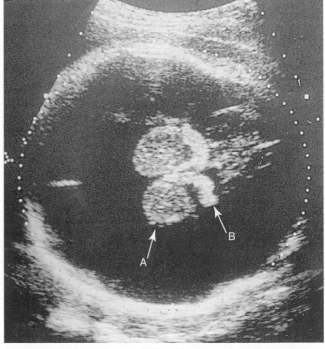

FIG. 37

Using Figure 35, answer questions 120 and 121.

120. The arrow in this sonogram identifies:
   a. single choroid plexus
   b. fused thalamic cerebri
   c. stenosis of the fourth ventricle
   d. compressed echogenic brain tissue

121. This abnormality is commonly associated with which of the following syndromes?
   a. Down
   b. Patau
   c. Turner
   d. Eagle-Barrett

Using Figure 36, answer question 122.

122. A patient presents in the first trimester of pregnancy with a history of hyperemesis and small for dates. Based on this clinical history, the sonogram most likely displays a(n):
   a. molar pregnancy
   b. endometrial polyp
   c. incomplete abortion
   d. degenerating fibroid

Using Figure 37, answer question 123.

123. Arrow A identifies which of the following structures?
   a. thalamus
   b. cerebellum
   c. choroid plexus
   d. corpus striatum

124. Arrow B identifies which of the following structures?
   a. thalamus
   b. choroid plexus
   c. corpus callosum
   d. sylvian fissure

125. Fetuses of diabetic mothers have an increased risk of developing:
   a. macrosomia
   b. fetal hydrops
   c. nuchal edema
   d. hyperechoic bowel

126. Hands should be scrubbed a minimum of:
   a. 15 seconds
   b. 20 seconds
   c. 30 seconds
   d. 45 seconds

127. Which of the following syndromes is associated with an extra set of chromosomes?
   a. Turner
   b. Edward
   c. triploidy
   d. Arnold-Chiari

128. Visualization of a fractured fetal femur is most suspicious for:
   a. achondroplasia
   b. achondrogenesis
   c. diastrophic dysplasia
   d. osteogenesis imperfecta

129. A cystic teratoma is most commonly located:
   a. in the lateral adnexa
   b. inferior near the cervix
   c. lateral to the uterine isthmus
   d. superior to the uterine fundus

130. Second trimester ultrasound examinations are best in determining fetal:
   a. age
   b. viability
   c. position
   d. anatomy

131. Which of the following structures allow communication between the right and left atria?
   a. atrial septum
   b. foramen ovale
   c. ductus venosus
   d. ductus arteriosus

132. Precocious puberty may indicate the possible presence of a mass of the:
   a. liver, kidneys, or pituitary gland
   b. gonads, kidneys, or thyroid gland
   c. pituitary gland, kidneys, or gonads
   d. hypothalamus, gonads, or adrenal gland

133. A unilocular thin-walled cystic structure is identified adjacent to a normal-appearing ovary. This mass is most suspicious for a(n):
   a. cystadenoma
   b. hydrosalpinx
   c. cystic teratoma
   d. parovarian cyst

134. The most common gynecological malignancy in the United States involves the:
   a. ovary
   b. cervix
   c. vagina
   d. endometrium

135. A bicornuate uterus is a congenital anomaly resulting from a(n):
   a. septum between the müllerian ducts
   b. absence of the caudal müllerian ducts
   c. incomplete fusion of the müllerian ducts
   d. complete failure of the müllerian ducts to fuse

136. In ectopic pregnancy, serial human chorionic gonadotropin levels are expected to:
   a. increase rapidly
   b. decrease rapidly
   c. abnormally increase
   d. abnormally decrease

137. The fallopian tube is divided into which of the following sections?
   a. fimbria, isthmus, cornua, ampulla
   b. isthmus, ampulla, cornua, interstitial
   c. ampulla, infundibulum, fimbria, isthmus
   d. interstitial, isthmus, ampulla, infundibulum

138. Which endometrial phase demonstrates the greatest dimension?
   a. early secretory
   b. late menstrual
   c. early menstrual
   d. late proliferative

139. Fertilization of the ovum occurs in the:
   a. endometrium
   b. uterine cornua
   c. distal fallopian tube
   d. proximal fallopian tube

140. Which of the following structures is responsible for the secretion of follicle-stimulating hormone?
   a. ovary
   b. hypothalamus
   c. thyroid gland
   d. pituitary gland

141. The normal endometrium of a postmenopausal patient not receiving hormone replacement therapy is expected to appear:
   a. multilayered
   b. thin and echogenic
   c. thick and echogenic
   d. thin and hypoechoic

142. Cystic structures located within the choroid plexus:
   a. are associated with skeletal dysplasia
   b. are associated with Dandy-Walker syndrome
   c. should normally regress by 26 weeks' gestation
   d. are frequently associated with chromosomal abnormalities

143. Which biometric parameter is most widely used to determine gestational age in the early second trimester?
   a. long bone length
   b. crown–rump length
   c. biparietal diameter
   d. abdominal circumference

144. Which of the following neoplasms is most likely associated with Meigs syndrome?
   a. fibroma
   b. cystic teratoma
   c. theca lutein cysts
   d. polycystic ovarian disease

Using Figure 38, answer question 145

145. This endovaginal sonogram is demonstrating which of the following?
   a. adenomyosis
   b. intramural fibroid
   c. submucosal fibroid
   d. endometrial polyp

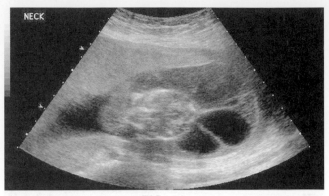

FIG. 39

Using Figure 39, answer question 146.

146. What chromosomal abnormality is most likely associated with this second trimester fetus?
   a. triploidy
   b. Trisomy 13
   c. Turner syndrome
   d. Arnold-Chiari syndrome

Using Figure 40, answer question 147.

147. This sagittal image of the lower fetal spine is most suspicious for which abnormality?
   a. encephalocele
   b. choriocarcinoma
   c. myelomeningocele
   d. sacrococcygeal teratoma

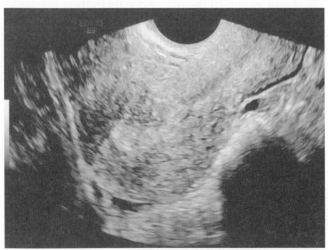

FIG. 38

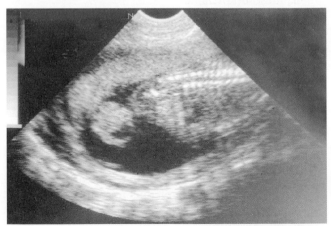

FIG. 40

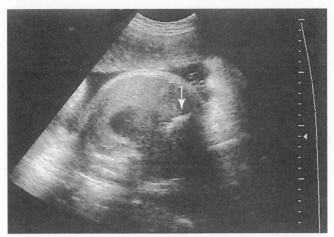

FIG. 41

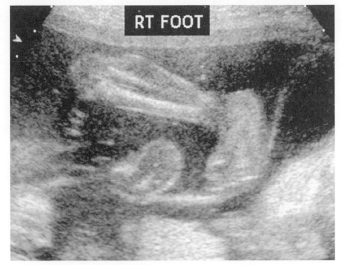

FIG. 43

Using Figure 41, answer question 148.

148. This cross-sectional image of the fetal abdomen is most suspicious for:
- **a.** cholelithiasis
- **b.** nephrolithiasis
- **c.** meconium ileus
- **d.** duodenal atresia

Using Figure 42, answer question 149.

149. This cross-sectional image of the umbilical insertion is most suspicious for which of the following abnormalities?
- **a.** gastroschisis
- **b.** omphalocele
- **c.** umbilical hernia
- **d.** meconium peritonitis

Using Figure 43, answer question 150.

150. This late second trimester sonogram of the right foot demonstrates a:
- **a.** clubfoot
- **b.** normal foot
- **c.** rocker bottom foot
- **d.** metatarsal fracture

Using Figure 44, answer question 151.

151. This four-chamber view of the fetal heart displays a(n):
- **a.** normal heart
- **b.** open foramen ovale
- **c.** atrioventricular defect
- **d.** ventriculoseptal defect

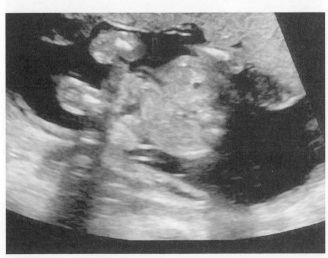

FIG. 42

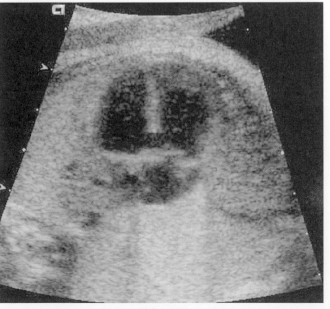

FIG. 44

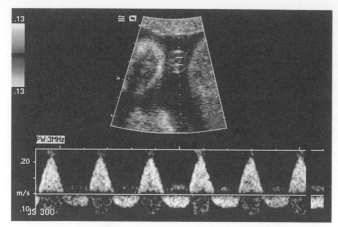

FIG. 45

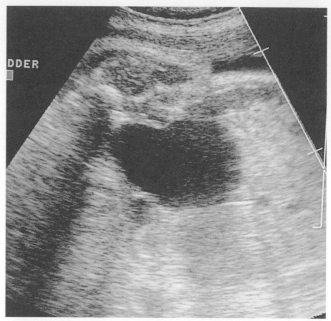

FIG. 46

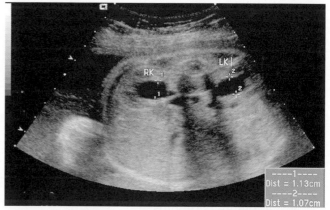

FIG. 47

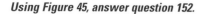

Using Figure 45, answer question 152.

152. This spectral analysis of the umbilical artery of a 32-week fetus demonstrates:
    a. absent diastolic flow
    b. a critical spectral waveform
    c. a normal spectral waveform
    d. a slightly abnormal spectral waveform

Using Figure 46, answer question 153.

153. This coronal image of the fetal bladder is most suspicious for which of the following abnormalities?
    a. urachal cyst
    b. bladder exstrophy
    c. bladder diverticulum
    d. posterior urethral valve obstruction

Using Figure 47, answer question 154.

154. This cross-sectional image of a third trimester fetal abdomen is most suspicious for:
    a. prominent renal pelvis
    b. bilateral hydronephrosis
    c. fetal ascites
    d. bilateral renal cysts

Using Figure 48 (and Color Plate 13), answer question 155.

155. A patient presents with a history of abnormal vaginal bleeding. She states she suffered a first trimester miscarriage followed by a dilation and curettage 5 months earlier. Based on this clinical history, the sonogram most likely demonstrates which of the follow abnormalities?
    a. endometritis
    b. trophoblastic disease
    c. arteriovenous fistula
    d. retained products of conception

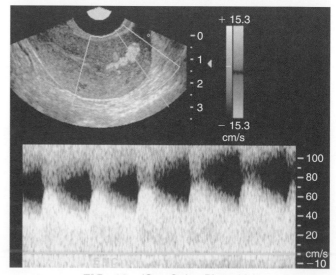

FIG. 48 (See Color Plate 13.)

156. The door should be closed for four hours after a patient with a(n):?
    a. contact pathogen
    b. droplet pathogen
    c. airborne pathogen
    d. droplet and airborne pathogens

157. Which portion of the primitive brain displays as a prominent cystic structure?
    a. diencephalon
    b. prosencephalon
    c. mesencephalon
    d. rhombencephalon

158. The maternal side of the developing placenta is termed decidua:
    a. basalis
    b. parietalis
    c. capsularis
    d. frondosum

159. The purpose of the cephalic index is to determine:
    a. fetal weight
    b. gestational age
    c. fetal well-being
    d. normalcy of head shape

160. Normal fetal lung development is dependent on the:
    a. length of the umbilical cord
    b. efficiency of the placental circulation
    c. exchange of amniotic fluid within the lungs
    d. ability of the fetus to move within the amniotic cavity

161. Which term refers to midcycle or ovulatory pain?
    a. menorrhea
    b. dyspareunia
    c. dysmenorrhea
    d. Mittelschmerz

162. Which of the following is a sonographic finding associated with trisomy 21?
    a. microcephaly
    b. dolichocephaly
    c. clenched hands
    d. duodenal atresia

163. A rapid increase in serial human chorionic gonadotropin levels is associated with:
    a. ectopic pregnancy
    b. trophoblastic disease
    c. heterotopic pregnancy
    d. anembryonic pregnancy

164. Which pelvic mass is commonly displayed in a normal first trimester pregnancy?
    a. leiomyoma
    b. cystadenoma
    c. corpus luteal cyst
    d. theca lutein cysts

165. Which of the following is caused by the presence of one defective gene?
    a. triploidy
    b. monosomy X
    c. autosomal recessive
    d. autosomal dominant

166. A lemon-shaped cranium is more commonly associated with:
    a. duodenal atresia
    b. ventriculomegaly
    c. myelomeningocele
    d. infantile polycystic disease

167. Visualization of the distal femoral epiphysis documents a fetus with an approximate gestational age of:
    a. 28 weeks
    b. 32 weeks
    c. 35 weeks
    d. 37 weeks

168. A fixed, small, hyperechoic focus within the left ventricle is most likely the:
    a. mitral valve
    b. ductus venosus
    c. bicuspid valve
    d. papillary muscle

169. The normal diameter of the lateral ventricle atria should not exceed:
    a. 6 mm
    b. 8 mm
    c. 10 mm
    d. 12 mm

170. The apex of the fetal heart is normally positioned toward the:
    a. left side of the body at 45 degrees
    b. left side of the body at 65 degrees
    c. right side of the body at 40 degrees
    d. right side of the body at 65 degrees

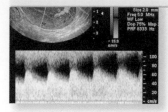

Physics Answers

Chapter 1 Clinical Safety

1. **c.** Transient and stable are the two types of cavitation. Stable cavitation involves microbubbles already present in the tissues.
2. **d.** Spatial average–temporal average (SATA) has the lowest output intensity.
3. **a.** There are no confirmed significant biological effects in mammalian tissue for exposures below 1 W/cm² for focused or 100 mW/cm² for unfocused transducers.
4. **b.** SPPA denotes spatial peak pulse average or the peak intensity of the pulse, averaged over the pulse duration.
5. **c.** Pulse Doppler generates the highest output intensity. Continuous-wave and color Doppler have slightly lower intensities compared with pulse wave.
6. **d.** After each patient, transducers used during the examination should be cleaned and disinfected. Cleaning of the keyboard after each patient is encouraged.
7. **d.** Plant studies are useful for understanding cavitation effects on living tissues.
8. **d.** Almost 90% of sonographers have some form of work-related musculoskeletal disorder (WRMSD), with the highest percentage of injuries in the upper extremity and neck. Although the thumb is part of the upper extremity, it is not the best answer.
9. **b.** Epidemiology studies various factors determining the frequency and distribution of diseases in the human community. Biological effects describe the effect of ultrasound waves on living organisms, including their composition, function, growth, origin, development, and distribution.
10. **a.** Mechanical index indicates the likelihood of cavitation occurring with diagnostic ultrasound, and thermal index relates to the heating of tissue.
11. **b.** Spatial peak–temporal average is used when researching and reporting possible biological effects of diagnostic ultrasound.
12. **b.** Clinical trials and animal testing are forms of in vivo research. In vivo refers to experimentation done in or on the living tissue as a whole. Ex vivo refers to experimentation done in or on living tissue in an artificial environment outside the organism.
13. **c.** Temporal peak is the greatest intensity during the pulse. Spatial peak is the greatest intensity across the beam.
14. **c.** Pulse average is defined as the average intensity over the duration of a pulse (pulse duration).
15. **d.** Cavitation is the interaction of the sound wave with microscopic bubbles found in tissues.
16. **c.** Proper handwashing is the best protection to stop the spread of disease.
17. **c.** The American Institute of Ultrasound in Medicine (AIUM) recommends prudent use of ultrasound in the clinical environment. Examinations solely for sex determination are discouraged. Biological effects are dependent on the output intensity and duration of exposure.
18. **c.** Cavitation is the result of pressure changes in soft tissue causing the formation of gas bubbles. Contrast agents have a potential for cavitational changes in soft tissue from the introduction of bubbles into the tissues and circulation.
19. **b.** Absorption of the sound beam is highest in bone, especially in the fetus.
20. **c.** Thermal index in soft tissue is proportional to the operating frequency. Increasing the frequency will increase the thermal index.
21. **d.** The sonographer's shoulder is abducted greater than 30 degrees. Lowering the chair or raising the table will correct this improper position. The sonographer must also position the patient closer to the edge of the table to reduce further both abduction of the shoulder and reaching of the arm.
22. **a.** Work-related musculoskeletal disorders (WRMSDs) are defined as injuries that involve musculoskeletal symptoms that remain for 7 days or longer.
23. **b.** de Quervain's disease is a specific type of tendonitis involving the thumb that can result from gripping the transducer.
24. **d.** The mechanical index is used as an indicator of the likelihood that cavitation will occur. Thermal index relates to the heating of tissues.
25. **a.** Spatial peak is the greatest intensity across the sound beam.
26. **c.** Research has revealed a rapid increase in the temperature of the cranium when using TCD.
27. **a.** As a form of energy, ultrasound has a small potential to produce a biological effect. Contrast agents may increase the risk of cavitation.
28. **b.** Biological studies of the cytoskeleton have shown ultrasound induced changes are nonspecific and temporary.
29. **b.** The introduction of bubbles into the tissues and circulation from contrast agents increase the risk of cavitation.
30. **c.** The ALARA principle encourages prudent and conservative use of ultrasound exercised by minimizing exposure time and output intensity.
31. **d.** Ex vivo refers to experimentation done on living tissue in an artificial environment outside the organisms. In vitro refers to the technique of performing a given

experiment in a controlled environment outside a living organism.

32. **c.** Heat is most dependent on the SATA intensity. SPTA is used when researching and reporting biological effects of diagnostic ultrasound.

33. **d.** The sonographer is demonstrating proper ergonomics. The examination table is at the correct height with the patient close enough to avoid bending and reaching. The monitor is directly in front of the sonographer at a height so her eyes are even with the top of the monitor. An ergonomic chair is being used with neutral neck and back position. Her elbow is close to her body with shoulder abduction less than 30 degrees. Her scanning wrist is in a neutral position.

34. **a.** Focused transducers require higher intensities to produce biological effects.

35. **c.** To avoid WRMSD, the elbow should be kept close to the body with shoulder abduction less than or equal to ($\leq$) 30 degrees.

36. **d.** There are no confirmed significant biological effects in mammalian tissue for exposures below 100 mW/cm^2 for unfocused *or* 1 W/cm^2 for focused transducers.

37. **b.** Temporal average is the average intensity during the PRP. Pulse average is the average intensity over the pulse duration. The average intensity within the beam from the beginning of one pulse to the beginning of the next pulse defines SATA intensity.

38. **d.** Proper ergonomic positioning of the monitor is at a height so the eyes are even with the top of the monitor.

39. **a.** Awkward or static posture may result in development of spinal degeneration.

40. **c.** Repeated twisting of the forearm may result in cubital tunnel syndrome and epicondylitis.

41. **b.** Pulse average is the average (common) intensity over the duration (extent) of a pulse.

42. **d.** In situ, temperatures greater than 41° C are dangerous to the fetus. Higher than 39° C, biological effects are determined by the temperature and exposure time.

43. **b.** Epidemiology studies of the bioeffects of diagnostic ultrasound have determined there are no significant biological differences between exposed and unexposed patients.

44. **a.** Cavitation is a result of pressure changes in soft tissue causing formation of gas bubbles.

45. **a.** When pressure is applied, microbubbles will expand and collapse.

46. **b.** Low acoustic output and limited exposure time are consistent with the ALARA principle of achieving information with the least amount of energy exposure to the patient.

47. **c.** Use of ultrasound is *only* recommended when medically indicated.

48. **b.** The rate at which work is performed or the rate at which energy is transmitted into the body defines power.

49. **b.** Animal testing and clinical trials are examples of in vivo research. Test-tube research is a form of in vitro testing.

50. **b.** The intensity of M-mode imaging is greater than the intensity of gray-scale imaging.

Chapter 2 Physics Principles

1. **d.** In soft tissue, propagation speed is influenced by the stiffness and density of the medium. A change in frequency will not affect the propagation speed.

2. **b.** Bandwidth is the range of frequencies found within a pulse of ultrasound. Harmonics frequencies are even and odd multiples of the fundamental frequency generated as sound travels through tissues. Duty factor is the fraction of time that pulse ultrasound is transmitting.

3. **a.** Sonography generally uses 2 to 3 cycles per pulse, whereas Doppler imaging uses 5 to 30 cycles per pulse.

4. **c.** Audible frequencies range between 20 Hz and 20,000 Hz (20 kHz).

5. **c.** The stiffness and density of a medium determine the propagation speed of the sound wave. The amount of reflection and transmission occurring as a wave propagates through tissue is determined by the impedance differences between the media.

6. **c.** Acoustic variables include pressure, density, and particle motion (distance and temperature were previously included).

7. **c.** Short pulse lengths improve image quality.

8. **b.** Increasing the stiffness of a medium increases the propagation speed (e.g., bone). Increasing the density will decrease the propagation speed.

9. **c.** The length of a pulse from the beginning to end is termed the *spatial pulse length*. Wavelength is the length of a cycle. Pulse duration and pulse repetition period correlate with the time of a pulse and the time from the start of one pulse to the next, respectively.

10. **b.** Stiff structures (bone) increase the propagation speed of a sound wave.

11. **c.** When penetration depth is increased, pulse repetition frequency will decrease, pulse repetition period and spatial pulse length will increase. Changes in imaging depth does not affect propagation speed.

12. **b.** The intensity of a sound wave is equal to the amplitude squared. If the amplitude doubles (2×) then the intensity will quadruple (2^2).

13. **b.** Pulse duration is the amount of time for one pulse to occur. Pulse repetition period is the time from the start of one pulse to the beginning of the next pulse. Duty factor defines the amount of time pulse ultrasound is transmitting.

14. **a.** Bandwidth is the range of frequencies contained in a pulse. Widening the bandwidth improves image quality (lower Q-factor) and shortens the spatial pulse length.

15. **c.** Sound waves contain regions of high pressure or density (compressions) and regions of low pressure and density (rarefactions).

16. **b.** Duty factor equals the amount of time the ultrasound transducer is emitting sound. DF = PD/PRP.

17. **c.** Resistance to the propagation of a sound wave through soft tissue describes acoustic impedance. Attenuation is a weakening of sound as it propagates through a medium.

18. **b.** Pascal is the unit used to quantify pressure.

19. **d.** Reducing the gain setting by one-half is equal to a 3-dB reduction in amplitude.

New gain setting = 36 dB − 3 dB = 33 dB

20. **a.** Attenuation occurring with each centimeter that sound travels through soft tissue defines the attenuation coefficient. Attenuation

coefficient is equal to one-half of the operating frequency (MHz).

21. **c.** Spatial relates to space whereas temporal relates to time.

22. **b.** Attenuation is measured in decibels (dB). Attenuation coefficient (dB/cm) measures the attenuation occurring with each centimeter traveled. Impedance is measured in rayls whereas intensity is measured in mW/cm^2.

23. **c.** If frequency increases, period decreases, reducing the pulse duration.

24. **d.** Giga is the metric prefix designated to represent one billion.

25. **b.** The number of pulses per second defines the pulse repetition frequency (PRF) The unit of measurement for the PRF is kHz.

26. **d.** Density and propagation speed determine the impedance of a medium. Impedance is equal to the density of the medium multiplied by the propagation speed of the medium.

27. **c.** Attenuation is the weakening of a sound wave as it travels through a medium. Acoustic impedance is the resistance to sound traveling through a medium. Scattering and reflection redirect the sound wave.

28. **b.** Specular reflections occur when a sound wave strikes a smooth large surface at a perpendicular angle. Specular reflections are angle dependent, make up the boundaries of organs, and reflect sound in only one direction. Nonspecular reflections (scatter) occur when the reflector is smaller, irregular, or rough.

29. **c.** Ninety-nine percent of the incident beam transmits to the next medium with perpendicular incidence.

30. **d.** Amplitude is the maximum variation occurring in an acoustic variable. Acoustic variables include density, pressure, and particle motion. Units will vary with each acoustic variable.

31. **b.** The duty factor defines the percent of time that pulse ultrasound is transmitting. Increasing the pulse repetition frequency (PRF) will increase the duty factor, because there is less "silence" between pulses. PRF is inversely proportional to the penetration depth, spatial pulse length, and pulse repetition period.

32. **d.** Propagation speed depends on the stiffness and density of the medium. Increasing the density of the medium will decrease the propagation speed of a wave. Increasing the stiffness of the medium will increase propagation speed.

33. **c.** For short pulses (fewer number of cycles), the Q factor is equal to the number of cycles in a pulse. The lower the Q factor, the better the image quality.

34. **d.** The positive and negative halves of a pressure wave correspond to the compression and rarefaction of the wave, respectively.

35. **a.** Definity, Imagent and Optison are contrast agents approved for use in the United States. Echovist, Lenovist, and Sonovue are contrast agents approved for use in Canada, Europe, and Japan.

36. **b.** Redirection or bending of the transmitting sound beam after it passes through one medium to the next describes refraction. Scattering is a redirection of the sound beam in several directions on encountering a rough surface. Multiple reflections occurring between the transducer and a strong reflector describe reverberation.

37. **c.** Attenuation is a result of absorption (most common), reflection, and scattering.

38. **a.** Half-value layer is the depth of penetration required to reduce the intensity of the sound beam by one-half. A 3-dB reduction (-3 dB) decreases the intensity of the sound beam by one-half.

39. **b.** Propagation speed is directly related to the stiffness of the medium and inversely related to the density of the medium.

40. **b.** Impedance is proportional to the propagation speed and density of the medium. Impedance determines how much of the incident beam will reflect and how much will transmit from one medium to the next.

41. **b.** Decibel is a unit used to compare the ratio of amplitudes or intensities of two sound waves or two points along the wave path. Attenuation occurring with each centimeter of travel is measured in dB/cm.

42. **a.** Attenuation is proportional to the frequency of the sound.

43. **c.** A difference in impedance between two media determines how much of the incident beam reflects from the first medium and how much transmits into the second medium.

44. **c.** Dissipation of heat in a medium primarily in the form of heat describes absorption.

45. **d.** Contrast harmonics are created during receiving and tissue harmonics are created during transmission. Harmonic imaging improves lateral resolution and degrades axial resolution. Harmonic imaging is nonexistent in the near field and is weaker than fundamental sound beams.

46. **b.** Snell's law determines the refraction of the sound wave at an interface. The difference in acoustic impedance between two structures and the angle of incidence determines the reflection and transmission of a sound wave.

47. **b.** Reflection angle, incidence angle, and angle of incidence are terms used to describe the direction of the incident beam with respect to the media boundary. The transmission angle depends on the propagation speeds of the media.

48. **c.** Specular reflections make up the boundaries of organs and reflect sound in only one direction. Specular reflections are angle dependent.

49. **b.** An angle of incidence where there is no transmission and 100% reflection describe the critical angle. Transmission angle at this time is 90 degrees.

50. **b.** The greater the impedance differences between the media, the greater the reflection.

Chapter 3 Ultrasound Transducers

1. **d.** The sound beam diverges (widens) in the Fraunhofer (far) zone. In the Fresnel (near) zone, the sound beam tapers as it nears the focal point.

2. **c.** Grating lobes are secondary weak sound beams emitted from a multielement transducer. Side lobes are associated with single-element transducers.

3. **d.** The thickness and propagation speed of the active element determines the fundamental (operating) frequency of a pulse wave. For a continuous wave, the frequency of the sound wave is equal to the electrical frequency of the ultrasound system.

4. **d.** Heat sterilization exceeds the Curie point, resulting in the loss of piezoelectric properties of the crystal.

5. **b.** Continuous-wave ultrasound does not use pulses to transmit the sound beam. Damping reduces the duration of the pulse. Two piezoelectric elements are located in one transducer assembly with continuous-wave ultrasound. One element operates transmission of the sound source, and the other element receives the returning echo reflections.

6. **a.** The width of the sound beam determines lateral resolution. Spatial pulse length determines axial resolution.

7. **c.** Dynamic damping is an electronic means to suppress the element from ringing.

8. **b.** More frequencies (bandwidth) and wavelengths are present in shorter pulses.

9. **d.** Diagnostic ultrasound transducers operate on the piezoelectric effect or principle. Huygens principle states: "…points on a wave front are the point source for the production of secondary wavelets." Snell's law determines the amount of refraction at an interface.

10. **b.** The width of the sound beam at the focal point is equal to one-half of the transducer diameter.

11. **d.** Constructive interference occurs when two waves in phase with each other create a new wave with amplitude greater than the original waves. Destructive interference occurs when two waves out of phase with each other create a new wave with amplitude less than the original waves.

12. **c.** The matching layer reduces the impedance difference between the active element and the skin. Aqueous gel is not a component of the transducer assembly. Damping (backing) layer reduces the number of cycles in each pulse.

13. **a.** The sound beam is more uniform in intensity in the far zone (Fraunhofer zone). Intensity variations are greatest in the near zone (Fresnel zone). Maximum intensity of the sound beam occurs at the focal point (focus).

14. **d.** Depth of field is also known as focal zone length or field length. Depth of field is the distance between equal beam widths that are some multiples of the minimum value (at the focus).

15. **c.** Decreasing the frame rate will increase temporal resolution. This can be accomplished by decreasing the number of focal zones, imaging depth, and beam width. Decreasing persistence will also decrease the frame rate, improving temporal resolution.

16. **d.** Multizone focusing decreases frame rate (temporal resolution).

17. **d.** Both linear sequenced array and linear phased array transducers demonstrate a rectangular shape.

18. **c.** The distance from the transducer face to the point of spatial peak intensity (focal point) is termed the *focal* or *near zone length.*

19. **c.** The focal point (focus) is the narrowest and most intense portion of the sound beam. The focal zone is the region or area of the focus.

20. **c.** Multiple transducer elements with individual wiring and system electronics describes channels.

21. **c.** The diameter at the focal point is equal to one-half of the transducer diameter. Axial resolution is equal to one-half of the spatial pulse length. Thickness and propagation speed of the element determine the operating frequency of the transducer.

22. **b.** The impedance of the damping layer is similar to that of the element. The impedance of the matching layer is between that of the element and skin.

23. **d.** Backing (damping) reduces the number of cycles in a pulse, pulse duration, and spatial pulse length. Damping increases the bandwidth and axial resolution.

24. **b.** Vector, sequenced, and phased are types of transducer operation. Linear, convex, and annular are types of transducer construction.

25. **b.** Lateral resolution varies with distance and is directly related to the diameter of the sound beam. Focusing (narrowing) the sound beam improves lateral resolution. Axial resolution does not vary with depth and is directly related to the operating frequency.

26. **d.** The ultrasound system alters the electronic excitation of the elements, steering the beam in various directions. Delays in the reflected echoes also occur.

27. **d.** Exceeding the Curie point of a transducer element will result in a loss of all piezoelectric properties (e.g., heat sterilization).

28. **c.** Axial resolution is equal to one-half of the spatial pulse length.

29. **b.** Increasing compression (dynamic range) increases contrast resolution (increases the range of gray scale). Postprocessing maps, increasing operating frequency and decreasing the beam width are additional techniques to optimize contrast resolution.

30. **b.** Temporal resolution is the ability to separate two points in time, and it is determined by the frame rate. Beam width determines lateral resolution. Operating frequency relates to axial resolution.

31. **c.** To improve posterior acoustic shadowing (axial resolution) in this image the sonographer should decrease the imaging depth and depth of focus. Increasing operating frequency and number or focal zones are additional techniques to optimize axial resolution.

32. **d.** A linear sequenced array transducer applies voltage pulses to groups of linear elements in succession. Phased array transducers operate by applying voltage pulses to most or all of the elements using minor time differences.

33. **c.** Focusing of the sound beam is only accomplished within the near zone.

34. **b.** At one near zone length (focal point), the diameter of the sound beam is one-half of the original transducer diameter.

35. **d.** Azimuthal (lateral) resolution is the ability to distinguish two structures in a path perpendicular to the sound beam.

36. **d.** Lead zirconate titanate (PZT) is the most common piezoelectric element used in ultrasound transducers.

37. **b.** Beam steering is accomplished mechanically in an annular array transducer.

38. **c.** Diagnostic frequencies presently range between 2.0 and 20.0 MHz.

39. **b.** Increasing transducer frequency and the number of focal zones, and decreasing the beam width and imaging depth, improve axial resolution.

40. **d.** Diagnostic ultrasound transducers convert electrical energy into acoustic energy during transmission

and acoustic energy into electrical energy for reception.

41. d. The piezoelectric principle states that some materials produce a voltage when deformed by an applied pressure. Ohm's acoustic law states, "Musical sound is perceived by the ear as the sum of the number of cycles of pure harmonic tones."

42. b. Damping reduces the sensitivity of the pulse while increasing the bandwidth and axial resolution. A low-quality factor is a good thing.

43. c. Doppler imaging uses 5 to 30 cycles per pulse, whereas real-time imaging generally uses 2 to 3 cycles per pulse.

44. c. Electronic focusing allows the operator to determine the depth and number of focal zones. Internal focus, external focus, and acoustic mirrors are predetermined and are out of the operator's control.

45. c. The impedance of the matching layer is less than that of the crystal and greater than the impedance of the skin.

46. b. Vector array transducers convert the format of a linear array into a trapezoidal image. Vector array transducers combine linear sequential and linear phase array technologies.

47. c. The ability to differentiate similar or dissimilar tissues describes contrast resolution. Contrast resolution is directly related to both axial and lateral resolution (detail resolution).

48. b. Section thickness (z-axis) is related to the beam thickness and is determined by the transducer.

49. d. Operating frequency is directly related to the propagation speed of the element and inversely related to the element thickness.

50. c. The matching layer is composed of an aluminum powder in an epoxy resin. Damping is composed of metal powder and an epoxy.

Chapter 4 Pulse-Echo Instrumentation

1. c. Real-time imaging is a two-dimensional display demonstrating motion of moving structures. Static imaging does not demonstrate motion. M-mode is a one-dimensional display. Temporal resolution is the ability to position a moving structure precisely.

2. a. The vertical or y-axis represents the penetration depth in a B-mode display. The horizontal or x-axis represents the side-to-side or superior-to-inferior aspect of the body.

3. a. The number of images (frames) per second is termed the *frame rate.* The pulse repetition frequency determines the number of scan lines per frame.

4. d. Increasing or decreasing the imaging depth will change the frame rate. The sonographer can also modify the frame rate by adjusting the number of focal zones.

5. d. Decreasing imaging depth, placing the focus higher (more superficial), and decreasing overall gain. are the most likely techniques used to improve this sagittal image of the left upper quadrant. The image demonstrates an adrenal adenoma medial to the spleen and left kidney.

6. c. A-mode (amplitude mode) demonstrates the strength of the echo along the vertical (y) axis. Depth of penetration is displayed on the y-axis in B-mode imaging.

7. d. Frame rate is determined by the propagation speed of the medium and penetration depth. Frame rate is proportional to PRF and determines temporal resolution.

8. a. Frame rate and temporal resolution are inversely related to the line density. Increasing the line density will decrease the frame rate and temporal resolution. Line density is directly related to the pulse repetition frequency and spatial resolution.

9. a. Propagation speed of the medium limits the penetration depth. Harmonic frequencies are determined by the fundamental (operating) frequency. Temporal resolution is determined by the frame rate.

10. c. Functions of the imaging processor include persistence, pre- and postprocessing, storing image frames, gray scale, color scale, analog-to-digital converter and 3-D acquisition and presentation. Filtering, detection, and compression are functions of the signal processor.

11. d. Propagation speed artifacts include mirror image, comet tail, grating lobes, range ambiguity, refraction, reverberation, ringdown, slice thickness, acoustic speckle, and speed error.

12. a. Line density is directly related to the pulse repetition frequency (PRF). Imaging depth and operating frequency are inversely related to the PRF.

13. b. Signal-to-noise ratio is proportional to the output of the ultrasound machine. Increasing the output by 3 dB will increase the signal-to-noise ratio and double the acoustic intensity.

14. c. The T/R switch protects the amplifier components from the large driving voltage of the pulse. The transducer delivers electrical voltages to the memory. The pulser adjusts the PRF with changing imaging depth. Focusing controls the width of the sound beam.

15. a. Subdicing reduces grating lobes by dividing the elements into smaller pieces.

16. a. An increase in the intensity of the sound beam is identified in the area of the focal zones. Decreasing the number of focal zones and smoothing out the TGC can reduce the effects of this artifact.

17. d. Time-gain or depth-gain compensation is offset for attenuation by boosting the amplitudes of deep reflections and suppressing superficial reflections.

18. b. The transducer receives returning echo reflections, producing an electrical voltage, and it delivers this voltage to the memory.

19. d. The knee of the time-gain compensation curve is the deepest region in which attenuation compensation can occur. The area of maximum amplification describes the far zone.

20. a. When imaging depth is changed, the pulser will readjust the pulse repetition frequency.

21. c. The T/R switch is part of the beam former. It directs the driving voltage from the pulser to the transducer and the returning echo voltage from the transducer to the signal processor.

22. d. An independent pulse delay and element combination constitutes a transmission channel. Each independent element, amplifier, analog-to-digital converter, and delay path constitutes a reception channel.

23. c. The sonogram demonstrates ringdown (reverberation), posterior enhancement and edge shadowing artifacts.

24. b. Harmonic imaging reduces slice thickness artifact.

25. **b.** Code excitation uses a series of pulses and gaps allowing for multiple focal zones and harmonic frequencies. Controlling the characteristics of the sound beam is directly related to the number of channels used.

26. **a.** Cine loop is a postprocessing feature that stores the last several frames of a real-time imaging display. 3-D acquisition is a preprocessing attribute whereas 3-D presentation is a postprocessing function.

27. **b.** Binary number 0110010 is equal to $0 + 32 + 16 + 0 + 0 + 2 + 0 = 50$.

28. **c.** A 6-bit memory is equal to 2 to the sixth power $= 2 \times 2 \times 2 \times 2 \times 2 \times 2 = 64$.

29. **d.** A voxel is the smallest picture element in a 3-D image.

30. **c.** Decreasing the overall gain would improve this sagittal image of the right upper quadrant. An additional decrease of the near field TGC may also be necessary. Focal placement appears appropriate for imaging to the level of the most posterior structure (diaphragm). Changes in all TGC slide controls could also be used to achieve the same effect.

31. **a.** Harmonic imaging will improve resolution of the echogenic debris in the posterior portion of the urinary bladder as well as decrease the reverberation in the near field. Spatial compounding reduces speckle and noise and is a great tool to improve visualization beneath a highly attenuating structure, which is not displayed in this image.

32. **b.** Read magnification is a postprocessing feature that displays only the original data. The number of pixels or scan lines is the same as the original image.

33. **d.** Hyperechoic is a comparative term to describe an increase in echogenicity when compared to surrounding structures or the normal expected echo pattern of a structure.

34. **b.** Increasing or decreasing the pixel density has a direct relationship to the spatial resolution of the image. The number of gray shades relates to the number of memory bits.

35. **a.** Storage of the last several real-time frames describes a postprocessing feature, cine-loop. Freeze frame displays a single real-time frame.

36. **d.** This is the best answer. Matrix denotes the rows and columns of pixels in a digital image. The number of picture elements in a digital image describes pixel density.

37. **b.** B-color presents different echo intensities in various color shades improving contrast resolution. Rejection suppresses weak intensities without affecting the intense amplitudes. Persistence reduces noise and smoothes the image.

38. **d.** Write magnification rescans only the area of interest, increasing the number of pixels or scan lines in the image.

39. **d.** Improper location of a true reflector is displayed with range ambiguity, propagation-speed error, refraction, grating lobes, side lobes, and multipath artifacts. Reverberation, comet-tail, and mirror-image artifacts display additional false reflectors. Focal banding demonstrates improper brightness in the focal zone(s).

40. **b.** Doppler gain set too high will most likely demonstrate a mirror-image artifact. Acoustic speckle is a gray-scale interference artifact. Aliasing relates to a pulse repetition frequency set too low. Range ambiguity relates to a pulse repetition frequency set too high.

41. **d.** A pulse repetition frequency set too high results in range ambiguity. Decreasing the PRF will decrease the likelihood of range ambiguity.

42. **c.** The ultrasound system assumes sound travels directly to and from a reflector. Other assumptions include: sound travels in a straight line and at a constant speed in soft tissue, echoes only originate from the central sound beam, intensity of the echo corresponds to the strength of a reflector, the imaging plane is thin, and distance to the reflector is proportional to the time it takes an echo to return.

43. **c.** Shadowing is a reduction (weakening) of echoes distal to a strongly attenuating or reflecting structure. Enhancement describes an increase in echo amplitude distal to a weakly attenuating structure.

44. **d.** Increasing the time-gain compensation in the near field would improve the diagnostic quality of the left lobe of the liver. The far field could be slightly decreased to

remove artifactual echoes in the IVC and aorta.

45. **c.** Enhancement of displayed reflectors occurs posterior to a weakly attenuating structure, resulting in false brightness to distal reflections.

46. **c.** A change in direction of the sound beam is more commonly a result of the sound wave striking a boundary at an oblique angle. A resonance phenomenon is associated with ring-down artifact.

47. **d.** Grating lobes are a result of the spacing between the active elements of an array transducer. They produce minor secondary sound beams that travel in directions different than the primary central beam.

48. **c.** Distance to a reflector is proportional to the time it takes for an echo to return. The ultrasound machine assumes the propagation speed of the medium is a constant 1.54 mm/ms.

49. **c.** Imaging a surgical clip will most likely demonstrate a comet-tail reverberation artifact. A surgical clip may cause acoustic speckle.

50. **c.** Shadowing and enhancement are useful artifacts caused by a strong or weakly attenuating structure, respectively.

Chapter 5 Doppler Instrumentation and Hemodynamics

1. **a.** Blood flows into the left atrium through the pulmonary veins.

2. **a.** Bruits are auscultory consequences or products of turbulent blood flow. Turbulent or disturbed flow is a consequence of arterial narrowing.

3. **d.** Hemodynamics is the science or the physical principles concerned with the study of blood circulation.

4. **a.** Plug flow, found in large arteries such as the aorta, displays a constant flow velocity across the entire vessel.

5. **c.** Microcirculation consists of the arterioles, capillaries, and venules.

6. **d.** Zero Doppler shift (zero velocity; baseline) is assigned the color black. True flow reversal will demonstrate black between the red and blue colors assigned to flow toward the transducer and away from the transducer respectively.

7. **d.** Decreasing the depth to the sample volume increases the pulse

repetition frequency, allowing for a larger display of Doppler shifts. Increasing the pulse repetition period decreases the pulse repetition frequency. Increasing the operating frequency increases sensitivity of low-flow velocities.

8. **c.** A positive Doppler shift occurs when the received frequency is greater than the transmitted frequency. A positive Doppler shift displays above the baseline.

9. **c.** Increasing the operating frequency increases system's sensitivity of the Doppler shifts. Increasing the Doppler angle decreases the Doppler shift and can bring it down below the Nyquist limit.

10. **a.** Doppler shifts do not occur when the received and transmitted frequencies are equal.

11. **c.** The ability to measure high velocities is a major advantage of CW Doppler. Aliasing is not an issue with continuous-wave Doppler. Interrogation of multiple vessels simultaneously is a disadvantage. Small probe size maybe an advantage but is not the best answer.

12. **d.** The Doppler equation determines the Doppler shift (change in the transmitted and reflected frequencies). Poiseuille's equation determines the volume flow rate.

13. **d.** A Reynolds number greater than 2000 consistently predicts the onset of turbulent flow.

14. **c.** A difference in pressure is necessary for flow to occur. The circulatory system creates hydrostatic pressure.

15. **c.** Blood flow velocity is dependent on left ventricular output, resistance of the arterioles, vessel course, and cross-sectional area.

16. **b.** Venous pressure is lowest when the patient is lying flat (supine or prone). Venous pressure is the highest when the patient is standing.

17. **c.** The greatest portion of circulating blood is located in the venous system. Veins accommodate larger changes in blood volume with little change in pressure.

18. **d.** Parabolic flow is an uncommon type of laminar flow where the average flow velocity is equal to one-half the maximum flow speed in the center. Laminar flow demonstrates a maximum flow velocity in the center of the artery and minimum flow velocity near the arterial wall.

19. **a.** Phasic flow describes the normal respiratory variations in venous blood flow. Bidirectional or pulsatile flow is a normal finding in the hepatic veins and proximal inferior vena cava. Unprompted venous flow is termed spontaneous.

20. **a.** Duplex imaging requires a decrease in the imaging frame rate to allow for interlaced acquisition of the Doppler information. Duplex imaging can use high operating frequencies.

21. **b.** Clutter is noise within the Doppler signal that is generally a result of high-amplitude Doppler shifts. Flash is an extension of color Doppler outside of the vessel wall caused by motion.

22. **b.** Pressure is the driving force of blood flow. Velocity is the speed at which RBCs travel in a vessel. Volume flow rate is the quantity of blood moving through a vessel per unit of time.

23. **c.** Observed frequency changes of moving structures most accurately defines Doppler *effect*. Doppler shift is the actual change in frequency equal to the reflected intensity minus the transmitted frequency.

24. **d.** The Nyquist limit is equal to one-half of the pulse repetition frequency.

25. **c.** Disturbed flow may demonstrate spectral broadening.

26. **c.** Thickening of the spectral trace is a result of an increase in the range of Doppler shift frequencies.

27. **d.** Spectral broadening describes a vertical thickening of the spectral trace caused by an increase in the range of Doppler shift frequencies. Clutter is a result of high-amplitude Doppler shifts.

28. **d.** The gate length, beam diameter, and emitted pulse length determine the size of the sample volume (gate).

29. **c.** Spectral analysis uses a fast Fourier transfer (FFT) to convert Doppler shift information into a visual spectral display. Autocorrelation is necessary for color flow Doppler.

30. **c.** Packet describes the multiple sample gates positioned in the area of interest in color Doppler imaging. Pixels are the smallest elements of a digital image.

31. **c.** The color Doppler image of a pseudoaneurysm is demonstrating aliasing. Methods to overcome aliasing include increasing the pulse repetition frequency (scale), increasing the Doppler angle, adjusting baseline to zero (move down), and decreasing the operating frequency and imaging depth.

32. **c.** Blood flows from the higher pressure to the lower pressure. A difference in pressure is required for flow to occur.

33. **d.** Increasing operating frequency will increase the sensitivity to low Doppler shifts. Decreasing operating frequency may overcome aliasing.

34. **b.** The color Doppler image is demonstrating color Doppler extending beyond the region of true blood flow. Decreasing the color gain is the most likely change to improve this image.

35. **d.** The pressure gradient is proportional to the flow rate (volume of blood flow).

36. **d.** Resistance to blood flow is proportional to the length of the vessel and inversely proportional to the blood flow volume.

37. **c.** During inspiration, abdominal pressure increases, and thoracic pressure decreases.

38. **d.** Continuous wave is the simplest form of Doppler.

39. **d.** The vertical axis of a spectral analysis represents the frequency shift or velocity. The horizontal axis represents time.

40. **c.** Velocity is defined as the rate of motion with respect to time. Acceleration is an increase in velocity.

41. **d.** Poiseuille's equation predicts flow volume in a cylindrical vessel. Reynolds number predicts the onset of turbulent flow.

42. **d.** Pulse wave Doppler uses a minimum of 5 cycles per pulse and a **maximum** of 30 cycles per pulse.

43. **c.** Autocorrelation is necessary for rapid obtainment of color Doppler frequency shifts. Fast Fourier transfer converts Doppler shift information into a visual spectral display.

44. **a.** Wall filter settings that are too high eliminate low-flow velocities. The spectral display of a low-resistance artery does not touch baseline, a common appearance when the wall filter is set too high.

45. **a.** Color Doppler is commonly used to demonstrate nonvascular motion (e.g., ureteral jets).

46. c. Power Doppler displays the amplitude or z-axis of the signal. Spectral analysis displays the frequency shift (velocity).

47. b. Spectral analysis of the artery demonstrates a mirror image of the blood flow. Decreasing the Doppler gain and/or changing the angle of insonation can eliminate this artifact. Decreasing the PRF will not change the mirroring of the spectral display.

48. b. Increasing the Doppler angle is a method of overcoming aliasing. Changing the Doppler angle may overcome a mirror image.

49. b. Smaller arteries commonly display laminar flow whereas larger arteries display plug flow.

50. b. Increasing the packet size of the color Doppler will decrease the frame rate and temporal resolution. Sensitivity and accuracy are increased.

Chapter 6 Quality Assurance, Protocols, and New Technologies

1. a. The number of correct test results divided by the total number of tests determines test accuracy. Registration accuracy is the ability to place echoes in proper location when imaging from different orientations.

2. b. Specificity is the ability of a test to detect the absence of disease. Sensitivity is the ability of a test to detect disease.

3. b. A hydrophone measures acoustic output. Beam profiler measures transducer characteristics.

4. d. The most accurate definition of quality assurance. QA is the routine, periodic evaluation of the ultrasound system including transducers.

5. d. The beam profiler is a testing device that measures transducer characteristics. A hydrophone measures acoustic output.

6. b. Image performance is determined primarily by detail resolution, contrast resolution, penetration, dynamic range, time gain compensation, and accuracy of depth and distance measurements.

7. d. Registration accuracy is the ability to place echoes in proper position when imaging from different acoustic windows. Accuracy in this chapter pertains to the number of correct test results divided by the total number of tests.

8. b. Elastography depicts tissue stiffness by the relative displacement before and during compression.

9. a. *Phantom* is the most common term used to illustrate a tissue-equivalent device.

10. d. The American Institute of Ultrasound Medicine (AIUM) and the American College of Radiology (ACR) have adapted universal scanning protocols for medical sonography examinations.

11. b. The AIUM 100 test object cannot evaluate compression (dynamic range), gray-scale, or penetration. The test object provides measurement of system performance and evaluates dead zone, axial and lateral resolution, vertical and horizontal calibration, and compensation.

12. b. Record keeping for each ultrasound unit is necessary for hospital and outpatient clinic accreditation. Record keeping aids in detection of gradual or sporadic changes in the system and in scheduling the next preventive maintenance service.

13. c. American College of Radiology (ACR) requires a minimum of semi-annual quality control testing.

14. d. The positive predictive values are calculated by dividing the true positive tests by the sum of the true and false positive tests.

15. b. AIUM test object evaluates system sensitivity. Contrast resolution, gray-scale characteristics, direction of blood flow, and sample volume location are evaluated by tissue and Doppler phantoms.

16. a. A hydrophone uses a small transducer element mounted on the end of a hollow needle or a large piezoelectric membrane with small electrodes on each side.

17. a. Quality assurance programs provide assessment of image quality and consistency.

18. d. A tissue-equivalent phantom is used in many quality-assurance programs.

19. c. System sensitivity measures how weak a reflection the system can display.

20. d. The hydrophone measures acoustic output, period, pulse repetition period, and pulse duration.

21. c. The number of true positive test results divided by the sum of the true positive and false negative tests yields the sensitivity of the test.

22. c. Fusion imaging pair ultrasound images with another imaging modality (MRI, CT) to enable a direct comparison.

23. c. The AIUM 100 test object, tissue-equivalent, and Doppler phantoms evaluate the operation of the ultrasound system. Beam former, hydrophone, and force-balance systems evaluate the acoustic output of the ultrasound system.

24. c. Acoustic output testing evaluates the safety and biological effects of ultrasound and Doppler imaging.

25. a. Negative predictive value is the ability of a diagnostic test to predict normal findings (how often is correct when negative for disease). Identifying the true absence of disease defines specificity.

26. b. The output of the hydrophone evaluates the pressure or intensity of the sound beam. A testing device measures acoustic output. Acoustic exposure is dependent on the acoustic output and exposure time.

27. c. Parallel processing technique enables rapid image acquisition and very high frame rates.

28. a. The hydrophone evaluates the relationship between the acoustic pressure and the voltage produced. Hydrophones measure the acoustic output, period, pulse repetition period, and pulse duration of an acoustic wave.

29. b. Elastography is an imaging version of palpation.

30. c. Tissue-mimicking phantom can evaluate penetration, compression, lateral resolution, and system sensitivity. Doppler phantoms can evaluate flow direction.

31. c. Acoustic output testing requires specialized equipment and considers only the beam profiler and transducer.

32. a. Quality control is a testing used to collect data on the operation and acoustic output of the ultrasound system.

33. b. Quality assurance programs ensure diagnostic image quality and consistency from routine assessment of the ultrasound system. Developing a quality assurance program does not ensure lab accreditation.

34. d. Positive predictive value is equal to the number of true positive tests

(20) divided by the sum of the true positive (20) and false positives (5).

$$\frac{20}{20+5}=\frac{20}{25}=0.8\times100=80\%$$

35. **d.** Test sensitivity is equal to the true positives (20) divided by the sum of the true positive (20) and false negative (0).

$$\frac{20}{20+0}=\frac{20}{20}=1.0\times100=100\%$$

36. **c.** Overall test accuracy is equal to the sum of the true positive tests (20) and true negative tests (75) divided by the total amount tested (100).

$$\frac{95}{100}=0.95\times100=95\%$$

37. **d.** Negative predictive value is equal to true negative tests (75) divided by the sum of the true negative (75) and false negative tests (0).

$$\frac{75}{75+0}=\frac{75}{75}=1.0\times100=100\%$$

38. **c.** Positive predictive value measures how often the test is correct when positive for disease. Sensitivity is the ability of a test to detect disease.

39. **a.** Dead zone is the region closest to the transducer face in which imaging cannot be performed.

40. **b.** Test sensitivity is defined as the ability of a diagnostic technique to identify the presence of disease when disease is actually present.

41. **a.** A large piezoelectric membrane with small metallic electrodes centered on each side is a type of hydrophone.

42. **b.** Blood mimicking Doppler phantoms simulate clinical conditions.

43. **d.** Negative predictive value measures how often the test is correct when negative for disease. Specificity is the ability of a test to detect the absence of disease.

44. **b.** Accuracy measures the percentage of examinations that agree with the gold standard.

45. **d.** Accuracy is the quality of being near to the true value. It is equal to the number of correct test results divided by the total number of tests.

46. **b.** Parallel processing uses a broad pulse.

47. **b.** The beam profiler plots 3-D reflection amplitudes received by the transducer to evaluate the characteristics of the transducer.

48. **c.** Moving string Doppler phantom scatters the sound beam and can produce pulsatile and retrograde flow.

49. **a.** The hydrophone evaluates the relationship between the amount of acoustic pressure and the voltage produced.

50. **c.** Accuracy is equal to the number of correct test results divided by the total number of tests.

$$\text{Accuracy}=\frac{18}{20}=0.9=90\%$$

Physics Mock Exam

1. **d.** Prudent use of sonographic imaging (as low as reasonably achievable) is the mission of the ALARA principle.

2. **b.** Spatial pulse length is proportional to the number of cycles in a pulse and the wavelength. Operating frequency is proportional to the thickness of the crystal. Pulse repetition frequency is proportional to the duty factor.

3. **d.** The Doppler shift frequency is proportional to the velocity of the reflector and is dependent on the Doppler angle and transducer frequency.

4. **a.** The beam width diverges in the Fraunhofer (far) zone and the intensity becomes more uniform.

5. **c.** Reverberation artifact displays as equally spaced reflections of diminishing amplitude with increasing depth.

6. **d.** Enhancement describes the increase in reflection amplitude from structures beneath a weakly attenuating structure. Shadowing occurs beneath a strongly attenuating structure.

7. **c.** Dynamic range (compression) describes the ratio of the largest power to the smallest power the ultrasound system can handle. Bandwidth is the range of frequencies found in pulse ultrasound.

8. **d.** Axial resolution is directly related to the operating frequency and inversely related to the spatial pulse length and penetration depth.

9. **d.** The crystal will increase or decrease according to the polarity of the applied voltage.

10. **c.** The resistance of the arterioles accounts for about one-half of the total resistance in the systemic system.

11. **d.** Rayleigh scattering occurs when the sound wave encounters a reflector much smaller than the wavelength of the sound beam (e.g., red blood cells).

12. **d.** The color black always represents the baseline (zero Doppler shift) in color Doppler imaging.

13. **c.** Frequency is equal to the number of complete cycles in a wave occurring in one second. Pulse repetition frequency is the number of pulses occurring in 1 second.

14. **b.** Fusion imaging pairs ultrasound images with another imaging modality to enable direct comparison

15. **d.** Grating lobes are additional weak beams caused by the regular periodic space of the elements in array transducers.

16. **a.** Clutter is noise in the Doppler signal caused by high-amplitude Doppler shifts. Increasing the wall filter can reduce clutter in the Doppler signal.

17. **d.** Compressions are regions of high pressure or density in a compression wave.

18. **d.** Compression is measured in decibels. Units for amplitude vary with the acoustic variable.

19. **c.** Impedance determines how much of a sound wave will transmit to the next medium or reflect back toward the transducer. Impedance is the product of the density and propagation speed of the medium.

20. **b.** Focusing of the sound beam improves lateral resolution and creates a tapering of the near zone (Fresnel zone). The focal point exhibits the maximum intensity of the sound beam.

21. **d.** Increasing the diameter of the transducer will increase the near zone length and decrease the divergence of the sound beam in the far field.

22. **d.** Freeze frame holds and displays a single image of sonographic information. Cine loop stores the last several frames of information.

23. **b.** Binary number 0010011 = 0 + 0 + 16 + 0 + 0 + 2 + 1 = 19

24. **d.** The thickness of the matching layer is equal to one fourth of the wavelength of the transducer crystal.

25. **d.** The priority Doppler control adjusts gray-scale strength below which color will be shown.
26. **c.** A high resistance waveform demonstrates a tall, sharp, narrow upstroke with reversed, absent or low forward flow velocities in diastole.
27. **c.** Heat sterilization of ultrasound transducers will raise the temperature of the element above the Curie point, losing its piezoelectric properties.
28. **b.** Intensity is zero between pulses. Intensity varies across the sound beam and within a pulse.
29. **c.** The Fresnel or near zone is the region between the transducer and focal point.
30. **d.** Volumetric flow rate must remain constant because blood is neither created nor destroyed as it flows through a vessel (continuity rule).
31. **b.** The greater the impedance difference between two structures, the greater the reflection.
32. **a.** The greatest Doppler shift occurs parallel with the blood flow at a 0-degree angle.
33. **c.** Increasing transducer frequency increases image quality, sensitivity to Doppler shifts, and attenuation of the sound beam.
34. **d.** Shorter pulse lengths, increasing the operating frequency, and decreasing the beam width will improve image quality.
35. **b.** Damping material reduces the number of cycles in each pulse, pulse duration, spatial pulse length, and sensitivity. Matching layer diminishes the reflections near the transducer face and improves sound transmission into the body.
36. **a.** The pulser generates the electric pulses to the crystal producing pulsed ultrasound waves. The master synchronizer instructs the pulser to send a pulse to the transducer.
37. **c.** The beam former determines the firing sequence, delay patterns, and delays during reception.
38. **b.** Stiffness and density of the medium determine the propagation speed of a tissue or structure.
39. **a.** Shifting the baseline may eliminate aliasing. Other methods include increasing the Doppler angle or pulse repetition frequency and decrease imaging depth or transducer frequency.

40. **c.** Focal banding is a product of horizontal enhancement or increase in intensity at the focal zone.
41. **a.** Duplex imaging permits switching between gray-scale imaging and Doppler functions several times per second, decreasing the imaging frame rate and temporal resolution. Aliasing may occur for Doppler shifts with high-peak velocities.
42. **c.** Heat is most dependent on SATA intensity.
43. **a.** Duty factor (transmitting time) is proportional to the pulse duration and pulse repetition frequency and inversely proportional to the pulse repetition period and penetration depth.
44. **a.** Depth or time-gain compensation offsets attenuation by boosting the amplitudes of deep reflections and suppressing superficial reflections.
45. **b.** The Reynolds number predicts the onset of turbulent flow. A vessel with a Reynolds number of 2000 or greater will demonstrate turbulence. Nyquist limit predicts the onset of aliasing.
46. **a.** Axial resolution depends on the operating frequency and is equal to one-half the spatial pulse length. Lateral resolution depends on the beam width, and temporal resolution depends on the frame rate.
47. **d.** The function of the matching layer is to reduce the impedance difference between the element and skin, improving sound transmission across the tissue boundary. Damping reduces the number of cycles in each pulse, pulse duration, and spatial pulse length.
48. **c.** The number of memory bits is equal to 2n. 128 shades of gray = $2 \times 2 \times 2 \times 2 \times 2 \times 2 \times 2 = 128$ or 2^7 (to the seventh power).
49. **b.** Read magnification is a postprocessing function that magnifies and displays stored data. Write magnification is a preprocessing function that increases the number of pixels per inch, improves spatial resolution, and acquires and magnifies new information.
50. **b.** Persistence is a preprocessing, sonographer adjustable function that changes imaging frame rates.
51. **c.** In areas of stenosis, flow speed increases, resulting in a decrease in pressure (Bernoulli effect).

52. **d.** Reducing the gain setting by one-half (-3 dB) would display a new gain setting of 27 dB.
53. **b.** Attenuation is a progressive weakening of the intensity or amplitude of the sound beam as it travels through soft tissue, resulting from absorption, reflection, and scattering of the sound wave.
54. **d.** The sound beam diverges (widens) in the far zone (Fraunhofer) and tapers in the near zone toward the focal point.
55. **b.** Specificity defines the ability of a diagnostic technique to identify correctly the absence of disease (normalcy).
56. **d.** No confirmed significant biological effects exist in mammalian tissue for exposures less than 100 mW/cm^2 with unfocused and 1 W/cm^2 with focused transducers.
57. **c.** Intensity ranges from smallest to highest are SATA (smallest), SPTA, SATP, and SPTP (highest).
58. **c.** Diagnostic ultrasound transducers operate on the piezoelectric effect or principle.
59. **a.** The sound beam is more uniform in intensity in the far field. Maximum intensity occurs at the focal point. Intensity variations are greatest in the near field.
60. **d.** Output or power functions control the intensity of both the transmitted and received signals. The amplifier increases small electric voltages received from the transducer to a level suitable for processing.
61. **d.** Volume flow rate is equal to the average flow speed across the vessel multiplied by the cross-sectional area of the vessel.
62. **d.** Line density is directly related to the pulse repetition frequency and spatial resolution and inversely related to temporal resolution and frame rate.
63. **c.** 4, 6, and 8 MHz are even harmonic frequencies of a 2.0 MHz fundamental frequency.
64. **d.** Range ambiguity is most likely a result of a pulse repetition frequency set too high. Aliasing is a result of a pulse repetition frequency set too low. Decreasing amplification can overcome acoustic speckle and flash artifacts.
65. **d.** Raising the baseline and decreasing the sweep speed will improve the evaluation of this spectral analysis

waveform. Decreasing the PRF after changing the baseline and sweep speed may improve evaluation of the spectral display. A slight decrease in the overall gain could be implemented to improve the spectral mirror image. The wall filter is adjusted appropriately. Priority control is used mainly with color Doppler to help demonstrate blood flow.

66. **b.** Mirror image is duplication of a structure on the opposite side of a strong reflector. Impedance difference determines how much of the incident beam will reflect and transmit at a media boundary.

67. **a.** With perpendicular incidence and different impedances, 99% of the sound beam is transmitted leaving 1% of the sound beam reflecting backing to the transducer.

68. **d.** Distance to a reflector (placement of an echo) is dependent on the round-trip time and propagation speed of the medium.

69. **d.** The low-flow velocities are missing in the spectral display because of a high wall filter setting. Decreasing the wall filter and the pulse repetition frequency will improve the spectral display. The Doppler gain is set appropriately.

70. **d.** The pulse repetition frequency determines the number of scan lines per frame. Contrast resolution is dependent on the number of bits per pixel.

71. **d.** A change in propagation speed as a sound wave travels through a medium does not affect the frequency of the wave.

72. **c.** Arterial diastolic flow shows the state of downstream arterioles. Flow reversal is a characteristic of a high resistance waveform and indicates high-resistance distally.

73. **d.** Decreasing the number of focal zones, imaging depth, beam width, and persistence improves temporal resolution.

74. **d.** Linear phased array transducers contain a compact line of elements about one fourth of a wavelength wide. Linear sequenced array transducers demonstrate a straight line of rectangular elements about one wavelength wide.

75. **c.** Color blossoming or color bleeding is a result of a color gain set too high. Decreasing the color gain should eliminate this color Doppler artifact.

76. **a.** The Nyquist limit predicts the onset of aliasing. A Reynolds number of 2000 or greater predicts the onset of turbulent flow.

77. **d.** Specular reflections occur when the sound wave strikes a smooth large surface perpendicularly.

78. **d.** Increasing the number of focal zones and resonant frequency will improve lateral resolution. Decreasing the imaging depth and beam width will also improve lateral resolution.

79. **c.** Decreasing the imaging depth, lowering the focal zone, and increasing the overall gain will improve this sonogram.

80. **d.** Propagation speed and thickness of the element determine the operating frequency.

81. **b.** Duty factor is the fraction of time pulse ultrasound is transmitting. Period is the time to complete one cycle.

82. **d.** Unprompted venous flow is termed spontaneous. Phasic flow demonstrates respiratory variations. Continuous flow is monophasic and generally indicates obstruction proximally and sometimes distally to the site of Doppler sampling.

83. **d.** Increasing the packet size will decrease the frame rate and temporal resolution.

84. **d.** The spectral display demonstrates a mirror-image artifact from a Doppler gain that is set too high.

85. **b.** Compression is the ratio of the largest to smallest amplitudes the ultrasound system can display.

86. **a.** Imaging depth determines the frame rate.

87. **b.** Apodization reduces grating lobes using a varying excitation of the elements in an array. Subdicing divides each element into small pieces to reduce grating lobes.

88. **d.** The near zone is under gained. Increasing the time-gain compensation in the near field is the first option for the sonographer to improve this image. The focal zone is placed appropriately. Increasing the number of focal zones or decreasing the imaging depth would not increase the near field gain.

89. **d.** Mechanical index is inversely proportional to the operating frequency and proportional to the acoustic output.

90. **a.** A linear phased array sweeps the ultrasound beam electronically by applying voltage pulses to most or all of the elements using minor time differences (delays).

91. **b.** Pulse inversion is a harmonic imaging technique using two pulses per scan line with the second pulse an inversion of the first.

92. **d.** Dynamic focusing uses a variable receiving focus that follows the changing position of the pulse as it propagates through tissue.

93. **a.** The spectral display demonstrates turbulent flow (arteriovenous fistula) with a mirror image spectral artifact. Increasing the PRF (scale), raising the baseline and decreasing the Doppler gain will improve this spectral display.

94. **a.** Nyquist limit is the highest frequency in a sampled signal represented unambiguously and is equal to one-half the pulse repetition frequency.

95. **d.** Compensation provides equal amplitude for all similar structures regardless of the depth.

96. **c.** Spatial compounding directs scan lines in multiple directions improving visualization of structures beneath a highly attenuating structure.

97. **c.** When flow speed increases, pressure energy decreases (Bernoulli effect).

98. **b.** Frequency is proportional to image quality and attenuation. Wavelength, period, and penetration depth are inversely proportional to frequency.

99. **c.** The posterior portion of the far field is under gained. Increasing the time-gain compensation in the far field will improve this sonogram. Raising the focal zone may also help to improve this transverse image of the femoral artery and vein. Increasing the imaging depth would not improve the diagnosis of this image

100. **a.** Plug flow is found in larger arteries and demonstrates a constant velocity across the entire vessel. Parabolic flow is a type of laminar flow where the average flow velocity is equal to one-half of the maximum flow speed at the center.

101. **b.** The intensity of a sound wave is equal to the amplitude squared. If the amplitude is doubled, then the intensity will quadruple.

102. **d.** *Hypoechoic* is a comparative term used to describe a decrease in echogenicity when compared to the surrounding structures or compared to that normally expected for the structure.

103. **c.** Oblique incidence and a change of velocity or propagation speed between the media *must* take place for refraction to occur.

104. **b.** Power Doppler imaging has an increased sensitivity to Doppler shifts (presence of flow), but it is unable to display flow direction, velocity, or characteristics.

105. **d.** Line density directly relates to the pulse repetition frequency and spatial resolution. Frame rate and temporal resolution relates inversely to the line density.

106. **c.** A hydrophone measures acoustic output. Beam profiler measures transducer characteristics.

107. **b.** A rise in tissue temperature is significant when it exceeds 2° C.

108. **c.** Frequency compounding separates the received radiofrequencies into sub-bands. Each sub-band creates an image that are combined into one assimilated image being created with different frequency transducers.

109. **c.** Comet-tail artifact displays a series of closely spaced reverberation echoes behind a strong reflector.

110. **c.** Angling the color Doppler box to the right or left changes the Doppler shift.

111. **a.** Slower propagation speeds will place a reflector deeper than it is actually located.

112. **d.** To overcome range ambiguity, the pulse repetition frequency should be reduced.

113. **d.** Altering the electronic excitation of the elements steers the beam in various directions.

114. **c.** Spectral analysis allows visualization of the Doppler signal providing quantitative data, including peak, mean, and minimum flow velocities, flow direction, and flow characteristics.

115. **b.** Air has the highest attenuation coefficient when compared to fat, liver, kidney, and muscle. Bone has a higher attenuation coefficient when compared to air.

116. **b.** Bandwidth is the range of frequencies found within a pulse.

117. **a.** Infrasound is below human hearing with a frequency range below 20 Hz.

118. **d.** Continuous wave (CW) uses separate transmit and receiver elements housed in a single transducer assembly.

119. **b.** Assumptions about the ultrasound system are the most likely cause of sonographic artifacts.

120. **c.** Structures within the focal zone may display an improper brightness (focal banding).

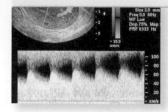

Abdomen Answers

Chapter 7 Liver

1. **c.** The hepatic artery should demonstrate a low resistance waveform with a sharp systolic upstroke and continuous antegrade flow during diastole.

2. **b.** Portal hypertension is associated with compression or occlusion of the portal veins. Sonographic findings may include: hepatomegaly, splenomegaly, hepatofugal flow in the main portal vein, increased resistance in the hepatic artery, formation of venous collaterals, and an increase in diameter of the main portal, splenic, and superior mesenteric veins. Echogenicity of the liver parenchyma is generally hyperechoic. Hypoechoic liver parenchyma is more commonly associated with hepatitis.

3. **a.** Gain settings should display the normal liver parenchyma as a medium shade of gray. The liver is hyperechoic to the normal renal cortex. The normal spleen is actually iso- to hyperechoic to the liver. The impression the spleen is slightly hypoechoic to the liver is due to the larger number of vessels within the liver parenchyma.

4. **b.** A smooth circular or oval-shaped hyperechoic mass is the *most* common sonographic appearance of a cavernous hemangioma. A complex appearance attributed to necrosis or hemorrhage is less common. A hypoechoic mass is suspicious for an adenoma, normal liver tissue with associated fatty infiltration, or malignancy.

5. **c.** The ligamentum of venosum separates the left lobe from the caudate lobe of the liver. The coronary ligament separates the subphrenic space from Morison pouch. The falciform ligament divides the subphrenic space into right and left compartments. The hepatoduodenal ligament connects the liver to the duodenum.

6. **c.** Cirrhosis is a general term used for chronic and severe insult to the liver cells leading to fibrosis and regenerating nodules. Alcohol abuse and hepatitis C are the *most common* cause of cirrhosis in the United States. Worldwide, hepatitis B is the most common cause of cirrhosis. Other etiologies may include: biliary obstruction, viral hepatitis, Budd-Chiari syndrome, nutritional deficiencies, or cardiac disease.

7. **d.** Patients presenting with hepatocellular carcinoma (hepatoma) may demonstrate a decrease in serum albumin, suggesting a decrease in protein synthesis. Additional clinical findings of a hepatoma may include: abdominal pain, palpable mass, weight loss, hepatomegaly, jaundice, unexplained fever, elevated AST, ALT and alkaline phosphatase, and positive alpha-fetoprotein.

8. **c.** In the United States, ascending cholangitis is the most common cause of a hepatic abscess. Additional etiologies may include: recent travel abroad, biliary infection, appendicitis, or diverticulitis. Pseudocyst formation is the most common complication associated with acute pancreatitis. Biliary obstruction is not directly linked with hepatic abscess formation.

9. **c.** The left lobe of the liver is separated from the right lobe by the middle hepatic vein superiorly and the main lobar fissure inferiorly. The left hepatic vein separates the left lobe into medial and lateral segments. The ligamentum venosum separates the caudate and left lobes of the liver.

10. **c.** The right hepatic vein divides the right lobe of the liver into anterior and posterior segments. The middle hepatic vein divides the right lobe from the left medial lobe. Portal veins course within the liver segments (intrasegmental), whereas the hepatic veins course between the liver segments (intersegmental).

11. **a.** An accumulation of triglycerides in the hepatocyte is found in hepatic steatosis (fatty infiltration). Excessive deposition of glycogen is found in glycogen storage disease.

12. **b.** Hepatitis B increases a patient's risk for developing cirrhosis or a hepatoma. Focal nodular hyperplasia and cavernous hemangioma are vascular malformations not related to hepatitis B. Adenomas are related to the use of oral contraceptives.

13. **d.** A "daughter cyst" is defined as a cyst containing smaller cysts. This finding is associated with an echinococcal cyst. A cystadenoma appears as a multiloculated cystic mass. An adenoma demonstrates as a solid hypoechoic mass, whereas a fungal abscess typically demonstrates a complex appearance.

14. **c.** The hepatic veins course between the lobes of the liver *(interlobar)*. The portal veins, hepatic arteries, and biliary ducts generally course parallel with one another within the lobes of the liver *(intralobar)*.

15. **a.** Flow in the main portal vein varies with respiration and is termed *phasic flow*. Blood courses into the liver (hepatopetal) at a low velocity (10 to 30 cm/s). Continuous flow does not vary with respiration. Multiphasic (pulsatile) flow is demonstrated in the hepatic veins.

16. **d.** The hypoechoic area represents normal liver tissue surrounded by fatty infiltration. These focal areas of normal parenchyma are most commonly located anterior to the porta hepatis or near the inferior

vena cava. An enlarged lymph node is a possible differential but not as likely a diagnosis. Nodular fibrosis is related to cirrhosis.

17. **c.** The liver parenchyma appears hyperechoic. The intrahepatic vessel walls are difficult to distinguish but course in a straight pattern. This is most consistent with fatty infiltration.

18. **c.** A solitary hyperechoic mass demonstrating smooth wall margins is most suspicious for a cavernous hemangioma.

19. **b.** The main portal vein should demonstrate flow into the liver (hepatopetal; above baseline). In this duplex image, the main portal vein is demonstrating flow away from the liver (hepatofugal; below baseline). Hepatofugal flow is *most commonly* associated with portal hypertension. When hepatofugal flow is encountered, the sonographer should evaluate for splenic enlargement and venous collaterals. Budd-Chiari syndrome is associated with thrombosis of the hepatic veins. Portal vein thrombosis will demonstrate a minimum or an absence of hepatopetal flow.

20. **c.** The image demonstrates the hepatic veins entering the inferior vena cava. The arrow identifies the hepatic lobe located between the left and middle hepatic veins. The left and middle hepatic veins border the medial left lobe. The left hepatic vein divides the medial and lateral segments of the left lobe. The middle hepatic vein divides the medial left lobe from the anterior right lobe. The right hepatic vein divides the right lobe into anterior and posterior segments.

21. **c.** Extension of the liver anterior and inferior to the right kidney is *most likely* a nonpathological Reidel lobe.

22. **b.** A *single* anechoic area demonstrating posterior acoustic enhancement is identified in the area in question. This finding is most consistent with a simple hepatic cyst. A biloma is associated with recent biliary surgery. A resolving hematoma can appear anechoic but is not as likely a diagnosis as a simple cyst. An echinococcal cyst demonstrates a septated appearance.

23. **c.** A hyperechoic focus demonstrating strong posterior acoustic shadowing is identified in the gallbladder. These are characteristic sonographic findings of cholelithiasis. A small echogenic focus demonstrating a comet tail reverberation artifact is identified in the anterior gallbladder wall consistent with adenomyomatosis. Posterior acoustic enhancement is demonstrated posterior to the hepatic cyst, falsely increasing the echogenicity of the liver tissue.

24. **b.** Candidiasis is a rare fungal infection found in immune-compromised patients. Hypoechoic or target lesions may develop in the liver parenchyma. Hepatic adenomas are associated with the use of oral contraceptives. Echinococcal cysts are associated with recent travel to an underdeveloped country. Immune-suppressed patients are not at an increased risk for developing polycystic disease.

25. **b.** Metastatic lesions involving the liver *most commonly* originate from a malignant neoplasm of the colon. Metastatic neoplasms of the pancreas, breast, and lung can also metastasize to the liver.

26. **b.** The right coronary ligament serves as a barrier between the subphrenic and subhepatic spaces (bare area). Fluid cannot directly ascend from the Morison pouch into the right subphrenic space. The falciform ligament separates the subphrenic space into two compartments. The gastrohepatic and hepatoduodenal ligaments attach the liver to the stomach and duodenum, respectively.

27. **b.** Varix is the most common term used to describe a dilated vein. Aneurysm is more commonly used to describe a focal arterial dilatation. Shunt or stent describes a type of passageway between two structures. Perforator veins connect the superficial and deep venous systems.

28. **b.** Traditional lobar anatomy divides the liver into the right, left, caudate, and quadrate lobes. Functional lobar or segmental anatomy divides the liver into three lobes: left, right, and caudate. Couinaud anatomy divides the liver into eight segments using an imaginary "H" pattern.

29. **a.** Cirrhosis is a general term used to describe chronic and severe insult to the liver cells leading to inflammation of the parenchyma and subsequent necrosis. Portal hypertension is generally a secondary pathology caused by underlying liver disease (e.g., cirrhosis). Budd-Chiari syndrome is associated with thrombosis of the hepatic veins. Focal nodular hyperplasia is considered a congenital vascular malformation.

30. **c.** Von Gierke disease is the most common type of glycogen storage disease (Type I). Patients have a predisposing factor for developing a hepatic adenoma. Schistosomiasis is caused by a parasite. Cirrhosis is not related to Von Gierke disease.

31. **b.** Prominence of the wall margins of the portal veins, or "star effect," is characteristic with hepatitis. In cases of cirrhosis, and glycogen storage disease, the liver demonstrates an increase in parenchymal echogenicity decreasing the distinction of the portal veins, hepatic veins, and biliary ducts.

32. **a.** The TIPS is *commonly* placed between the right portal and right hepatic veins. The purpose of the shunt is to bypass blood from the engorged portal venous system directly into the hepatic venous system.

33. **d.** The paraumbilical vein courses within the falciform ligament from the umbilicus to the left portal vein. Recanalization of the paraumbilical vein is caused by an increase in venous pressure within the portal circulation.

34. **b.** The right hepatic artery lies between the right portal vein and common hepatic duct

35. **d.** The subphrenic space is located superior to the liver and inferior to the diaphragm. The pleura is located superior to the diaphragm. The subhepatic space is located inferior to the liver. The lesser sac is located anterior to the pancreas and posterior to the stomach.

36. **a.** The caudate lobe has a unique blood supply that is routinely spared from disease. Enlargement of the caudate lobe is *most commonly* associated with cirrhosis. The caudate lobe isn't always enlarged in cases of portal hypertension.

37. c. Hepatic veins demonstrate a multiphasic or pulsatile blood flow pattern, coursing away from the liver toward the inferior vena cava (hepatofugal). In laminar flow, the fastest flow is located in the center of the lumen, and slowest flow is located near the lumen walls (e.g., common carotid artery). Parabolic or plug flow demonstrates a steady flow pattern with variable speeds across the vessel lumen (e.g., aorta).

38. b. The falciform ligament attaches the liver to the *anterior* abdominal wall and separates the right and left subphrenic spaces. The right coronary ligament attaches the liver to the lateral abdominal wall. The triangular ligament is the most lateral portion of the coronary ligament.

39. d. The middle hepatic vein is antegrade (blue), flowing toward the inferior vena cava (IVC), whereas the left hepatic vein is retrograde (red), flowing away from the IVC.

40. c. The caudate lobe is located posterior to the ligamentum venosum and porta hepatis, anterior and medial to the inferior vena cava, and lateral to the lesser sac.

41. b. Multiple engorged vessels in the left upper quadrant. This finding is most suspicious for gastric varices.

42. c. A decrease in prothrombin time is associated with subacute or acute cholecystitis, internal biliary fistula, gallbladder carcinoma, injury to the bile ducts, and prolonged extrahepatic bile duct obstruction. Cirrhosis, malignancy, malabsorption of vitamin K, and clotting failure are associated with elevation of prothrombin time.

43. c. Severe abdominal pain and loss of appetite are the *most common* symptoms associated with portal vein thrombosis. Weight loss is precipitated by a loss of appetite. Tachycardia and lower extremity edema are more commonly associated with pulmonary embolism and deep vein thrombosis of the lower extremity.

44. c. After placement of a TIPS, the main portal vein should have demonstrated turbulent hepatopetal flow. The right and left portal veins should demonstrate hepatofugal flow. The velocities within the shunt range from 65 cm/s to 225 cm/s.

45. a. A long history of oral contraceptive use is a predisposing factor for developing a hepatic adenoma. A hypoechoic liver mass demonstrating a hypoechoic halo is identified in the right lobe of the liver. This is characteristic of an adenoma. Focal nodular hyperplasia is influenced by hormones but presents as (a) well-defined isoechoic or hyperechoic mass(es). A hepatoma could be a differential consideration but not a likely diagnosis in this case. Cavernous hemangiomas can undergo degeneration, changing the echo pattern, but are not associated with a hypoechoic halo. Adenoma is the most likely diagnosis for this liver mass with these sonographic findings and clinical history.

46. d. The liver parenchyma appears heterogeneous, demonstrating multiple hyperechoic masses throughout the right lobe. This is most consistent with liver metastasis. Cirrhosis is associated with a hyperechoic liver parenchyma irregular nodular contour, and the inability to distinguish portal vein wall margins. Hypoechoic or target lesions are characteristic of candidiasis.

47. d. A small fluid collection is identified inferior to the diaphragm (hyperechoic linear structure) and superior to the liver in the right subphrenic space. The pleura is located superior to the diaphragm. The subhepatic space and right paracolic gutter are located inferior to the liver.

48. b. A well-defined anechoic structure demonstrating posterior acoustic enhancement is documented anterior to the porta hepatis. This mass most likely represents a simple hepatic cyst.

49. c. The falciform ligament attaches the liver to the anterior abdominal wall, extending from the diaphragm to the umbilicus. The ligamentum venosum separates the left lobe of the liver from the caudate lobe. The triangular ligament is the most lateral portion of the coronary ligament, which connects the liver to the diaphragm.

50. b. The liver parenchyma appears slightly hypoechoic with prominent portal veins (star effect). These sonographic findings are most suspicious for acute hepatitis. Candidiasis demonstrates as uniform hypoechoic lesions on ultrasound.

Chapter 8 Biliary System

1. d. A malignant neoplasm located at the junction of the right and left hepatic ducts is termed a Klatskin tumor. A biloma is an extrahepatic collection of extravasated bile. Extension of pancreatic inflammation into the peripancreatic tissues describes a phlegmon. Caroli disease demonstrates a saccular or beaded appearance to the intrahepatic biliary tree on ultrasound.

2. d. Supine, left posterior oblique, and left lateral decubitus positions are routinely used in abdominal imaging. The cystic duct is not routinely visualized in these positions. Trendelenburg or right lateral decubitus positions may aid in visualization of the cystic duct. A prone position helps in visualizing some retroperitoneal structures.

3. a. A fold or septation located between the neck and body of the gallbladder describes a junctional fold. Hartmann pouch is a small posterior pouch located near the neck of the gallbladder. A phrygian cap describes a fold in the gallbladder fundus.

4. b. Demonstration of a focal hyperechoic gallbladder *wall* with *marked* posterior acoustic shadowing is characteristic of a porcelain gallbladder. Emphysematous cholecystitis appears as an echogenic focus in the gallbladder wall or lumen with *ill-defined* posterior acoustic shadowing. Cholelithiasis is an intraluminal abnormality. Mirizzi syndrome is a condition caused by a lodge stone in the neck of the gallbladder or cystic duct.

5. c. Nonshadowing, low amplitude echoes located in the dependent portion of the gallbladder describes biliary sludge. The key words in this question are: dependent and nonshadowing. This implies the echoes are mobile and do not demonstrate posterior acoustic shadowing. Mobile echoes rule out adenomyomatosis and polypoid masses. Nonshadowing echoes rules out cholelithiasis. Cholecystitis describes an inflammatory process affecting the gallbladder.

6. **d.** Cholesterolosis is an accumulation of triglycerides and esterified sterols in the wall of the gallbladder caused by a local disturbance in cholesterol metabolism. There are two types of cholesterolosis: cholesterosis and cholesterol polyps. Cholesterolosis is not associated with serum cholesterol levels.

7. **a.** The spiral valves of Heister are located in the cystic duct. These valves make visualization difficult on ultrasound.

8. **b.** Localized thickening of the gallbladder wall in a patient with a positive Murphy sign (extreme pain over the gallbladder fossa) is most consistent with acute cholecystitis. Cholelithiasis does not generally demonstrate a positive Murphy sign without gallbladder inflammation. Irregular thickening of the gallbladder wall is seen in cases of gallbladder carcinoma but doesn't typically present with a positive Murphy sign. Adenomyomatosis is not associated with a positive Murphy sign.

9. **d.** A hyperechoic focus demonstrating posterior acoustic shadowing is identified in the *common bile duct* consistent with choledocholithiasis. Cholangiocarcinoma appears as a *nonshadowing* intraluminal echogenic focus. Thickening of the bile duct walls is consistent with cholangitis.

10. **a.** Complications associated with choledocholithiasis may include biliary obstruction, cholangitis, and pancreatitis. Choledocholithiasis is not a precipitating factor of portal hypertension or lymphadenopathy.

11. **c.** A *nonvascular* tubular structure is identified posterior to the gallbladder in the porta hepatis in a neonate. This is most suspicious for a choledochal cyst. Duplication of the gallbladder or hepatic cyst in a neonate is not as likely.

12. **a.** An anechoic structure contiguous with the gallbladder fundus is demonstrated on this sonogram. This is most likely a fold in the gallbladder fundus, termed a *phrygian cap*. A junctional fold and Hartman's pouch are located near the neck of the gallbladder.

13. **b.** A refractive artifact is demonstrating a "shadow" posterior and medial to the phrygian cap of the gallbladder. Sound is refracted in a lateral direction from the projected path, leaving weak echoes to return from the expected path. This causes a shadow appearance. Refraction occurs at the edge of generally round or oval-shaped structures and is commonly termed an *edge artifact*. Grating lobes are additional, weaker sound beams traveling in different directions from the primary beam. Reverberation demonstrates multiple equally spaced echoes. Slice thickness artifact decreases detail resolution.

14. **d.** The biliary system has three main functions: (1) transport bile to the gallbladder through the biliary ducts; (2) store and concentrate bile in the gallbladder; and (3) transport bile through the bile ducts from the gallbladder to the duodenum to aid in the digestion of fats.

15. **b.** Biliary sludge is not necessarily a pathological condition. It may be demonstrated in patients with abnormal eating patterns or prolonged fasting. Cholelithiasis and cholangitis are related to biliary stasis but are not as likely to occur as biliary sludge. Polypoid or malignant lesions are unrelated to episodes of fasting.

16. **a.** The gallbladder wall is composed of four layers: (1) outer serosal, (2) subserosal, (3) muscular, and (4) inner epithelial.

17. **c.** The CBD courses inferiorly through the head of the pancreas terminating in the descending portion of the duodenum at the ampulla of Vater. The superior portion of the common bile duct is located near the hepatic hilum and neck of the gallbladder.

18. **b.** The common hepatic duct lies anterior to the main portal vein and lateral to the proper hepatic artery in the region of the porta hepatis.

19. **d.** Right upper quadrant pain, postprandial pain, elevated liver function tests, fatty food intolerance, or a positive Murphy sign are common indications for a biliary sonogram. Tenderness over the McBurney point is a clinical sign of appendicitis.

20. **d.** The release of cholecystokinin stimulates gallbladder contraction and secretion of pancreatic enzymes. Cholecystokinin is released when food reaches the duodenum. Gastrin stimulates the secretion of gastric acids. Amylase and bilirubin are not hormones.

21. **b.** The normal fasting adult gallbladder measures 8 to 12 cm in length and 4 cm in diameter. Diameters exceeding 4 cm are considered enlarged or hydropic.

22. **c.** The sonogram is demonstrating a *fluid/fluid layer* within the gallbladder lumen. The fluids consist of echogenic biliary sludge in the dependent portion of the gallbladder and the less dense anechoic bile. The layering effect of the two types of fluid rules out an intraluminal mass.

23. **c.** The hyperechoic linear structure extends from the right portal vein (echogenic walls) to the gallbladder fossa. This is most consistent with the main lobar fissure. The main lobar fissure is an *inter*segmental boundary between the right and left lobes of the liver. The ligamentum of venosum separates the caudate and left lobes of the liver. The ligamentum of Teres and falciform ligament are located in the left lobe.

24. **b.** The main lobar fissure is a boundary between the left and right lobes of the liver and is routinely used as a sonographic landmark for locating the gallbladder fossa. The ligamentum venosum is a sonographic landmark used to locate the caudate lobe. The falciform ligament and ligamentum of Teres are sonographic landmarks used for locating the superior portion of the paraumbilical vein.

25. **a.** Multiple small echogenic foci are located in the dependent portion of the gallbladder. Acoustic shadowing is demonstrated posteriorly. These sonographic findings are most consistent with cholelithiasis. The gallbladder wall appears thin and smooth, ruling out adenomyomatosis, porcelain gallbladder, and acute cholecystitis as differential considerations. Tumefactive sludge is generally irregular in shape, slow moving, and nonshadowing.

26. **d.** Changing the patient position will document mobility of the echogenic foci consistent with cholelithiasis. An intercostal approach or deep inspiration may increase resolution of the foci but would not

demonstrate mobility. Ingestion of water aids in visualization of the pancreas.

27. **a.** Low-level echoes in the bile duct that are mobile with patient position changes are most suspicious for hemobilia. A Klatskin tumor is not gravity dependent.

28. **b.** Alkaline phosphatase is an enzyme produced primarily by the liver, bone, and placenta and excreted via the bile ducts. Marked elevation is associated with obstructive jaundice. ALT is an enzyme found in high concentrations in the liver and lower concentrations in the heart, muscle, and kidneys. AST is an enzyme present in many types of tissue.

29. **a.** Under normal conditions, the common bile duct will decrease in size or remain unchanged after ingestion of a fatty meal. Enlargement is associated with biliary disease.

30. **a.** In the fasting state, the gallbladder wall usually measures 1 to 2 mm in thickness and should not exceed 3 mm.

31. **b.** Dilatation of only the intrahepatic ducts suggests obstruction within the liver (intrahepatic). A Klatskin tumor is an intrahepatic tumor located at the junction of the left and right hepatic ducts. Cholangitis, choledocholithiasis, and pancreatic neoplasm are generally extrahepatic pathologies.

32. **c.** Older diabetic patients have an increased risk for developing gangrenous cholecystitis and perforation of the gallbladder.

33. **d.** The intrahepatic biliary tree, hepatic arteries, and portal venous system course adjacent with one another. Progressive dilatation of the bile ducts compresses and flattens the portal veins. A beaded appearance to the intrahepatic biliary ducts is characteristic of Caroli disease.

34. **b.** The transverse diameter of the normal gallbladder should not exceed 4 cm. A diameter exceeding 4.0 cm is termed *hydrops*. The gallbladder in this sonogram measures 7.6 cm in transverse diameter with normal wall thickness.

35. **a.** The gallbladder is demonstrating the wall-echo-shadow (WES) sign consistent with a stone-filled gallbladder.

36. **c.** Multiple solid, immobile, non-shadowing echogenic masses are demonstrated in an asymptomatic patient. This is most suspicious for multiple adenomas (polyps). Adenomyomatosis lesions demonstrate a comet tail-shadowing artifact not seen in these masses. Metastatic lesions are not the most likely answer in an asymptomatic patient.

37. **b.** Hyperechoic foci demonstrating posterior acoustic shadowing in a patient with a previous history of biliary surgery is most suspicious for pneumobilia. Surgical clips following cholecystectomy are generally located near the porta hepatis. Calculus within a bile duct and arterial calcifications are not as likely a diagnosis as pneumobilia.

38. **d.** Multiple hyperechoic foci are identified in the anterior gallbladder *wall*. Comet-tail reverberation artifact is demonstrated posterior to the foci. These sonographic findings are characteristic of adenomyomatosis. Chronic or acute cases of cholecystitis generally demonstrate a thickened gallbladder wall. Gallstones are typically gravitationally dependent.

39. **a.** A form of reverberation, the comet-tail artifact occurs with marked impedance changes. It appears as a dense, tapering trail of echoes just distal to a strongly reflecting structure. This type of artifact is characteristic in adenomyomatosis. Refraction occurs at the edge of generally round or oval-shaped structures and is commonly termed an *edge artifact*. Mirror image is a form of reverberation artifact where structures that exist on one side of a strong reflector are also identified on the opposite side.

40. **b.** A small posterior pouch near the neck of the gallbladder describes Hartmann pouch. A junctional fold is defined as a septation or fold near the gallbladder neck. Morison pouch is located in the lateral subhepatic space. Choledochal cysts do not involve the neck of the gallbladder.

41. **a.** Imaging of dilated intrahepatic ducts parallel with the associated portal vein is termed *parallel channeling*, *double channel sign*, or *shotgun sign*. Prominence of the portal veins is seen in hepatitis and is

termed the *star effect*. A color Doppler twinkle sign is an artifactual Doppler signal found in adenomyomatosis.

42. **a.** Bilirubin is a product of the breakdown of hemoglobin in old red blood cells. AST, ALT, and alkaline phosphatase are liver enzymes. Alpha-fetoprotein is a protein normally synthesized by the fetus.

43. **d.** Risk factors include: family history of gallstones, fair complexion, female gender, fertility, obesity, pregnancy, diabetes mellitus, estrogen replacement therapy, prolong fasting, abnormal hemolysis, and alcohol cirrhosis. Hepatitis and cirrhosis are not predisposing factors associated with the development of cholelithiasis. Biliary disease is the most common cause of pancreatitis.

44. **c.** Increasing the transducer frequency increases the axial resolution necessary to demonstrate shadowing posterior to small gallstones. Decreasing overall gain and number of focal zones will not increase the image's axial resolution.

45. **c.** Ascariasis is caused by the ingestion of contaminated water or food especially in the southern gulf states of the United States, Africa, Asia, and South America.

46. **d.** Pneumobilia generally demonstrates as a hyperechoic focus with posterior acoustic shadowing. A surgical clip, stent, calculus, or vascular calcification can appear on ultrasound as a hyperechoic focus with or without posterior acoustic shadowing. A hemangioma appears as a nonshadowing, hyperechoic, or complex mass.

47. **b.** The solid gallbladder mass is immobile (image annotation states decubitus position). Adenomas and malignant neoplasms are immobile lesions. Tumefactive sludge, although slow moving, is generally mobile.

48. **d.** Sonographic and clinical findings are most consistent with metastatic gallbladder disease. Metastasis to the gallbladder is a likely diagnosis with the following criteria: (1) focal intraluminal masses, (2) history of pancreas neoplasm, and (3) no associated cholelithiasis. The patient has a history of pancreatic cancer. The

gallbladder demonstrates immobile echogenic masses without associated gallstones.

49. b. Two nonconnecting sonolucencies are identified in the *gallbladder fossa*. This is most suspicious for gallbladder duplication. The gallbladders are located in the gallbladder fossa. Strawberry gallbladder is a sonographic appearance in cholesterosis.

50. b. Acute cholecystitis is the most likely diagnosis with a history of acute right upper quadrant pain and a thickened hyperemic gallbladder wall. The patient will likely demonstrate a positive Murphy sign.

Chapter 9 Pancreas

1. d. Annular pancreas is a congenital anomaly in which the head of the pancreas surrounds the duodenum. This may result in obstruction of the biliary tree or duodenum. Pancreas divisum is an anomaly of the pancreatic ducts. Phlegmon is a complication of acute pancreatitis.

2. c. Clinical findings associated with acute pancreatitis include an abrupt onset of epigastric pain (typically severe), nausea/vomiting, elevation in serum amylase and lipase, and paralytic ileus.

3. d. Trypsin is a highly digestive enzyme that breaks down proteins into amino acids. Amylase breaks down carbohydrates, and lipase breaks down fats. Gastrin is a hormone.

4. c. The uncinate process, a medial portion of the pancreatic head, is located directly posterior to the superior mesenteric vein and anterior to the inferior vena cava. The uncinate process is located posterior and medial to the gastroduodenal artery and main portal vein.

5. c. Pseudocyst formation is the most common complication of acute pancreatitis. Additional complications may include: phlegmon, hemorrhage, abscess formation, or duodenal obstruction.

6. b. Islet cells of Langerhans secrete hormones directly into the bloodstream. These hormones include: glucagon (alpha cells), insulin (beta cells), and somatostatin (delta cells).

7. c. In a Whipple procedure (pancreatoduodenectomy) normal pancreatic tissue is attached to the duodenum. The gallbladder is removed, if present. The common bile duct is anastomosed to the duodenum distal to the pancreas, and the stomach is anastomosed to the duodenum distal to the common bile duct.

8. c. A phlegmon is an extension of pancreatic inflammation into the peripancreatic tissues. A pseudocyst is a collection of fluid caused by a leakage of pancreatic enzymes. Annular pancreas is a congenital anomaly. An abscess is a collection of a purulent substance.

9. b. Biliary disease is the most common cause of acute pancreatitis followed by alcohol abuse. Additional etiologies may include: trauma, peptic ulcer disease, and hyperlipidemia.

10. c. The sonogram demonstrates a complex mass near the lesser sac and anterior pararenal space. The complex appearance may be related to hemorrhage or necrosis. Pseudocyst formation is the most common complication in acute pancreatitis and the *most likely* diagnosis with this clinical history. A phlegmon is an extension of the inflammation into the peripancreatic tissues and generally appears as a solid hypoechoic mass. A biloma is typically located in the region of the porta hepatis. A mass identified in the sonogram located in the left upper quadrant is more consistent with the stomach and not the duodenal region

11. b. An anechoic tubular structure is located anterior to the splenic vein within the body of the pancreas. This is most consistent with the main pancreatic duct (duct of Wirsung). The splenic artery courses superior to the body of the pancreas. The common bile duct courses through the posterior lateral portion of the pancreatic head. The gastroduodenal artery is located in the anterior lateral portion of the head of the pancreas.

12. a. The arrow is identifying an anechoic structure located anterior to the spine, lateral to the inferior vena cava, and posterior to the pancreas, left lobe of the liver, superior mesenteric artery, and portosplenic confluence. This is most consistent with the abdominal aorta.

13. c. A hypoechoic mass is identified in the head of the pancreas most suspicious for a malignant neoplasm.

14. b. An anechoic tubular structure is identified anterior to the splenic vein within the body of the pancreas. This is *most likely* a dilated pancreatic duct secondary to compression from the neoplasm. A tortuous splenic artery is a *possible* consideration. Doppler imaging would help to differentiate between a vascular or nonvascular structure. Before color Doppler imaging, anatomical landmarks and real-time imaging were used to differentiate between a vascular and nonvascular structure.

15. a. A pseudocyst is most *often* located in the lesser sac followed by the anterior pararenal space. Because it does not contain a lining membrane, it will conform to the surrounding space(s).

16. c. Lipase is an enzyme responsible for changing fats into fatty acids and glycerol. Amylase is an enzyme that breaks down carbohydrates. Trypsin is an enzyme that breaks down proteins into amino acids. Gastrin and secretin are hormones.

17. d. The pancreas lies in a transverse oblique plane with the tail portion located most superiorly and the uncinate process most inferiorly. The body is considered the most anterior portion of the pancreas.

18. d. A congenital anomaly, ectopic pancreatic tissue may be located in the stomach, duodenum, or small or large intestines.

19. a. The pancreas and surrounding vascular landmarks should be examined from the level of the celiac axis (superior to the pancreas) to below the renal veins (inferior to the pancreas).

20. d. Microcystic cystadenomas account for 50% of cystic neoplasms involving the pancreas, with the majority located in the body or tail. It generally appears as an echogenic or complex mass because of multiple small cystic structures.

21. a. Pancreatic enzymes, amylase, and lipase are associated with acute pancreatitis. Amylase and lipase rise at a similar rate, but the elevation in lipase persists for a longer period.

22. b. The pancreatic duct is routinely visualized in the body of the pancreas. A tortuous splenic artery may be mistaken as the pancreatic duct. The common bile duct is visualized in the posterior lateral portion of the pancreatic head.

23. **a.** Ninety percent of nonfunctioning islet cell tumors are malignant and appear as a small, well-defined hypoechoic mass. Islet cell tumors are most commonly located in the tail or body of the pancreas. A nonfunctioning tumor would not be related to insulin levels.

24. **d.** Sonographic findings associated with chronic pancreatitis include: atrophy, hyperechoic parenchyma, prominent pancreatic duct, parenchymal calcifications, irregular borders, and/or pseudocyst formation.

25. **c.** Clinical findings associated with pancreatic carcinoma may include: weight loss, severe back pain, abdominal pain, painless jaundice, anorexia, thrombophlebitis of the lower extremities, or *new onset of diabetes*. Weight gain, fatty food intolerance, and chest pain are not commonly associated with pancreatic carcinoma.

26. **c.** The sonogram demonstrates a small, well-defined mass in the tail of the pancreas. History of elevating insulin levels and a solid hypoechoic mass in the tail of the pancreas are most suspicious for a functioning islet cell tumor (insulinoma). Adenocarcinoma and focal pancreatitis are differential considerations but not as likely a diagnosis with a clinical history of elevating insulin levels.

27. **d.** The tail of the pancreas is demonstrating a cobblestone appearance, a common variant in normal pancreatic parenchyma.

28. **a.** An anechoic circular structure is located in the posterolateral portion of the pancreatic head. This is most likely the common bile duct. The gastroduodenal artery is located in the anterolateral portion of the head of the pancreas.

29. **c.** Endocrine functions of the pancreas include secretion of insulin, glucagon, and somatostatin. Exocrine functions include: secretion of enzymes (amylase, lipase, and trypsin) and the release of hormones (gastrin and secretin).

30. **b.** The celiac axis is the first branch of the abdominal aorta located

superior to the pancreas. The splenic vein and superior mesenteric artery are used as landmarks for locating the body of the pancreas. The pancreas should be evaluated from the celiac axis (superior to the pancreas) to below the renal veins (inferior to the pancreas).

31. **b.** The tail of the pancreas *generally* extends toward the splenic hilum and *occasionally* extends toward the left renal hilum.

32. **c.** The splenic vein is a vascular landmark used for locating the tail of the pancreas. The tail of the pancreas courses parallel with the splenic vein.

33. **b.** The diameter of a normal pancreatic duct in the head/neck region should not exceed 3 mm. The normal diameter in the body should not exceed 2 mm. The hyperechoic walls should also appear smooth coursing parallel with each other.

34. **b.** Acinar cells are responsible for the secretion of highly digestive pancreatic enzymes via the pancreatic duct. Alpha and beta cells are hormones secreted by the islet cells of Langerhans directly into the bloodstream.

35. **c.** The neck is located between the body and head of the pancreas directly anterior to the superior mesenteric vein and portosplenic confluence. The celiac axis is located superior to the pancreas. The uncinate process lies directly posterior to the superior mesenteric vein.

36. **a.** The head is involved in 70% of cases of malignant neoplasms involving the pancreas, whereas 20% involve the body.

37. **a.** Islet cell tumors are more commonly located in the body and tail of the pancreas. Adenocarcinoma most commonly involves the pancreatic head.

38. **c.** The duct of Santorini is the secondary secretory duct of the pancreas. The duct of Wirsung is the primary secretory duct of the pancreas.

39. **d.** The normal *adult* pancreas appears isoechoic to hyperechoic compared to the normal liver parenchyma.

40. **c.** The letter D identifies the superior mesenteric vein (SMV). The SMV courses parallel with the superior mesenteric artery (B) and the aorta (A).

41. **a.** The letter A identifies the abdominal aorta. The abdominal aorta lies posterior to the SMA (D).

42. **b.** The letter B identifies the superior mesenteric artery. The SMA lies posterior to the SMV (D) and anterior to the abdominal aorta (A).

43. **d.** This vascular structure is a common sonographic landmark used in locating the pancreas. The hyperechoic echoes surrounding this vessel and location are characteristic of the superior mesenteric artery.

44. **c.** The vascular structure is located in the hepatic hilum consistent with the main portal vein. The hepatic veins converge on the inferior vena cava.

45. **a.** The majority of cystadenomas involving the pancreas are located in the body and tail.

46. **c.** The body is the largest and most anterior section of the pancreas. The tail lies most superior.

47. **a.** Multiple cysts in the pancreas might signify polycystic disease. The liver, spleen, and kidneys should be evaluated for evidence of polycystic disease.

48. **c.** Rapid progression of pancreatic inflammation describes a phlegmon. A phlegmon may cause necrosis or hemorrhage and is considered a complication of acute pancreatitis.

49. **c.** The sphincter of Oddi is a sheath of muscle fibers surrounding the distal common bile and pancreatic ducts as they cross the wall of the duodenum through the ampulla of Vater.

50. **c.** Leakage of pancreatic enzymes into the surrounding peritoneal space describes a pseudocyst. Phlegmon is an extension of pancreatic inflammation into the surrounding tissues. Abscess is a collection of a purulent substance.

Chapter 10 Urinary System

1. **a.** The medullary pyramids commonly appear anechoic in the neonate. The renal cortex generally appears moderate to highly echogenic. A sparse amount of perinephric fat makes it difficult to distinguish the renal capsule or the renal sinus.

2. **c.** A decrease in BUN is associated with liver failure, overhydration, pregnancy, smoking, and decreases in protein intake.

3. **b.** The right renal artery arises from the anterolateral aspect, and the left renal artery arises from the posterolateral aspect of the abdominal aorta. The celiac axis and gonadal, superior, and inferior mesenteric arteries arise from the anterior aspect of the abdominal aorta.

4. **a.** The basic functional unit of the kidney is the nephron. The glomerulus is a structure composed of blood vessels or nerve filters. Loop of Henle is the "U"-shaped portion of a renal tubule. Collecting tubules funnel urine into the renal pelvis.

5. **d.** The quadratus lumborum is a muscle of the posterior abdominal wall located posterior and medial to each kidney. The transversus abdominis muscle is located in the anterolateral wall.

6. **b.** A variant of the horseshoe kidney, a cake or lump kidney demonstrates fusion of the medial aspects of both kidneys. Fusion of both kidneys within the same quadrant in the body describes crossed fused ectopia. Fusion of the superior pole of one kidney to the inferior pole of the contralateral kidney is termed a sigmoid or "S"-shaped kidney.

7. **d.** A hypertrophied column of Bertin extends from the cortex into the medullary pyramids. This anatomical variant may mimic a renal duplication. Fetal lobulation and dromedary hump are variants associated with the outer renal contour. Congenital variation in the fusion of the superior and inferior poles of the kidney is termed a *junctional fold defect*. It is identified on sonography as a triangular hyperechoic focus in the anterior aspect of the kidney.

8. **b.** Patients on dialysis are at increased risk for developing a renal cyst, renal adenoma, and renal carcinoma. Nephrocalcinosis is associated with hyperparathyroidism, hypercalcemia, and hypercalciuria.

9. **a.** Fifty percent of patients older than 55 years demonstrate a simple renal cyst.

10. **c.** A staghorn calculus is a large stone forming in the renal pelvis and extending into some or all of the calyces.

11. **c.** A circular anechoic structure with a distinct linear echo (catheter) is identified in an empty urinary bladder. A ureterocele is a possible differential consideration but not as likely as a catheter balloon. Residual urine is neither typically circular in shape nor demonstrated in catheterized patients. A bladder diverticulum is defined as an outpouching of the bladder wall.

12. **c.** Anechoic appearance of the medullary pyramids is a normal sonographic finding in a neonatal kidney and may be mistaken for hydronephrosis. Arcuate vessels are peripherally located. A hyperechoic appearance to the kidneys is typically seen with infantile polycystic disease.

13. **d.** Dilatation of the renal calyces is identified. This is most suspicious for Grade 3 hydronephrosis. Pelviectasis (Grade 1) does not involve the calyces. Pyelonephritis may demonstrate prominent medullary pyramids. Nephrolithiasis is a possible cause for the hydronephrosis but would appear as a hyperechoic focus(i).

14. **d.** Obstruction of the urinary tract is the most common cause of hydronephrosis. The cause of the obstruction will vary (e.g., ureteral stone, congenital anomaly). Urinary stasis is a predisposing factor for developing a urinary tract infection.

15. **d.** The sonogram demonstrates an irregular contour to the urinary bladder. An anechoic outward pedunculation in the wall is identified. This is most consistent with a bladder diverticulum. . The urethra is a midline structure, and the sonogram is imaged to the right of midline (image annotation and caption). Ureterocele is a bladder abnormality within the bladder at the ureteric orifice.

16. **a.** The glomerulus is composed of blood vessels or nerve fibers. Loop of Henle is a portion of the renal tubule. The renal pyramids contain tubules and loops of Henle.

17. **a.** Renal colic describes sharp, severe flank pain that radiates to the groin. It is considered a clinical symptom of nephrolithiasis. Dysuria and dyspareunia describe painful urination and intercourse, respectively. *Mittelschmerz* is a term used to describe pain during ovulation.

18. **d.** Contained within the renal *sinus* is the major and minor calyces, peripelvic fat, fibrous tissues, segmental arteries, segmental veins, lymphatics, and part of the renal pelvis. The renal artery, renal vein, and ureter are located in the renal *hilum*. *Perinephric* fat surrounds the kidney.

19. **d.** The transversus abdominis muscle is located lateral to each kidney. The psoas muscle lies posterior to the inferior pole of the kidney. The quadratus lumborum muscle lies posterior and medial to the kidney.

20. **d.** A triangular shaped hyperechoic focus located in the *anterior* renal cortex most likely represents a junction parenchymal defect. Renal calculus is a possible differential *but not the most likely* consideration. An adenoma generally appears as a well-defined hypoechoic mass.

21. **b.** Postvoid urine volume will vary from case to case but should not exceed 20 mL in the adult patient to be considered within normal limits.

22. **a.** Generalized swelling of the kidney characterized by well-defined (prominent) renal pyramids is most consistent with pyelonephritis.

23. **b.** Renal biopsy procedures are generally performed with patients lying on their stomachs in the prone position. A pillow, sponge, or towels may be placed under the abdomen.

24. **b.** Ureteric orifices appear as small echogenic protuberances located on the posterior aspect of the urinary bladder on ultrasound. Hydroureters, bladder diverticula, and arcuate vessels generally appear anechoic on ultrasound.

25. **b.** Patients with adult polycystic renal disease have an increased incidence of developing renal calculi and infection.

26. **d.** An isoechoic mass extends from the renal cortex into the medullary pyramids. This is most consistent with a hypertrophied column of Bertin. This anatomical variant may be mistaken for a renal duplication or neoplasm. Junctional parenchymal defect appears as a small triangular hyperechoic mass on ultrasound. Cross-fused ectopia is a congenital anomaly.

27. **a.** Perinephric fat varies with each patient. Obese patients commonly demonstrate an increased amount of perinephric fat.

28. c. A hypoechoic mass with internal blood flow is extending from the renal parenchyma. This is most suspicious for renal cell carcinoma. Dromedary hump is a possible differential but not the most likely diagnosis with this clinical history. Angiomyolipoma may demonstrate gross hematuria but appears on ultrasound as a hyperechoic mass. A hematoma or hemorrhagic cyst would not demonstrate internal blood flow.

29. b. A circular anechoic area is noted *within* the urinary bladder in the area of the right ureteric orifice. This is most consistent with an ureterocele. A catheter balloon would demonstrate an echogenic linear echo (catheter) within the anechoic balloon. A diverticulum is an outward pedunculation of the urinary bladder.

30. c. Parapelvic cysts are located within the renal sinus. The renal pelvis *extrudes* from the renal hilum with an extrarenal pelvis. Neither a hydroureter nor hydronephrosis is identified in this sonogram.

31. a. Mesoblastic nephroma is a benign pediatric tumor occurring during the first year of life in the majority of cases (90%).

32. d. Angiomyolipoma is a benign tumor composed of blood vessels *(angio)*, muscle *(myo)*, and fat *(lipoma)*.

33. a. Fibromuscular hyperplasia is associated with stenosis in the mid- to distal portion of the main renal artery.

34. c. A peak systolic velocity exceeding 180 cm/s suggests the possibility of renal artery stenosis.

35. d. Painless hematuria is *most* likely associated with renal cell carcinoma or transitional cell carcinoma of the urinary bladder. Careful evaluation of the urinary tract is warranted with this finding. An angiomyolipoma may cause hematuria but is not the *most likely* condition associated with painless hematuria.

36. b. Nephrolithiasis is a condition most frequently associated with urinary stasis. Chronic renal failure is more frequently associated with an inflammatory or vascular condition than urinary stasis from chronic hydronephrosis.

37. c. Sigmoid kidney, or S-shaped kidney, is a variant of the horseshoe kidney. This congenital anomaly presents as a fusion of the superior pole of one kidney with the inferior pole of the contralateral kidney. Fusion of the medial surfaces of both kidneys describes a cake kidney. Crossed fused ectopia demonstrates fused kidneys located in the same body quadrant.

38. b. The normal renal cortex in adult patients should measure a minimum of 1 cm. Thinning of the renal cortex raises suspicion of chronic renal disease.

39. b. Renal failure is defined as the complete inability of the kidneys to excrete waste, concentrate urine, and conserve electrolytes. Renal insufficiency is defined as partial kidney function failure characterized by less than normal urine output. Renal colic is a clinical symptom associated with passage of a renal calculus. Renal obstruction may be a predisposing factor of renal failure.

40. b. The medullary pyramids appear hyperechoic, most suspicious for nephrocalcinosis. Metastatic disease is more likely to demonstrate hyperechoic and hypoechoic mass(es) within the renal parenchyma. Angiomyolipomas are located in the renal cortex. Glomerulonephritis is characterized by enlarged kidney(s) demonstrating a hyperechoic renal cortex.

41. d. The superior pole of the left kidney is fused to the inferior pole of the right kidney consistent with a sigmoid or S-shaped kidney. Fusion of the medial aspect of both kidneys is termed a *cake* or *lump* kidney. Duplication involves two distinct collecting systems within one kidney. Dromedary hump is an anatomical variant of the lateral cortex.

42. d. A tubular structure extends from the apex of the bladder to the umbilicus. The sonographic and clinical findings in this case are most consistent with a urachal sinus. Meckel diverticulum is an anomalous sac protruding from the ileum.

43. c. A hyperechoic renal cortex in a patient with proteinuria is most suspicious for glomerulonephritis. Acute tubular necrosis demonstrates a normal renal cortex with hyperechoic medullary pyramids. Renal sinus lipomatosis demonstrates thinning of the renal cortex and an increase in echogenicity of the renal sinus. Pyelonephritis may demonstrate renal enlargement but does not increase the echogenicity of the renal parenchyma.

44. c. Multiple small cysts are located throughout the right kidney, decreasing identification of the renal parenchyma. These findings are most suspicious for polycystic renal disease. . A nephroblastoma demonstrates as a solid, well-defined renal mass on ultrasound. Renal sinus lipomatosis demonstrates an increase in the echogenicity of the renal sinus.

45. c. A solid mass demonstrating internal blood flow is demonstrated in an elderly patient's urinary bladder. This is most suspicious for bladder malignancy. Bladder adenoma is a possible differential consideration but not as likely in an elderly patient.

46. c. When encountering a mass within the urinary bladder, the sonographer should ask the patient whether he or she has noticed any blood in the urine (hematuria). Painless hematuria is a common clinical indication in bladder carcinoma.

47. b. Motion in the area of the right ureteric orifice is most suspicious for a ureteral jet.

48. b. The renal cortex is demonstrating a lobulated appearance with similar echogenicity throughout, most consistent with fetal lobulation.

49. d. Vessels located near the cortical periphery are most likely arcuate vessels. Without spectral analysis, it is difficult to evaluate whether these are arcuate arteries or veins or both.

50. c. A calcified mass conforming to the renal pelvis and calyces with posterior acoustic shadowing is most suspicious for a staghorn calculus. Nephrocalcinosis may demonstrate calcifications within the medullary pyramids.

Chapter 11 Spleen

1. c. Accessory spleens are commonly located medial to the splenic hilum. The tail of the pancreas may extend toward the splenic or left renal hilum.

2. d. The normal splenic parenchyma is generally considered to be isoechoic to slightly hypoechoic to the normal liver, when in fact the normal adult spleen is actually iso- to slightly hyperechoic when compared to the normal liver parenchyma. This impression is due to the large number of vessels within the normal liver parenchyma. The normal renal cortex is hypoechoic to the liver and spleen.

3. **d.** The spleen is an intraperitoneal organ *predominantly* located in the left hypochondriac region with the superior aspect extending into the epigastric region.

4. **d.** The cavernous hemangioma is the *most common benign neoplasm* of the spleen. Cysts and cystadenomas involving the spleen are uncommon findings. An accessory spleen is considered a congenital anomaly.

5. **c.** Hematocrit is the percentage of red blood cells in the blood. Hemoglobin is the oxygen-carrying pigment of the red blood cell. Platelets are formed in the bone marrow, and some are stored in the spleen.

6. **a.** Anemia is the *most* common clinical finding associated with a hemangiosarcoma involving the spleen. Other symptoms may include: left upper quadrant pain, weight loss, and leukocytosis.

7. **b.** Metastasis to the spleen is rare. Metastatic disease involving the spleen most commonly originates from melanoma. Other primary neoplasms metastasizing to the spleen may arise from the breast, lung, ovary, stomach, colon, kidney, and prostate.

8. **b.** Patients with a history of multiple splenic infections are at an increased risk for developing candidiasis. This condition is most commonly found in autoimmune-compromised patients. An embolism originating from the heart is the most common cause of splenic infarction. Calcifications in the spleen are more commonly caused by granulomatosis or infarction.

9. **b.** Patients with a history of polycythemia vera can demonstrate splenomegaly with the possibility of splenic thrombosis and/or infarct.

10. **a.** Hemangiosarcoma is a rare primary malignant neoplasm of the spleen that frequently metastasizes to the liver.

11. **b.** This sonogram demonstrates an enlarged spleen measuring 19.4 cm in length (normal ≤12 cm in length). Lymphoma may demonstrate splenomegaly but is *not the most likely* differential in this case.

12. **b.** In cases of splenomegaly, the liver should be evaluated for associated liver disease (e.g., portal hypertension).

13. **c.** A smooth, solid mass is identified in medial to inferior portion of the spleen and left kidney. This mass demonstrates an echo pattern similar to the spleen (isoechoic). These sonographic findings are most consistent with an accessory spleen. An adrenal adenoma is a possibility, but the mass is isoechoic to the spleen and the sonogram appears to be at level to inferior for the adrenal gland. An enlarged lymph node appears as an oval-shaped hypoechoic mass with a prominent hyperechoic fatty center.

14. **a.** Smooth, thin wall margins are identified along with posterior acoustic enhancement. This is most consistent with a splenic cyst. A chronic hematoma could appear anechoic with posterior enhancement but not the most likely choice. Cystic lymphangioma demonstrates a multilocular cystic mass appearance.

15. **b.** Formation of a splenic abscess is most commonly associated with infective endocarditis. Infarction of the spleen may be caused by emboli from the heart, subacute bacterial endocarditis, leukemia, sickle cell anemia, metastasis, or pancreatitis. Hematomas are generally associated with trauma. Hamartomas are composed of lymphatic tissue.

16. **c.** The spleen is an intraperitoneal structure located lateral to the pancreas, anterior to the left kidney, inferior to the left hemidiaphragm, and lateral to the stomach and left adrenal gland.

17. **d.** Factors associated with an increased risk for developing an aneurysm of the splenic artery include: female prevalence, trauma, atherosclerosis, infection, and portal hypertension.

18. **c.** Polysplenia is associated with multiple small spleens, two left lungs, and congenital anomalies of the gastrointestinal tract, cardiovascular

system, and biliary system. Asplenia syndrome is associated with two right lungs, gastrointestinal and urinary anomalies, and a midline placement of the liver. Accessory spleen and wandering spleen are not associated with additional anomalies.

19. **b.** The celiac axis (trunk) is the first branch of the abdominal aorta. The celiac axis trifurcates into the splenic, left gastric, and common hepatic arteries. Branches of the superior mesenteric artery supply the head of the pancreas and portions of the small and large intestine.

20. **c.** The majority of patients with a history of splenic infarction are asymptomatic but may demonstrate left upper quadrant (LUQ) pain.

21. **c.** Hyperechoic foci within the parenchyma are *most* suspicious for splenic calcifications. Calcifications are generally an incidental finding commonly associated with granulomatosis. Other etiologies may include splenic infarction, calcified cyst, or abscesses. Pneumobilia is associated with air in the biliary tree.

22. **b.** Splenic calcifications are generally an incidental finding. Follow-up is typically recommended only if clinically indicated. Splenic calcifications are most commonly associated with granulomatosis or in response to infection.

23. **a.** A cystic mass in a patient with a history of abdominal trauma most likely represents an intraparenchymal hematoma. Pseudocyst formation is a complication of acute pancreatitis. A loculated abscess is an unlikely diagnosis in an afebrile patient.

24. **c.** Cavernous hemangiomas are common benign masses that may develop in the splenic parenchyma. Hemangiomas are the most common benign solid mass, and they are the most likely diagnosis of this hyperechoic intraparenchymal mass. Lipoma is a differential consideration but not a common finding within the splenic parenchyma.

25. **b.** In a patient with a history of leukemia, the parenchymal nodules most likely represent primary malignant tumors. Leukemia may demonstrate hypoechoic or hyperechoic splenic masses on ultrasound.

Metastatic disease to the spleen most commonly originates from melanoma or malignancy of the breast, lung, or pancreas. Candidiasis and multiple splenic abscesses are unlikely in an afebrile patient.

26. **d.** Hemoglobin carries carbon dioxide from the cells back to the lungs. Platelets are essential for the coagulation of blood and the maintenance of hemostasis. Hematocrit is the percentage of red blood cells in the blood. Lymphocytes and leukocytes are associated with infection.

27. **b.** A hemangiosarcoma located in the spleen appears on ultrasound as a hyperechoic or complex mass. Frequently metastatic lesions are discovered in the liver.

28. **a.** Indications for an ultrasound of the spleen may include: chronic liver disease, infection, leukocytosis, leukopenia, abdominal or left upper quadrant mass, fatigue, leukemia, lymphoma, or trauma.

29. **b.** Granulomatosis is defined as an abnormal increase in the total number of granulocytes in the blood. Granulomatosis occurs in response to infection. Calcifications within the splenic parenchyma are associated with granulomatosis.

30. **b.** Splenomegaly is the most common sonographic finding associated with portal hypertension. Other findings may include hepatomegaly, diameter enlargement of the main portal, splenic, and/or superior mesenteric veins, development of portosplenic collaterals, and changes in the flow or direction pattern of the portal circulation.

31. **d.** Leukocytosis is defined as a white blood count *above* 20,000. Normal serum levels range between 4500 and 11,000 mm³.

32. **c.** A subcapsular hematoma is located between the splenic capsule and parenchyma. It most commonly appears on ultrasound as a crescent-shaped fluid collection inferior to the diaphragm.

33. **a.** Splenic candidiasis and metastatic lesions most commonly demonstrate a "wheel within a wheel" or target pattern on ultrasound. A hemangiosarcoma generally appears on ultrasound as a hyperechoic or complex mass. Infarction may appear hypoechoic when acute or hyperechoic in chronic cases.

Cystic lymphangiomatosis demonstrates as a multiloculated cystic mass.

34. **a.** An embolism originating in the heart is the most common source of a splenic infarction.

35. **a.** Elevation in hematocrit may be related to infection, dehydration, shock, and polycythemia vera. Decreases are associated with hemorrhage, anemia, and leukemia.

36. **a.** Arrow A identifies the superior medial portion of the spleen.

37. **c.** Arrow B identifies the midportion of the spleen known as the splenic hilum.

38. **b.** Arrow C identifies the inferior lateral portion of the spleen.

39. **d.** The sonogram demonstrates the length of the left kidney. The spleen and kidney lie closest to the transducer footprint, and the spinous processes lie furthest from the transducer footprint. These findings are most consistent with a coronal plane. There are three basic scanning *planes:* sagittal, transverse, and coronal.

40. **a.** Anechoic free fluid is identified inferior to the diaphragm and superior to the spleen. This sonographic finding is most suspicious for ascites.

41. **d.** The possibility of internal hemorrhage is a concern for the emergency department physician in cases involving trauma. Ultrasound is a portable imaging tool used to evaluate quickly the abdominal and pelvic cavity for hemoperitoneum.

42. **b.** Sickle cell anemia will demonstrate splenomegaly as a child with atrophy later in life.

43. **c.** The main portal vein is formed at the junction of the splenic and superior mesenteric veins.

44. **a.** Leukopenia is defined as a white blood count below 4000 mm³. Normal serum levels range between 4500 and 11,000 mm³.

45. **d.** The spleen is a major destruction site of old red blood cells. The red blood cells are removed, and the hemoglobin is recycled into iron.

46. **c.** A decrease in leukocytes may be associated with viral infections, leukemia, hypersplenia, aplastic anemia, and diabetes mellitus. Leukemia may also demonstrate an increase in leukocytes. Anemia is

defined as a decrease in hemoglobin levels.

47. **c.** Normal hemoglobin levels vary between males and females but should not exceed 20 g/dl. Hemoglobin is developed in the bone marrow and is the oxygen-carrying pigment in the blood.

48. **c.** In adults, splenomegaly is suggested after the length of the spleen exceeds 13 cm. The normal spleen measures approximately 10 to 12 cm in superior-inferior length, less than 4 cm in width, and less than 8 cm in anteroposterior diameter.

49. **b.** Accessory spleens are rarely a source of a patient's clinical symptoms. They are considered an incidental finding.

50. **c.** A hamartoma is a benign neoplasm composed of lymphoid tissue. A lipoma is composed of fatty tissue. An adenoma is an epithelial neoplasm. A cavernous hemangioma is a benign tumor consisting of a mass of blood vessels.

Chapter 12 Retroperitoneum

1. **c.** Glucocorticoids (cortisol) modify the body's response to inflammation. Aldosterone helps maintain the body's fluid and electrolyte balance. Norepinephrine modifies blood pressure. Epinephrine increases in times of excitement or emotional stress.

2. **c.** Rhabdomyosarcoma is a highly malignant neoplasm derived from striated muscle. Leiomyosarcoma contains smooth muscle. Pheochromocytoma is a rare vascular tumor of the adrenal medulla. A myxoma is a benign retroperitoneal neoplasm.

3. **a.** Gastrohepatic lymphadenopathy is associated with stomach, esophageal, and pancreas carcinoma, lymphoma, and metastatic disease.

4. **d.** Adrenal hyperplasia is typically demonstrated in both adrenal glands (bilaterally). On occasion, bilateral adrenal hemorrhage may be seen in the neonattypically

5. **c.** Lymph nodes filter the lymph of debris and organisms. Lymphocytes and antibodies are produced in response to an infection. Glucocorticoids modify the body's response to inflammation. Aldosterone regulates

sodium and water levels, which affects blood volume and pressure.

6. **b.** Symptoms associated with adrenocortical carcinoma include: hypertension, weakness, weight loss, abdominal pain, and weakening of the bones. Severe anxiety is a symptom associated with pheochromocytoma (vascular tumor of the adrenal medulla).

7. **a.** Adrenal adenoma is the most common cause of Conn syndrome (70%) and approximately 30% by adrenal hyperplasia. Conn syndrome is rarely caused by carcinoma.

8. **b.** Liposarcomas and fibrosarcomas are malignant neoplasms likely to infiltrate surrounding structures and tissues.

9. **c.** A urinoma is most likely to develop in the perinephric space. A urinoma is defined as a urine-filled cystic mass adjacent to or within the urinary tract.

10. **a.** Liposarcoma is the most common neoplasm located in the retroperitoneum.

11. **d.** The superior suprarenal artery arises from the inferior phrenic artery. The middle suprarenal artery arises from the aorta, and the inferior suprarenal artery arises from the renal artery. The medulla comprises 10% of the gland. The cortex secretes gonadal hormones, and norepinephrine is secreted by the medulla.

12. **b.** The anterior pararenal space is located between the posterior peritoneum and Gerota's fascia. Although the anterior pararenal space does lie between the anterior abdominal wall and the psoas muscle, this is *not the best* choice in defining the most accurate location.

13. **c.** Neuroblastoma is an adrenal neoplasm most commonly found in young children. Wilms' tumor (nephroblastoma) is a malignant tumor of the kidney. Liposarcoma is the most common retroperitoneal neoplasm.

14. **c.** The posterior parietal peritoneum forms the anterior border of the retroperitoneum. The diaphragm and pelvic rim form the superior and inferior borders of the retroperitoneum, respectively. The posterior abdominal wall muscles form the posterior border of the retroperitoneum.

15. **a.** An enlarged irregular lymph node demonstrating a round appearance is most consistent with an underlying malignancy.

16. **b.** The anterior pararenal space is located between the posterior peritoneum and Gerota's fascia and includes pancreas, descending portion of the duodenum, ascending and descending colon, superior mesenteric vessels, and inferior portion of the common bile duct. The kidneys, adrenal glands, and inferior vena cava are located in the perirenal space.

17. **b.** Pheochromocytoma is a rare vascular tumor of the adrenal medulla. It is associated with hypertension, sweating, tachycardia, chest or epigastric pain, headache, palpitations, severe anxiety, and elevation in epinephrine and norepinephrine levels.

18. **c.** Visceral lymph nodes are located in the peritoneum and course along the vessels supplying the major organs. Parietal nodes are located in the retroperitoneum and course along the prevertebral vessels. The adrenal glands are retroperitoneal structures.

19. **b.** The adrenal glands are located anterior, medial, and superior to the kidneys. *The right adrenal gland* is located posterior and lateral to the IVC.

20. **d.** Clinical findings in Addison disease may include: elevation in serum potassium, decrease in serum sodium and glucose, anorexia, chronic fatigue, dehydration, bronze skin pigmentation, hypotension, gastrointestinal disorders, salt cravings, and emotional changes. Cushing disease and hyperaldosteronism may demonstrate a decrease in serum potassium.

21. **c.** Risk factors associated with development of an adrenal adenoma include diabetes mellitus, obesity, hypertension, and the elderly population.

22. **d.** Enlarged lymph nodes posterior to the aorta displaces the aorta anteriorly giving the impression that the aorta is floating above the spine. Enlarged lymph nodes surrounding the aorta and possible IVC is termed the "donut-ring" appearance.

23. **d.** The adrenal gland is located superior and medially to the upper pole of the kidney. An adrenal mass would displace the upper pole of the kidney lateral and caudally.

24. **b.** The adrenal medulla secretes epinephrine and norepinephrine hormones. The adrenal cortex secretes cortisol, androgens, estrogens, progesterone, and aldosterone.

25. **b.** Addison disease is caused by complete or partial failure of the adrenocortical function. Also known as adrenocortical insufficiency. Overproduction of cortisol is found in Cushing disease. Conn syndrome may cause hyperaldosteronism. Graves disease involves the thyroid glands.

26. **d.** The adrenal glands are prominent in the neonate demonstrating a hypoechoic outer cortex and a central hyperechoic medulla. The arrow identifies the normal medulla. An adrenal hemorrhage may occur following a traumatic or hypoxic birth. Hemorrhage generally appears as an anechoic or complex adrenal mass.

27. **a.** The anechoic structure is most suspicious for an adrenal cyst. An adrenal cyst may cause hypertension. A pheochromocytoma may cause hypertension but generally presents as a solid homogeneous mass. Liver cysts are not linked to hypertension. A retroperitoneal hemorrhage generally demonstrates as a hypoechoic mass on ultrasound and is not likely to cause hypertension.

28. **b.** An adrenal cyst is considered a rare finding. A cyst in the liver is a common incidental finding. Hemorrhage may result from trauma. Pheochromocytoma is considered a rare vascular tumor of the adrenal medulla.

29. **b.** Hypoechoic masses are identified in the paraaortic region. Lymphadenopathy is the most likely consideration for the hypoechoic masses. Retroperitoneal fibrosis could be a differential consideration, although not as likely. The hypoechoic masses do not appear to connect decreasing the likelihood of a horseshoe kidney.

30. **c.** Hydronephrosis is the most likely complication of retroperitoneal fibrosis. Fibrotic masses may place pressure on the ureter(s), ultimately causing an obstruction.

31. c. An enlarged lymph node demonstrating a normal oval shape and smooth wall margins is most consistent with an underlying infection. A round shape or irregular margins is suspicious for an underlying malignancy.

32. c. A urinoma develops in the first few weeks after renal transplant surgery. It demonstrates a rapid increase in size on serial examinations.

33. d. Mesotheliomas are caused by an abnormal growth of epithelial cells. A myxoma consists of connective tissue, a lipoma consists of fat, and a teratoma consists of different types of tissue.

34. c. Leiomyosarcoma is a malignant neoplasm containing large spindle cells of smooth muscle. Fibrosarcomas contain fibrous connective tissue, and a liposarcoma is a malignant growth of fat cells.

35. b. A liposarcoma is a malignant growth of fat. A hyperechoic mass with thick wall margins is the most common sonographic appearance.

36. c. Identification of a homogeneous, echogenic adrenal mass in a neonatal patient is most likely an adrenal hemorrhage. This image does not demonstrate the normal hyperechoic inner medulla surrounded by the hypoechoic outer cortex of the normal adrenal gland. Adrenal adenomas are more commonly identified in the elderly patient.

37. c. A hypervascular complex mass superior and medial to the right kidney is suspicious for an adrenal mass. A solid mass of the adrenal gland in a toddler is most suspicious for a neuroblastoma. Nephroblastoma is a renal neoplasm. Adrenal hemorrhage would not demonstrate internal blood flow.

38. c. Oval-shaped hypoechoic masses with a hyperechoic center are identified in the left groin. These are most likely prominent lymph nodes. Lymph nodes are common incidental findings in the groin region. The echo pattern is well defined, which is uncharacteristic of a complex hematoma.

39. d. The cortex is the outer portion of the adrenal gland, which comprises 90% of the total gland. The medulla, or inner portion, comprises the other 10%.

40. c. *Suprarenal glands* are another term used to describe the adrenal glands.

41. c. The right suprarenal vein empties directly into the inferior vena cava. The left suprarenal vein drains into the left renal vein.

42. c. Epinephrine is secreted by the adrenal medulla during times of excitement or emotional stress. Also known as adrenaline and "fight-or-flight" hormone. Norepinephrine affects blood pressure. Cortisol modifies the body's response to infection, surgery, or trauma. Aldosterone helps to maintain the body's fluid and electrolyte balance.

43. a. Sodium is a major component in determining blood volume. Potassium is essential to the normal function of every organ. Vitamin K is related to normal clotting times. Calcium aids in the transportation of nutrients through the cell membranes.

44. c. Predisposing factors of developing an adenoma of the adrenal gland include: obesity, hypertension, diabetes mellitus, and the elderly population.

45. d. Adrenocorticotrophic hormone is produced by the pituitary gland. Epinephrine and aldosterone are produced by the adrenal glands.

46. a. Producing hormones is a function of the adrenal glands. The release of secretin hormones is an exocrine function of the pancreas. Regulation of serum electrolytes is a function of the kidneys. The release of glycogen as glucose is a function of the liver.

47. d. Pheochromocytoma is a rare vascular tumor of the adrenal gland. Rhabdomyosarcoma is a neoplasm derived from striated muscle.

48. d. The medulla is the inner portion and the cortex is the outer portion of the adrenal glands. The inner lining of a blood vessel composed of a single layer of cells describes the tunica intima. A hilum is described as a recess at the portion of an organ where vessels and nerves enter.

49. d. The left adrenal gland is located posterior and medial to the splenic artery, posterior to the stomach, lesser sac, and tail of the pancreas and lateral to the abdominal aorta. The adrenal glands lie anterior and medial to the superior border of each kidney.

50. b. The *most common* etiology of Cushing disease is a pituitary mass. Other causes may include: an adrenal mass, polycystic ovarian disease, and an excessive amount of glucocorticoid hormone.

Chapter 13 Abdominal Vasculature

1. b. The diameter of the abdominal aorta must reach a minimum diameter of 3.0 cm to be considered a true abdominal aortic aneurysm. An ectatic aneurysm describes an arterial dilatation that measures larger than a more proximal segment but less than 3.0 cm in diameter.

2. b. A fusiform aneurysm is characterized by a uniform dilatation of the arterial walls. An arterial dilatation characterized by a focal outpouching of one arterial wall describes a saccular aneurysm. Dilatation of an artery when compared to a more proximal segment describes an ectatic aneurysm.

3. b. The celiac axis is the first *visceral* branch of the abdominal aorta. The celiac artery courses approximately 1 to 3 cm before trifurcating into the splenic, left gastric, and common hepatic arteries. Inferior phrenic arteries are the first parietal branches of the abdominal aorta.

4. d. The left renal vein receives the left suprarenal vein superiorly and the left gonadal vein inferiorly. The coronary vein enters the superior portion of the portosplenic confluence and the inferior mesenteric vein enters the inferior portion of the portosplenic confluence.

5. c. The main portal vein bifurcates at the hepatic hilum into the right and left portal veins. The left portal vein subdivides into the medial and lateral left portal veins. The right portal vein subdivides into the anterior and posterior right portal veins.

6. d. Normal compression from the mesentery may cause dilatation of the left renal vein. Renal veins demonstrate a spontaneous phasic flow pattern. The left renal artery is located posterior to the left renal vein. The superior mesenteric artery courses anterior to the left renal vein.

7. d. The head of the pancreas lies anterior to the inferior vena cava. The psoas muscles, right adrenal gland, and diaphragmatic crura are located posterior to the inferior vena cava.

8. **c.** The abdominal aorta bifurcates into the right and left common iliac arteries at the level of the fourth lumbar vertebra (umbilicus). The inferior vena cava is formed at the level of the fifth lumbar vertebra.

9. **d.** The celiac axis branches into the common hepatic, left gastric, and splenic arteries.

10. **d.** A palpable vibration ("thrill") within an artery is highly suspicious for an arteriovenous fistula.

11. **b.** Saccular-shaped aneurysms are most often caused by an infection or trauma. A mycotic aneurysm generally demonstrates a focal outpouching of one arterial wall. Small saccular aneurysms primarily affecting the cerebral arteries are termed *berry* aneurysms. Fusiform aneurysms are the most common type of true abdominal aortic aneurysms.

12. **b.** The gonadal arteries arise from the anterior aspect of the abdominal aorta inferior to the renal arteries and superior to the lumbar arteries.

13. **b.** The gastroepiploic artery is a branch of the splenic artery.

14. **d.** Hepatic veins course between the segments of the liver toward the inferior vena cava. The middle hepatic vein divides the liver into right and left segments.

15. **c.** The diameter of the main portal vein should not exceed 1.3 cm in diameter in adults older than 20 years, 1.0 cm in diameter between 10 and 20 years of age, and 0.85 cm in diameter younger than 10 years.

16. **b.** Based on a history of pulmonary embolism, the echogenic mass is most suspicious for a thrombus. The majority of pulmonary embolisms propagate from the lower extremities through the IVC to the lungs.

17. **d.** A cross sectional image of a vascular structure is identified posterior to the inferior vena cava. This most likely represents the right renal artery.

18. **b.** An *anechoic* structure is identified adjacent to the main lobar fissure in the region of the gallbladder fossa.

19. **b.** Arrow A identifies a proximal anterior branch of the aorta. The celiac axis is the first visceral branch

of the abdominal aorta. The inferior phrenic artery is the first parietal branch of the abdominal aorta.

20. **c.** An anechoic tubular structure is branching from the anterior aspect of the abdominal aorta. Arrow B identifies the superior mesenteric artery, a common sonographic landmark. The renal arteries arise from the lateral aspect of the abdominal aorta.

21. **c.** Approximately 25% of patients with a popliteal aneurysm demonstrate a coexisting abdominal aortic aneurysm.

22. **c.** Arteriosclerosis is the most common predisposing factor for developing an abdominal aortic aneurysm. Pathological thickening, hardening, and loss of wall elasticity allow the weakened arterial walls to stretch.

23. **c.** A mycotic aneurysm is usually caused by a recent bacterial infection.

24. **d.** The inferior vena cava usually measures less than 2.5 cm and is considered enlarged after the diameter exceeds 3.7 cm.

25. **a.** Development of an arteriovenous fistula may be congenital or caused by trauma, surgery, inflammation, or a neoplasm.

26. **c.** Neoplasms from the kidney extend into the renal vein and may infiltrate the inferior vena cava. The liver and adrenal gland are possible differentials but not the most likely origin of an IVC neoplasm. The portosplenic venous system does not directly empty into the inferior vena cava.

27. **b.** *Direct* extension of thrombus into the inferior vena cava most commonly originates from the lower extremity (femoral) but may also originate from the iliac, renal, hepatic, or right gonadal veins.

28. **b.** Berry aneurysms are small saccular aneurysms (1.0 to 1.5 cm) primarily affecting the cerebral arteries. The carotid and vertebral arteries are considered extracranial structures.

29. **c.** The mesenteric vessels include the celiac axis, superior mesenteric artery, and the inferior mesenteric artery. Diagnosis of mesenteric ischemia is made when a minimum of two mesenteric vessels demonstrate stenosis.

30. **b.** Hypovolemic shock is a clinical finding in patients with a history of ruptured aortic aneurysm. Marfan syndrome is associated with aortic dissection.

31. **d.** The clinical history includes: leukocytosis and an enlarging pulsatile abdominal mass. The distal aorta measures 5 cm in height and 6 cm in width. Complex intraluminal echoes are also identified. Based on the clinical history, the sonographic findings are most suspicious for a mycotic abdominal aortic aneurysm.

32. **b.** The vascular structure identified by arrow A courses in a transverse plane, anterior to the superior mesenteric artery and posterior to the body of the pancreas. This is most consistent with the splenic vein.

33. **d.** Arrow B identifies a vascular structure located posterior to the body of the pancreas and is surrounded by a thick hyperechoic rim. These findings are most consistent with the superior mesenteric artery.

34. **d.** A complex aortic aneurysm demonstrating smooth wall margins is identified in this sonogram of the abdominal aorta. The anechoic area represents the lumen of the aorta, and the complex area represents chronic changes in intraluminal thrombus. Chronic thrombus within an aneurysm may demonstrate a complex appearance mimicking a dissection or rupture.

35. **d.** Vessel A is located in the upper abdomen and courses in a transverse plane, posterior to the liver toward the right renal hilum. Arrow A is most likely the right renal vein.

36. **b.** Vessel B courses in a sagittal plane directly posterior to the liver. This is most consistent with the inferior vena cava. Arrow C identifies the abdominal aorta.

37. **c.** A pseudoaneurysm is defined as a dilatation of an artery caused by damage to one or more layers of the arterial wall. Trauma and aneurysm rupture are the most common etiologies.

38. **c.** Aortic ectasia (arteriomegaly) demonstrates diffuse enlargement of the abdominal aorta without distal tapering. An ectatic aneurysm is a dilatation of an artery when compared with a more proximal segment.

39. b. The right renal artery is a common sonographic landmark coursing posterior to the inferior vena cava.

40. d. The gastroduodenal artery lies between the superior portion of the duodenum and the anterior aspect of the pancreatic head. It is visualized routinely in the anterolateral portion of the head of the pancreas.

41. d. The left renal artery courses posterior to the splenic vein, left renal vein, and the tail of the pancreas. Duplication of the main renal arteries is found in 33% of the population. Both main renal arteries are located anterior to the crus of the diaphragm.

42. d. The inferior mesenteric artery supplies the left transverse colon, descending colon, upper rectum, and sigmoid.

43. c. Marfan syndrome is a musculoskeletal condition that affects the elastic fibers in the media of the aorta, increasing the risk for developing an aneurysm.

44. b. 15% of abdominal aortic aneurysms measuring 6.0 cm in diameter will rupture within 5 years.

45. d. Approximately 70% to 75% of the blood supplied to the liver is from the portal venous system, whereas the hepatic artery supplies approximately 25% to 30%.

46. c. The left renal vein courses anterior to the aorta and left renal artery and posterior to the superior mesenteric artery (SMA). The splenic vein courses anterior to the SMA.

47. a. The inferior mesenteric vein usually drains into the splenic vein but may enter at the inferior border of the portosplenic confluence.

48. c. The splenic artery is a tortuous branch of the celiac axis and is most commonly mistaken as a dilated pancreatic duct.

49. c. An ectatic aneurysm is a dilatation of an artery when compared with a more proximal segment. In cases of abdominal aortic aneurysms, the ectatic dilatation does not exceed 3.0 cm in diameter.

50. d. Decreasing the time gain compensation at the level of the abdominal aorta will decrease the artifactual echoes *only* within the abdominal aorta. Overall gain, dynamic range, and postprocessing change all the echo amplitudes within the sonographic image.

Chapter 14 Gastrointestinal Tract

1. a. The esophagus begins at the pharynx, courses through the esophageal hiatus of the diaphragm, and terminates at the cardiac orifice of the stomach.

2. d. Male infants have an increased risk for developing infantile hypertrophied pyloric stenosis.

3. c. Clinical symptoms of acute appendicitis may include: periumbilical or right lower quadrant pain, fever, nausea/vomiting, leukocytosis, and a positive McBurney sign.

4. b. Rugae describe the ridges and folds found in the mucosal layer of the stomach. The recesses found in the walls of the colon are termed *haustra*.

5. c. Bilious vomiting is a symptom of intussusception and volvulus. Projectile vomiting is a symptom of hypertrophied pyloric stenosis.

6. c. The duodenum secretes large quantities of mucus to protect the small intestines from the strong stomach acids. The stomach secretes pepsin. Bacteria in the colon produce vitamin K and some B complex vitamins.

7. b. Crohn disease is a chronic inflammation of the intestines most commonly occurring in the ileum.

8. c. Intussusception occurs when one section of bowel has prolapsed into the lumen of an adjacent section of bowel. An ileus may be a complication of intussusception. Volvulus is the abnormal twisting of a portion of the intestines or bowel, which can impair the blood flow.

9. a. The gastroesophageal junction is located anterior to the aorta, posterior to the left lobe of the liver, inferior to the diaphragm, and superior to the celiac axis.

10. a. Twisting of a portion of the bowel describes volvulus. Volvulus may be caused by a congenital malrotation of the bowel. In cases of intussusception one segment of the bowel prolapses into the lumen of an adjacent segment of bowel.

11. c. The right margin of the esophagus is contiguous with the lesser curvature of the stomach. The left margin of the esophagus is contiguous with the greater curvature of the stomach.

12. d. The colon demonstrates haustral wall markings.

13. d. The small intestines extend from the pyloric opening of the stomach to the junction of the ileum and cecum (ileocecal valve).

14. c. Thickness of the pyloric muscle is the most accurate measurement when evaluating for hypertrophied pyloric stenosis.

15. c. The normal adult appendix should not exceed 6 mm in diameter or 2 mm in wall thickness.

16. c. Extreme pain or tenderness over the McBurney point is most commonly associated with acute appendicitis. Positive Murphy sign correlates to extreme pain over the gallbladder fossa consistent with acute cholecystitis.

17. b. Fifty percent of cases of carcinoma involving the colon are located in the rectum. Twenty-five percent are located in the sigmoid portion of the colon.

18. b. The descending portion (second portion) of the duodenum receives bile from the common bile duct. The duodenum is divided into the superior, descending, transverse, and ascending portions.

19. c. Patients may experience gastritis following an episode of excessive alcohol consumption. Ileus is more likely related to acute pancreatitis.

20. c. The stomach is considered the principal organ of digestion. The majority of food absorption occurs in the small intestines. The mouth, pharynx, and esophagus allow ingestion of food.

21. b. The walls of the stomach contain two individual layers of muscle. The five individual layers include the serosal, muscularis propria, submucosal, muscular, and mucosal layers.

22. c. The McBurney point is located midway between the umbilicus and the right iliac crest.

23. b. The duodenum is divided into the superior, descending, transverse, and ascending portions.

24. b. The descending portion (second portion) of the duodenum is located posterior to the transverse colon and common bile duct. The transverse portion is located anterior to the great vessels and posterior to the superior mesenteric artery and vein.

25. c. The sonogram demonstrates an outpouching in the wall of the colon most suspicious for a diverticulum.

26. **c.** The length of the pyloric canal and thickness of the pyloric wall exceed the normal limits, most consistent with hypertrophied pyloric stenosis.

27. **b.** A blunt ended dilated tubular structure in the right lower quadrant is most suspicious for an inflamed appendix (appendicitis).

28. **d.** The sonogram demonstrates multiple circular rings of bowel with one segment of bowel prolapsed into the lumen of an adjacent segment of bowel consistent with intussusception.

29. **d.** A target mass is demonstrated in this **midline** sonogram of the upper abdomen. This is most suspicious for the gastroesophageal junction. The pyloric canal is typically located to the right of midline near the porta hepatis and gallbladder fossa.

30. **c.** Crohn disease is a chronic disease affecting the small intestines. Clinical symptoms may include: abdominal cramping, blood in stool, diarrhea, fever, decreased appetite, and weight loss. This sonogram of the small intestines demonstrates a thick, *matted loop of bowel* most suspicious for Crohn disease.

31. **d.** The recesses demonstrated in the walls of the *ascending* colon are most suspicious for normal haustral wall markings in a fecal-filled colon. Transducer pressure on a fecal-filled section of intestines may cause abdominal or pelvic discomfort.

32. **c.** The mucosal layer is the layer of the duodenum nearest the lumen, demonstrating a thin, hyperechoic, linear appearance.

33. **b.** A Meckel diverticulum is usually located slightly to the right of the umbilicus.

34. **b.** Wall thickness of the pyloric canal should not exceed 3 to 4 mm to be considered within normal limits.

35. **d.** Hypertrophied pyloric stenosis most commonly develops in infants between 2 to 10 weeks of age.

36. **c.** The lesser curvature of the stomach is the most common location for gastric ulcers to develop.

37. **a.** Fluid- or air-filled loops of small intestines with hypoactive or absent peristalsis describes an ileus. Crohn disease generally demonstrates as *thick* or *matted* loops of small bowel.

38. **b.** Graded compression is a technique commonly used when evaluating the appendix for appendicitis.

39. **b.** Chyme is a semiliquid composed of food and gastric juices. The duodenum secretes a large amount of mucous, protecting the small intestines from the acidic chyme. The stomach secretes pepsin.

40. **d.** The ileum is the distal portion of the small intestines, extending from the jejunum to the junction with the cecum (ileocecal junction).

41. **c.** The small intestines are responsible for the majority of food absorption. The stomach is responsible for digestion.

42. **b.** Pepsin is a protein-digestive enzyme produced in the stomach. Gastrin is a hormone released by the stomach that stimulates secretion of gastric acids.

43. **d.** Peristalsis is the forward movement of intestinal contents through the digestive tract through serial rhythmic contractions of the intestinal walls. Pylorospasm is associated with pyloric stenosis.

44. **c.** Clinical symptoms in this nonpregnant patient include fever, periumbilical pain, and vomiting. Based on this clinical presentation, the referring physician should order an abdominal ultrasound to rule out appendicitis.

45. **c.** The anal canal extends upward and forward then turns backward and follows the sacral canal.

46. **d.** Right posterior oblique position will place fluid in the pylorus of the stomach. Right lateral decubitus position will place fluid in the superior duodenum. Semi-Fowler position will place fluid in the body of the stomach. Supine position will place fluid in the fundus of the stomach.

47. **c.** The superior portion (first portion) of the duodenum is located anterior to the common bile duct, gastroduodenal artery, head of the pancreas, common hepatic artery and portal vein and posterior to the liver and gallbladder.

48. **c.** Gastritis is not associated with the formation of a mucocele. Mucoceles are distensions of the appendix or cecum with mucous fluid. Inflammatory scarring involving the large intestines is the most common cause of a mucocele. Other etiologies may include neoplasm, fecalith, or polyp.

49. **b.** The colon demonstrates the largest lumen diameter in the cecum and gradually decreases in size as it nears the rectum.

50. **a.** A polyp is the most common tumor of the stomach. It appears on ultrasound as a hypoechoic mass protruding from of stomach wall. Cases of gastric polyps are generally asymptomatic.

Chapter 15 Abdominal Wall, Musculoskeletal, and Pediatric Hip Review

1. **a.** A direct inguinal hernia arises inferior and medial to the inferior epigastric artery. An indirect inguinal hernia arises superior and lateral to the inferior epigastric artery.

2. **d.** The muscles and joints of the shoulder allow a full range of motion (360 degrees) in the sagittal plane. The shoulder can abduct and adduct, extend in front, behind, above the torso, as well as rotate. This remarkable range of motion makes the shoulder the most mobile joint in the body. The hip is a multiaxial joint, producing motion in more than one axis.

3. **b.** Risk factors associated with an increase risk in developmental dysplasia of the hip (DDH) include breech presentation, female infant, oligohydramnios during pregnancy, foot deformity that requires further treatment, family history of DDH, and infant torticollis.

4. **b.** A positive Tinel's and Phalen's sign is associated with carpal tunnel syndrome of the wrist.

5. **b.** The transversus abdominis muscle is located posterior to both the internal and the external oblique muscles.

6. **d.** Place the patient in a prone position on a stretcher or kneeling in a chair with the foot overhanging the stretcher or chair.

7. **c.** Anisotropy can be a problem in musculoskeletal imaging. It is associated with a false hypoechoic area within the tendon. This occurs when the ultrasound beam is not perpendicular with a tendon's fibers.

8. **b.** The patient is position sitting with the arm behind their back, as if placing their hand in the opposite back pocket when evaluating the supraspinatus muscle.

9. **c.** Hyperemia is found in the early stages of rheumatoid arthritis.

Tendon disease (tenosynovitis, tendinosis, and tear) is found in the late stages of rheumatoid arthritis.

10. **d.** The triradiate cartilage separates bony ossifications centers in the ilium, ischium, and pubis to form the acetabulum. It is located medial to the femoral head.

11. **c.** An indirect inguinal hernia arises superior and lateral to the inferior epigastric artery (IEA). A direct inguinal hernia arises inferior and medial to the IEA.

12. **d.** A *normal* infant hip demonstrates an alpha angle of 60 degrees or greater and beta angle less than 55 degrees.

13. **a.** Bursae appear as thin, hypoechoic structures that merge with the surrounding fat in the sagittal plane. It is difficult to visualize bursae in the transverse plane.

14. **a.** The ilium is identified by the letter A.

15. **b.** The labrum is identified by the letter B.

16. **d.** The acetabular roof is identified by the letter C.

17. **c.** The triradiate cartilage is identified by the letter D.

18. **d.** An increase in distance between the rectus abdominis muscles is a sonographic finding associated with diastasis recti abdominis.

19. **c.** Flattening of the medial nerve at the level of the hamate bone, bulging flexor retinaculum, fat layer or large fluid collection around the tendon, and decrease movement of the nerve through the tunnel when the finger is flexed are sonographic findings associated with carpal tunnel syndrome.

20. **c.** An abdominal wall *defect* allows extension of the intestines and/or omentum.

21. **c.** The Thompson test (pointing the toes while squeezing the calf) is used to check the integrity of the Achilles tendon. A positive Thompson test is suspicious for a ruptured Achilles tendon.

22. **d.** The patient is sitting with arm resting close to the body and palm facing up.

23. **c.** Anechoic fluid within a tendon sheath is a sonographic finding of acute tenosynovitis.

24. **a.** Tendons attach muscles to bone with bands of dense fibrous connective tissue. A flexible band of fibrous tissue binding joints together defines a ligament. A fibril is a small filamentous fiber. A fibrous sac found between a tendon and bone defines a bursa.

25. **d.** Rheumatoid arthritis is an autoimmune disorder affecting the lining of joints.

26. **c.** A hypoechoic mass within the rectus sheath is identified in the left lower quadrant. A rectus sheath hematoma may develop with severe or chronic coughing. A urachal sinus connects the apex of the bladder with the umbilicus.

27. **b.** An anechoic fluid collection is identified in the medial portion of the popliteal fossa or knee joint. This is most suspicious for a synovial (Baker) cyst.

28. **a.** A focal disruption of the gastrocnemius muscle is identified in the upper calf most suspicious for a muscle tear.

29. **c.** A defect is identified in the anterior abdominal wall allowing extension of the omentum and intestines. This is most consistent with a hernia. A urachal sinus connects the apex of the bladder with the umbilicus.

30. **c.** Tendinosis is a termed used to describe degenerative changes in a tendon without signs of inflammation and is associated with over usage injuries.

31. **d.** The femoral head is located lateral to a dysplastic hip joint most consistent with a hip dislocation.

32. **d.** The supraspinatus tendon is located superior to the humeral head under the acromion. the infraspinatus tendon is located lateral and posterior to the shoulder.

33. **a.** The anterior recess of the left hip joint is significantly thicker in diameter when compared to the contralateral right hip. Asymmetry exceeding 2 mm in diameter is considered abnormal. This is most suspicious for a hip joint effusion.

34. **c.** The hyperechoic structure is most suspicious for a foreign body. Fascial planes appear as a continuous hyperechoic line. Ligaments bind joints together.

35. **a.** Sonographic findings include a homogeneous Achilles tendon demonstrating smooth margins. The thickness of the tendon does not exceed 5 mm. These findings are most consistent with a normal Achilles tendon. Focal disruption is generally identified in a complete or incomplete tear of the tendon. Tendonitis demonstrates a thickening in the tendon.

36. **d.** A femoral hernia protrudes through the femoral canal superior to the saphenofemoral junction, inferior to the inguinal canal and medial to the common femoral vein.

37. **c.** Thickness of a normal Achilles tendon should not exceed 7 mm. Tendonitis is suggested after the thickness exceeds 7 mm in diameter.

38. **c.** An anechoic, smooth wall mass that demonstrates posterior acoustic enhancement is identified near the tendon connection to the carpal bone. This is most suspicious for a ganglion cyst. A Baker cyst is located in the medial popliteal space.

39. **b.** The linea alba is a midline tendon extending from the xiphoid process to the symphysis pubis. The rectus abdominis muscles are located lateral to the linea alba and extend the entire length of the anterior abdominal wall.

40. **b.** The fascial interface of the anterior abdominal wall is located directly anterior to the peritoneum. The linea alba, rectus abdominis muscles, and the subcutaneous fat are located anterior to the fascial plane.

41. **c.** The Valsalva maneuver is a common technique used when evaluating the anterior abdominal wall, groin, or lower-extremity venous system.

42. **c.** A *nonvascular* hypoechoic mass following a recent *injury* is most suspicious for a hematoma. Baker cysts are caused by chronic conditions of the knee joint.

43. **c.** An anterior approach to the hip is used when evaluating for hip effusion. A lateral approach is used when evaluating for developmental dysplasia of the hip.

44. **a.** The Graf technique is used to evaluate for developmental dysplasia of the hip.

45. **d.** A Morton neuroma appears as a hypoechoic intermetatarsal mass on ultrasound. Patients will complain of sharp pain in the foot radiating toward the toes.

46. **b.** The Achilles tendon should be measured in the transverse plane. The position of the patient is irrelevant.

47. d. A complete tear of the Achilles tendon is most commonly located in the distal portion of the tendon approximately 2 to 6 cm from the calcaneus (inferior insertion).

48. c. The rectus abdominis *muscles* extend the entire length of the anterior abdominal wall. The linea alba is a tendon not a muscle.

49. c. The inferior epigastric artery is the key vascular landmark use to identify the inguinal canal and aides in determining a direct from an indirect inguinal hernia.

50. d. An abdominal wall lipoma most commonly appears on ultrasound as an isoechoic to hypoechoic superficial mass.

Chapter 16 Male Pelvis

1. b. A hydrocele is defined as an abnormal fluid collection between the two layers of the tunica vaginalis. The tunica vaginalis covers the anterior and lateral portions of the testis and epididymis. The tunica albuginea is a fibrous sheath enclosing each testis. The spermatic cord is located on the posterior border of the testes.

2. c. "Bell clapper" is another term used to describe testicular torsion. Twisting of the spermatic cord on itself gives the appearance that the testis is dangling, similar to the clapper in a bell.

3. a. The testes generally descend into the scrotal sac during the third trimester of pregnancy. Normal testes will descend into the scrotal sac by 6 months of age.

4. b. The peripheral zone comprises approximately 70% of the glandular tissue of the prostate gland and is the most common site of prostatic carcinoma.

5. c. Focal hyperechoic thickening, echogenic plaque or calcifications located in the tunica albuginea are the common sonographic findings in Peyronie's disease.

6. c. The tunica albuginea is a fibrous sheath enclosing each testis. The tunica vaginalis is a two-layered serous membrane covering the anterior and lateral borders of the testis and epididymis.

7. d. Functions of the prostate gland include: secretion of an alkaline fluid to aid in the transport of sperm, production of ejaculation fluid, and production of prostate-specific antigen.

8. d. The mediastinum testis is the thickened portion of the tunica albuginea. The mediastinum testis appears as a hyperechoic linear structure in the medial and posterior aspect of the testis.

9. c. The spermatic cord supports the posterior border of the testes and courses superiorly through the inguinal canal. The rete testis connects the epididymis with the superior portion of the testis. The epididymis carries sperm from the testis to the vas deferens.

10. d. The verumontanum divides the urethra into proximal and distal segments.

11. c. A cystic structure arising from the rete testis describes a spermatocele. Dilatation of an epididymal tubule describes an epididymal cyst.

12. b. A scrotal pearl is generally an incidental finding demonstrating as a mobile hyperechoic focus on ultrasound.

13. a. The spermatic vein generally measures 1 to 2 mm in diameter. It is considered dilated after the diameter exceeds 2 mm.

14. a. The scrotum is divided into two separate compartments by a medium raphe or septum.

15. b. A complex mass is identified within the inferior portion of the left testis. This is most suspicious for a malignant neoplasm. Epididymitis, and acute orchitis frequently cause scrotal pain. Scrotal herniation is an extratesticular abnormality.

16. d. An echogenic mass is identified superior to the epididymis. This is most suspicious for herniation of the bowel into the scrotal sac.

17. c. Midline hyperechoic foci are identified at the base of the prostate gland consistent with the central zone. The peripheral zone occupies the posterior, lateral, and apical regions of the prostate gland. Seminal vesicles lie superior to the prostate gland.

18. c. Dilated anechoic tubular structures are identified inferior to the testis. This is most suspicious for a varicocele (enlarged spermatic veins). Veins will increase in size with the Valsalva maneuver.

19. a. Varicoceles are the most common cause of male infertility.

20. a. An anechoic fluid collection is identified superior and anterior to the testis most consistent with a hydrocele.

21. d. The solid structure superior to the testis most likely represents an appendix testis or possibly the head of the epididymis

22. c. A lower urinary tract infection is the most common cause of epididymitis.

23. c. Benign prostatic hypertrophy (BPH) is a noninflammatory enlargement of the prostate usually occurring in the transitional zone of the gland. The majority of carcinoma occurs in the peripheral zone.

24. d. Twisting of the spermatic cord leads to obstruction of the blood vessels supplying the testis and epididymis leading to torsion of the testis. Spermatocele is a retention cyst arising from the rete testis.

25. d. Chlamydia is the most common cause of orchitis. Orchitis can be secondary to epididymitis.

26. d. A sudden onset of severe scrotal pain in an *adolescent* patient is most suspicious for testicular torsion. Adolescents are at an increased risk for developing testicular torsion. A sudden onset of scrotal pain in an adult is most suspicious for epididymitis.

27. c. The rete testis is a network of ducts formed in the mediastinum testis connecting the epididymis to the superior portion of the testis. Vas deferens transport sperm from the testis to the prostatic urethra.

28. a. The corpus spongiosum is located in the midline of the penis anterior to the paired corpus cavernosum. A cavernous artery is located within each corpus cavernosum.

29. b. Two-thirds of the blood supplied to the prostate gland is through the capsular artery. The urethral artery supplies one-third of the blood into the prostate gland.

30. c. An enlarged hypoechoic epididymis is identified posterior and inferior to the left testis. This is most suspicious for epididymitis.

31. c. The structure is contiguous with the body of the epididymis and superior to the testis most consistent with the head of the epididymis.

32. d. A cystic mass is identified in the region of the mediastinum testis. This most likely represents tubular ectasia of the rete testis. *Chronic* orchitis may demonstrate complex areas of necrosis.

33. d. Tubular ectasia of the rete testis is usually a bilateral condition.

34. d. A cystic structure superior to the testis is most consistent with a spermatocele or epididymal cyst. Spermatoceles arise in the rete testis and do not compress the testicle. An epididymal cyst may compress the testicle.

35. d. A small hypoechoic mass is identified by the calipers in the peripheral zone. The peripheral zone comprises approximately 70% of the glandular tissue and occupies the posterior, lateral, and apical regions of the prostate gland.

36. c. A hypoechoic oval mass is identified in the inguinal canal of a male infant. This is most likely an undescended testicle (cryptorchidism). An enlarged lymph node is a possibility, but a fatty hyperechoic hilum is not identified in this mass.

37. b. Normal monoclonal levels of PSA should not exceed 4 ng/mL. Elevation of 20% or an increase of 0.75 ng/mL within 1 year is indicative of carcinoma.

38. d. Decreased urinary output is most commonly associated with benign hypertrophy of the prostate gland (BPH).

39. c. The epididymis lies posterior and lateral to the testis.

40. c. The cremasteric and deferential arteries supply blood to the epididymis, scrotal tissue, and testis. Two-thirds of the blood supply to the prostate gland is through the capsular artery. The testicular artery courses along the periphery of the testicle.

41. a. The left testicular vein empties into the left renal vein. The inferior vena cava receives the right testicular vein.

42. c. All of the conditions may cause scrotal pain. Epididymitis is the *most* common cause of *acute* scrotal pain in the adult patient.

43. c. The seminal vesicles appear hypoechoic on ultrasound and are located superior to the prostate gland, posterior to the urinary bladder, and lateral to the vas deferens. The ducts of the seminal vesicles enter the central zone of the prostate gland.

44. a. The cremasteric and deferential arteries are contained in the spermatic cord.

45. d. Clinical symptoms of BPH include urinary frequency, decrease in urinary output, dysuria, and urinary tract infection.

46. c. Patients with an undescended testis are at an increased risk for developing testicular torsion, malignancy, and infertility.

47. c. The transitional zone comprises only 5% of the glandular tissue of the prostate gland. The periurethral glands comprise approximately 1% of the glandular tissue.

48. c. The periurethral glands line the tissue of the prostatic urethra. The verumontanum divides the urethra into proximal and distal segments.

49. d. The prostate gland consists of five lobes: the anterior, middle, posterior, and two lateral lobes. It is also divided into the central, peripheral, and transitional *zones.*

50. a. The mediastinum testis appears as a hyperechoic linear structure located in the posterior medial aspect of each testis.

Chapter 17 Neck and Salivary Glands

1. c. The superior and middle thyroid veins empty directly into the internal jugular vein. The external jugular empties into the subclavian vein. The vertebral vein empties into the brachiocephalic (innominate) vein.

2. b. Thyroid stimulating hormone (TSH) controls the secretion of thyroid hormones. TSH is produced by the anterior pituitary gland. The hypothalamus activates, controls, and integrates the peripheral autonomic nervous system, endocrine processes, and many somatic functions.

3. c. Symptoms associated with *hyper*thyroidism may include: nervousness, weight loss, exophthalmos, increased heart rate, heat intolerance, palpitations, and diarrhea. Weight gain, skin dryness, and constipation are associated with hypothyroidism.

4. c. Hashimoto disease is often painless and is considered the most common cause of hypothyroidism. Graves disease is most commonly associated with hyperthyroidism.

5. d. The parathyroid glands maintain homeostasis of blood calcium concentrations. The thyroid glands secrete calcitonin. The kidneys regulate serum electrolytes. Producing hormones is a function of the adrenal glands.

6. b. The right and left vertebral arteries ascend through the vertebral processes and join at the base of the skull, forming the basilar artery.

7. c. A superficial cystic structure lying directly below the angle of the jaw is most likely a brachial cleft cyst. A thyroglossal cyst is located between the isthmus of the thyroid gland and the tongue.

8. b. A pyramidal lobe is a congenital anomaly associated with a third thyroid lobe arising from the superior portion of the isthmus and ascending to the level of the hyoid bone.

9. a. A 5.0-MHz to 12-MHz linear transducer is recommended for imaging the adult thyroid gland. When encountering a dense or enlarged thyroid gland, a 3.5-MHz curvilinear transducer may be necessary for measuring the length of an enlarged thyroid lobe(s).

10. c. A decrease in the thyrotropin (TSH) level is the *first* indication of thyroid gland failure. A decrease in thyroxine is an indication of thyroid disease or a nonfunctioning pituitary gland. Hashimoto thyroiditis is associated with a decrease in triiodothyronine (T3).

11. b. A thyroid mass demonstrating a prominent hypoechoic peripheral "halo" is most consistent with an adenoma.

12. a. The parotid gland is the only salivary gland with intraparenchymal lymph nodes.

13. b. Clinical findings associated with thyroiditis may include hyperthyroidism followed by hypothyroidism, fever, leukocytosis, neck pain, and dysphagia. The thyroid gland generally demonstrates diffuse enlargement with an increase in vascular blood flood within the gland. Goiters and hyperplasia generally demonstrate multiple solid nodules within an enlarged thyroid gland.

14. c. A thyroglossal cyst is located between the isthmus of the thyroid gland and tongue.

15. **c.** The main blood supply to the eyes and brain is through the internal carotid artery. The internal carotid artery may remain patent with occlusion of the ipsilateral common carotid artery by collateral flow through the ipsilateral external carotid artery or through the circle of Willis.

16. **b.** An anechoic structure is identified posterior and slightly lateral to the thyroid lobe. A symmetrical structure is identified on the contralateral side. This most likely represents the carotid artery.

17. **c.** An isoechoic echogenic "bridge" is identified between the left and right thyroid lobes consistent with the isthmus.

18. **b.** The strap muscles are a group of muscles located anterior and lateral to the thyroid lobes. The strap muscles appear hypoechoic compared to the adjacent thyroid parenchyma. The superficial sternocleidomastoid muscle lies lateral to the strap muscles. The longus colli muscle is located posterior to the thyroid lobe. The trachea is located posterior to the isthmus of the thyroid gland.

19. **c.** The thyroid lobe appears slightly enlarged and hypoechoic without any evidence of a focal or discrete mass. Hypervascular flow is identified within the thyroid lobe on color Doppler imaging. Thyroiditis (Hashimoto disease or de Quervain syndrome) is the most likely diagnosis with these sonographic findings and a clinical history of fatigue following an infection. Patients with Graves disease more commonly complain of palpitations, nervousness, and an increase in heart rate. The thyroid gland generally enlarges and demonstrates multiple solid nodules in Graves disease.

20. **b.** Hashimoto disease is the most common cause of *hypo*thyroidism. Fatigue, sore throat, dyspnea, and dysphagia are symptoms associated with hypothyroidism. Graves disease is associated with hyperthyroidism. Increases in calcium may be related to an underlying malignancy, hyperthyroidism, or hyperparathyroidism.

21. **b.** A smooth heterogeneous mass is identified within the thyroid lobe. A prominent hypoechoic peripheral "halo" is demonstrated around the majority of the mass most suspicious for an adenoma. Chronic adenomas may undergo degeneration and demonstrate a heterogeneous echo pattern.

22. **c.** A *midline* anechoic mass superior to the thyroid gland is most suspicious for a thyroglossal cyst. A brachial cleft cyst is located directly below the angle of the mandible.

23. **c.** Approximately 80% of the population has two *paired* (4), bean-shaped parathyroid glands located posterior to the thyroid glands.

24. **b.** The ophthalmic artery is the first branch of the internal carotid artery. The superior thyroid artery arises from the external carotid artery. The internal carotid artery terminates at the circle of Willis.

25. **d.** Clinical symptoms of hypercalcemia may include: abdominal pain, formation of stones, weight loss, anorexia, confusion, gout, arthritis, bone demineralization, muscle pain, and weakness. Hyperparesthesia of the hands, feet, lips, and tongue are symptoms of hypocalcemia. Fatigue and weight gain are symptoms of hypothyroidism. Palpitations are a symptom of hyperthyroidism.

26. **b.** Clinical symptoms of pancreatitis, hypertension, *and* hypercalcemia, are related to the development of an adenoma of a parathyroid gland. Other symptoms may include formation of calculi or a decrease in serum phosphorus levels.

27. **d.** The parathyroid glands are located posterior to the thyroid lobe and anterior to the longus colli muscle.

28. **c.** An inadequate drainage of lymph fluid into the jugular vein or an increase in secretion from the epithelial lining of the neck are the most common causes of a cystic hygroma. An impaired synthesis of thyroid hormones is related to development of a goiter.

29. **c.** The internal carotid artery terminates at the circle of Willis. The left common carotid generally arises directly from the aortic arch. The ECA courses medial to the ICA. The ICA generally courses posterior to the ECA.

30. **d.** Subacute thyroiditis secondary to a viral infection defines de Quervain syndrome. Graves disease is a multisystemic autoimmune disorder characterized by pronounced hyperthyroidism. Caroli and Mirizzi syndromes involve the biliary tree.

31. **c.** The longus colli muscles are located posterior to the thyroid lobes. The sternocleidomastoid muscles are located lateral to the thyroid lobes. The strap muscles (omohyoid, sternothyroid, and sternohyoid) are located anterior and lateral to the thyroid lobes.

32. **c.** The most common thyroid neoplasm is an adenoma.

33. **d.** Exposure to ionizing radiation is a predisposing factor for development of a parathyroid adenoma.

34. **a.** Primary thyroid carcinoma is *known* to extend to the cervical lymph nodes, lung, bone, and larynx. The majority of metastatic lesions in the liver are extensions of primary carcinoma in the colon, pancreas, breast, and lung.

35. **b.** Hashimoto disease is associated with an increased risk for developing a malignancy of the thyroid gland.

36. **c.** A normal adult thyroid lobe measures approximately 4.0 to 6.0 cm in length, up to 1.8 cm in height (AP), and up to 2.0 cm in width.

37. **b.** 100 to 200 mg of iodide must be ingested per week for normal thyroxine production.

38. **c.** Chronic sialadenitis is associated with parotitis. Sialolithiasis is associated with an infection in fifty percent of cases.

39. **c.** Clinical symptoms related to hypothyroidism may include: arthritis, muscle cramps, weight gain, skin dryness, physical lethargy, constipation, slow metabolic rate, and a decrease in heart rate. Tremors, weight loss, and exophthalmos are clinical symptoms associated with hyperthyroidism.

40. **c.** The superior thyroid artery is the first branch of the external carotid artery. The ascending pharyngeal is the second branch followed by the lingual and facial arteries.

41. **b.** Serial imaging of a multinodular goiter should include the overall measurements of the thyroid lobe along with measurements of the *largest* nodules.

42. **a.** Sixty percent of thyroid nodules identified on ultrasound are benign lesions.

43. **a.** Graves disease typically demonstrates multilocular nodules within the thyroid gland. de Quervain syndrome and Hashimoto disease demonstrate a generalized enlargement of the thyroid gland without specific evidence of a nodule(s).

44. **c.** Hyperparathyroidism is a precipitating factor in the development of osteoporosis and nephrolithiasis.

45. **a.** Sonographic findings associated with thyroid carcinoma include: hypoechoic mass, irregular borders, microcalcifications, and a thick incomplete peripheral "halo."

46. **c.** The parathyroid glands lie posterior to the thyroid lobes and anterior to the longus colli muscles.

47. **b.** The platysma muscles are located in the lateral neck just beneath the subcutaneous tissues. The strap muscles consisting of the sternohyoid, omohyoid, and sternothyroid muscles are located posterior to the platysma muscles.

48. **c.** The longus colli muscles are most often affected by a whiplash injury.

49. **c.** Pronounced swelling of the neck is most commonly caused by an enlarging thyroid gland.

50. **b.** In 80% of cases, hyperparathyroidism is caused by an adenoma of a parathyroid gland. Other etiologies may include: renal disease or a deficiency in calcium or vitamin D.

Chapter 18 Peritoneum, Noncardiac Chest, and Invasive Procedures

1. **d.** An intraabdominal fluid collection (subphrenic) following a recent trauma most likely represents blood within the peritoneal cavity (hemoperitoneum).

2. **d.** Infectious or inflammatory conditions of the lungs and cardiovascular disease are predisposing factors for developing a pleural effusion.

3. **d.** The subhepatic space is the most common site for ascites to collect, followed by the Morison pouch and paracolic gutters.

4. **b.** The peritoneum is an extensive serous membrane lining the abdominal cavity. The lesser and greater omentum are part of the peritoneum. The mesentery is a double layer of peritoneum suspending the intestines from the posterior abdominal wall.

5. **b.** The patient is generally placed in a sitting position, bent slightly forward at the waist during a thoracentesis procedure.

6. **d.** The lesser sac communicates with the subhepatic space through the foramen of Winslow. Foramen of Monro is located between the third and lateral ventricles in the brain. Foramen ovale is located between the atrium of the heart. The common bile duct enters the descending portion of the duodenum through the ampulla of Vater.

7. **a.** Organs contained within the peritoneum include the liver, spleen, stomach, gallbladder, uterine body, and portions of the small and large intestines. The pancreas, kidneys, and adrenal glands lie within the retroperitoneum.

8. **c.** A collection of chyle and emulsified fats in the peritoneal cavity (chylons ascites) is most commonly associated with an abdominal neoplasm.

9. **c.** The paracolic gutters are located lateral to the intestines. The retrovesical pouch is located posterior to the urinary bladder and anterior to the rectum.

10. **c.** A lymphocele is an accumulation of lymphatic fluid more commonly occurring following a renal transplant. Lymphoceles are usually located medial to a renal transplant.

11. **d.** Paracentesis is an invasive procedure where fluid is withdrawn from the abdominal cavity for diagnostic or therapeutic purposes. Biopsies remove a small portion of living tissue.

12. **a.** Peritoneal ascites is associated with malignancy, postsurgery, postovulation, chronic liver disease, cardiovascular disease, infection, and inflammation. Pneumonia is more likely to cause a pleural effusion rather than peritoneal ascites.

13. **c.** A decrease in hematocrit is suspicious for hemorrhage.

14. **d.** The greater omentum is a double fold of peritoneum that spreads like an apron over the transverse colon and small intestines. The mesentery suspends the intestines from the posterior abdominal wall. The perineum supports and surrounds the distal portions of the urogenital and gastrointestinal tracts of the body.

15. **c.** The peritoneum extends from the diaphragm to the deep pelvic spaces and from the anterior abdominal wall to the retroperitoneum and paraspinal tissues.

16. **b.** The vesicouterine pouch or anterior cul de sac is located anterior to the uterus and posterior to the urinary bladder. The retropubic and prevesical spaces are located anterior to the urinary bladder and posterior to the symphysis pubis.

17. **a.** The pleura is a fine, delicate, serous membrane composed of visceral and parietal layers.

18. **b.** On ultrasound, visualization of the biopsy needle is obtained in a plane *parallel with the needle path.*

19. **b.** The bare area (lacking peritoneum) is a triangular space located between the two layers of the right coronary ligament.

20. **d.** Fine-needle aspiration (FNA) uses a thin needle and gentle suction to obtain tissue samples for pathological testing.

21. **c.** The arrow identifies a space posterior to the right lobe of the liver and superior and lateral to the right kidney. This is most consistent with Morison pouch. Pouch of Douglas is located anterior to the rectum in the posterior pelvis.

22. **b.** The liver is located in the peritoneal cavity. The pancreas, kidneys, and great vessels are located within the retroperitoneum.

23. **c.** Arrow A identifies a hyperechoic linear structure extending from the liver to the undersurface of the diaphragm. This is most consistent with the coronary ligament. The right coronary ligament serves as a barrier between the right subphrenic space and the Morison pouch.

24. **c.** Arrow B identifies an anechoic area posterior to the diaphragm and anterolateral to the liver. This is most consistent with free fluid (ascites) in the right subphrenic space. Blood typically demonstrates internal echoes.

25. **c.** Arrow C identifies a peritoneal space posterior to the liver and lateral to the gallbladder. This is most consistent with the subhepatic space.

26. **c.** Ascites is identified adjacent to hyperechoic bowel in the right paracolic gutter. The retrovesical pouch is located posterior to the

urinary bladder and anterior to the rectum. Space of Retzius is located anterior to the urinary bladder and posterior to the symphysis pubis.

27. **a.** A fluid collection is identified above (superior) the diaphragm consistent with a pleural effusion. Subphrenic ascites would be located below (inferior) the diaphragm.

28. **b.** Free fluid is identified posterior to the uterus and anterior to the rectum consistent with the pouch of Douglas posterior cul de sac, or retrouterine pouch.

29. **a.** The pancreas is identified in this transverse sonogram of the upper abdomen. The lesser sac separates the pancreas from the stomach.

30. **b.** A *large* core needle is identified consistent with a core needle biopsy. A slender needle is used in fine-needle aspiration procedures.

31. **c.** The peritoneum secretes serous fluid to reduce friction between organs. It also enfolds and suspends peritoneal organs. The coronary ligament serves as a barrier between the subphrenic and subhepatic spaces.

32. **b.** Vital signs include pulse, temperature, respiration, and blood pressure.

33. **b.** The falciform ligament divides the subphrenic space into right and left sides. The crura of the diaphragm extend from the diaphragm to the vertebral column.

34. **d.** The lungs are *separated* into right and left hemispheres by the pleural membrane. The heart is located between the inferior borders of the lungs. The pleural cavity is a space within the thorax that contains the lungs. The sternum is the middle portion of the anterior thorax.

35. **b.** An intercostal (between the ribs) approach is typically used in noncardiac imaging of the chest. Intracoastal pertains to the inner surface of the rib. Subcostal and suprasternal are used in cardiac imaging.

36. **b.** Omental cysts are small cystic structures developing adjacent to the stomach or lesser sac (pancreas).

37. **b.** Patients are typically placed in the supine position for a paracentesis procedure. Renal biopsies are generally performed with the patient in a prone position.

38. **a.** The prevesical space is located in the pelvis, lying anterior to the

urinary bladder and posterior to the symphysis pubis. It is also known as the retropubic space.

39. **d.** Palsy of the phrenic nerve is associated with diaphragmatic paralysis.

40. **a.** The greater omentum has the potential to seal off infections or hernias within the peritoneal cavity. The greater omentum spreads like an apron covering most of the abdominopelvic cavity.

41. **a.** The pouch of Douglas (retrouterine pouch) is located in the most posterior portion of the pelvis. The inferior portion of the parietal layer of the peritoneum forms it.

42. **c.** The paracolic gutters are located in the lateral portions of the abdominopelvic cavity and serve as conduits between the upper abdomen and the deep pelvis.

43. **c.** Blood in the peritoneal cavity (hemoperitoneum) can be associated with trauma, rupture of an abdominal blood vessel, postsurgical complication, ectopic pregnancy, fistulas, and necrotic neoplasms.

44. **a.** Congenital failure of the mesentery to fuse is a congenital anomaly associated with development of an omental cyst. Mesentery cysts are related to the Wolffian or lymph ducts.

45. **b.** The "sandwich sign" (anechoic mass with a hyperechoic center) is the most common term used to describe the sonographic appearance of mesenteric lymphomatous.

46. **c.** The inferior end of the esophagus is enclosed by the lesser omentum. The lesser omentum extends from the portal fissure of the liver to the diaphragm.

47. **d.** Hand washing of a minimum of 20 seconds is the best defense against the spreading of pathogens.

48. **c.** Exudative ascites is defined as an accumulation of fluid, pus, or serous fluid in the peritoneal cavity. Transudative ascites contains small protein cells. Chylous ascites contains chyle and emulsified fats. Peritonitis is an inflammation of the peritoneal cavity.

49. **a.** A biopsy removes a small piece of living tissue for microscopic analysis. Surgical incision of a tumor without removal of surrounding tissue describes a lumpectomy.

Fine-needle aspiration uses a thin needle and suction to obtain tissue sampling for pathological testing.

50. **d.** When localizing a fluid collection for a paracentesis procedure, the sonographer must align the transducer perpendicular to the table or floor. Care should be taken to use minimal transducer pressure for accurate depth measurement.

Abdomen Mock Exam

1. **b.** The main lobar fissure is a sonographic landmark used to locate the gallbladder fossa. It extends from the right portal vein to the gallbladder fossa. It is also considered a boundary between the left and right lobes of the liver.

2. **b.** Biliary disease is the most common cause of acute pancreatitis followed by alcohol abuse. Other etiologies may include trauma, peptic ulcer disease, and hyperlipidemia. Occasionally acute pancreatitis is idiopathic.

3. **c.** Gerota's fascia provides a protective covering around the kidneys. The liver is covered by Glisson's capsule, and the spleen is covered by the peritoneum.

4. **c.** Increased pressure within the portosplenic venous system will most likely lead to portal hypertension. Fatty infiltration may compress or occlude the portal veins causing an increase in venous pressure

5. **c.** The diameter of the main portal vein varies with respiration and fasting state but should not exceed 1.3 cm to be considered within normal limits in the adult patient

6. **c.** The Thompson test (pointing the toes while squeezing the calf muscles) checks the integrity of the Achilles tendon.

7. **c.** Chronic pancreatitis is associated with atrophy of the pancreas and hyperechoic parenchyma.

8. **c.** Endocrine glands release hormones and include the pituitary gland, thyroid gland, parathyroid glands, adrenal glands, pancreas, ovaries, and testes.

9. **d.** A septated cystic (honeycomb) mass is a sonographic finding of an echinococcal cyst. The five patterns of liver metastasis include: (1) bull's eye or target lesions, (2) hyperechoic masses, (3) cystic masses,

(4) complex masses, and (5) diffuse pattern.

10. **d.** Risk factors for developing cholangiocarcinoma include a history of cholangitis, ulcerative colitis or choledochal cyst, and male gender.

11. **b.** A Baker cyst is a synovial cyst located in the posterior medial portion of the popliteal fossa.

12. **a.** Liver length should be measured at the midclavicular level.

13. **a.** Budd-Chiari syndrome is a life-threatening condition associated with thrombosis of the hepatic veins. The sonographer should thoroughly evaluate the liver.

14. **c.** The left lobe of the liver is divided into medial and lateral segments by the left hepatic vein and the ligamentum of Teres. Ligamentum of venosum separates the caudate lobe from the left lobe of the liver.

15. **d.** Cholecystokinin is stimulated after food reaches the duodenum causing the secretion of pancreatic enzymes and contraction of the gallbladder.

16. **c.** The gallbladder lies medial and anterior to the right kidney, lateral to the IVC, and inferior to the main lobar fissure.

17. **c.** The thickness of the pyloric muscle is the most important measurement when evaluating for pyloric stenosis and should not exceed 3 mm to maintain normal limits. The pyloric canal should not exceed 17 mm in length to be considered within normal limits.

18. **c.** Clinical symptoms of severe back pain, weight loss, and painless jaundice are most suspicious for a malignant neoplasm in the pancreas.

19. **d.** Currant jelly stool (a mixture of mucous and blood) is a clinical finding associated with intussusception.

20. **d.** Glisson's capsule surrounds the liver. Gerota's fascia surrounds each kidney.

21. **d.** Mirizzi syndrome results in jaundice caused by compression of the common hepatic duct from an impacted stone in the cystic duct or neck of the gallbladder. Courvoisier sign results in painless jaundice and a hydropic gallbladder secondary to an obstruction of the distal common bile duct by an external mass (e.g., pancreatic neoplasm).

22. **a.** Nonshadowing spaghetti-like echogenic structure(s) within a bile duct describe sonographic findings in ascariasis. Schistosomiasis demonstrates thick hyperechoic portal veins on ultrasound. Clonorchiasis demonstrates dilated intrahepatic ducts.

23. **c.** Gallbladder wall thickening is not a sonographic finding in hyperalbuminemia. Gallbladder wall thickening is a sonographic finding in nonfasting patients, patients with benign ascites, cirrhosis, congestive heart failure, hypoalbuminemia, and acute hepatitis.

24. **c.** The Whipple procedure (pancreatoduodenectomy) is a surgical resection of the pancreatic head or periampullary region area. Resection will relieve a biliary obstruction often caused by a malignant tumor of the pancreas.

25. **a.** A fluid collection caused by extravasated bile is termed a *biloma.* Seroma is a collection of serous fluid.

26. **c.** Spontaneous separation of the intima and media layers of an artery describes a dissection.

27. **d.** Free fluid most commonly accumulates in the subhepatic space.

28. **c.** The pancreas, descending duodenum, ascending and descending colon, superior mesenteric vessels, and the inferior portion of the common bile duct lie within the anterior pararenal space.

29. **d.** The crura of the diaphragm lie superior to the celiac axis, posterior to the inferior vena cava, and anterior to the abdominal aorta.

30. **c.** Splenomegaly is a consistent finding in cases of portal hypertension. Hepatocellular carcinoma and Budd-Chiari syndrome (thrombosed hepatic veins) may demonstrate splenomegaly secondary to liver congestion (e.g., portal hypertension).

31. **d.** Direct extension of carcinoma into the gallbladder may originate in the pancreas, stomach, or bile duct. Indirect extension may originate in the lung, kidney, esophagus, or skin (melanoma) via the lymphatic system or bloodstream.

32. **c.** Obstruction of the common bile duct by a distal external neoplasm instigating enlargement of the gallbladder is termed *Courvoisier sign.*

33. **a.** The superior and inferior borders of the retroperitoneum are defined by the diaphragm and pelvic rim, respectively.

34. **c.** Elevation in prostatic-specific antigen is a clinical finding suspicious for carcinoma of the prostate gland.

35. **c.** Budd-Chiari syndrome is a rare life-threatening condition associated with thrombosis of the hepatic veins. Caroli disease involves the biliary tree.

36. **b.** Left untreated, obstruction of the cystic duct eventually initiates an episode of acute cholecystitis.

37. **a.** A dilated renal vein, hydroureter, or parapelvic cyst may be mistaken as an extrarenal pelvis.

38. **c.** A febrile patient demonstrating an irregular complex liver mass is most suspicious for a hepatic abscess. A "honeycomb" cystic mass is generally identified with echinococcal cysts.

39. **a.** Varix or varicose vein is a common term to describe an abnormally enlarged or dilated vein. An aneurysm is an abnormally enlarged artery.

40. **d.** Ascending cholangitis is the most common cause of a hepatic abscess. Other etiologies may include: recent travel abroad, biliary infection, appendicitis, and diverticulitis.

41. **c.** The gastroduodenal artery lies in the anterolateral portion of the pancreatic head, whereas the common bile duct lies in the posterolateral portion.

42. **c.** An echogenic mass demonstrating a prominent hypoechoic halo is most consistent with an adenoma of the thyroid gland. Carcinoma demonstrates an irregular peripheral halo surrounding a hypoechoic mass.

43. **a.** The liver manufactures heparin and glycogen, releases glycogen as glucose, breaks down red blood cell–producing bile pigments, secretes bile into the duodenum, and converts amino acids into urea and glucose. Production of antibodies and lymphocytes is a function of the spleen.

44. **c.** A normal adult spleen measures 12 cm or less in length and should not exceed 13 cm in length to be considered within normal limits.

45. b. Mycotic aneurysms develop secondary to an underlying bacterial infection. A dissecting aneurysm is the result of a tear in the intimal lining.

46. b. Pepsin is a protein-digesting *enzyme* produced by the stomach. Gastrin is a *hormone* produced by the stomach. Amylase is an enzyme produced by the pancreas. Cholecystokinin is a hormone produced by the small intestines.

47. c. The McBurney point is located between the umbilicus and right iliac crest. Rebound pain at the McBurney point (McBurney sign) is most commonly associated with appendicitis.

48. d. Frequent hand washing is the best defense against the spread of disease.

49. d. Severe abdominal pain is the most common symptom associated with portal vein *thrombosis.*

50. c. The urethral orifice indicates the neck of the bladder.

51. d. A nonshadowing, smooth hyperechoic neoplasm located in the renal cortex is most suspicious for an angiomyolipoma.

52. b. The prominence of the collecting system may signify Grade 2 hydronephrosis (dilation of the renal sinus and some of the calyces.

53. b. The distal abdominal aorta demonstrates an abnormal increase in diameter compared to a more proximal portion. A measurement of 2.8 cm is consistent with an ectatic abdominal aortic aneurysm. A true abdominal aortic aneurysm measures a minimum of 3.0 cm in diameter.

54. c. The right renal artery courses posterior to the inferior vena cava and is a common sonographic landmark used in abdominal and retroperitoneal scanning.

55. c. The gallbladder demonstrates a smooth, thick edematous wall with a coexisting gallstone(s) most consistent with acute cholecystitis. Carcinoma of the gallbladder demonstrates gallstone(s) and a thick, irregular gallbladder wall in the majority of cases.

56. a. An anechoic fluid collection is identified anterior and lateral to the right testis. This is most consistent with a hydrocele.

57. c. The anechoic structure measured is located in the body of the pancreas. This is most consistent with a pancreatic duct.

58. c. A diffuse increase in liver echogenicity is identified consistent with fatty infiltration. A hypoechoic "mass" anterior to the portal hepatis (arrow) in a fatty liver is most likely normal liver parenchyma.

59. b. The arrows in the walls of the transverse colon identify comma-like recesses. These saccular indentations are consistent with haustral wall markings found in the ascending and transverse colon. Haustra are located approximately 3 to 5 cm apart.

60. d. A cavernous hemangioma is the most common benign neoplasm of the spleen and appears as a well-defined hyperechoic mass on ultrasound.

61. d. The spleen measures approximately 18 cm in length in a patient with a history of alcohol abuse. Based on the clinical history, the sonogram is most consistent with splenomegaly.

62. d. Splenomegaly in a patient with a history of alcohol abuse is suspicious for portal hypertension. The sonographer should document the flow direction of the main portal vein and evaluate for venous collaterals.

63. c. A hyperechoic focus with posterior acoustic shadowing is identified in the distal common bile duct (choledocholithiasis). Courvoisier sign (painless jaundice, hydropic gallbladder, and obstruction of the distal common bile duct) cannot be determined by this image alone.

64. d. An outpouching of the bladder wall is most consistent with a bladder diverticulum. A ureterocele appears as a hyperechoic septation within the urinary bladder at the ureteric orifice.

65. b. A complex mass is identified in the posterior renal cortex most suspicious for renal malignancy. Symptoms of renal cell carcinoma include uncontrolled hypertension, painless hematuria, and headaches.

66. c. Mild dilatation of the renal calyces is identified consistent with hydronephrosis.

67. b. Multiple lobulations are identified in the renal contour. This is consistent with fetal lobulation. A solitary cortical bulge on the lateral aspect of the kidney describes a dromedary hump.

68. d. A complex lesion demonstrated in the region of the mediastinum testis is suspicious for tubular ectasia of the rete testis. This lesion is typically bilateral and asymptomatic.

69. d. An extratesticular anechoic structure is identified superior to the testis in the region of the epididymal head. This is most suspicious for an epididymal cyst or possibly a spermatocele.

70. c. Two distinct collecting systems are demonstrated in this elongated kidney most consistent with a renal duplication.

71. c. Based on the **cortical thickness**, thinning of the renal cortex in this sonogram is most likely associated with chronic renal disease.

72. c. The inferior pole of the right kidney is fused with the superior pole of the left kidney. This is most consistent with a sigmoid kidney. A horseshoe kidney more commonly demonstrates fusion of the inferior poles Even though a sigmoid kidney is a form of a horseshoe kidney the best answer to this question is sigmoid kidney.

73. a. Anechoic fluid is identified within the superficial echogenic cellular tissue most consistent with superficial skin edema. The best answer for this question is cellulitis.

74. b. Ascites is identified superior to the liver and inferior to the diaphragm consistent with the right subphrenic space. Fluid is also demonstrated inferior to the gallbladder in the subhepatic space.

75. d. The presence of a thick hyperechoic gallbladder wall surrounded by benign free fluid is most consistent with a noninflammatory condition of the gallbladder. Note the thickness of the gallbladder wall adjacent to the liver is within normal limits. This area would likely be thickened in cases of acute cholecystitis.

76. d. The ligamentum venosum separates the caudate lobe from the left lobe of the liver. The falciform ligament divides the subphrenic space. The main lobar fissure is considered a boundary between the left and right hepatic lobes.

77. c. The anterior right hepatic lobe is bordered by the middle and right hepatic veins. The middle hepatic vein separates the left medial lobe from the right anterior lobe. The right hepatic vein separates the anterior and posterior right lobes.

78. **a.** A smooth circular anechoic renal mass is most likely a simple cyst. An extrarenal pelvis would not displace the renal calyces.

79. **b.** The urinary bladder should be evaluated for evidence of a ureter or bladder outlet obstruction when hydronephrosis is identified. A neoplasm, calculus, or stricture of the distal ureter or urethra may cause the obstruction.

80. **a.** Omental cysts generally develop adjacent to the stomach or lesser sac.

81. **c.** Increasing axial resolution by increasing the transducer frequency may aid in the demonstration of posterior acoustic shadowing.

82. **d.** A superficial cystic mass located just beneath the angle of the mandible is most likely a brachial cleft cyst.

83. **d.** A phlegmon is associated with acute pancreatitis and is defined as an extension of pancreatic inflammation into the peripancreatic tissues.

84. **d.** The normal inferior vena cava generally measures less than 2.5 cm in diameter. The inferior vena cava is considered dilated after the diameter exceeds 3.7 cm.

85. **d.** Levels of aldosterone are most commonly associated with abnormalities of the adrenal gland(s).

86. **b.** A round, solid, homogeneous mass near the splenic hilum is most likely an accessory spleen.

87. **a.** The small and tortuous splenic artery is the most common vascular structure mistaken as the pancreatic duct.

88. **b.** Cortical thickness of the normal adult kidney will vary but should measure a minimum of 1.0 cm.

89. **b.** Addison disease is associated with a partial or complete failure of the adrenocortical function. Cushing disease is a metabolic disorder resulting from chronic and excessive production of cortisol.

90. **d.** The main renal arteries arise from the lateral aspect of the aorta approximately 1.0 to 1.5 cm below the inferior margin of the superior mesenteric artery.

91. **c.** A decrease in hematocrit is associated with hemorrhage. Hemoglobin carries oxygen from the lungs to the cells and returns carbon dioxide back to the lungs.

92. **b.** Hepatic veins course away from the liver toward the inferior vena cava, termed *hepatofugal flow*. Hepatic veins demonstrate spontaneous multiphasic (pulsatile) flow.

93. **b.** The "olive sign" is a clinical finding associated with hypertrophied pyloric stenosis.

94. **b.** A thoracentesis is typically performed with the patient in a sitting position, slightly bent forward at the waist, with the arms leaning on a table.

95. **d.** Hypertrophied column of Bertin is the most common structure frequently mistaken as a renal neoplasm. A junctional parenchymal defect is less frequently mistaken as a lipoma or angiomyolipoma.

96. **b.** Elevation in indirect or nonconjugated bilirubin is associated with a prehepatic or hepatic abnormality (nonobstructive jaundice).

97. **b.** The neck is the most superior portion of the gallbladder.

98. **c.** Hashimoto disease is an inflammatory condition of the thyroid gland(s) associated with an increased risk in developing a thyroid malignancy.

99. **a.** A core biopsy uses a large-core needle to remove a small piece of living tissue for microscopic analysis.

100. **a.** A pancreatic pseudocyst most commonly develops in the lesser sac followed by the anterior pararenal space.

101. **c.** Elevated serum lipase in a patient with severe left upper quadrant pain is suspicious for acute pancreatitis. Biliary disease is the most common cause of acute pancreatitis.

102. **b.** A cortical bulge on the lateral aspect of the kidney describes a dromedary hump. Fetal lobulation demonstrates multiple indentations in the contour of the renal cortex. Hypertrophied column of Bertin extends from the cortex into the medullary pyramids.

103. **d.** Fusion of both kidneys within the same body quadrant describes a congenital anomaly termed *cross fused ectopia*.

104. **c.** Color Doppler imaging demonstrates turbulent or swirling arterial blood flow within a fluid collection adjacent to the common femoral artery following an invasive procedure. A pseudoaneurysm is associated with trauma to the arterial wall, permitting the escape of blood into the surrounding tissues.

105. **b.** A transverse color Doppler image to include the inferior epigastric and external iliac arteries should be included in all ultrasound examinations evaluating for an inguinal hernia.

106. **b.** Removal of foreign material from the blood is a function of the spleen. Other functions include initiating an immune reaction resulting in production of antibodies and lymphocytes, reservoir for blood, destruction site of old red blood cells, and recycling hemoglobin.

107. **b.** "Comet-tail" reverberation artifact is a characteristic sonographic finding of adenomyomatosis. Pneumobilia may demonstrate an imprecise posterior acoustic shadow but is not an abnormality of the gallbladder wall.

108. **c.** Transplant kidneys are more commonly placed superficially in the right lower quadrant.

109. **c.** Meckel diverticulum is a congenital anomaly of the yolk stalk. On ultrasound, the diverticulum appears as an anechoic or complex mass, slightly to the right of the umbilicus.

110. **d.** *Tendinosis* is a term used to describe noninflammatory degenerative changes in a tendon. Pain related to a tendon describes tenaglia and tenodynia.

111. **a.** There is a 5% risk that an abdominal aortic aneurysm measuring 5 cm in diameter will rupture within 5 years. An aneurysm measuring 7 cm has a 75% risk factor for rupture within 5 years.

112. **d.** The inferior mesenteric artery is the last major *visceral* branch of the abdominal aorta in advance of the bifurcation into the right and left common iliac arteries. The median sacral artery is the last main parietal branch of the abdominal aorta.

113. d. Twenty-five percent of popliteal aneurysm cases demonstrate a co-existing abdominal aortic aneurysm. Deep vein thrombosis is a possible complication of popliteal aneurysm.

114. c. The subphrenic space is located superior to the liver and inferior to the diaphragm.

115. d. Hepatitis B carriers have a predisposing risk for developing hepatocellular carcinoma (hepatoma). Hepatitis C carriers may develop portal hypertension because of an increased risk for developing cirrhosis.

116. c. The majority of metastatic lesions in the liver originate from colon carcinoma. Pancreas, breasts, and lungs are additional primary sites commonly metastasizing to the liver.

117. c. The common bile duct joins the duct of Wirsung before passing through the ampulla of Vater to enter the duodenum. The sphincter of Oddi is a sheath of muscle fibers surrounding the distal common bile and pancreatic ducts as they cross the wall of the duodenum.

118. c. Hashimoto disease is the most common cause of hypothyroidism. Hyperthyroidism is a common symptom in Graves disease.

119. b. The pyramidal or third lobe arises from the superior aspect of the isthmus and ascends the neck to the level of the hyoid bone.

120. c. Under normal conditions, the internal carotid arteries supply the majority of blood to the brain and eye. The subclavian arteries supply the vertebral column, spinal cord, ear, and brain. Blood to the neck, scalp, and face is supplied through the external carotid arteries.

121. a. A ureterocele is defined as a prolapse of the distal ureter into the urinary bladder caused by a congenital obstruction of the ureteric orifice.

122. b. Postvoid residual in an adult urinary bladder should not exceed 20 mL to be considered within normal limits.

123. c. Fifty percent of all malignant neoplasms involving the colon are located in the rectum and 25% in the sigmoid colon.

124. c. The left renal vein courses posterior to the superior mesenteric artery (SMA) and anterior to the abdominal aorta. The splenic vein and splenic artery course anterior to the SMA. The superior mesenteric vein courses parallel with the SMA.

125. a. On ultrasound, visualization of a biopsy needle is obtained at a plane parallel to the needle path. Perpendicular incidence is used in gray-scale imaging.

126. b. A diffuse heterogeneous parenchyma containing multiple echogenic foci is identified in this transverse sonogram of the liver. This is most suspicious for metastatic liver lesions.

127. b. A round anechoic structure demonstrating posterior acoustic enhancement is visualized within the hepatic parenchyma. This most likely represents a simple hepatic cyst.

128. b. A large gallstone within a contracted gallbladder demonstrating strong posterior acoustic shadowing is an excellent example of the wall-echo-shadow (WES) sign.

129. d. A hyperechoic linear structure is identified posterior to the left lobe and anterior to the caudate lobe of the liver. This is most consistent with the ligamentum venosum.

130. b. Patients with a history of hepatitis B are at an increased risk for developing hepatocellular carcinoma (HCC; hepatoma). Variable echogenicity in a solid hepatic mass surrounded by a hypoechoic halo are common sonographic findings for a hepatoma.

131. b. Caroli disease is characterized by a segmental, saccular, or beaded appearance to the intrahepatic ducts.

132. a. Renal cysts are frequent incidental findings in middle-aged and elderly patients. The sonographic findings are characteristic of a renal cyst.

133. d. Chronic intraluminal thrombus commonly appears complex secondary to degenerative changes. In this sonogram, the lumen of the distal aorta is surrounded by complex intraluminal thrombus. In many cases, rupture of an aortic aneurysm will demonstrate blood within the peritoneum and a normal caliber aorta.

134. b. An oval hypoechoic mass demonstrating a prominent hyperechoic center and hilar blood flow are common sonographic findings of a normal lymph node.

135. d. The length of the kidney states 6.0 cm, which would be the size of a normal infant kidney. In the infant kidney, the renal sinus is barely visible and is surrounded by prominent anechoic medullary (renal) pyramids and a moderately echogenic renal cortex. This image demonstrates the typical appearance of a normal neonatal kidney.

136. a. A hyperechoic septation identified within the urinary bladder is identified near the ureteric orifice. This most likely represents a ureterocele.

137. d. Carcinoma of the gallbladder is the fifth most common malignancy. Ninety percent of cases are associated with cholelithiasis and may demonstrate on ultrasound as an irregular, immobile intraluminal mass(es). Absence of cholelithiasis is more commonly associated with metastatic lesions involving the gallbladder. Comet-tail reverberation artifact is a characteristic sonographic finding in adenomyomatosis.

138. c. A smooth, hyperechoic hepatic mass identified in an asymptomatic thin female patient is most suspicious for a cavernous hemangioma. Hepatic adenomas generally demonstrate as solid, slightly hypoechoic masses. Fatty infiltration is unlikely in a thin patient with normal laboratory values.

139. b. Equally spaced reflections of diminishing amplitude with increases in imaging depth describes reverberation artifact.

140. a. Hyperechoic echogenic focus demonstrating posterior acoustic shadowing is demonstrated in the neck of the gallbladder.

141. d. Calculus appears to be nonmobile within the neck of the gallbladder (patient is in the left lateral decubitus position). This finding increases the risk for the patient to develop acute cholecystitis.

142. b. A hyperechoic focus demonstrating posterior acoustic shadowing is identified near the corticomedullary junction of the right kidney. This is most suspicious for a renal calculus.

143. **a.** The gallbladder demonstrates multiple intraluminal, hyperechoic, nonshadowing, immobile foci most consistent with gallbladder polyps (adenomas).

144. **a.** Changes in the patient position will demonstrate mobility of the intraluminal foci, narrowing down the differential considerations.

145. **b.** According to the color legend the blood is flowing away from the transducer (hepatofugal flow).

146. **d.** Retrograde flow in the main portal vein (hepatofugal) is a sonographic finding associated with portal hypertension.

147. **c.** The pyloric wall exceeds 3 mm in thickness, and the stomach is still distended with fluid.. This is most consistent with stenosis of the pyloric canal.

148. **d.** The head/neck regions of the pancreas appear hypoechoic and enlarged, suspicious for a solid mass. A mass in the head of the pancreas is most suspicious for a malignant neoplasm.

149. **c.** The coronary ligament forms the anterior and posterior borders of the bare area.

150. **a.** Fluid collections are identified superior to the diaphragm bilaterally, consistent with bilateral pleural effusions.

151. **a.** A solid structure is located medial to the spleen. This mass is isoechoic to the splenic parenchyma. This is most suspicious for an accessory spleen.

152. **c.** A solid bladder mass is most suspicious for bladder carcinoma. Sludge is gravity dependent.

153. **d.** A large anechoic structure is located anterior to the main portal vein. With a history of jaundice, choledochal cyst is the most likely diagnosis. Bilomas are generally associated with trauma, surgery, or gallbladder disease. A hepatic cyst is not likely in an infant and generally not the source of jaundice.

154. **c.** The sonogram demonstrates pancreatic calcifications and an irregular dilated pancreatic duct is most suspicious for chronic pancreatitis. The head of the pancreas appears hypoechoic because of the posterior shadowing caused by the calcifications.

155. **a.** The ultrasound demonstrates a nodular contour to the liver periphery and an enlarged caudate lobe. In a patient with known alcohol abuse, this is most suspicious for cirrhosis.

156. **c.** A hyperechoic focus with posterior acoustic shadowing is demonstrated in the distal portion of the right ureter.

157. **b.** The distal right collecting system appears obstructed by the ureteral stone and is likely to cause ipsilateral hydronephrosis.

158. **b.** The sonogram demonstrates marked prominence of the biliary tree. Based on a clinical history of fever, fatigue, and marked elevation in AST, ALT, and bilirubin, the sonogram most likely demonstrates acute hepatitis. Peliosis hepatitis is a rare disorder occurring in chronically ill patients.

159. **d.** The renal cortex is extending to the renal pyramids, characteristic of a hypertrophied column of Bertin. Duplication of the left kidney is unlikely, because the length of the kidney is within normal limits for an adult. An outward cortical bulge is characteristic of a dromedary hump.

160. **c.** A solid mass is identified medial to the left kidney in a patient with a complex hypervascular testicular mass. With a history of left testicular carcinoma, the retroperitoneal mass is most suspicious for metastatic disease.

161. **b.** A complex mass anterior and medial to the right kidney in a 13-month-old child is most suspicious for a neuroblastoma (adrenal). The right kidney appears within normal limits in this image,

which would rule out a nephroblastoma.

162. **b.** A midline anechoic structure is demonstrated superior to the thyroid gland, characteristic of a thyroglossal cyst. A brachial cleft cyst is located laterally, directly below the angle of the mandible.

163. **a.** Hyperechoic foci with comettail reverberation artifact postcholecystectomy are most likely a result of air within the biliary tree (pneumobilia).

164. **d.** A supraumbilical abdominal wall defect with extension of the omentum is identified characteristic of an abdominal wall hernia.

165. **c.** Annular pancreas describes a congenital anomaly where the head of the pancreas surrounds the duodenum. This anomaly may result in obstruction of the biliary tree or duodenum. In pancreas divisum, there is abnormal fusion of the pancreatic ducts.

166. **b.** Biliary sludge appears on ultrasound as nonshadowing, low amplitude internal echoes that layer in the dependent portion of the gallbladder. Tumefactive sludge resembles a polypoid mass (sludge ball).

167. **a.** The tail of the pancreas is the most superior portion of the pancreas lying anterior and parallel with the splenic vein. The body is the most anterior portion, and the uncinate process is the most inferior portion of the pancreas.

168. **c.** Polycystic disease is an inherited disorder, and multicystic dysplasia is a noninherited disorder of the kidney.

169. **d.** Renal dialysis patients have an increased risk for developing a renal cyst, adenoma, or carcinoma.

170. **c.** An anterior approach is used when evaluating the pediatric hip for effusion. A lateral approach is used when evaluating for developmental dysplasia of the hip.

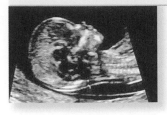

Obstetrics and Gynecology Answers

Chapter 19 Pelvic Anatomy

1. **d.** The ovarian ligament extends from the cornua of the uterus to the medial aspect of the ovary. The round ligament arises in the cornua of the uterus and extends to the pelvic sidewalls.
2. **b.** Arcuate vessels are commonly visualized near the periphery of the uterus as anechoic circular structures. Adenomyosis may demonstrate anechoic areas within the myometrium.
3. **c.** The interstitial segment of the fallopian tube extends laterally from the uterine wall and may be visualized in normal conditions as an echogenic tenuous structure.
4. **b.** *Adnexa* is the term used to describe the region of the ovary and fallopian tube. The one fimbriae attached to the ovary is termed the *fimbriae ovarica.*
5. **c.** The interstitial segment of the fallopian tube passes through the cornua of the uterus. The infundibulum is the most lateral segment of the oviduct.
6. **d.** The flanged portions of the iliac bones and the base of the sacrum form the posterior boundary of the false pelvis.
7. **d.** The fallopian tubes are covered by peritoneum and contained within the superior portion of the broad ligament. They are derived from the nonfused cranial portion of the müllerian ducts.
8. **b.** Only the functional layer (echogenic) is included when measuring endometrial thickness. The hypoechoic basal layer or fluid within the endometrial cavity is *not* included when measuring the thickness of the endometrium.
9. **d.** The suspensory ligaments extend from the lateral aspect of the ovary to the pelvic sidewalls. The broad ligaments extend from the lateral aspect of the uterus to the pelvic sidewalls.
10. **d.** *Failure* of the müllerian ducts to fuse will result in uterine didelphys. *Partial failure* of these ducts to fuse will result in a bicornuate uterus.
11. **c.** The anterior–posterior dimension of the endometrium is *only* measured in the sagittal plane.
12. **c.** The external or serosal layer of the uterus is termed the *perimetrium.*
13. **b.** The ovaries receive blood primarily from the ovarian arteries and secondarily through the uterine arteries. The uterine arteries arise from the hypogastric (internal iliac) arteries.
14. **b.** The vesicouterine pouch (anterior cul de sac) is located anterior to the uterus and posterior to the urinary bladder. The retrouterine space (posterior cul de sac) is located posterior to the uterus and anterior to the rectum.
15. **c.** The cervix is twice as large as the corpus during premenarche. The cervix-to-corpus ratio is 2:1.
16. **d.** The cervix and corpus (uterine body) appear equal in size (1:1). This is most consistent with a postmenopausal uterus. The corpus portion of the menarche uterus is twice the size of the cervix.
17. **a.** The uterus bends slightly anterior (forward), characteristic of anteversion. A hyperechoic linear echo is demonstrated in the endometrium representing an IUD.
18. **b.** The levator ani and piriformis muscles form the pelvic floor and lie posterior to the vagina. Obturator internus and iliopsoas muscles are located in the lateral true pelvis.
19. **c.** Fluid is demonstrated posterior to the uterus in the pouch of Douglas. The vesicouterine pouch is located anterior to the uterus.
20. **a.** The uterus is lying in the anteverted position.
21. **d.** An L-shaped homogeneous ovarian contour is a normal anatomical variant.
22. **d.** The uterus displays myometrial tissue between two individual endometrial cavities. This is *most* consistent with a bicornuate uterus. Uterine didelphys demonstrates a wide separation between two distinct uterine fundi.
23. **c.** Evenly spaced, hypoechoic or anechoic, circular structures identified in the outer portion of the myometrium *most* likely represent arcuate veins. Uterine arteries are located in the broad ligament lateral to the uterus.
24. **b.** The hyperechoic linear structure extends from the uterus to the *pelvic sidewall.* This is most consistent with the broad ligaments. The fallopian tubes are tortuous and do not attach to the pelvic sidewall.
25. **d.** The obturator internus muscles abut the lateral walls of the urinary bladder. Levator ani muscles lie lateral to the vagina.
26. **d.** Two distinct endometrial cavities are identified with myometrial tissue between the cavities and a single uterine cervix consistent with a bicornuate uterus. Uterine didelphys demonstrates two individual endometrial cavities and cervixes.
27. **c.** Free fluid is identified anterior and posterior to the uterus in the vesicouterine and retrouterine spaces. The small anechoic area represents a small amount of urine in an otherwise empty bladder.
28. **d.** The uterus displays a posterior tilt and the cervix forms an angle less than 90° to the vaginal canal, characteristic of retroversion.
29. **d.** An anechoic pedunculation of the urinary bladder describes a diverticulum. A ureterocele is a prolapse of the distal ureter into the bladder.

30. **a.** A 3D rendering of the uterus demonstrates a separation within the endometrium consistent with septate or subseptus uterus. Bicornuate uterus demonstrates two distinct endometriums separated by a small amount of myometrial tissue.

31. **b.** The ovaries attach to the mesovarian portion of the broad ligament. The tunica albuginea is an outer covering of the ovary.

32. **a.** Ovarian volume is lowest during the luteal phase and highest during the periovulatory phase.

33. **d.** The segments of the fallopian tube include the interstitial, isthmus, ampulla, and infundibulum.

34. **b.** Pelvic ligaments are not routinely visualized. With the presence of intraperitoneal fluid, pelvic ligaments appear as thin, hyperechoic linear structures.

35. **c.** The cornua are the lateral funnel-shaped horns of the uterus located between the uterine fundus and fallopian tube.

36. **c.** The spiral artery arises from the radial arteries (a branch of arcuate artery) and is the primary blood supply to the functional layer of the endometrium.

37. **b.** Coexisting renal anomalies occur in 20% to 30% of patients with a congenital uterine anomaly.

38. **a.** The septate or subseptus uterus is *most* likely to display a **slight** indentation to the fundal contour.

39. **c.** It is common to visualize a small amount of free fluid in the retro-uterine space (posterior cul de sac).

40. **c.** Premenarche is the portion of time before the onset of menstruation. Puberty is the physical process of changing into an adult body capable of reproduction.

41. **c.** Situated between the symphysis pubis and coccyx, the perineum is located below the pelvic floor.

42. **a.** An arcuate uterus is most likely to display a normal uterine contour. Bicornuate, unicornuate, and didelphys demonstrate an abnormal contour to the uterine fundus.

43. **a.** The uterus is derived from the fused caudal portion of the paired müllerian ducts. The fallopian tubes are derived from the nonfused cranial portion of the müllerian ducts.

44. **c.** The iliopectineal line is a bony ridge on the inner surface of the ilium and pubic bones that divides the true from the false pelvis. The iliopsoas muscles are lateral landmarks of the true pelvis, coursing anterior and lateral through the false pelvis.

45. **d.** Pelvic ligaments and muscles form the pelvic floor.

46. **b.** The uterosacral ligament extends from the superior cervix to the lateral margins of the sacrum.

47. **c.** The junctional zone is the innermost layer of the myometrium. The functional and basal layers are the inner and outer layers of the endometrium, respectively.

48. **c.** In the *menarche* patient, the endometrial thickness should not exceed 14 mm.

49. **b.** The ovaries are the only abdominopelvic organ *not* lined by peritoneum. A thin layer of germinal epithelium covers each ovary.

50. **d.** Periovulatory phase exhibits the highest ovarian volume, and the luteal phase shows the lowest volumes.

Chapter 20 Physiology of the Female Pelvis

1. **a.** Progesterone levels increase in the endometrial secretory phase and the ovarian luteal phase.

2. **d.** During the early proliferation or late menstrual phases, the endometrial lining is thin, typically measuring 2 to 3 mm.

3. **a.** Estradiol levels reflect the activity of the ovaries. Luteinizing hormone reflects ovulation. Progesterone levels increase after ovulation. Follicular stimulating hormone initiates follicular growth.

4. **b.** Postmenopausal patients may display simple ovarian cysts. Simple cysts <5.0 cm is most likely benign. Visualization of a simple cyst in postmenopausal or premenarche patients is not a rare finding.

5. **d.** If fertilization does not occur, the corpus luteum will regress, and progesterone levels will decrease. When anticipating fertilization, the corpus luteum may increase in size and may secrete some estrogen and an increasing amount of progesterone.

6. **c.** The endometrium demonstrates a triple-line appearance during the late proliferation phase (days 10–14).

7. **b.** The cumulus oophorus appears as a hyperechoic focus within a mature follicle. Ovulation generally will occur within the next 36 hours.

8. **b.** A corpus luteum originates from a ruptured graafian follicle. Corpus luteal cysts are common in early pregnancy but do not indicate that fertilization has occurred.

9. **b.** Dysmenorrhea is termed used to describe painful menses. Abnormal pain during sexual intercourse is termed dyspareunia.

10. **d.** The anterior pituitary gland secretes luteinizing hormone. The hypothalamus produces luteinizing hormone releasing factor.

11. **d.** Adrenal glands, liver, and the breasts produce small amounts of estrogen.

12. **c.** Luteinizing hormone stimulates ovulation. Follicular stimulating hormone initiates follicular growth and stimulates maturation of the graafian follicle.

13. **c.** Fluid within the endometrial cavity is not included when measuring the endometrial thickness. Granulosa cells produce fluid in the follicular cyst.

14. **b.** Mittelschmerz (middle pain) is a local effect of the enlarging graafian follicle before ovulation.

15. **c.** Dyspareunia is a termed used to describe abnormal pain during sexual intercourse.

16. **b.** During the late menstrual and early proliferative phases, anechoic areas within the ovary most likely represent functional, follicular, or physiological cysts. This follicle does not appear large enough for a graafian follicle.

17. **b.** Scarring from a previous corpus luteal cyst (corpus albicans) displays as a hyperechoic focus within the ovary and is the *most* likely diagnosis for this hyperechoic focus. An early cystic teratoma (dermoid) is a possible differential consideration.

18. **b.** The secretory phase demonstrates the greatest endometrial thickness. The functional layer appears thick and hyperechoic. The ovarian luteal phase coincides with the secretory phase of the endometrium.

19. **a.** In a patient in the late menstrual phase, an anechoic 2.9-cm ovarian mass demonstrating smooth, thin walls and posterior enhancement *most* likely represents a simple cyst. In a menarche patient, a simple cyst is the failure of a dominant follicle to rupture.

20. **d.** The ovaries display multiple small follicles *most* consistent with the early proliferation phase of the endometrium. Five to eleven follicles typically begin to develop in the early follicular phase of the ovary.

21. **d.** A thin endometrial cavity is *most* likely demonstrated in the late menstrual or early proliferative phases. Don't be fooled by the free fluid in the posterior cul de sac.

22. **d.** Strong hyperechoic linear echoes within the endometrial cavity most likely represent an IUD.

23. **c.** The cervix is larger than the corpus most consistent with a premenarche uterus.

24. **b.** An 18-mm anechoic structure with an intraluminal echogenic focus (posterior wall), in a menarche patient, is *most* consistent with a graafian follicle.

25. **d.** An echogenic focus projected within a graafian follicle is most consistent with a cumulus oophorus.

26. **d.** Thick, hypoechoic functional layers between the endometrial cavity with a hyperechoic basal layer are characteristic of the late proliferation phase. Endometrial phases include menstrual, proliferation, and secretory.

27. **c.** Triple line or trilaminar echo pattern describes a characteristic sonographic finding during the late proliferative phase.

28. **c.** A slightly irregular anechoic structure with prominent peripheral flow, in the luteal stage of the cycle (LMP 3 weeks earlier) is *most likely* a corpus luteal cyst. Ectopic pregnancies are generally adnexal in location. Nondominant follicles generally do not demonstrate prominent peripheral flow.

29. **b.** A thin, hyperechoic endometrial cavity is *most* consistent with the late menstrual or early proliferation phases. The adjacent left ovary displays small physiological cysts.

30. **d.** The endometrium is thick, demonstrating a hyperechoic functional layer and a hypoechoic basal layer, most consistent with the secretory phase. The secretory phase of the endometrium coincides with the luteal phase of the ovary. Normal, small, regressing follicles or a corpus luteal cyst is the most likely ovarian mass demonstrated during the secretory or luteal phase.

31. **c.** Menorrhagia defines abnormally heavy or long menses. Dysmenorrhea defines painful menses. Menoxenia defines any abnormality relating to menstruation.

32. **b.** Levels of follicular stimulating hormone begin declining in the late follicular phase and demonstrate a slight increase in the late luteal phase.

33. **d.** Estradiol levels normally range between 200 and 400 pg/mL in the ovulatory phase. Follicular phase ranges between 30 and 100 pg/mL, and luteal phase ranges between 50 and 140 pg/mL. These levels are important when monitoring ovulation induction therapy.

34. **c.** The follicular phase of the ovary coincides with the proliferation phase of the endometrium.

35. **d.** Corpus albicans is a scar from a previous corpus luteal cyst. It appears as a hyperechoic ovarian mass on ultrasound.

36. **c.** In asymptomatic postmenopausal patients *without* hormone replacement therapy, the endometrium should not exceed 8 mm or 5 mm in patients with vaginal bleeding to be considered within normal limits.

37. **d.** Follicular stimulating hormones can be slightly higher after menopause. Progesterone and estrogen levels decrease after menopause.

38. **d.** During the late proliferation phase, the endometrium demonstrates a triple line appearance or a thick, *hypoechoic functional* layer and a *hyperechoic basal* layer. During the secretory phase, the functional layer becomes hyperechoic and the basal layer becomes hypoechoic.

39. **b.** *Mittelschmerz* (middle pain) is a term used to describe acute pelvic pain before ovulation. It is thought to be a result of the increasing size of the graafian follicle.

40. **c.** Preparing and maintaining the endometrium for possible implantation of a blastocyst is a function of progesterone. Estrogen promotes endometrial growth.

41. **d.** Developing graafian follicles secrete estrogen. The corpus luteum produces progesterone. The anterior portion of the pituitary gland produces luteinizing and follicular stimulating hormones.

42. **c.** The typical length of a menstrual cycle is 28 days but can normally range between 21 and 35 days.

43. **b.** A rise in hormone levels associated with precocious puberty may be a result of a neoplasm of the hypothalamus, gonads, or adrenal glands.

44. **a.** Increasing levels of estrogen regenerate and promote growth of the functional layer of the endometrium.

45. **b.** During the secretory phase, the endometrium measures 7 to 14 mm, 6 to 10 mm in the late proliferation phase, and 4 to 8 mm during the early menstrual phase.

46. **d.** A hypoechoic ovarian mass in a patient with a history of *acute* lower quadrant pain is most suspicious for a hemorrhagic cyst outlined by circle D.

47. **c.** The corpus luteum will continue to secrete progesterone if fertilization occurs. The trophoblastic tissue of the blastocyst secretes human chorionic gonadotropin (hCG).

48. **a.** A thin echogenic line is the most common endometrial appearance with oral contraceptive use.

49. **d** An intrauterine device should be located in the center of the endometrium at the level of the fundus and superior portion of the endometrium.

50. **a.** Decreases in estrogen in postmenopause patients can shorten the vagina and decrease cervical mucus.

Chapter 21 Uterine and Ovarian Pathology

1. **d.** Abnormal accumulation of blood within the vagina is termed *hematocolpos*. Hematometra defines an abnormal accumulation of blood in the endometrial cavity

2. **b.** Postmenopausal women are at risk for developing endometrial carcinoma. Other risk factors include obesity, diabetes mellitus, and nulliparity.

3. **a.** Inflammation of the endometrium (endometritis) will likely demonstrate an increase in internal blood flow. Hyperplasia is a noninflammatory process not likely to increase internal vascular flow.

4. **c.** Dysgerminoma is the most common ovarian malignancy in childhood and is a possible cause for precocious puberty. Fibroma, thecoma, Brenner tumor, and granulosa cell tumor are benign neoplasms.

5. **d.** Uterine tenderness during a physical exam, especially during menstruation, is a classic symptom of adenomyosis. Other symptoms include pelvic pain, menorrhagia,

dysmenorrhea, uterine enlargement, pelvic pain, or cramping.

6. **a.** A large multilocular adnexal mass *most* likely represents a serous or mucinous cystadenoma. A less likely differential, theca lutein cysts, can demonstrate a multilocular appearance.

7. **c.** Uterine fibroids are commonly located within the myometrium (intramural).

8. **c.** Scarring from a previous endometrial infection or invasive procedure adheres and ablates the endometrial cavity (Asherman syndrome). Ovulatory disorders are the most common cause of female infertility.

9. **c.** A coexisting adnexal mass is *commonly associated* with torsion of the ovary. Ectopic pregnancies are generally located in the adnexa, but not typically associated with ovarian torsion.

10. **d.** A side effect of tamoxifen therapy is an increase in endometrial thickness. Special attention to the endometrial thickness is necessary in tamoxifen patients.

11. **b.** A complex adnexal mass with diffusely bright internal echoes with or without posterior shadowing is most suspicious for a cystic teratoma (dermoid).

12. **c.** Cystic teratomas (dermoids) are commonly located superior to the uterine fundus. They arise from the wall of a follicle and may contain fat, hair, skin, and teeth.

13. **a.** Nabothian cysts can result from obstruction of an inclusion cyst. Serous cystadenomas are epithelial neoplasms.

14. **d.** A submucosal fibroid distorts the endometrium and will most likely cause bleeding irregularities. The location of cervical fibroid in relation to the endometrial canal will determine clinical symptoms.

15. **c.** Polycystic ovary disease can result from an endocrine imbalance causing chronic anovulation. Endometrial abnormalities can result from unopposed estrogen.

16. **d.** Antiestrogen medication used in treating breast cancer may cause side effects to the endometrium. These may include endometrial polyps, carcinoma, or hyperplasia.

17. **a.** A homogeneous hypoechoic uterine mass in a *premenarche* 13-year-old

patient is most suspicious for hematometra. An accumulation of blood in the vagina defines hematocolpos.

18. **c.** The arrow is pointing to a hypoechoic mass extending from the uterine serosa. Subserosal fibroid is the most likely diagnosis for the anterior hypoechoic uterine mass.

19. **c.** A small amount of free fluid is demonstrated posterior to the uterus in the retrouterine space.

20. **b.** A dense, hypoechoic, ovarian mass with diffusely bright internal echoes is identified in a menarche patient. Based on this clinical history, the mass is *most* suspicious for a cystic teratoma (dermoid). Severe acute pelvic pain is generally associated with hemorrhagic cysts. This patient is expressing a history of *chronic* pelvic pain.

21. **b.** The uterus is enlarged and demonstrates striated edge shadowing (venetian-blind). The MRI demonstrates low signal intensities in the myometrium adjacent to the endometrium. These findings are most suspicious for adenomyosis.

22. **b.** Clinical findings associated with adenomyosis include: dysmenorrhea, menorrhagia, uterine enlargement, uterine tenderness, pelvic pain, or cramping.

23. **a.** Leiomyomas are the most common uterine mass. This isoechoic mass is compressing the endometrial cavity.

24. **b.** A **submucosal** leiomyoma is *most* likely associated with menorrhagia. Dysmenorrhea is a possible clinical finding but not the most likely.

25. **b.** Two contiguous masses are distorting the outer portion of the uterus. In an asymptomatic patient, this is most consistent with two adjacent subserosal fibroids.

26. **a.** The uterine and cervix display a posterior tilt consistent with a *retroverted* position. The subserosal fibroids are located on the anterior surface of a retroverted uterus.

27. **b.** The presence of multiple small follicles around the periphery of the ovary is *most* suspicious for polycystic ovarian disease.

28. **c.** Clinical findings in polycystic ovary disease include irregular menses, hirsutism, obesity, and infertility.

29. **a.** A small cystic structure in the cervix demonstrating posterior acoustic enhancement is most likely a nabothian cyst. A gartner duct cyst is located in the vagina.

30. **b.** A multilocular complex mass demonstrating smooth, thick wall margins is *most* suspicious for a mucinous cystadenoma. Cystadenocarcinoma is a differential consideration. Small clusters of cysts are the typical sonographic findings in surface epithelial cysts.

31. **c.** The hyperechoic mass is identified within the endometrium, most suspicious for an endometrial polyp.

32. **c.** Asherman syndrome is a result of adhesions within the endometrial cavity making it difficult to distinguish the endometrium on ultrasound. Bright endometrial echoes within the endometrium are also associated with Asherman syndrome.

33. **d.** A coexisting adnexal or ovarian mass is commonly associated with ovarian torsion. Other sonographic findings include decreased or absent blood flow to the ovary and a large heterogeneous ovarian mass.

34. **d.** Polycystic ovarian disease is a result of an endocrine imbalance causing chronic anovulation. Clinical findings include hirsutism, irregular menses, infertility, and obesity.

35. **b.** Serous and mucinous cystadenomas are a common cause of a rapid increasing pelvic mass. A rapid increase in a leiomyoma is highly suspicious for malignancy.

36. **c.** Surface epithelial cysts arise from the cortex of the ovary, appearing on ultrasound as a small cluster of ovarian cysts.

37. **d.** Submucosal fibroids distort the endometrium and are most likely to cause menstrual abnormalities and infertility.

38. **b.** Sonographic characteristics of a fibroma are similar to those of a leiomyoma.

39. **c.** Multiple serpentine vascular structure *within* the myometrium following a dilation and curettage (D&C) are most suspicious for an arteriovenous abnormality. Risk factors for development of an AV fistula of the uterus include pelvic surgery, pelvic trauma, gestational trophoblastic disease, and malignancy.

40. **a.** Ovarian carcinoma generally appears as an irregular hypoechoic ovarian mass on ultrasound.

41. **c.** An endometrial thickness of 2 cm is abnormal regardless of the menstrual status and is suspicious for proliferation of the endometrium.

42. **b.** Cystic teratomas (dermoids) arise from the wall of a follicle and may contain fat, hair, skin, and bone.

43. **a.** Multiparity, elevated estrogen, and aggressive curettage are risk factors associated with development of adenomyosis. Polycystic ovary disease is a result of an endocrine imbalance causing chronic anovulation.

44. **b.** A benign stromal mass, the thecoma appears as a hyperechoic ovarian mass with prominent posterior acoustic shadowing. Fibromas *may* demonstrate posterior shadowing.

45. **c.** An intramural fibroid distorts the myometrium, and a submucosal fibroid distorts the endometrium.

46. **c.** A small cyst within the vagina is termed a *gartner duct cyst*. Nabothian cysts are cervical in location.

47. **c.** A heterogeneous *intrauterine mass* in a patient with postmenopausal bleeding is suspicious for a uterine malignancy.

48. **c.** The cystic teratoma (dermoid) is the most common benign neoplasm of the ovary. The serous cystadenoma is the second most common benign ovarian neoplasm.

49. **c.** An *ill-defined*, multilocular, complex ovarian mass is *most* suspicious for a cystadenocarcinoma. Cystadenomas generally demonstrate smooth wall margins.

50. **a.** *Meigs syndrome* is a term used to describe a combination of a pleural effusion, ascites, and an ovarian mass, which resolve after surgical removal of the mass. Stein-Leventhal syndrome is a polycystic ovarian disease.

Chapter 22 Adnexal Pathology and Infertility

1. **c.** Krukenberg tumors are metastatic lesions most commonly resulting from primary gastric carcinoma. Other primary structures may include breast, large intestine, and appendix.

2. **c.** Paraovarian cysts are typically located in the broad ligament. The fallopian tube is contained within the superior portion of the broad ligament.

3. **d.** Endometriosis is a condition occurring when functional endometrial tissue invades the peritoneal cavity. Endometriomas are collections of extravasated endometrial tissue.

4. **c.** Infertility is suggested when conception does not occur within 1 year.

5. **c.** Multiple embryos are transferred to the endometrial cavity, increasing the likelihood of multiple gestations and decreasing the likelihood of ectopic pregnancy.

6. **d.** An *ill-defined*, complex adnexal mass in a patient with symptoms of an infection is most suspicious for a tubo-ovarian abscess.

7. **d.** Peritoneal inclusion cysts are caused by adhesions trapping normal secretions produced by the ovary. Clinical symptoms include lower abdominal pain and a palpable pelvic mass. Septated fluid collections *surrounding* a normal-appearing ovary are a common sonographic finding of a peritoneal inclusion cyst.

8. **c.** The GIFT technique transfers oocytes and sperm into the fallopian tube. ZIFT transfers a zygote to the fallopian tube. In vitro fertilization transfers embryos to the endometrial cavity.

9. **b.** Estradiol levels reflect the maturity of the stimulated follicles. The size and number of follicles, along with the estradiol level, determine when ovulation is induced.

10. **d.** Metastatic lesions in the adnexa (Krukenberg tumors) are more commonly associated with a primary malignancy of the gastrointestinal tract.

11. **b.** Hydrosalpinx is a common consequence of pelvic inflammatory disease. Parovarian cysts are typically located in the broad ligament and are mesothelial in origin.

12. **c.** A full luteal is expected if the endometrium is at least 11 mm in thickness in the midluteal phase. Endometrial thickness not exceeding 8 mm during the menstrual cycle is associated with a decrease in fertility.

13. **c.** GIFT, or gamete intrafallopian transfer, mixes oocytes with sperm added to the fallopian tube. ZIFT places a zygote in the fallopian tube. IVF places embryos in the endometrium.

14. **d.** Ovarian hyperstimulation syndrome is the *most* likely complication associated with ovulation induction therapy. Ultrasound examinations monitor the size and number of maturing follicles to prevent hyperstimulation and to aid in the timing of ovulatory medication.

15. **a.** Theca lutein cysts result from elevated levels of hCG and are associated with hyperstimulation of the ovaries during infertility induction therapy.

16. **b.** A circular anechoic mass is identified contiguous with the right ovary located between the uterus and ovary. This is most suspicious for a simple ovarian cyst versus paraovarian cyst.

17. **c.** Repeating the pelvic sonogram in 6 to 8 weeks is the *most* likely follow-up care on this patient. This will allow enough time for regression of a simple cyst. The size of a paraovarian cyst would remain unchanged. This cystic structure regressed and was no longer apparent in a follow-up sonogram 8 weeks later.

18. **a.** A complex mass located in the adnexa *adjacent to a normal ovary* is most suspicious for an endometrioma. Cystic teratomas involve the ovary.

19. **b.** A tubular anechoic structure courses directly to the left ovary. In a patient with a *previous* history of an infection following an appendectomy, this sonographic finding is most suspicious for a hydrosalpinx.

20. **c.** An "L-shaped" ovary is a normal anatomic ovarian variant. This irregular contour can be misdiagnosed as an isoechoic ovarian or adnexal mass.

21. **d.** The presence of five large follicles increases the likelihood of medical stimulation. In polycystic ovarian disease, the follicles are typically smaller than those identified in this sonogram.

22. **d.** Endometrial tissue within the peritoneal cavity describes endometriosis. An accumulation of ectopic endometrial tissue describes an endometrioma.

23. **a.** A hypoechoic adnexal mass in a patient with a history of endometriosis is most likely an endometrioma.

24. **d.** Massive, *bilateral* enlargement of the ovaries or adnexae should raise the suspicion of Krukenberg tumors (metastatic lesions). Primary ovarian malignancies are rarely solid.

25. **c.** A round anechoic structure is identified between the left and right ovaries. There is a separation between the mass and left ovary. These sonographic findings are

most suspicious for a paraovarian cyst. A simple ovarian cyst is a possible differential consideration.

26. **d.** Adhesions can trap fluid normally produced by the ovary. A septated fluid collection (arrowheads) surrounding an ovary is most suspicious for a peritoneal inclusion cyst.

27. **c.** An ill-defined adnexal mass in a patient with severe pelvic pain and fever is *most* suspicious for a tubo-ovarian abscess. The patient has a negative pregnancy test, making an ectopic pregnancy an unlikely differential consideration.

28. **b.** The image demonstrates a septation in the fundal portion of the endometrium with a normal appearing uterine contour consistent with a subseptate uterus. The fundal contour of the uterus appears smooth and regular, ruling out a submucosal fibroid.

29. **b.** An anechoic tubular structure contiguous with the right ovary is most suspicious for a hydrosalpinx.

30. **a.** Ascites and pleural effusion are additional findings associated with ovarian hyperstimulation syndrome.

31. **c.** Pelvic inflammatory disease (PID) is a general classification for inflammatory conditions of the cervix, uterus, ovaries, fallopian tubes, and peritoneal surfaces. It can be a result of a bacterial infection, diverticulitis, or appendicitis. Tubo-ovarian abscess is commonly a result of sexually transmitted diseases and pelvic infections.

32. **b.** During ovarian induction therapy, only follicles greater than 1 cm are measured.

33. **c.** Nabothian cysts are a common finding in the uterine cervix and would not likely cause infertility. A submucosal leiomyoma could cause infertility.

34. **b.** Paraovarian cysts are not affected by cyclic changes in hormone levels and will generally remain the same size on serial examinations.

35. **c.** Dysmenorrhea is a *common* symptom associated with endometriosis. Other symptoms may include pelvic pain, irregular menses, dyspareunia, and infertility.

36. **d.** A peritoneal inclusion cyst is a result of adhesions trapping fluid normally secreted by the ovary, creating a septated fluid collection around the ovary.

37. **d.** A hypoechoic, homogeneous adnexal mass is the most common sonographic appearance associated with an endometrioma. Other findings may include fluid/fluid levels and internal solid components.

38. **b.** Salpingitis is a result of a pelvic infection causing inflammation within the fallopian tube.

39. **d.** Under normal circumstances, a surge in luteinizing hormone stimulates ovulation. With ovarian induction therapy, intramuscular injection of human chorionic gonadotropin (hCG) triggers ovulation.

40. **b.** Scarring within the endometrium caused by a previous D&C or spontaneous abortion is termed *synechiae*.

41. **b.** Fixation of the ovaries posterior to the uterus is a sonographic finding in cases of endometriosis.

42. **d.** Depending on the severity of the infection, a tubo-ovarian abscess may present as a total breakdown of normal adnexal anatomy.

43. **a.** Inflammation of the endometrium is an *acquired* cause of infertility. Other acquired conditions include endometriosis, pelvic inflammatory disease, and Asherman syndrome. Congenital uterine anomalies are not acquired conditions.

44. **d.** Synechiae are a result of scarring caused by previous D&C or spontaneous abortion, and they demonstrate as a bright band of echoes within the endometrium.

45. **d.** A baseline study before starting ovarian induction therapy is performed to assess the ovaries for an ovarian cyst or dominant follicle and the uterus for anomalies or abnormalities.

46. **c.** A *focal* hypoechoic adnexal mass describes the sonographic appearance of an endometrioma. Sonographic findings in pelvic inflammatory disease can vary from a normal-appearing pelvis to an ill-defined multilocular adnexal mass.

47. **b.** Endometriomas are collections of ectopic endometrial tissue. Endometriosis is an acquired condition occurring when active endometrial tissue invades the peritoneal cavity (ectopic location of functional endometrial tissue). Endometrial tissue will attach to the fallopian tubes, ovaries, colon, and urinary bladder. Adenomyosis is ectopic endometrial tissue within the myometrium.

48. **d.** A submucosal fibroid distorts the endometrial cavity and is a possible cause of female infertility.

49. **a.** Sonographic findings in salpingitis include a thick wall and a nodular tubular adnexal mass demonstrating posterior acoustic enhancement. Pyosalpinx attenuates the sound wave.

50. **d.** Ovarian hyperstimulation syndrome demonstrates as a multicystic ovarian mass generally measuring greater than 5 cm in diameter.

Chapter 23 Assessment of the First Trimester

1. **c.** Ninety-five percent of ectopic pregnancies are located in the fallopian tube with the majority in the ampullary portion. Approximately 3% are located in the ovary and 2% in the cornua of the uterus.

2. **d.** Within the fallopian tube, cells of the zygote multiply, forming a cluster of cells termed the *morula*. Fluid rapidly fills the morula, forming a *blastocyst*. The blastocyst implants into the endometrium.

3. **d.** Trophoblastic tissue secretes human chorionic gonadotropin (hCG). Decidua basalis and decidua parietalis describe portions of the endometrium in relation to the implanting blastocyst.

4. **a.** Measurement of nuchal translucency is most accurate from the gestational age of 11 weeks and 0 days to 13 weeks and 6 days. Measurement exceeding 3 mm is abnormal and suspicious for fetal chromosomal abnormalities. The larger the measurement, the higher the probability that an abnormality exists.

5. **d.** The amnion attaches to the embryo at the umbilical cord insertion.

6. **b.** Measurement of gestational age begins with the mean sac diameter. After an embryo is evident, crown–rump length is the measurement of choice for determining *gestational age*. The yolk sac is the first structure visualized within the gestational sac but not used to measure gestational age.

7. **d.** Gestational weeks 6 to 10 constitute the embryonic phase or period. Weeks 11 and 12 are part of the fetal phase. The first trimester

extends through the twelfth week of pregnancy.

8. **c.** The double decidua sign is composed of the decidua capsularis and decidua parietalis, giving the appearance of a thick, hyperechoic rim surrounding an intrauterine pregnancy.

9. **b.** A *rapid* decline in serial hCG levels is most likely associated with a spontaneous abortion (miscarriage). The gestational sac will continue to expand in a blighted ovum, keeping hormone levels elevated.

10. **b.** Visualization of the amnion without a coexisting embryo is an abnormal finding. The rhombencephalon displays as a prominent cystic structure in the posterior portion of the brain during the first trimester. Prior to 6 weeks' gestation, a fetal heart rate of 100 to 115 bpm in within normal limits.

11. **b.** Implantation of the blastocyst into the endometrium may result in a low-grade hemorrhage between the uterine wall and chorionic cavity. This may result in a miscarriage but more likely will resolve over time. Vaginal spotting is the most common clinical finding.

12. **b.** The decidua parietalis (decidua vera) is the decidua exclusive of the area occupied by the implanted conceptus.

13. **c.** Mean sac diameter (MSD) is calculated by adding the length, height, and width of the gestational sac and dividing this total by three.

14. **c.** The amnion expands with the growth of the fetus and accumulation of fluid. By the sixteenth gestational week, the amnion should obliterate the chorionic cavity.

15. **c.** Hyperemesis is a common clinical finding associated with trophoblastic disease (molar pregnancy). Multifetal gestations (e.g., twins) are another consideration for hyperemesis.

16. **d.** An anechoic structure with a double decidua sign is identified in the fundal portion of the endometrium consistent with an early intrauterine pregnancy. The gestational sac is too small to considered a blighted ovum.

17. **c.** A prominent hyperechoic linear structure is identified inferior to the gestational sac consistent with an intrauterine device.

18. **d.** A normal yolk sac within the gestational sac is demonstrated in an early intrauterine pregnancy.

19. **d.** A cystic midline uterine mass in a patient with dramatic elevation in hCG levels is most suspicious for gestational trophoblastic disease (hydatidiform mole).

20. **a.** Theca lutein cysts are associated with rapidly increasing hormone levels. Approximately 40% of molar pregnancies demonstrate theca lutein cysts.

21. **a.** Hyperemesis is a common clinical symptom of rapidly increasing hormone levels associated with molar pregnancies, multiple gestation, and ovarian hyperstimulation.

22. **c.** A midline, echogenic fluid collection is identified inferior to an intrauterine pregnancy. This is most suspicious for a subchorionic hemorrhage.

23. **c.** The double decidual sign is characteristic of an intrauterine pregnancy. Myometrium surrounds the entire gestational sac, ruling out a possible cornual pregnancy.

24. **b.** The amnion displays as a thin, hyperechoic linear structure surrounding the developing embryo. This is a normal sonographic finding for an 8-week gestation.

25. **c.** An extrauterine gestational sac (double decidua sign) demonstrated in the right adnexa is most suspicious for an ectopic pregnancy.

26. **c.** Ectopic pregnancies demonstrate an abnormal rise in hCG levels.

27. **c.** The sonogram demonstrates a large intrauterine gestational sac without evidence of a yolk sac or embryo. An anembryonic pregnancy, or blighted ovum, occurs when a blastocyst implants into the endometrium, and the inner cell mass does not develop into an embryo. Pseudogestational sacs are typically much smaller.

28. **d.** A complex endometrial cavity following a therapeutic abortion, in an afebrile patient is most suspicious for retained products of conception.

29. **d.** A cystic structure in the posterior cranium between 7 and 10 gestational weeks is most likely the developing rhombencephalon. This structure will ultimately contribute to the fourth ventricle, brain stem, and cerebellum. It can be confused

with a Dandy-Walker cyst, hydrocephalus, or subarachnoid cyst.

30. **b.** The amnion obliterates the chorionic cavity by the sixteenth gestational week. The hyperechoic structure is most likely the normal amnion. An abnormal nuchal translucency is a differential consideration.

31. **a.** Nuchal translucency measuring 3 mm is a normal finding between 11 weeks and 0 days to 13 weeks and 6 days. Measurements exceeding 3 mm in thickness are abnormal, suggesting additional testing.

32. **b.** An hCG level of 750 mIU/mL 2nd IS lies within the discriminatory zone for visualization of a small normal gestational sac when using transvaginal imaging.

33. **b.** *Normal* hCG levels should double every 48 hours. Normal and abnormal levels can increase every 24 hours. Levels peak at the tenth gestational week and then begin to decline until the eighteenth week, where they level out for the duration of the pregnancy.

34. **b.** Transvaginally, failure to identify cardiac activity in a gestational sac with a mean sac diameter >16 mm is an abnormal finding. Under normal circumstances, cardiac activity should be evident with a maximum mean sac diameter of 16 mm with transvaginal imaging. Failure to identify cardiac activity in a gestational sac with an MSD of 25 mm or greater is an abnormal finding in transabdominal imaging.

35. **a.** Failure to visualize the amnion surrounding an embryo is a normal finding. Visualizing an amnion without identifying an embryo is an abnormal finding.

36. **b.** When using a transvaginal approach, failure to demonstrate a yolk sac within a mean sac diameter of >8 mm is an abnormal sonographic finding and is suspicious for an embryonic pregnancy.

37. **a.** The early gestational sac should be measured from the inner border to the inner border (anechoic area) in three planes (mean sac diameter).

38. **b.** The secondary yolk sac is located in chorionic cavity and provides nutrition to the developing embryo. Trophoblastic tissue secretes hCG.

39. **b.** *Initial* visualization of the hyperechoic choroid plexuses is expected near the tenth gestational week.

40. **c.** Vascular flow near the junction of the interstitial portion of the fallopian tube and the cornua of the uterus is increased when compared to other areas in the female pelvis. An ectopic pregnancy in this location can become life threatening.

41. **b.** Trophoblastic disease (molar pregnancy) can be attributed to trophoblastic changes in retained placental tissue or hydatid swelling in an anembryonic pregnancy (blighted ovum).

42. **d.** A heterotopic pregnancy describes the coexistence of both an extrauterine and intrauterine pregnancy. This is a rare dizygotic pregnancy. An increase in the size of an adnexal mass on serial sonograms with a coexisting intrauterine pregnancy should raise suspicion of a heterotopic pregnancy.

43. **a.** The amnion is an extraembryonic membrane that lines the chorion and contains the fetus and amniotic fluid.

44. **c.** The term *embryo* is used to describe a developing zygote through the tenth gestational week and fetus beginning in the eleventh gestational week.

45. **b.** A solid mass of cells formed by the cleavage of a fertilized ovum (zygote) is termed the *morula*. Fluid rapidly enters the morula, forming a blastocyst. The blastocyst implants into the endometrium approximately 5 to 7 days after fertilization.

46. **c.** The chorionic villi become more prolific near the implantation site, and areas away from implantation become smooth. The chorionic villi and decidua basalis form the placenta.

47. **c.** The cardiovascular system is the first to function in the developing embryo. Fluid in the fetal stomach is identified around the twelfth gestational week.

48. **c.** A hypervascular peripheral rim is displayed in both the trophoblastic tissue of an ectopic pregnancy and a corpus luteal cyst termed *ring of fire*.

49. **d.** The discriminatory zone is the threshold amount of hCG present at which there should be sonographic evidence of a gestational sac.

50. **c.** The crown–rump length is the most accurate measurement for determining gestational age.

Chapter 24 Assessment of the Second Trimester

1. **a.** The left atrium lies most posterior, closest to the fetal spine. The right ventricle lies most anterior, closest to the chest wall.

2. **a.** Abdominal circumference is measured slightly superior to the cord insertion at the junction of the left and right portal veins of the liver.

3. **a.** Cavum septum pellucidi is located in the midline portion of the anterior fetal brain, slightly inferior to the anterior horns of the lateral ventricles. It resolves approximately 2 years after birth.

4. **b.** Before 33 weeks' gestation, anterior–posterior diameter of the renal pelvis should not exceed 4 mm. After 33 weeks, normal diameter increases to 7 mm.

5. **b.** The third ventricle is visualized in the biparietal diameter along with the falx cerebri, thalamic nuclei, and the cavum septum pellucidi.

6. **b.** The umbilical arteries arise from the internal iliac (hypogastric) arteries. The placenta receives blood from the umbilical arteries.

7. **d.** Visualization of the gallbladder peaks around 20 to 32 gestational weeks and signifies the presence of a biliary tree. Normal liver function is not the sole responsibility of the biliary tree.

8. **d.** The cephalic index was devised to determine the normalcy of the shape of the fetal head. Biparietal diameter and head circumference do not account for changes in vertical cranial diameter. A normal cephalic index average just less than 80%.

9. **b.** The biparietal diameter is an accurate predictor of gestational age before 20 weeks. It is the most widely used biometric parameter for determining gestational age starting in the second trimester of pregnancy. The abdominal circumference is difficult to obtain and is a great predictor of fetal *growth*, not gestational age.

10. **c.** Choroid plexus cysts can be a normal finding and are typically identified between 16 and 23 gestational weeks. They should regress by 26 weeks' gestation. They can be associated with trisomy 18.

11. **c.** In the coronal plane, the normal fetal spine displays three parallel hyperechoic lines. Two curvilinear hyperechoic lines are demonstrated in the sagittal plane.

12. **b.** The normal cervical length ranges from 2.5 to 4.0 cm. In the second trimester, a cervical length less than 2.5 cm is worrisome for early cervical incompetence. Multiple measurements and imaging techniques should be used when evaluating cervical competence.

13. **d.** The ductus venosus, foramen Ovale, and the ductus arteriosus are fetal cardiac shunts. Foramen Monroe is part of the ventricular system connecting the third and paired lateral ventricles.

14. **c.** The lithotomy position is the preferred position for translabial and transvaginal imaging.

15. **a.** The foramen Ovale shunts blood between the atria of the fetal heart. The ductus arteriosus connects the main pulmonary artery with the descending aorta.

16. **d.** The arrow is pointing to a small midline "box" in the anterior portion of the fetal brain at the level of the thalami. This most likely represents the cavum septum pellucidi.

17. **b.** The sonogram displays a normal chest, abdomen, and diaphragm in a late second-trimester fetus. The image is off midline, displaying only a portion of the fetal heart.

18. **b.** An elongated anechoic structure is located in the right upper quadrant, posterior to the fetal liver and lateral to the umbilical vein. This is most consistent with a normal fetal gallbladder.

19. **b.** Arrow A points to one side of a dumbbell-shaped solid structure located in the posterior fossa. This is most consistent with a lateral horn of the cerebellum. The vermis is located between the cellebellar hemispheres.

20. **c.** Arrow B points to a fluid space between the cerebellum and calvarium. This is most consistent with the cisterna magna.

21. **b.** The arrow identifies a smooth, elongated solid structure inferior to the fetal stomach. This is most likely a normal left kidney.

22. **a.** A round anechoic structure is identified in the pelvic midline. This is most likely the urinary bladder.

23. **a.** Echogenic foci within the fetal stomach are normal incidental findings, thought to be a result of the fetus swallowing vernix in the amniotic fluid. It is associated in 30% of Down syndrome cases.

24. **d.** The sonogram displays a normal right ventricular outflow tract.

25. **b.** The calipers are measuring a dumbbell-shaped structure in the posterior fossa. This is most consistent with the normal cerebellum.

26. **b.** A low-lying placenta is located within 2 cm of the internal os. This placenta margin exceeds 2 cm.

27. **b.** The placenta is located on the anterior wall of the amniotic cavity and clear of the internal cervical os. A lateral placenta or anterior fundal placenta is possible, but the question states, "*This image* displays the location of the placenta . . ."

28. **a.** The arrow identifies a *round* anechoic structure in the upper fetal abdomen. This is most suspicious for the fetal stomach. Gallbladder displays an elongated shape.

29. **c.** The image displays three parallel hyperechoic lines in the lumbar portion of the spine consistent with a coronal imaging plane. The arrows identify the normal tapering of the vertebral ossification centers between the sacroiliac joints.

30. **d.** The normal fetal spine imaged in the transverse plane displays three equidistant ossification centers surrounding the spinal (neural) canal.

31. **d.** The abdominal circumference is measured slightly superior to the cord insertion at the junction of the left and right portal veins (hockey stick).

32. **b.** Elevation in maternal alpha-fetoprotein levels can be a result of an abdominal wall defect, underestimation of gestational age, multifetal gestations, open neural tube defect, fetal-maternal hemorrhage, and fetal demise.

33. **b.** The biparietal diameter (BPD) is measured in a transverse axial plane that includes the third ventricle, falx cerebri, thalamic nuclei, cavum septum pellucidi, and the antrum of the lateral ventricle.

34. **a.** The left ventricular outflow tract denotes the ascending aorta, and the right ventricular outflow tract denotes the pulmonary artery.

35. **d.** The fetus becomes the major producer of amniotic fluid by 16 weeks through swallowing and urine production. Amniotic fluid volume provides information regarding renal and placental function.

36. **c.** The atrium of the lateral ventricle should not exceed 10 mm throughout the pregnancy.

37. **b.** Low maternal AFP levels are associated with chromosomal abnormalities. Increases in AFP are suspicious for neural tube and abdominal wall defects.

38. **d.** The papillary muscle is commonly displayed in the left ventricle of the fetal heart as a small echogenic focus within the ventricle.

39. **b.** The umbilical cord inserts into the fetal abdomen at a level superior to the bladder and inferior to the liver and adrenal glands.

40. **c.** The length of the cervix determines cervical competence.

41. **b.** Ossification of the cranium begins around the ninth gestational week.

42. **b.** Oxygenated blood leaves the placenta and *enters the fetus* through the umbilical vein. After entering the fetal abdomen, blood courses through the ductus venosum to the right atrium of the heart.

43. **b.** Nuchal thickness is measured in the axial plane at a level to include the cerebellum, cisterna magna, and cavum septum pellucidi. Thickening is associated with aneuploidy and is accurate up to 20 weeks' gestation.

44. **b.** During the second trimester, the normal small bowel is moderately echogenic and hyperechoic compared to the normal liver and large intestines and is hypoechoic compared to fetal bone.

45. **b.** Swirling echogenic debris within the amniotic cavity (vernix) is a normal sonographic finding. Vernix can collect in the fetal stomach and demonstrate as a focal echogenic mass within the stomach.

46. **b.** The fetus *becomes* the major producer of amniotic fluid through swallowing and urine production after 16 weeks (early second trimester).

47. **d.** Presence of the cavum septum pellucidi excludes most central nervous anomalies.

48. **d.** Meconium is a material that collects in the intestines of the fetus, forming the first stool of a newborn.

49. **b.** The head circumference is measured in a plane that must include the cavum septum pellucidi and the tentorium.

50. **d.** Abdominal circumference is a better predictor of fetal *growth* than gestational age. Up to 20 weeks, biparietal diameter is a good predictor of gestational age.

Chapter 25 Assessment of the Third Trimester

1. **b.** Maternal hypertension increases the risk of intrauterine growth restriction by 25%. The fetus has major control over the amniotic fluid volume through swallowing and urine production.

2. **d.** An amniotic fluid index (AFI) exceeding 24 cm is termed *polyhydramnios*. AFI greater than 24 cm is consistently associated with co-existing fetal anomalies.

3. **c.** By 32 weeks' gestation, the distal femoral epiphysis is consistently visualized. A few weeks later, the proximal tibial epiphysis can be visualized.

4. **c.** By the third trimester, the fetus is the major producer of amniotic fluid. Decrease in urine production from genitourinary abnormalities is the most likely fetal contributor to oligohydramnios.

5. **d.** Maternal obesity and diabetes are common causes of macrosomia. Maternal hypertension and cigarette smoking can contribute to a reduction in normal fetal growth.

6. **c.** Amniotic fluid volume is a chronic marker of fetal hypoxia. Acute markers of fetal hypoxia include fetal breathing movement, fetal tone, nonstress test, and fetal movement.

7. **d.** When measuring amniotic fluid volume, the transducer must remain *perpendicular* to the maternal *coronal* plane and *parallel* to the maternal *sagittal* plane.

8. **d.** A gestation greater than 42 weeks is considered postterm. The third trimester covers weeks 27 to 42.

9. **a.** *Symmetrical* IUGR is a result of *embryologic* disturbance. Asymmetrical IUGR is associated with maternal hypertension and placental insufficiency.

10. **d.** The systolic-to-diastolic ratio of the umbilical artery can evaluate fetal well-being after 30 weeks' gestation.

A ratio greater than 3.0 is abnormal. Absence or reversal of the diastolic component is also abnormal.

11. **c.** Macrosomia is a condition in which accelerated fetal growth results in an infant with a birth weight greater than 4000 grams in a nondiabetic mother or greater than 4500 grams in a diabetic mother or a fetal weight above the 90th percentile for gestational age.

12. **d.** Fetal tone is one of five parameters included in a biophysical profile. One complete episode of flexion to extension and back to flexion documents fetal tone. Three separate fetal movements document fetal movement.

13. **c.** Frank breech describes a fetal position in which both the head and feet are located in the uterine fundus with the buttocks as the presenting part. Footling or incomplete breech demonstrate one or both feet as the presenting part. With a complete breech position, the knees are bent with the feet down near the buttocks.

14. **b.** Maternal hypertension is defined as a systolic pressure above 140 mm Hg or a diastolic pressure above 90 mm Hg.

15. **b.** An amniotic fluid index (AFI) below 5 cm or a single largest pocket below 2 cm defines oligohydramnios.

16. **b.** This single image displays an excessive amount of amniotic fluid in relation to the fetus. This is most suspicious for polyhydramnios.

17. **a.** The image is taken in the maternal transverse plane. The fetus displays a cross-section image in this plane. Therefore, the fetus is lying spine down, parallel with the maternal sagittal plane. Breech versus cephalic presentation can be determined by the fetal heart. The apex of the fetal heart points to the left side of the body. The left side of the fetus is lying on the left side of the mother. In order for the fetus to lie supine with the left side of the body on the maternal left, the head must be located in the superior portion of the uterus breech.

18. **a.** Severe oligohydramnios is present in this third-trimester gestation.

19. **d.** In the third trimester, premature rupture of membranes is a probable cause of severe oligohydramnios.

Genitourinary abnormalities can cause oligohydramnios, but multicystic renal dysplasia is typically a unilateral disease that does not generally affect amniotic fluid production.

20. **a.** The placenta is located on the anterior surface of the gestational sac.

21. **a.** A slight increase in amniotic fluid is present in this one image. The sonographer needs to evaluate and document the amniotic fluid index to rule out polyhydramnios.

22. **b.** Determining the fetal gender is not an indication for a third trimester ultrasound.

23. **c.** During the late second trimester and early third trimester, the circumference of the fetal head is slightly larger than the circumference of the abdomen. During the late third trimester, with the increase of fetal body fat, the abdominal circumference is typically equal to or slightly larger than the head circumference.

24. **d.** Placental insufficiency is the most *common* cause of intrauterine growth restriction (IUGR). Other factors associated with IUGR include maternal hypertension, chromosomal abnormalities, and uterine infection.

25. **b.** Abdominal circumference, biparietal diameter and femur length are the most common biometric measurements used to calculate estimated fetal weight.

26. **b.** The liver is one of the most severely affected fetal organs. Decrease in liver size results in a decrease in abdominal circumference.

27. **c.** The amniotic fluid index (AFI) is a technique for assessing amniotic fluid volume by using the sum of four equal quadrants.

28. **c.** The abdominal circumference is the *single* most sensitive indicator of intrauterine growth restriction (IUGR).

29. **a.** Fetuses with macrosomia have an increased incidence of morbidity and mortality resulting from head injuries and cord compression during delivery.

30. **b.** Of all the techniques to assess amniotic fluid volume, the amniotic fluid index (AFI) is both valid and reproducible.

31. **c.** The umbilical cord and fetal lungs produce and remove amniotic fluid.

32. **c.** Complete extension and flexion of both lower extremities (2 points). Minimum of three separate fetal movements (2 points). Amniotic fluid volume above 5 cm (2 points). Normal nonstress test (2 points). No fetal breathing movement (0 points).

33. **d.** The gastrointestinal tract is the primary source of amniotic fluid removal through swallowing and fluid absorption in the intestines.

34. **c.** A decrease in the growth of the abdominal circumference with appropriate growth of the fetal head circumference and femur length on serial examinations is the expected sonographic finding in asymmetrical IUGR cases.

35. **d.** A fetal weight at or below the 10th percentile for gestational age defines IUGR.

36. **d.** Evaluation of the amniotic fluid volume, estimated fetal weight, and maternal blood pressure has the best diagnostic accuracy in determining intrauterine growth restriction.

37. **b.** Placenta previa is a possible cause of a transverse fetal lie in the late third trimester. Polyhydramnios typically allows free fetal movement.

38. **d.** Incomplete or footling breech places the fetal foot as the presenting part and places the greatest risk for cord prolapse.

39. **c.** A biophysical profile is a sonographic method for evaluating fetal well-being by displaying specific movements, responses, and amount of amniotic fluid.

40. **d.** The fetal genitourinary system helps to regulate the amount of amniotic fluid surrounds the fetus. Amniotic fluid volume may decrease with certain types of genitourinary abnormalities (renal agenesis) or remain within normal limits (multicystic dysplastic disease).

41. **c.** Maternal risk factors for developing intrauterine growth restricted fetus include hypertension, poor nutrition, and drug or alcohol abuse.

42. **a.** A minimum of 7 days (1 week) between sonographic evaluations is necessary to determine interval fetal growth.

43. **c.** Proteins, calcium, iron, and carbohydrates are stored in the placenta and released into the fetal circulation. The amniotic fluid protects the fetus from injury, allows the fetus

free movement within the amniotic cavity, promotes lung growth and development maintains intrauterine temperature, and prevents adherence of the amnion to the fetus.

44. **c.** The biparietal diameter continues appropriate growth whereas the abdominal circumference demonstrates a decrease in growth in cases of asymmetrical intrauterine growth restriction (IUGR). A small placenta, oligohydramnios, and normal femur growth are additional sonographic findings associated with asymmetrical IUGR.

45. **b.** The kidneys are the primary source of amniotic fluid production.

46. **d.** The abdominal circumference is probably the single most useful parameter for assessing fetal *growth*.

47. **b.** Presentation of the fetal head in the uterine fundus and the lower extremities or buttocks in the lower uterine segment describes a breech presentation.

48. **b.** Breech presentation in the third trimester may increase cranial pressure, resulting in an elongated appearance to the pliable fetal cranium (dolicocephalic).

49. **d.** A transverse fetal presentation is perpendicular to the maternal sagittal plane.

50. **d.** The proximal tibial epiphysis is first visualized around 35 gestational weeks. Visualization of the distal femoral epiphysis first occurs near 32 gestational weeks.

Chapter 26 Fetal Abnormalities

1. **b.** Ebstein anomaly is a congenital defect in which the septal and posterior leaflets of the tricuspid valve are displaced toward the apex of the right ventricle of the heart.

2. **b.** *Unilateral demonstration* of multiple renal cysts is most suspicious for a multicystic dysplastic kidney. With infantile polycystic disease, multiple cysts are too small to visualize, giving the kidneys an enlarged hyperechoic appearance.

3. **c.** The dilated stomach and proximal duodenum found in duodenal atresia produces a sonographic sign termed the *double bubble sign.*

4. **b.** Both Dandy-Walker syndrome and arachnoid cysts will splay the hemispheres of the cerebellum. Dandy-Walker syndrome additionally displays a complete or partial

absence of the vermis, whereas an arachnoid cyst demonstrates a normal cerebellar vermis.

5. **d.** Agenesis of the corpus callosum (midline structure) demonstrates a dilation of the third ventricle and outward angling of the frontal and lateral horns on ultrasound. Holoprosencephaly displays a large, single central ventricle with an absence of the midline structures including the third ventricle.

6. **a.** Marked increases in maternal alpha-fetoprotein levels are expected in cases of gastroschisis.

7. **d.** Thanatophoric dysplasia is a lethal skeletal dysplasia demonstrating severe rhizomelia, bell-shaped chest, and a cloverleaf skull.

8. **c.** A crescent-shaped cerebellum (banana sign) raises suspicion of spina bifida and signals the sonographer to give additional evaluation and documentation of the fetal spine.

9. **d.** Abdominal calcifications with associated dilated bowel and polyhydramnios are suspicious for meconium peritonitis.

10. **b.** Anencephaly is the *most common* neural tube defect.

11. **c.** Protrusion of the forehead (frontal bossing) is most likely associated with hydrocephalus. The forehead is absent in anencephaly, and an encephalocele is more commonly located in the occipital region of the head.

12. **a.** An encephalocele is defined as the extension of a brain-filled sac through a bony calvarium defect.

13. **b.** Facial abnormalities frequently affect the ability of the fetus to swallow, resulting in polyhydramnios.

14. **d.** Osteogenesis imperfecta is a collagen disorder leading to brittle bones and bone fractures.

15. **c.** A large central single ventricle is most suspicious for alobar holoprosencephaly. Hydranencephaly is an abnormality of the brain tissue.

16. **b.** The lateral ventricle measures 1.1 cm, consistent with mild ventricular enlargement. The occipital horn is generally the first portion to dilate.

17. **d.** A solid mass is extending from the posterior buttock. The sacrum and skin line appear normal. This is most suspicious for a sacrococcygeal teratoma.

18. **c.** A sacrococcygeal teratoma demonstrates a normal spine and may extend into the pelvis and abdomen, displacing the urinary bladder and resulting in hydronephrosis.

19. **c.** An enlarged hyperechoic kidney is present, most suspicious for infantile polycystic kidney disease.

20. **d.** Infantile polycystic disease demonstrates severe oligohydramnios and the absence of urine in the fetal bladder.

21. **b.** An anechoic renal pelvis is *most* suspicious for hydronephrosis, likely a result of ureteropelvic junction obstruction. Renal cysts are uncommon findings.

22. **a.** The fetal forehead is present. Fetal brain is present above the orbits, but the calvarium does not appear calcified. This is most suspicious for acrania.

23. **a.** An open spinal defect is displayed in the sacral portion of the fetal spine. An anechoic mass extending from the defect is most likely a myelocele.

24. **c.** A multilocular cystic cervical mass is contiguous with the posterior surface of the fetal head and neck. This is most suspicious for a cystic hygroma.

25. **d.** A cystic hygroma is a classic sonographic finding in Turner syndrome (chromosomal abnormality).

26. **b.** The cerebrum and skull are absent with the presence of orbits and brainstem most suspicious for anencephaly. Microcephaly relates to the overall size of the cranium. Acrania will eventually result in anencephaly from exposure of the brain tissue to the amniotic fluid.

27. **d.** Anencephaly is the most common neural tube defect and typically demonstrates elevation in maternal alpha-fetoprotein levels.

28. **d.** An abnormal formation of the bronchial tree replaces normal pulmonary tissue with cysts. On ultrasound, a cystic mass identified in the fetal chest is most suspicious for cystic adenomatoid malformation.

29. **c.** A large single ventricle with fused thalami is most suspicious for holoprosencephaly. Hydranencephaly is a destruction of brain tissue, not a congenital malformation.

30. **d.** Demonstration of multiple *unilateral* renal cysts is most suspicious for a multicystic dysplastic kidney.

Hydronephrosis is a differential consideration but not the most likely diagnosis. Additional congenital renal anomalies occur in up to 40% of cases.

31. c. Lateral ventricular enlargement exceeding 10 mm defines ventriculomegaly (hydrocephalus).

32. d. Caudal regression syndrome is a neural tube defect seen almost exclusively in diabetic patients. Fetuses demonstrate fusion of the pelvis with short legs.

33. c. Cystic hygroma is the most common fetal neck mass caused by an obstruction of the lymphatic system.

34. c. Holoprosencephaly is the most likely abnormality to demonstrate a proboscis or cyclopia.

35. a. Pulmonary hypoplasia is a lethal condition associated in cases of oligohydramnios, genitourinary abnormalities, diaphragmatic hernia, skeletal dysplasia, and chromosomal abnormalities.

36. d. Diagnosis of clubfoot (talipes) is made with persistent abnormal inversion of the foot at an angle perpendicular to the lower leg.

37. a. Gastroschisis is a defect involving all layers of the anterior abdominal wall. Small bowel herniates through the defect, floating freely within the amniotic cavity. Gastroschisis is not typically associated with other fetal anomalies.

38. a. Achondroplasia is a nonlethal skeletal dysplasia with abnormal cartilage deposits at the long bone epiphysis. Diastrophic dysplasia is a very rare autosomal-recessive disorder characterized by micromelia, talipes, cleft palate, and hand abnormalities.

39. d. An obstruction at the ureteropelvic junction (UPJ) is the most common cause for hydronephrosis in utero and in the neonate.

40. b. The contents of an omphalocele are covered by a membrane consisting of the amnion and peritoneum.

41. c. Presence of a posterior fossa cyst and *agenesis of the cerebellar vermis* is characteristic of Dandy-Walker malformation.

42. d. Common causes of hydrocephalus include spina bifida, encephalocele, Dandy-Walker malformation, agenesis of the corpus callosum, holoprosencephaly, and aqueduct stenosis.

43. b. Replacement of *brain tissue* with anechoic masses is most suspicious for hydranencephaly. Hydranencephaly results from vascular compromise or congenital infection.

44. d. Failure of the callosal fibers to form a normal connection result in agenesis of the corpus callosum. Outward angling of the frontal and lateral horns of the lateral ventricles (steer sign) is a characteristic sonographic finding associated with agenesis of the corpus callosum.

45. b. Pelviectasis greater than or equal to 10 mm is consistent with mild hydronephrosis. An anterior–posterior diameter of less than 4 mm before 33 weeks' gestation and less than or equal to 7 mm after 33 weeks is within normal limits.

46. c. The fetus is the major producer of amniotic fluid after 16 weeks' gestation. Renal agenesis is generally bilateral and results in severe oligohydramnios.

47. a. Multicystic renal dysplasia is generally a unilateral disease presenting as multiple renal cysts of varying sizes.

48. c. Demineralization of the bone or abnormal limb length or shape may not be apparent before 24 weeks' gestation.

49. b. Type II is most severe, demonstrating hypomineralization, a thin cranium, bell-shaped chest, significant bone shortening, and multiple fractures involving the long bones, ribs, and spine.

50. c. Esophageal atresia is difficult to diagnose with sonography. Absence of the fetal stomach or a consistently small fetal stomach on serial sonograms is suspicious for esophageal atresia especially when accompanied by polyhydramnios.

Chapter 27 Complications in Pregnancy

1. c. Eighty percent of Edward syndrome cases (trisomy 18) are associated with a clenched fetal fist. Clinodactyly is associated with Down syndrome.

2. c. Generalized massive edema (anasarca) is often seen in cases of fetal hydrops.

3. c. Sonographic findings associated with Beckwith-Wiedemann syndrome include macroglossia, omphalocele, and hemihypertrophy.

4. b. Eagle-Barrett syndrome (prune belly) is associated with hydronephrosis, megaureter, and oligohydramnios.

5. c. A fetal weight discordance of ≥20% defines twin–twin transfusion syndrome. The donor twin may display oligohydramnios and IUGR whereas the receiving twin may display polyhydramnios and fetal hydrops.

6. b. Duodenal atresia is associated in approximately 30% of Down syndrome cases.

7. d. *Fetal papyraceous* is a term used to describe a twin pregnancy in which one twin has died and is too large to reabsorb.

8. d. In twin–twin transfusion syndrome, *arterial* blood from the *donor* twin pumps into the venous system of the *receiving* twin.

9. b. Syndactyly describes a fusion of the fingers or toes. The prefix *syn* defines the joining or union of structures.

10. b. Meckel-Gruber syndrome is associated with infantile polycystic disease, nonvisualization of the fetal bladder, *encephalocele*, and polydactyly.

11. a. IUGR is the most common cause of a discordant growth in dichorionic multifetal gestation. Twin–twin transfusion syndrome is the most common cause of discordant growth in monochorionic twin gestation.

12. b. VACTERL is associated with maternal diabetes and lead exposure.

13. b. Inward curving of the fifth finger (clinodactyly) is associated with Down syndrome. Polydactyly is associated with Patau (trisomy 13) and Meckel-Gruber syndromes.

14. c. VATER is a group of complex anomalies: vertebral defects, anal atresia, tracheoesophageal fistula and renal anomalies.

15. a. Trisomy 13 is also known as Patau syndrome. Edward syndrome is also known as trisomy 18. Triploidy demonstrates three complete sets of chromosomes.

16. c. Both twins are viable with Twin 2 (left of screen) demonstrates a poorly developed upper body consistent with an acardiac twin pregnancy (twin-reversal arterial perfusion TRAP).

17. a. Separation of the big toe from the other digits is a sonographic finding termed *sandal toe.*

18. c. "Sandal toe" is a sonographic finding associated with trisomy 21 (Down syndrome).

19. d. A single anechoic cyst is located within each choroid plexus.

20. b. Choroid plexus cysts are generally incidental findings that resolve by 23 gestational weeks. Occasionally, these cysts are associated with trisomy 18.

21. d. A multilocular cervical mass demonstrating a thin membrane extends from the posterior neck of the fetus. This most likely represents a cystic hygroma.

22. b. Cystic hygroma is a common sonographic finding in Turner syndrome. Turner syndrome can elevate the maternal alpha-fetoprotein levels. Meckel-Gruber syndrome is associated with an encephalocele and infantile polycystic renal disease.

23. c. This sonogram demonstrates fetal hydrops and anasarca. Identification of intraabdominal fluid (ascites) is a sonographic finding in fetal hydrops.

24. c. The anterior abdominal walls of this twin pregnancy are conjoined. Because *this* image is at the abdominal level, diagnosis of acardiac twin is not possible.

25. a. A membrane is present between the two fetuses (diamniotic). It is too early to determine placenta number and location (dichorionic).

26. d. Nuchal thickness greater than 6 mm is abnormal and suspicious for Down syndrome (trisomy 21). Measurement of nuchal thickness is accurate up to 20 weeks' gestation.

27. d. Approximately 30% of trisomy 21 cases are associated with duodenal atresia.

28. b. Holoprosencephaly and polydactyly are findings associated with trisomy 13. Other abnormalities include microcephaly, enlarged cisterna magna, agenesis of the corpus callosum, omphalocele, bladder exstrophy, and echogenic bowel

29. a. Clubfoot or rocker bottom feet are associated with trisomy 13.

30. b. Preeclampsia is an abnormal condition of pregnancy characterized by the onset of acute hypertension after the 24th week of gestation. The classic triad of symptoms includes maternal hypertension, proteinuria, and edema. The cause of the condition is unknown.

31. d. Preterm labor is the onset of labor before the 37th gestational week. A full-term pregnancy ranges between 37 and 42 gestational weeks.

32. d. Division of the zygote 4 to 8 days after fertilization will demonstrate two amnions (two gestational sacs) and one chorion (one shared placenta).

33. c. In twin–twin transfusion syndrome, the arterial blood of the donor twin shunts into the venous system of the recipient twin.

34. b. The recipient twin receives too much blood and may acquire hydrops fetalis, placentomegaly, and polyhydramnios. The donor twin may display IUGR and oligohydramnios.

35. d. Two individual amnions will demonstrate two separate gestational sacs. Monoamniotic pregnancies can demonstrate two allantoic ducts, yolk sacs, and embryos. Dichorionic pregnancies will demonstrate two individual placentas.

36. d. Fetal hydrops is an abnormal accumulation of fluid in the body cavities and soft tissue of the fetus. This can result in anasarca, scalp edema, pleural effusion, abdominal ascites, and pericardial effusion. Additional findings include placenta edema and polyhydramnios.

37. c. Fetal hydrops resulting from fetal *tachycardia* will commonly demonstrate a fetal heart rate of 200 to 240 beats per minute. Normal fetal cardiac rhythm ranges from 120 to 160 beats per minute.

38. c. Fraternal or dizygotic twins arise from separate ova that are individually fertilized.

39. b. Amniotic bands are fibrous strands of sticky amnion that may entangle fetal parts causing amputations or malformations of the fetus.

40. d. The ruptured sticky amnion entangles fetal parts resulting in amputation.

41. d. Beckwith-Wiedemann syndrome demonstrates a normal karyotype and is associated with hemihypertrophy, macroglossia, and omphalocele.

42. a. Two zygotes will always demonstrate dichorionic/diamniotic gestational sacs.

43. b. Eclampsia is the gravest form of pregnancy-induced maternal hypertension, characterized by seizures, proteinuria, edema, and coma.

44. c. Premature rupture of membranes (PROM) is defined as the leakage of part or all of the amniotic fluid.

45. a. Acardiac twin is a rare anomaly of a monozygotic pregnancy. The acardiac twin demonstrates a poorly developed upper body and an absent or rudimentary heart and receives blood through the normal twin gestation.

46. c. Eagle-Barrett syndrome (prunebelly) is manifested by dilatation of the renal collecting system. Sonographic findings include hydronephrosis, megaureter, oligohydramnios, small thorax, large abdomen, scoliosis, hip subluxation or dislocation, and cryptorchidism.

47. a. Acardiac twins shunt blood from the vein of one twin to the other or from one artery to the other. Twin–twin transfusion syndrome demonstrates an arteriovenous anastomosis.

48. c. Holoprosencephaly is a common abnormality associated with trisomy 13. Other associated abnormalities include microcephaly, polydactyly, echogenic kidneys, facial anomalies, cardiac defects, intrauterine growth restriction, abnormal cisterna magna, and echogenic cardiac focus.

49. b. Pentalogy of Cantrell is a congenital disorder characterized by two major defects—ectopia cordis and an abdominal wall defect.

50. b. Inward curving of the fifth finger (clinodactyly) is associated with Down syndrome.

Chapter 28 Placenta and Umbilical Cord

1. c. Placenta accreta describes a condition where the chorionic villi of the placenta are in direct contact with the superficial myometrium.

2. a. In a low-lying placenta, the edge of the placental margin lies within 2 cm of the internal os. With a marginal placenta previa, the edge of the placenta abuts the cervical os.

3. c. Focal dilatation of the umbilical *vein* is commonly located in an *extrahepatic* portion of the fetal abdomen.

4. a. The umbilical cord is *covered* by the amnion, and Wharton's jelly *surrounds* the vessels within the umbilical cord.

5. **a.** *Battledore placenta* is a term used to describe an umbilical cord insertion into the end margin of the placenta.

6. **b.** Placenta accreta is a condition where the chorionic villi growth invades the superficial layer of the myometrium, disrupting the normal uteroplacental vessels and myometrial border (retroplacental complex).

7. **a.** The cervical canal extends from the internal os to the uterus. The external os extends to the vagina.

8. **c.** The length of the umbilical cord during the first trimester is equal to the crown–rump length of the fetus.

9. **b.** Clinical findings associated with placental abruption include severe pelvic pain and vaginal bleeding. Painless vaginal bleeding is a classic symptom of placenta previa.

10. **a.** The umbilical arteries arise from the hypogastric arteries of the fetus. Each hypogastric artery courses alongside the fetal bladder and returns venous blood from the fetus back to the placenta.

11. **d.** Placenta percreta is a condition where the chorionic villi of the placenta encroach through the myometrial and serosal layer of the uterus into the adjacent organs (maternal urinary bladder).

12. **d.** The chorion frondosum develops into the fetal side of the placenta. Chorionic villi are the vascular projections of the chorion at the placental site.

13. **d.** Circumvallate placenta is a condition in which the chorionic plate is smaller than the basal plate, resulting in attachment of the placental membrane to the fetal surface of the placenta.

14. **c.** A true nuchal cord demonstrates *two* or *more* complete loops of umbilical cord *around* the fetal neck. This is can be a significant finding during the late third trimester or in cases of oligohydramnios.

15. **c.** A marginal placenta previa abuts but does not cross the internal cervical os. A low-lying placenta lies close to but does not border the cervix.

16. **b.** The placenta is completely covering the internal cervical os. The hypoechoic area is the retroplacental complex, not infiltration of the placenta into the myometrium demonstrated with placenta accreta.

17. **d.** Painless vaginal bleeding is the most common clinical finding associated with placenta previa, especially during the third trimester. A transverse fetal presentation can be associated with placenta previa.

18. **a.** The image is sagittal and the placenta is located within the most superior portion of the uterine fundus.

19. **a.** A circular homogeneous hypoechoic placental mass is most likely a chorioangioma arising from the amnion surface of the placenta.

20. **b.** A small piece of solid tissue, similar in echogenicity to the placenta, lies adjacent to the primary anterior placenta. This is most suspicious for a succenturiate placenta.

21. **c.** Two vessels of similar size are contained within the umbilical cord. This is consistent with a single umbilical artery.

22. **c.** Cases of single umbilical arteries are more common in multifetal gestations. In this case, the umbilical cord demonstrated both two umbilical arteries and one umbilical artery within the same cord. A single umbilical artery is associated with malformations of all major organ systems and chromosomal abnormalities.

23. **d.** A shortening of the cervical length is consistent with an incompetent cervix. A small amount of amniotic fluid is funneling within the dilated cervix.

24. **c.** Placental abruption often presents with severe pelvic pain and bleeding. The hemorrhage is located between the uterine wall and retroplacental complex (retroplacental hemorrhage).

25. **b.** The distance from the end margin of the placenta to the internal cervical os is 2.55 cm. A low-lying placenta lies *within* 2 cm of the internal os.

26. **a.** The placenta is completely covering the internal cervical os, consistent with a complete placenta previa.

27. **d.** Painless vaginal spotting or bleeding is the most common clinical symptom associated with placenta previa.

28. **b.** An abnormal increase in placental thickness is present in this sonogram, consistent with placentomegaly. Placentomegaly in this case is a result of Rh sensitivity.

29. **b.** Placentomegaly is associated with maternal diabetes mellitus, anemia, and intrauterine infection.

30. **c.** *Velamentous* umbilical cord inserts into the amniochorionic membrane of the gestational sac adjacent to the placenta.

31. **a.** Placenta previa is the most common cause of *painless* bleeding during the third trimester. Placenta abruption is generally associated with severe pelvic pain.

32. **c.** A battledore placenta refers to the insertion of the umbilical cord into the end margin of the placenta. Circumvallate placenta demonstrates an abnormal placental shape.

33. **b.** In a marginal placenta previa, the end margin of the placenta abuts or encroaches on the internal cervical os. A complete previa will completely cover the internal cervical os.

34. **a.** Chorionic villi are the vascular projections at the implantation site and the major functioning unit of the placenta.

35. **a.** Placenta increta demonstrates chorionic villi extension into the uterine myometrium. Chorionic villus in direct contact with the maternal urinary bladder is consistent with placenta *percreta*.

36. **c.** Coiling of the cord is a normal finding. Noncoiling is associated with fetal or cord abnormalities.

37. **b.** Fibrin deposits are found throughout the placenta but more commonly beneath the chorionic plate.

38. **d.** Primary causes of placentomegaly include maternal diabetes mellitus and Rh sensitivity. Placentomegaly is associated with maternal anemia, twin–twin transfusion syndrome, fetal anomalies, and intrauterine infection.

39. **b.** Complications of placenta previa include increased risk of intrauterine growth restriction, premature delivery, and life-threatening maternal hemorrhage, stillbirth, and placenta accreta.

40. **a.** Additional placental tissue adjacent to the main placenta is termed a succenturiate or accessory placenta. This accessory is a result of the inability of the chorionic villi to atrophy.

41. **d.** A circumvallate placenta demonstrates an abnormal shape presenting with an irregular rolled-up placenta edge. The upturned placenta may contain fluid or hemorrhage.

42. **d.** Placentomalacia is associated with intrauterine growth restriction (IUGR) and intrauterine infection. Rh sensitivity, maternal anemia, and twin–twin transfusion syndrome are associated with placentomegaly.

43. **b.** The decidua basalis (maternal side) and the decidua frondosum (fetal side) form the placenta.

44. **b.** Placenta thickness will vary with gestational age but generally measures around 2 to 3 cm in greatest thickness and should not exceed 4 cm in the second trimester and 6 cm in the third trimester.

45. **d.** Placentomalacia (small placenta) is associated with chromosomal abnormalities, intrauterine growth restriction, and intrauterine infection.

46. **a.** Vasa previa occurs when large fetal vessels coursing in the fetal membranes cross the internal cervical os, placing the patient and fetus at risk.

47. **a.** An increase in the length of the umbilical cord increases the risk of nuchal cord.

48. **b.** The presence of the umbilical cord before the presenting fetal part during the birthing process describes a prolapsed cord. Focal dilatation of an umbilical vessel describes an umbilical varix. A nuchal cord surrounds the fetal neck with more than one loop.

49. **a.** A succenturiate placenta is at an increased risk for a velamentous cord insertion and is a possible cause of a vasa previa.

50. **c.** The direction of umbilical coiling is of no clinical significance.

Chapter 29 Patient Care and Interventional Procedures

1. **b.** An advance directive is a legal document describing a patient's health-care wishes, if he or she is unable to communicate them.

2. **d.** The sonographer should introduce himself or herself to the patient and explain the requested sonogram before beginning the examination. Many patients are not sure why their doctor sent them for an ultrasound. Obtaining patient history and explaining the examination are important parts of the sonographers' health-care role.

3. **d.** HIPAA oversees many health-care functions, the primary being confidentiality. Breach in a patient's confidentiality can result in large federal fines to the health-care facility and/or employee.

4. **b.** A technical report is a private communication of the real-time examination between the sonographer and the interpreting physician. This is *not* an official report, and it is never shared with the patient.

5. **c.** Suppressing or inhibiting (subjugation) a patient's self-sufficiency (autonomy) is against the patient-care partnership.

6. **d.** On completion of the examination, the sonographer should inform the patient of the expected timeframe for examination results. Reviewing examination protocols generally occurs before the examination. Clinical information is more commonly obtained before and sometimes during the examination.

7. **a.** Clean and sterilize medical imaging transducers after each use according to the manufacturer's recommendation. Supervising sonographers and infectious control departments are generally involved in the decision, but typically follow the manufacturer's recommendation (warranty).

8. **c.** Amniocentesis for genetic testing is typically performed between 15 and 18 gestational weeks.

9. **b.** The Trocar technique is one of two techniques used for abscess drainage.

10. **b.** Adherence to moral and ethical principles describes integrity.

11. **a.** Availability of face masks, spatial spacing of patients a minimum of 3 feet apart, and posting signs, in languages appropriate to the population served, with instructions to patients and family members with respiratory infections to cover their noses/mouths when sneezing or coughing, prompt disposal of used tissues, and using surgical masks on the coughing person when tolerated are required of a medical facility to promote respiratory hygiene.

12. **d.** Illnesses associated with airborne pathogens include tuberculosis, chicken pox, varicella zoster, and severe acute respiratory syndrome.

13. **c.** Only patients with airborne pathogens are required to be placed in a private room with the door closed.

14. **b.** Hands, fingers, and nails should be scrubbed a minimum of 20 seconds.

15. **d.** Proper handwashing is the best protection against the spread of disease.

16. **a.** Gloves should be worn once and then discarded with all patient contact.

17. **d.** Transmission of severe acute respiratory syndrome (SARS) may occur through airborne, contact, and droplet exposure.

18. **d.** Retrieval of mature oocytes (follicular aspiration) occurs 30-34 hours after administration of hCG.

19. **c.** Chorionic villi sampling is typically performed between 10 and 12 gestational weeks.

20. **a.** The goal of intrauterine transfusion is to correct fetal anemia and suppress fetal erythropoiesis.

21. **c.** Glutaraldehyde is a common substance used to highly disinfect ultrasound transducers. Tegaderm and acetone should not be used on ultrasound transducers.

22. **d.** Maximizing benefits and minimizing possible harm describes beneficence.

23. **d.** Contaminated linens are always placed in a leak proof bag and placed in the appropriate linen bins.

24. **d.** Coughing etiquette is mainly targeted at patients and visitors. Health-care workers should already be educated in respiratory hygiene/coughing etiquette.

25. **a.** Truthfulness and honesty describe the term veracity.

26. **b.** Standard precautions are general measures taken to keep health-care workers, patients, and the surrounding environment clean to prevent the spread of germs. Standard precautions were formally known and universal precautions and body substance isolation.

27. **d.** Patient-care partnership is a standard describing patient health-care rights.

28. **b.** Transmission based precautions must be implemented based on clinical presentation and likely

pathogens. Test results can still be pending.

29. **d.** If a person faints the sonographer should lay the person down and elevate their legs.

30. **d.** Keeping the patient relaxed, safe, and comfortable is the sonographer's responsibility.

31. **c.** Except for educational purposes all ultrasound examinations should have an order with a proper indication for examination.

32. **b.** Accountability for professional judgment and decisions is an example of sonographer ethics.

33. **a.** Ethics is a system of valued behaviors and beliefs that govern proper conduct to ensure protection of an individual's rights.

34. **b.** Autonomy is the self-governing or self-directing freedom to choose and have one's choices respected.

35. **a.** The SDMS has developed and adopted clinical standards and a code of ethics specific for diagnostic medical sonographers. JRC-DMS and CAAHEP are organizations working together for accreditation of diagnostic medical sonography programs.

36. **d.** Washing of hands before and after an examination are examples of standard precautions.

37. **c.** Illnesses associated with droplet exposure included rubella, influenza, pneumonia, meningitis, pertussis, severe acute respiratory syndrome, rhinovirus, and streptococcal disease.

38. **d.** Automated disinfectant systems decontaminate ultrasound use hydrogen peroxide vapors to decontaminate ultrasound transducers.

39. **d.** Cardiac distress is most commonly caused by heart attack, respiratory arrest, and medication interaction.

40. **a.** Reviewing previous pertinent diagnostic studies and the ultrasound referral (order) should be completed prior to beginning the examination.

41. **c.** Hysterosalpingogram is a radiological procedure to evaluate extent of duplicated uterus, patency of fallopian tubes and localizes masses. Hysterosonogram is an ultrasound procedure that evaluates the endometrium

42. **d.** Protecting the patient's medical and personal privacy (confidentiality)

is a duty of all health-care professionals.

43. **a.** Transfusion is a therapeutic indication for cordocentesis. Fetal infection, fetal hematocrit and rapid karyotyping are diagnostic indications for cordocentesis.

44. **b.** CDC (Center for Disease Control) is a federal agency that protects America from health, safety, and security threats both foreign and in the United States.

45. **c.** Personal Protective Equipment includes gloves, gowns, masks, and face and eye shields.

46. **b.** Gloves should be long enough to cover the wrist.

47. **c.** When removing gloves, ensure the inside part is on the outside.

48. **d.** Agency for Healthcare Research and Quality (AHRQ) is a government agency looking to improve the quality, safety, efficiency, and effectiveness of American health care.

49. **d.** HIPAA stands for Health Insurance Portability and Accountability Act.

50. **b.** Hepatitis A is spread through contact.

Obstetrics and Gynecology Mock Exam

1. **d.** A cloverleaf shape to the skull is characteristic of skeletal dysplasia (thanatophoric dwarf).

2. **d.** The presence of valves within the *male* urethra results in a urinary obstruction demonstrating a dilated bladder and posterior urethra (keyhole sign).

3. **b.** The broad ligament provides a small amount of support for the uterus and contains the *uterine blood vessels and nerves*. The suspensory ligaments contain the ovarian vessels.

4. **a.** Placenta accreta is a condition where the chorionic villi invade the superficial layer of the uterine myometrium, obliterating the retroplacental complex.

5. **d.** Identification of the falx does not indicate the proper level for the biparietal diameter (BPD). Measurement of the BPD is at a level passing through the third ventricle, cavum septum pellucid and thalamic cerebri.

6. **c.** Crown–rump length during the first trimester is generally the best and most accurate method for measuring gestational age.

7. **a.** *Symmetric bilateral* pelvic masses are most likely pelvic muscles. Bilateral follicular cysts, theca lutein cysts, or uterine fibroids are not likely symmetrical.

8. **b.** A *hypoechoic* adnexal mass separate from the ovaries is most suspicious for an endometrioma. A complicated parovarian cyst is a differential consideration but is not the likely diagnosis.

9. **d.** HIPAA is a federal agency overseeing may health-care functions, the primary being patient confidentiality.

10. **b.** The biophysical profile is a sonographic evaluation of fetal well-being. It includes a specific time or number of fetal movements, breathing movements, fetal tone, amniotic fluid volume, and a nonstress test.

11. **b.** During the secretory phase, the functional layer of the endometrium continues to thicken and may demonstrate posterior acoustic enhancement. The luteal phase of the ovary corresponds with the secretory phase of the endometrium.

12. **d.** Normal serum maternal alpha-fetoprotein levels will vary with gestational age and number. Abnormal levels can be a result of improper estimation of gestational age.

13. **c.** A diamniotic/monochorionic twin pregnancy will demonstrate two gestational sacs (diamniotic) and one placenta (monoamniotic).

14. **a.** *Symmetrical* intrauterine growth restriction (IUGR) is generally a result of first trimester insult. *Asymmetrical* IUGR may be a result of placental insufficiency, chromosomal abnormality, uterine infection, or maternal hypertension.

15. **d.** The ductus arteriosus carries oxygenated blood from the pulmonary artery to the descending aorta (shunts blood away from the fetal lungs). The ductus venosus carries oxygenated blood from the umbilical vein to the inferior vena cava.

16. **b.** Twin–twin transfusion syndrome demonstrates an arteriovenous anastomosis. The arterial blood of the donor twin pumps into the venous system of the recipient twin. Acardiac twinning demonstrates a venous-to-venous or arterial-to-arterial anastomosis.

17. **a.** Thecomas are usually benign and unilateral, comprising 1% of

ovarian neoplasms with 70% occurring in postmenopausal women. Dysgerminoma is a malignant neoplasm in childhood. Fibromas also occur in postmenopausal women.

18. **c.** Hydranencephaly is a replacement of normal cerebral cortex with cerebrospinal fluid, resulting from vascular compromise or congenital infection of the fetal brain tissue.

19. **d.** Dandy-Walker syndrome is a malformation of the cerebellum and fourth ventricle. Sonographic findings include an enlarged posterior fossa, splaying of the cerebellar hemispheres, and complete or partial absence of the vermis.

20. **b.** Sonographic findings of adenomyosis include an inhomogeneous myometrium, diffuse uterine enlargement, poorly defined anechoic areas within the myometrium, and striated edge shadowing (venetian blind).

21. **c.** The arrow identifies an artifactual decrease in echogenicity of the uterine fundus. This is a refraction artifact (edge shadow) resulting from underdistention of the urinary bladder. Proper bladder distention extends slightly beyond the most superior portion of the uterus.

22. **a.** Hypoechoic ill-defined uterine masses are present in this sagittal sonogram of the uterus. Differential considerations would include uterine fibroids, leiomyosarcomas, adenomyosis, and peritoneal mass secondary to endometriosis.

23. **c.** A solid, predominately hypoechoic mass containing hyperechoic foci with acoustic shadowing is most suspicious for a cystic teratoma (dermoid). An endometrioma or hemorrhagic cyst generally does not demonstrate calcifications. Ectopic pregnancy is unlikely.

24. **b.** Absence of the cranial vault and underlying cerebral hemispheres is present in this 3D sonogram, most suspicious for anencephaly.

25. **b.** This image demonstrates a thin hyperechoic linear structure within the endometrium most consistent with an intrauterine contraceptive device (IUD).

26. **c.** Tamoxifen is an antiestrogen medication used in the treatment of primary breast carcinoma. Side effects of tamoxifen therapy include an endometrial neoplasm (polyp or carcinoma) or endometrial hyperplasia. Complex appearance to the endometrial cavity is a sonographic finding of the tamoxifen effect.

27. **a.** A large, hypoechoic midline mass in a patient with amenorrhea is most suspicious for hematometra (blood accumulation in the uterus). The anechoic area contiguous with the superior uterus is most likely dilatation of the uterine cornua.

28. **c.** The sonogram is annotated longitudinal stomach. The stomach is located within the chest cavity most suspicious for a diaphragmatic hernia.

29. **b.** The fetal cranium demonstrates a *calvarial defect* with a fluid-filled sac extending from the calvaria defect most suspicious for an encephalocele.

30. **d.** The sonogram demonstrates fluid dilation of the fetal bowel. This is most consistent with meconium peritonitis. It can be a result of bowel atresia or meconium ileus.

31. **b.** During the late menstrual phase, the endometrium lining demonstrates a thin 2 to 3 mm diameter. The endometrial lining measures approximately 4 to 6 mm during the early proliferation phase.

32. **d.** Physiological herniation of the fetal bowel into the umbilical cord permits development of the abdominal organs. Bowel herniation resolves by the eleventh gestational week and is abnormal if it persists after 12 gestational weeks.

33. **b.** Type II is the most lethal classification of osteogenesis imperfecta demonstrating hypomineralization, bell-shaped chest, and significant bone shortening.

34. **d.** A submucosal fibroid displaces and distorts the endometrial canal resulting in irregular or heavy uterine bleeding.

35. **d.** Cross-section measurement of the abdominal circumference is made slightly superior to the cord insertion at the junction of the left and right portal veins.

36. **b.** Influenza is transmitted through droplet exposure. Hepatitis A and shingles are transmitted through contact exposure. Tuberculosis is an airborne pathogen.

37. **b.** Normal nuchal translucency should not exceed 3 mm. Measurement of nuchal translucency is made between 11 weeks and 0 days to 13 weeks and 6 days.

38. **c.** Premature detachment of the placenta is a critical condition and an indication for immediate delivery. Placenta previa, vasa previa, and placenta accreta are conditions that will require a cesarean section but are not indications for immediate delivery.

39. **c.** Chorionic villus sampling is commonly performed between 10 and 12 gestational weeks. Scheduling of a genetic amniocentesis is generally between 15 and 18 gestational weeks and as early as 12 weeks.

40. **b.** A gartner duct cyst is located within the vagina. This is the most common cystic lesion of the vagina and is usually an incidental finding.

41. **c.** Hyperechoic bowel is associated with Down syndrome, cystic fibrosis, chromosomal abnormalities, and intrauterine growth restriction. When isolated, echogenic bowel is associated with a normal fetal outcome.

42. **d.** Clinodactyly is congenital, characterized by abnormal curvature of one or more digits.

43. **a.** Thickness of the postmenopausal endometrium is consistently benign when measuring 5 mm or less and should not exceed 8 mm.

44. **c.** Fluid within the endometrium is not included in the endometrial measurement. Fluid within the endometrial cavity is not always pathological in origin.

45. **d.** The premenarche cervix is twice the size of the uterine body (2:1). During the menarche phase, the cervix is one half the size of the corpus (1:2). The cervix and corpus are equal in size after menopause (1:1).

46. **c.** The failure of the corpus callosum to develop results in dilation of the third ventricle and outward angling of the frontal and lateral horns of the lateral ventricles.

47. **c.** As the narrowest portion of the fallopian tube, the interstitial segment passes through the highly vascular uterine cornua. Rupture in this area can cause severe internal hemorrhaging.

48. **b.** Esophageal atresia results from a congenital malformation of the foregut. Absence of the stomach or small stomach size in serial sonograms

with associated polyhydramnios are the most common sonographic findings in esophageal atresia.

49. b. The normal yolk sac should not exceed 6 mm in diameter. A yolk sac inner to inner diameter exceeding 7 mm is considered abnormal.

50. b. The external iliac vessels lie lateral to the ovaries. The internal iliac vessels lie posterior to the ovaries.

51. d. This sonogram demonstrates an enlargement of the posterior fossa and an absent vermis most consistent with Dandy-Walker syndrome. Dandy-Walker syndrome consists of variable degrees of cerebellar vermis agenesis, dilatation of the fourth ventricle, and enlargement of the posterior fossa. . Coexisting anomalies may include microcephaly, encephalocele, facial malformations, and polydactyly. An arachnoid cyst demonstrates a normal vermis with splaying of cerebellum hemispheres

52. d. An enlarged stomach and proximal duodenum (double bubble) are present in this sonogram, resulting from a duodenal obstruction. Duodenal atresia is associated with Down syndrome and cardiac and urinary anomalies.

53. c. Polyhydramnios is a common finding in cases of duodenal atresia.

54. b. Central *umbilical cord insertion* into a midline anterior abdominal wall mass is most suspicious for an omphalocele. The defect will contain varying amounts of abdominal contents and is covered by a membrane of peritoneum.

55. c. Normal or slightly elevated maternal serum alpha-fetoprotein (MSAFP) levels are typically observed in cases of omphalocele. Gastroschisis demonstrates a marked elevation in MSAFP levels.

56. c. The ovary is demonstrating multiple small follicles. This is a common feature in polycystic ovarian syndrome. A hydrosalpinx is also identified lateral and posterior to the ovary.

57. b. A small amount of fluid is identified in the pericardial sac consistent with a small pericardial effusion. A small amount of pericardial fluid (≤2 mm) can be a normal finding in the second trimester or can be associated with chromosomal abnormalities.

58. a. An avascular tubular adnexal mass demonstrating thin wall margins is identified in the left adnexa adjacent to a normal appearing left ovary. This is most suspicious for a hydrosalpinx.

59. a. A *hypoechoic* homogeneous *adnexal* mass demonstrating well-defined margins is most suspicious for an endometrioma. Paraovarian cysts typically are *anechoic* adnexal masses.

60. d. Bilateral enlarged multicystic ovaries in a patient undergoing ovulation induction therapy is most suspicious for ovarian hyperstimulation syndrome.

61. b. With this diagnosis, the sonographer should also evaluate Morison pouch and right paracolic gutter for ascites.

62. a. A thick membrane with a "V" shape called twin peak or lambda sign is identified in dichorionic-diamniotic twin pregnancies.

63. c. Proper handwashing is the best protection to stop the spread of disease.

64. c. When the edge of the placenta is a minimum of 2.0 cm from the internal cervical os, placenta previa is ruled out. A low-lying placental edge is located within 2.0 cm of the internal cervical os.

65. b. Dangling of the choroid plexus from gravitational forces is a sonographic finding in severe ventriculomegaly.

66. c. Developmental defect of the lymphatic system typically results in a cystic hygroma. In the early stages, nuchal thickness may appear increased.

67. c. Demonstration of a triple line appearance to the endometrial cavity occurs in the *late proliferation phase*. A thin echogenic endometrium occurs during the early proliferation phase.

68. b. The *external* iliac arteries course posterior to the ovaries and uterus and provide an imaging landmark for imaging of the ovaries.

69. a. The piriformis muscles form part of the pelvic floor and course posterior to the ovaries. The obturator internus muscles are located in the lateral portion of the true pelvis.

70. a. *Estrogen stimulates* proliferation of the endometrium, developing an environment for possible implantation.

71. d. The abdominal circumference measurement is the best predictor of fetal growth. The cephalic index is devised to determine the normality of the fetal head shape.

72. d. Extrauterine masses are most likely to develop on the broad ligament. The broad ligament is a wing-like fold of peritoneum draping over the fallopian tubes, uterus, ovaries, and blood vessels.

73. b. Graafian follicle describes a mature physiological cyst containing a cumulus oophorus.

74. a. The levator ani muscles along with the piriformis muscles form the pelvic floor supporting and positioning the pelvic organs. They are located posteriorly at the level of the vagina and cervix.

75. a. Nabothian cysts are a result of an obstructed inclusion cyst or a result of chronic cervicitis. Corpus albicans is a scar from a previous corpus luteal cyst. Theca lutein cysts are a result of ovarian hyperstimulation.

76. d. Encephaloceles are midline cranial defects that more commonly arise in the occipital portion of the fetal cranium.

77. a. Acrania is a condition where the brain tissue develops with a complete or partial absence of the cranial bones. Acrania may ultimately develop into anencephaly.

78. a. Anencephaly is the most common neural tube defect.

79. a. Holoprosencephaly is most often associated with trisomy 13 (Patau syndrome). Noonan syndrome is sometimes termed the male Turner syndrome because of their similarities, but it can occur in both genders.

80. b. An encephalocele is a spherical fluid-filled or brain-filled sac extending from a bony calvarial defect.

81. b. MSAFP levels generally remain normal in isolated cases of encephalocele. Cases of anencephaly, spina bifida aperta, multifetal gestation, and trophoblastic disease are likely to demonstrate elevated MSAFP levels.

82. b. The sonogram is demonstrating fluid in both lungs (bilateral pleural effusion). The pericardial sac appears within normal limits.

83. c. The arrow identifies an accessory or succenturiate placental lobe. The chorionic villi adjacent to the implantation site do not atrophy, resulting in additional placental tissue.

84. **c.** A cleft lip is demonstrated in this facial 3-D image of a second trimester fetus.

85. **b.** Difficulty in swallowing the amniotic fluid is associated with the fetus demonstrating a facial cleft lip resulting in polyhydramnios.

86. **d.** A well-defined hypoechoic ovarian mass displayed in the late proliferative and early secretory phases is most suspicious for a hemorrhagic corpus luteal cyst.

87. **d.** One vascular structure coursing along the lateral border of the normal fetal bladder is most suspicious for a single umbilical artery.

88. **c.** A large unilocular cystic structure in the right adnexa is most suspicious for a cystadenoma. Debris has accumulated in the inferior dependent portion of the mass.

89. **d.** A transabdominal image of the cervix demonstrates funneling of the amniotic fluid into the cervical canal, consistent with an incompetent cervix.

90. **a.** A thin, hyperechoic linear structure surrounds and extends past the posterior aspect of the fetus, most consistent with a normal amnion. The amnion and chorion are fused by 16 gestational weeks.

91. **d.** The placenta extends from the posterior wall completely across the internal cervical os consistent with a complete placenta previa.

92. **c.** Maximum placental thickness normally does not exceed 4 cm in the second trimester or 6 cm in the third trimester.

93. **d.** Intrauterine growth restriction (IUGR) is most likely associated with oligohydramnios. Facial cleft, anencephaly, duodenal atresia, and diaphragmatic hernia are conditions commonly associated with polyhydramnios.

94. **b.** The right atrium of the heart lies more anterior than the left atrium, or right and left ventricles.

95. **b.** Caudal regression is most commonly associated with maternal diabetes mellitus.

96. **c.** A surge of luteinizing hormone levels triggers ovulation and initiates the residual follicle into a corpus luteal cyst.

97. **d.** A cystic hygroma is often associated with chromosomal abnormalities (Turner syndrome) and does not demonstrate a cranial defect.

98. **a.** Nabothian cysts are common benign cystic structures located in the cervix.

99. **c.** The occipital horn of the lateral ventricle is the first to dilate in the majority of ventriculomegaly cases.

100. **c.** Theca lutein cysts are associated with marked increases in hormone levels, a clinical finding in trophoblastic disease.

101. **d.** Day 20 of the menstrual cycle falls within the secretory phase. The endometrium displays a hyperechoic functional layer and hypoechoic basal layer during the secretory phase of the menstrual cycle.

102. **d.** The chorion is formed by two layers: the embryonic mesoderm and a double layer of trophoblasts.

103. **a.** Thickness of the endometrium is directly related to hormone levels. Increasing estrogen levels regenerate and thicken the functional layer of the endometrium.

104. **b.** A focal collection of ectopic *endometrial* tissue is termed an *endometrioma* or "chocolate cyst."

105. **b.** Sonographic findings consistent with adenomyosis include an enlarged uterus demonstrating anechoic areas within the myometrium and a normal endometrial cavity.

106. **c.** The urinary bladder should display on the upper left portion of the *screen* in the sagittal plane.

107. **a.** Estradiol is an estrogen hormone that primarily reflects the *activity* of the ovary. Luteinizing hormone *triggers* ovulation and initiates the conversion of the residual follicle into a corpus luteum cyst.

108. **b.** During the late proliferative phase (day 10), the endometrium demonstrates as a "triple-line." The functional layer is thick and hypoechoic with a hyperechoic basal layer.

109. **c.** Decreases in estrogen can shorten the vagina and decrease cervical mucus. Ovaries atrophy and may be difficult to visualize.

110. **d.** The isthmus is the "narrow waist" of the uterus located between the cervix and corpus. The isthmus is termed the *lower uterine*

segment during pregnancy. The isthmus is located near the angle of the urinary bladder.

111. **b.** The suspensory ligaments extend from the lateral aspect of the ovary to the pelvic sidewalls. The broad ligament extends from the lateral aspect of the uterus to the pelvic sidewalls.

112. **a.** An anechoic *tubular adnexal mass* in an asymptomatic patient is most likely a hydrosalpinx. Questioning the patient about a previous history of pelvic surgeries, appendectomy, or pelvic infections may aid in the diagnosis.

113. **a.** A widening of the posterior ossification centers with an anechoic protrusion is most likely a sacral spina bifida.

114. **c.** A patient with a history of tamoxifen therapy demonstrating multiple small cystic structures within the endometrium is most suspicious for an endometrial polyp.

115. **a.** The endometrial cavity displays a hypervascular appearance. With a recent history of an endometrial invasive procedure, the sonogram most likely demonstrates endometritis from retained products of conception.

116. **c.** A gestational sac with an embryo is identified in the right adnexa in a patient with a last menstrual period 6 week earlier. This is most suspicious for an ectopic pregnancy.

117. **d.** A large empty gestational sac is present in the endometrial cavity, consistent with an embryonic pregnancy (blighted ovum).

118. **c.** Anechoic free fluid is identified posterior to the cervix and anterior to the rectum in the pouch of Douglas (retrouterine pouch). A hyperechoic IUD is also identified within the endometrial cavity.

119. **b.** Three normal-appearing functional cysts are present in this image of the left ovary.

120. **b.** The arrow identifies a single ventricle with fused thalamic cerebri, consistent with alobar holoprosencephaly.

121. **b.** Holoprosencephaly is commonly associated with Patau syndrome. Trisomy 13 is a fatal chromosomal abnormality associated with multiple severe malformations

including holoprosencephaly, cardiac defects, omphalocele, and infantile polycystic disease.

122. **a.** Small cystic structures are present in the endometrium of an early pregnancy. These sonographic findings in a patient with hyperemesis are most suspicious for a molar pregnancy (trophoblastic disease).

123. **a.** Arrow A identifies nonfused thalami identifies nonfused thalami.

124. **b.** Arrow B identifies the choroid plexus identifies the choroid plexus. Anechoic brain tissue, falx cerebri, nonfused thalami, and choroid plexus are most consistent with hydranencephaly.

125. **a.** Maternal diabetes mellitus and obesity are risk factors for a fetus developing macrosomia. Caudal regression is almost solely associated with maternal diabetes.

126. **b.** Hands should be scrubbed a minimum of 20 seconds.

127. **c.** In cases of triploidy, three complete sets of chromosomes are present. Most cases will abort spontaneously, occurring in 1 out of 5000 cases. Arnold-Chiari syndrome is an autosomal recessive condition affecting the posterior fossa and associated with ventriculomegaly and a myelomeningocele.

128. **d.** Osteogenesis imperfecta is a disorder of collagen production resulting in bones brittle to intrauterine fracture. Diastrophic dysplasia is a rare disorder characterized by micromelia, talipes, cleft palate, and hand abnormalities.

129. **d.** Cystic teratomas (dermoid cysts) are commonly located superior to the uterine fundus. They arise from the wall of the follicle and may contain fat, hair, skin, and teeth.

130. **d.** Second trimester ultrasound examinations are best for determining fetal anatomy. Determination of gestational age is most accurate in the first trimester and fetal weight in the third trimester.

131. **b.** The foramen ovale allows communication between the right and left atria in utero and closes after birth. The ductus arteriosus communicates between the pulmonary artery and the descending aorta, also closing after birth. The ductus venosus connects the umbilical vein to the inferior vena cava.

132. **d.** An early onset of puberty (precocious puberty) may be the result of a mass involving the hypothalamus, gonads (ovaries or testes), or adrenal glands.

133. **d.** A *unilocular, thin-walled* cystic structure is identified adjacent to a normal ovary. This is most consistent with a parovarian cyst. Differential consideration may include a cystadenoma, hydrosalpinx, or peritoneal cyst.

134. **d.** Endometrial carcinoma is the most common malignancy of the female pelvis.

135. **c.** A bicornuate uterus results from a partial fusion of the müllerian ducts. Complete failure of the müllerian ducts to fuse is associated with uterine didelphys.

136. **c.** Ectopic pregnancies demonstrate an abnormal rise in serial hCG levels.

137. **d.** The fallopian tube is divided into four sections: interstitial, isthmus, ampulla, and infundibulum.

138. **a.** The endometrium demonstrates the greatest thickness in the secretory phase, measuring between 7 and 14 mm.

139. **c.** Fertilization of the ovum occurs in the distal portion of the fallopian tube. Fertilization to endometrial implantation occurs in 5 to 7 days.

140. **d.** The anterior pituitary gland secretes follicular stimulating and luteinizing hormones. The hypothalamus produces follicular stimulating hormone releasing factor and luteinizing hormone.

141. **b.** In postmenopausal patients not receiving hormone replacement therapy, the normal endometrium is expected to appear as a thin echogenic line.

142. **c.** Choroid plexus cysts can be a normal finding, typically identified between 16 and 23 gestational weeks. They should regress by 26 weeks' gestation. They can be associated with trisomy 18.

143. **c.** The biparietal diameter is an accurate predictor of gestational age before 20 weeks. The crown–rump length is the most accurate parameter for measuring gestational age in the first trimester.

144. **a.** Meigs syndrome is a combination of a pleural effusion, ascites, and ovarian neoplasm that resolve after surgical removal of the ovarian mass

145. **c.** A small isoechoic submucosal fibroid is compressing the anterior border of the endometrium.

146. **c.** Demonstration of a cystic hygroma is a characteristic sonographic finding associated with Turner syndrome.

147. **d.** A solid and cystic mass is seen in the region of the fetal sacrum. The fetal skin line shows no evidence of a defect. This is most suspicious for a sacrococcygeal teratoma.

148. **a.** The arrow is identifying a hyperechoic focus in the right upper quadrant in the area of the gallbladder fossa. This is most suspicious for cholelithiasis.

149. **a.** An anterior abdominal wall defect is present to the right of a normal cord insertion characteristic of gastroschisis.

150. **a.** Persistent abnormal inversion of the fetal foot at an angle perpendicular to the lower leg is most suspicious for a clubfoot.

151. **d.** A ventriculoseptal defect (VSD) is the most common isolated congenital cardiac defect. It is essential to visualize the septum perpendicular to the sound beam.

152. **b.** Umbilical artery analysis is evaluated after 30 weeks' gestation. A reversal of diastolic flow in the umbilical artery is a critical finding.

153. **d.** Dilatation of the bladder and proximal urethra (keyhole sign) are most likely demonstrated in this image of the fetal bladder, consistent with posterior urethral valve obstruction.

154. **b.** Hydronephrosis demonstrates pelviectasis ≥10 mm (1.0 cm). The right renal pelvis measures 1.1 cm, and the left renal pelvis is 1.0 cm in diameter. Normal pelviectasis in a third trimester should not exceed 0.7 cm.

155. **c.** Abundant blood flow demonstrating a mosaic pattern on color Doppler and a high velocity, low resistant arterial flow coupled with venous component on spectral analysis is evident within the uterine myometrium. With a history of recent pelvic trauma (D&C), this sonogram is most suspicious for an arteriovenous fistula. This is an important diagnosis. A repeat D&C may lead to catastrophic hemorrhaging.

156. c. The door should be closed for 4 hours after a patient with an airborne pathogen has left the room.

157. d. The primitive hindbrain (rhombencephalon) demonstrates as a prominent cystic space in the posterior portion of the brain.

158. a. The decidua basalis forms the maternal side of the placenta, and the decidua frondosum forms the fetal side of the placenta. Decidua capsularis covers the surface of the implanted conceptus.

159. d. The cephalic index is devised to determine the normalcy of the fetal head shape.

160. c. Normal lung development depends on the exchange of amniotic fluid within the lungs.

161. d. Mittelschmerz is a term describing pelvic pain preceding ovulation.

162. d. Duodenal atresia is a sonographic finding associated in approximately 30% of Down syndrome cases. Other findings include macrocephaly, brachycephaly, sandal toe deformity, and clinodactyly.

163. b. Proliferation of the trophoblastic tissue results in dramatic increases in hCG levels. Vaginal bleeding and hyperemesis are additional clinical findings associated with gestational trophoblastic disease.

164. c. The corpus luteum is a physiological cyst that secretes progesterone early in pregnancy until the placenta develops.

165. d. Autosomal dominant is a disorder caused by the presence of one defective gene.

166. c. A lemon-shaped cranium and banana-shaped cerebellum are associated with a coexisting open neural tube defect (myelomeningocele).

167. b. The distal femoral epiphysis is visualized around 32 weeks and the proximal tibial epiphysis around 35 weeks' gestation.

168. d. A nonmobile hyperechoic focus within a ventricle is most likely the papillary muscle.

169. c. The atrium of the lateral ventricle normally measures between 6 and 10 mm throughout pregnancy and should not exceed 10 mm to remain within normal limits.

170. a. The apex of the fetal heart is normally positioned toward the left side of the body at about 45 degrees.

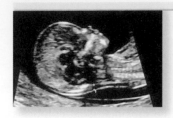

Bibliography

Burns J, Ladisa-Michalek, Willis A: *National certification exam review: abdominal sonography including superficial structures and musculoskeletal*, 2010, SDMS.

Cartensen EL: Biological effects of low-temporal, average-intensity, pulse ultrasound, *http://www.doi.wiley.com*, October 2005.

Curry RA, Tempkin BB: *Sonography introduction to normal structure and function*, ed 4, St Louis, 2016, Elsevier.

DeJong Jr., M Robert: *Craig's Essentials of Sonography and Patient Care*, St. Louis, 2018, Elsevier.

Gould BE: *Pathophysiology for the health profession*, ed 3, St Louis, 2006, Mosby.

Hagen-Ansert SL: *Textbook of diagnostic medical sonography*, ed 7, St Louis, 2012, Mosby.

Hedrick W: *Technology for diagnostic sonography*, St Louis, 2013, Mosby.

Henningsen C, Kuntz, K, Youngs, D: *Clinical guide to ultrasonography*, St Louis, 2014, Elsevier.

Hughes S: *National certification exam review: sonography principles and instrumentation*, 2009, SDMS.

Kremkau FW: *Diagnostic ultrasound: principles and instruments*, ed 9, Philadelphia, 2018, Elsevier.

Mosby's Medical Dictionary, St Louis, 2017, Elsevier.

Norton M, Scoutt, L., Feldstein, V: *Callen's ultrasonography in obstetrics and gynecology*, ed 6, Philadelphia, 2017, Elsevier.

Rumack CM, Levine, D: *Diagnostic ultrasound*, ed 5, Philadelphia, 2018, Elsevier.

Society of Thoracic Surgeons: *http://www.sts.org/aorticaneurysm*.

SonoWorld: *http://www.sonoworld.com*.

Tempkin BB: *Pocket protocols for ultrasound scanning*, ed 2, Philadelphia, 2007, Saunders.

Ultrasound Diagnosis of Hypertrophied Pyloric Stenosis: Thomas Ball, MD; *http://www.radiology.rsnajn/s.org.*

Young D, Praska K: *National certification exam review: obstetric and gynecologic sonography*, 2009, SDMS.

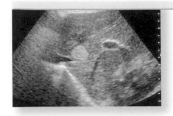

Illustration Credits

Anderhub B: General sonography: a clinical guide, St Louis, 1995, Mosby. Figs. 8.6, 11.6, 12.2, 12.3, 12.6, 19.15, 24.8, 24.11.

Curry RA, Tempkin BB: Sonography: introduction to normal structure and function, ed 4, Philadelphia, 2016, Elsevier. Figs. 11.1, 12.1, 13.1, 13.2, 16.1, 16.3.

Hagen-Ansert SL: Textbook of diagnostic ultrasonography, ed 6, St Louis, 2006, Mosby. Figs. 7.1, 7.2, 9.1, 14.1, 15.1, 15.2, 17.1, 18.1, 19.1, 19.2, 19.4, 19.5, 19.6, 22.12, 26.10.

Kremkau FW: Diagnostic ultrasound: principles and instruments, ed 9, Philadelphia, 2016, Saunders. Figs. 3.1, 3.2, 3.3, 3.4.

Norton M, Scoutt, L., Feldstein, V: *Callen's ultrasonography in obstetrics and gynecology,* ed 6, Philadelphia, 2017, Elsevier. Figs. 19.13, 19.18, 20.2 to 20.10, 20.20, 22.8, 23.1, 23.2, 23.12, 28.1.

Reuter KL, Babagbemi TK: Obstetric and gynecologic ultrasound, ed 2, St Louis, 2007, Mosby. Figs. 25.3, 25.5, 26.8, 26.9, 26.11, 27.8, 27.9, Obstetrics/Gynecology mock exam Figs. 12, 13, 15, 18, 20, 26, 35, 36, 37, 39, 40, 43 to 47, Color Plate 10.

Rumack CM et al: Diagnostic ultrasound, ed 4, St Louis, 2017, Elsevier. Figs. 7.9, 7.10, 8.13, 10.17, 10.18, 11.7, 14.2, 15.2, 28.6, 32.18, Physics mock exam Fig. 5.

Tempkin BB: Pocket protocols for ultrasound scanning, ed 3, Philadelphia, 2007, Saunders. Fig. 19.3.

Courtesies

Paul Aks, BS, RDMS, RVT. Figs. 7.10, 8.12, 10.11, 16.10, 18.4, 18.5, 19.10, 19.11, 19.17, 21.3, 21.4, 21.7, 23.3, 27.5, Abdomen mock exam Figs. 5, 15, 25, 34, Obstetrics/Gynecology mock exam Figs. 3, 19, 34, 40, 51.

Sharon Ballestero, RT, RDMS. Figs. 15.6, 16.9, 21.11, 27.1, 27.3, Obstetrics/Gynecology mock exam Fig. 30.

Carrie Bensen, RDMS. Figs. 13.4, 15.3.

Jeanette Burlbaw, BS RDMS, FSDMS, FAIUM. Fig. 23.5 Obstetrics/Gynecology mock exam Figs 4, 11.

Julie Camozzi, RDMS. Figs. 15.13, 15.14.

Diane Dlugos, BS, RDMS. Fig. 20.22, Obstetrics/Gynecology mock exam Fig. 27.

Ravi D Kadasne MD. Fig. 12.4

Jean Orpin, RT, RDMS. Fig. 28.6.

Lynne Ruddell, BS, RDMS. Figs. 10.15, 16.8.

Diane Short, RT, RDMS. Fig. 24.7.

Siemens Medical Solutions, Ultrasound Division. Figs. 10.4, 14.7, 16.5, 16.6, 16.11, 22.4, 24.2, 25.2, 28.2, 28.4, Abdomen mock exam Figs. 20, 26, 35, 36, 37, 40, Obstetrics/Gynecology mock exam Fig. 10.

B. Alex Stewart, RT, RDMS. Fig. 26.2.

Cover image of 3D fetal face. Courtesy Jeanette Burlbaw, BS, RDMS, FSDMS, FAIUM.

Cover image of hydronephrosis. Courtesy of Ravi D Kadasne, MD.

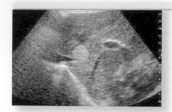

Index

A

A-mode. *See* Amplitude mode
Abdomen, fetal, 416–417t
Abdominal aorta
  anatomy, 208, 208f
  location, 214
  parietal branches of, 210
  pathology, 218t
  size, 214
  visceral branches of, 209–210
Abdominal aortic aneurysm, 207, 217–218t
Abdominal circumference (AC), 415, 427
Abdominal wall, 240–258
  anatomy, 241–242, 241f
  imaging technique, 245–252
  pathology, 249t
  physiology, 241
  sonographic appearance, 244
Abdominal wall hernia, 240
Abortion, 397, 405–406t
Abruptio placentae, 464
Abscess
  abdominal wall, 249t
  appendiceal, 233t
  diverticular, 233t
  drainage, 484t
  liver, 101–102t
  pancreatic, 142–143t
  peritoneal, 303–304t
  renal, 160–161t
  retroperitoneal, 200–201t
  splenic, 182–183t
  testicular, 271–272t
  tubo-ovarian, 388t
Absent isthmus, 284
Absorption, 15
AC. *See* Abdominal circumference
Acalculous cholecystitis, 127–128t
Acardiac twin, 457–458t
Accessory placenta, 467–469t
Accessory spleen, 177, 178–179t
Accountability, 479
Accuracy, 76
Acetabular labrum, 244
Acetabulum, 243
Achilles tendon, 240, 242, 243f, 250–251t
Achondrogenesis, 446–447t
Achondroplasia, 446–447t
Acini cells, 136
Acoustic, defined, 15
Acoustic exposure, 2, 5t
Acoustic impedance, 15
Acoustic output
  indexes, 8t
  labeling standards, 8
  quantities, 5t
  testing, 75–76
Acoustic speckle artifact, 52–53t
Acoustic variables, 15
ACR. *See* American College of Radiology
Acrania, 438–440t
Acromelia, 438
ACTH. *See* Adrenocorticotropic hormone
Acute cholecystitis, 127–128t

Acute tubular necrosis (ATN), 150, 160–161t
Addison disease, 191, 197–198t
Adenomas
  adrenal, 196t
  biliary, 116
  gallbladder, 125–127t
  hepatic, 103–105t
  kidney, 162–163t
  parathyroid, 288t
  thyroid, 288t
Adenomatoid tumor, 270t
Adenomyoma, 374
Adenomyomatosis, 116, 125–127t
Adenomyosis, 374, 375–376t
Adnexa, 336
Adnexal pathology, 387–388t, 387–396
Adrenal glands
  anatomy, 192, 192f
  disorders of
    benign pathology, 196t
    malignant pathology, 197t
    overview of conditions, 197–198t
  imaging technique, 193–195
  laboratory values, 195–198
  location, 192
  physiology, 191–192
  size, 192
  sonographic appearance, 193
Adrenaline, 192
Adrenocorticotropic hormone (ACTH), 195
Adrenogenital syndrome, 191, 197–198t
Adult polycystic kidney disease, 159–160t
Advance directive, 479
Afferent arteriole, 150
AFI. *See* Amniotic fluid index
Agency for Healthcare Research and Quality
  (AHRQ), 479
Agenesis
  corpus callosum, 438–440t
  ovarian, 346
  renal, 154–155t, 444–445t
  seminal vesicles, 265t
  uterine, 343–344t
AHRQ. *See* Agency for Healthcare Research
  and Quality
Airborne pathogen, 479, 481t
AIUM 100 test object, 75t
Alanine aminotransferase (ALT), 100, 122
ALARA (As Low As Reasonably Achievable)
  principle, 2, 4–5
Aldosterone, 191, 195
Aliasing, 60, 67t
Alimentary tract. *See* Gastrointestinal tract
Alkaline phosphatase (ALP), 99, 122
Allantoic duct, 464
Alpha-fetoprotein, 99, 414, 415
ALT. *See* Alanine aminotransferase
Amenorrhea, 358
American College of Radiology (ACR), 51
Amniocentesis, 484–485t
Amniochorionic separation, 467–469t
Amnion, 397, 398, 399f, 403–404t
Amniotic band syndrome, 455–456t
Amniotic fluid, 416–417t, 421t, 430–431, 431t

Amniotic fluid index (AFI), 431t
Amniotic fluid volume, 427, 431t
Amniotic sac, 399f
Amplifiers, 46
Amplitude, 15, 17t
Amplitude mode (A-mode), 42
Ampulla, 347t
Ampulla of Vater, 116, 136, 137f
Amylase, 136
  serum, 141
Anal canal, 226f, 228
Analog-to-digital converter, 46
Anasarca, 453
Androgens, 191
Anembryonic pregnancy, 405–406t
Anemia, 177
  sickle cell, 177, 182t
Anencephaly, 440–441t
Aneuploidy, 453
Aneurysms
  abdominal aortic, 207, 217–218t
  berry, 207
  ectatic, 207, 217–218t
  fusiform, 207
  mycotic, 207, 217–218t
  overview of, 207, 217–218t
  renal artery, 164t
  ruptured, 217–218t
  saccular, 207
  splenic artery, 177, 182–183t
  vein of Galen, 438–440t
Angiogenesis, 397
Angiomyolipoma, 150, 162–163t
Angiotensin, 150
Angle of divergence, 28
Angular resolution, 35–36t
Animal study, on bioeffects of ultrasound, 7t
Anisotropy artifact, 240
Annular array transducers, 31t
Annular pancreas, 138
Anophthalmia, 441–442t
Anterior cul de sac, 339t
Aortic dissection, 207
Aortic ectasia, 218t
Aperture, 28
Aplasia, 178–179t
Apodization, 41
Appendiceal abscess, 233t
Appendicitis, 233t
Appendix, anatomy, 226f, 228
Appendix testis, 259
Aqueduct of Sylvius, 438
Arachnoid cyst, 438–440t
Archive storage, 51
Arcuate arteries, 152t
Arcuate uterus, 343–344t
Arcuate veins, 152t
Arcuate vessels, 338t
Area, defined, 15
Arnold Chiari type II malformation, 438–440t
Array, 28
ART. *See* Assisted reproductive technologies
Arterial blood flow, types of, 63t
Arterial stenosis, 207